A Practical Approach to Orthopedic Medicine

A Practical Approach to Orthopedic Medicine

Edited by Marlow Coffey

hayle
medical
New York

Hayle Medical,
750 Third Avenue, 9th Floor,
New York, NY 10017, USA

Visit us on the World Wide Web at:
www.haylemedical.com

ISBN: 978-1-63241-479-3

The publisher's policy is to use permanent paper from mills that operate a sustainable forestry policy. Furthermore, the publisher ensures that the text paper and cover boards used have met acceptable environmental accreditation standards.

Printed in China.

Cataloging-in-Publication Data

A practical approach to orthopedic medicine / edited by Marlow Coffey.
p. cm.
Includes bibliographical references and index.
ISBN 978-1-63241-479-3
1. Orthopedics. I. Coffey, Marlow.
RD731 .P73 2018
617.3--dc23

Table of Contents

Preface

Orthopedic medicine studies the pathology, treatment and rehabilitation of traumatic injuries and disorders afflicting the musculoskeletal system. Sub-specialties of this particular branch of medicine include surgical sports medicine, pediatric orthopedics, shoulder and elbow surgery, spine surgery, hand surgery, etc. Internal and external implants are available for repairing severe injuries and biomaterials are especially used to avoid graft rejection of the device by the body. This book contains some path-breaking studies in the field of orthopedic medicine and surgery. Researchers and students in this field will be greatly assisted by this book.

The information shared in this book is based on empirical researches made by veterans in this field of study. The elaborative information provided in this book will help the readers further their scope of knowledge leading to advancements in this field.

Finally, I would like to thank my fellow researchers who gave constructive feedback and my family members who supported me at every step of my research.

Editor

The Spatiotemporal Role of COX-2 in Osteogenic and Chondrogenic Differentiation of Periosteum-Derived Mesenchymal Progenitors in Fracture Repair

Chunlan Huang[1], Ming Xue[1], Hongli Chen[1], Jing Jiao[2], Harvey R. Herschman[2], Regis J. O'Keefe[1], Xinping Zhang[1]*

1 Center for Musculoskeletal Research, University of Rochester, School of Medicine and Dentistry, Rochester, New York, United States of America, 2 Department of Molecular and Medical Pharmacology, David Geffen School of Medicine, University of California Los Angeles, Los Angeles, California, United States of America

Abstract

Periosteum provides a major source of mesenchymal progenitor cells for bone fracture repair. Combining cell-specific targeted *Cox-2* gene deletion approaches with *in vitro* analyses of the differentiation of periosteum-derived mesenchymal progenitor cells (PDMPCs), here we demonstrate a spatial and temporal role for Cox-2 function in the modulation of osteogenic and chondrogenic differentiation of periosteal progenitors in fracture repair. *Prx1Cre*-targeted *Cox-2* gene deletion in mesenchyme resulted in marked reduction of intramembraneous and endochondral bone repair, leading to accumulation of poorly differentiated mesenchyme and immature cartilage in periosteal callus. In contrast, *Col2Cre*-targeted *Cox-2* gene deletion in cartilage resulted in a deficiency primarily in cartilage conversion into bone. Further cell culture analyses using *Cox-2* deficient PDMPCs demonstrated reduced osteogenic differentiation in monolayer cultures, blocked chondrocyte differentiation and hypertrophy in high density micromass cultures. Gene expression microarray analyses demonstrated downregulation of a key set of genes associated with bone/cartilage formation and remodeling, namely *Sox9*, *Runx2*, *Osx*, *MMP9*, *VDR* and *RANKL*. Pathway analyses demonstrated dysregulation of the HIF-1, PI3K-AKT and Wnt pathways in Cox-2 deficient cells. Collectively, our data highlight a crucial role for Cox-2 from cells of mesenchymal lineages in modulating key pathways that control periosteal progenitor cell growth, differentiation, and angiogenesis in fracture repair.

Editor: Xing-Ming Shi, Georgia Regents University, United States of America

Funding: This study is supported by grants from the Musculoskeletal Transplant Foundation (XPZ), NYSTEM N08G-495 (XPZ) and N09G346 (XPZ), and the National Institutes of Health (R21 DE021513 to XPZ, RC1 AR058435 to XPZ, AR R01 AR048681 to XPZ and RJO, P50 AR054041 to RJO). The funders had no role in study design, data collection and analysis, decision to publish, or preparation of the manuscript.

Competing Interests: The authors have declared that no competing interests exist.

* Email: Xinping_Zhang@URMC.rochester.edu

Introduction

Fracture healing is a unique postnatal bone regeneration process that occurs as a cascade of well-orchestrated biological events leading to the restoration of bone tissue. Fracture healing requires the formation of an external bone callus, which is initiated primarily by the progenitor cells residing in the periosteum [1–4]. Analogous to embryonic skeletal development, periosteum-initiated fracture repair implicates endochondral and intramembranous bone formation, which proceed in a sequential and organized manner [5,6]. While adult bone repair recapitulates some essential regulatory mechanisms that occur in early skeletal development, repair is a unique bone morphogenetic process, orchestrated by an ensemble of genes distinct from early skeletal development [7]. Due to an inability to directly target the periosteum, the molecular mechanisms and the implicated molecular pathway(s) that control the differentiation program of periosteal mesenchymal progenitor cells in bone fracture repair remains poorly understood. Identifying the critical genes in periosteum-initiated bone repair, establishing their spatiotemporal expression, and elucidating their integrated roles will be essential to understand bone regeneration and to develop useful therapeutics to improve skeletal repair and reconstruction.

Cox-2 is the inducible isoform of cyclooxygenase, the enzyme responsible for a major control step in prostanoid biosynthesis pathway. Cox-2 plays an important role in cancer biology, in vascular pathophysiology, and in a variety of inflammatory disorders [8,9]. Global deletion of the *Cox-2* gene in mice does not affect overall skeletal development [10,11]. However, global absence of Cox-2 markedly impairs fracture healing [12,13]. An important role for Cox-2 in fracture healing has been shown in aged animals. Older mice have a marked reduction of *Cox-2* expression in the fracture callus, exhibiting delayed neovascularization and endochondral bone formation [14]. *In-situ* hybridization analyses demonstrate that *Cox-2* expression peaks at the early stage of intramembranous and endochondral stage of bone healing [15]. Elevated *Cox-2* expression is detected in chondroprogenitors and proliferating chondrocytes at days 5 and 7 post-fracture. Cox-2 expression is subsequently reduced in hypertrophic chondrocytes during the remodeling phase of healing, suggesting that Cox-2 expression is tightly regulated during fracture repair. In contrast to loss of Cox-2 function, Cox-2 gain of function by overexpression at the healing site accelerates fracture healing in animal models [16].

While an essential role of Cox-2 in fracture repair has been established, targeted tissues and implicated pathways remain unclear. Here we utilize two tissue-specific promoter driven-Cre transgenic mouse lines to delete the *Cox-2* gene in limb mesenchymal lineages (with Prx1Cre) and in chondrocytes (with Col2Cre), respectively. To determine the mechanistic involvement of Cox-2 in control of osteogenic and chondrogenic differentiation of periosteal mesenchymal progenitors, we further performed differentiation and gene expression profile analysis using periosteum-derived mesenchymal progenitor cells (PDMPCs) isolated from the healing periosteum of the mutant and control mice [17,18]. Our study established a critical role for Cox-2 in the differentiation paradigm of periosteal mesenchymal progenitor cell in fracture repair, underscoring the importance of spatial and temporal regulation of Cox-2 in bone repair and regeneration.

Materials and Methods

Animal models

To determine the gene recombination efficiency of Prx1Cre and Col2Cre lines in fracture callus, *Col2Cre; RosaR* and *Prx1Cre; RosaR* mice were generated and characterized for beta-galactosidase expression. Cox-2 conditional deletion (*Cox-2*$^{f/f}$) mice [19] were crossed with *Prx1-1Cre* or *Col2Cre* transgenic mice to produce *Cox-2*$^{f/f}$*; Prx1Cre* and *Cox-2*$^{f/f}$*; Col2Cre* mice. All studies and procedures were approved by the Institutional Animal Care and Use Committee at the University of Rochester. Littermates were used for analysis.

Fracture healing model

Closed stabilized femoral fractures were created in two month-old mice [14,15]. Mice were anesthetized with a mix of Ketamine and Xylazine. The skin and the underlying soft tissues over the knee were incised lateral to the patellar tendon. The tendon was displaced medially, and a small hole was drilled into the distal femur using a 26-gauge needle. A stylus pin from a 25G Type spinal needle (BD Medical Systems, Franklin Lakes, NJ) was inserted into the intramedullary canal and clipped. The wound was closed by suturing. Fractures were created at the diaphyseal region of mouse femurs using a three-point bending Einhorn device, as previously described [20]. Fracture healing was examined in gender and age-matched littermates. *Cox-2*$^{f/f}$*; Col2Cre* and *Cox-2*$^{f/f}$*; Prx1Cre* were compared with their respective Cre-negative *Cox-2*$^{f/f}$ littermate controls for analyses.

Micro-CT Imaging Analyses

Femurs were harvested at indicated time points and scanned using a Viva micro-CT system (Scanco Medical, Switzerland) at a voxel size of 10.5 μm to image bone. New bone formation was measured as previously described [21]. The threshold was chosen using 2D evaluation of several slices in the transverse anatomical plane. In this way, mineralized callus was identified while surrounding soft tissue was excluded. An average threshold of 220 was optimal and was used uniformly for all samples. Each sample was contoured around the external callus and along the edge of the cortical bone, excluding the marrow cavity. New bone volume was measured on the surface of fracture samples as previously described [15]. Gender and age matched littermates were used for analyses. Indices of cortical bone morphology from the diaphyseal tibia were assessed by micro-CT imaging as described previously [11]. Cortical bone morphology in male and female mice were analyzed separately and presented as gender-matched groups as indicated.

Histology and histomorphometric Analyses

Fractured femurs were harvested and processed for histological analyses as previously described [12]. Femurs were disarticulated from the hip and trimmed to remove excess muscle and skin. Specimens were stored in 10% neutral buffered formalin for 3 days. The tissues were infiltrated and embedded in paraffin. Sections were prepared and stained with Alcian blue/Hematoxylin as previously described [12]. Histomorphometric analyses were performed using Osteometrics software to determine the area of bone, cartilage, and mesenchyme (a subtraction of total callus from bone and cartilage tissue) by manual tracing. Pre-existing cortical bone was excluded from the analyses. The percent areas of bone, cartilage, and mesenchyme were used to illustrate the composition of the fracture callus. At least three nonconsecutive sections from each sample were used for histomorphometric analyses. The means of ten samples from each group were used for statistical analyses.

Isolation of periosteum-derived mesenchymal progenitors (PDMPCs) from autograft periosteum

We have previously devised a method which allows isolation of sufficient numbers of periosteum-derived mesenchymal progenitors (PDMPCs) from day 5 periosteum callus of autografts to perform *in vitro* differentiation analyses [17,18]. Briefly, autograft transplantations were performed in *Cox-2*$^{f/f}$*; Prx1Cre* mice and their Cre-negative control mice. Mice were anesthetized by peritoneal injection of a mix of Ketamine and Xylazine. A 7–8 mm long incision was made in hind limb, and the mid-shaft femur was exposed by blunt dissection of muscles without disturbing the periosteum. A 4-mm mid-diaphyseal segment was removed from the femur of the donor mice using a sharp diamond-cutting wheel attached to a cordless dremel. The same 4 mm cortical bone graft was then inserted back into the segmental defect and stabilized by a 22-gauge metal pin placed through the intramedullary marrow cavity (autograft transplantation). Donor bone autografts were collected at day 5 post-transplantation. Bone marrow inside the bone graft was removed and discarded by repeated flushing of the marrow cavities with serum-free α-MEM medium. Periosteum tissues were scraped off and pooled in a Petri dish. After digestion with Collagenase D (Roche Applied Science, Indianapolis, IN) at a concentration of 1 mg/ml for 1 hour, cells released from periosteal tissues were pooled and cultured in α-MEM medium containing 1% penicillin and streptomycin, 1% glutamine, and 20% fetal bovine serum (FBS). Once confluent, cells were trypsinized and further expanded in α-MEM medium containing 10% FBS. Periosteal cells from second and third passage were collected and used for all experiments.

For osteogenesis assays, cells isolated from Cox-2$^{f/f}$; Prx1Cre mice and their Cre-negative control mice were cultured as monolayers in fresh α-MEM media containing 1% penicillin and streptomycin, 1% glutamine, and 10% fetal bovine serum (FBS). Since PDMPCs can spontaneously differentiated into osteoblastic cells in regular media following 7 day culture, the basal level of differentiation was examined in control and KO cells in regular media. To examine osteogenic differentiation in response to BMP-2, identical amount of BMP-2 (100 ng/ml) was added to the control and KO culture. Cells were harvested on day 7 for Alkaline Phosphatase staining (ALP) staining and RNA analyses as previously described [17,18]. For chondrogenesis assays, 2×10^5 cells per well were seeded as micromass in a 24-well plate and cultured in DMEM media with 10% fetal bovine serum with or without identical amount of BMP-2 (100 ng/ml). Cell pellets were harvested on day 1 and 7 for Alcian Blue staining and gene expression analyses.

Real-Time PCR Analyses

Total RNA was prepared using a Qiagen RNA extraction kit. Exactly 0.5 μg of mRNA from 4 different samples was pooled and reverse transcribed to make single-strand cDNA, using a commercial first strand cDNA synthesis kit (Invitrogen). Quantitative RT-PCR reaction was performed using SyberGreen (ABgene, Rochester, NY) in a RotorGene real time PCR machine (Corbett Research, Carlsbad, CA). All genes were compared to a standard β-actin control. Data were assessed quantitatively using analysis of variance, comparing relative levels of transcript expression as a function of time. All primers used for the assessment can be found in previous publications [15,17,18] or listed in Table S2. Data are expressed as the means ± SEM. Statistical significance between experimental groups was determined using one-way ANOVA and a Tukey's posthoc test (GraphPad Prism, San Diego, CA). A P value <0.05 was considered statistically significant.

Western blot analyses

Cells were lysed in Golden lysis buffer supplemented with protease inhibitor (Roche Applied Science). The protein extracts (10 μg) were separated using NuPAGE BisTris gels (Invitrogen). Gels were transferred to a polyvinylidene difluoride membrane (PerkinElmer Life Sciences Waltham, MA) and probed with anti–Cox-2 (Cayman Chemical Inc, Ann Arbor, MI) and anti–β-actin monoclonal antibody (Sigma, St. Louis, MO).

Microarray analyses

For microarray analysis, a total of 24 RNA samples in 8 indicated groups (n = 3 per group) were prepared from micromass cultures of Cox-$2^{f/f}$; Prx1Cre or Cox-$2^{f/f}$ PDPMCs, with or without BMP-2 treatment, at day 1 and day 7. Total RNA from each sample was isolated using an RNeasy Mini extraction kit. RNA quality and purity were determined using a NanoDrop ND-1000 spectrophotometer (NanoDrop Technologies, Wilmington, DE, USA). RNA integrity was determined by the Agilent 2100 bioanalyser (Agilent Technologies, Palo Alto, CA, USA). Whole mouse gene expression microarrays (Ilumina, BD-202-0202), containing over 25,600 unique probes and over 19,100 unique genes, were used to detect the gene expression profile each sample. The raw data obtained from all 24 samples were normalized by applying a background correction (using the 'normexp' algorithm) followed by normalization of intensity distributions within and between arrays (using the 'quantile' algorithm). The resulting data were imported into Partek Genomics Suite (Partek Inc., St. Louis, MO) and log2 transformed for statistical processing and hierarchical clustering analyses. Differential gene expression and hierarchical clustering were generated from comparison between 8 different groups, using one-way ANOVA. Differentially expressed genes were selected with a p value less than 0.01 and a fold of change of more than 2 when comparing between groups. Heat maps were generated by Partek Genomics Suite software. All raw and processed data files have been deposited in the National Center for Biotechnology Information Gene Expression Omnibus dataset.

Biological processes, functional classifications and gene annotations were analyzed using Partek Genomics Suite associated with Kyoto Encyclopedia of Genes and Genomes (KEGG) pathway database (updated December 2013), as well as database for Annotation, Visualization and Integrated Discovery (DAVID) (http://david.abcc.ncifcrf.gov). To identify biological processes with significant enrichment, the distribution of genes from our data was compared with a reference annotation gene list for each gene ontology (GO) category. Fisher exact P values were used for gene enrichment analysis. The value ranges from 0 to 1, where value equal to zero represents perfect enrichment. P value less than or equal to 0.05 is considered significantly enriched in the annotation categories.

Results

Targeted Cox-2 gene deletion in cartilage or mesenchyme results in impaired fracture healing

To establish Cre-recombinase mediated gene targeting efficiency and specificity, femoral fractures were created in two-month-old *Prx1Cre; RosaR* and *Col2Cre; RosaR* mice. Prior to fracture in intact bone, intense LacZ staining was identified in all limb mesenchymal lineages, including strong staining in the periosteum of Prx1Cre; RosaR mice (Fig. 1A&B). Bone marrow and muscle were largely negative for LacZ staining. Following fracture, LacZ staining was observed in mesenchyme, chondrocytes and osteoblasts throughout the fracture callus in Prx1Cre; RosaR mice at day 7, indicating efficient gene recombination in all limb mesenchymal lineages (Fig. 1C–F). In *Col2Cre; RosaR* fracture callus, strong LacZ staining was observed as early as day 5 post-fracture, primarily in chondrocytes along the periosteal surface and within the bone marrow cavity, where endochondral bone formation takes place (Fig. 1G&H). Mesenchymal progenitors (Fig. 1I) at the fracture junctions and osteoblasts (Fig. 1J) at the distal flanking region of the callus remained negative for LacZ staining.

Long bone length and cortical bone morphology were examined in *Cox-$2^{f/f}$; Prx1Cre* mice and their littermate controls. No significant differences in long bone length or cortical bone thickness could be determined between *Cox-$2^{f/f}$* and *Cox-$2^{f/f}$; Prx1Cre* mice (Fig. S1), consistent with our previous findings in global Cox-$2^{-/-}$ mice [11]. Fracture healing was examined in both *Cox-$2^{f/f}$; Prx1Cre* and *Cox-$2^{f/f}$; Col2Cre* mice, along with gender and age-matched control Cre-negative *Cox-$2^{f/f}$* mice. Micro-CT analyses showed delayed bony union in both *Cox-$2^{f/f}$; Prx1Cre* and *Cox-$2^{f/f}$; Col2Cre* mice at day 14 post-fracture (Fig. 2A–F). Quantitative and volumetric analyses demonstrated a 47% and a 25% reduction of new bone callus in *Cox-$2^{f/f}$; Prx1Cre* and *Cox-$2^{f/f}$; Col2Cre* mice, respectively (Fig. 2G). Evaluation of new bone callus from individual micro-CT-images suggested that 80% of Cre negative mice demonstrated mature union with formation of a complete bridging callus on day 14. In contrast, only 10% of *Cox-$2^{f/f}$; Col2Cre* mice showed mature union and none of the *Cox-$2^{f/f}$; Prx1Cre* mice showed any evidence of bony union at day 14 post-fracture.

Histologic analyses showed mature bridging callus at day 14 in the *Cox-$2^{f/f}$* control mice of both groups, with only a small amount of residue cartilage present in the callus (Fig. 2H). In contrast, substantial amounts of cartilaginous tissue remained in the fracture callus of *Cox-$2^{f/f}$; Col2Cre* mice at day 14 (Fig. 2I). Cartilage conversion into bone was markedly reduced, yet intramembranous bone formation flanking the cartilaginous tissue (arrows in Fig. 2I) remained largely intact in these mice. Careful examination of the cartilaginous tissue showed that they were mostly mature chondrocytes (Fig. 2J) or less differentiated chondrocytes (Fig. 2K). In *Cox-$2^{f/f}$; Prx1Cre* fracture callus, where *Cox-2* is deleted in mesenchymal progenitors, severe reduction of bone formation at the periosteal sites was evident (Fig. 2L). Extensive mesenchyme (Fig. 2M) and poorly differentiated cartilage tissue (Fig. 2N) were observed throughout the fracture callus. Histomorphometric analyses revealed marked differences in callus composition among the three groups of mice at day 14 post-fracture (Fig. 2K). Compared to the Cre-negative controls which contained 8% mesenchyme, 9.9% mature cartilage and 0% immature

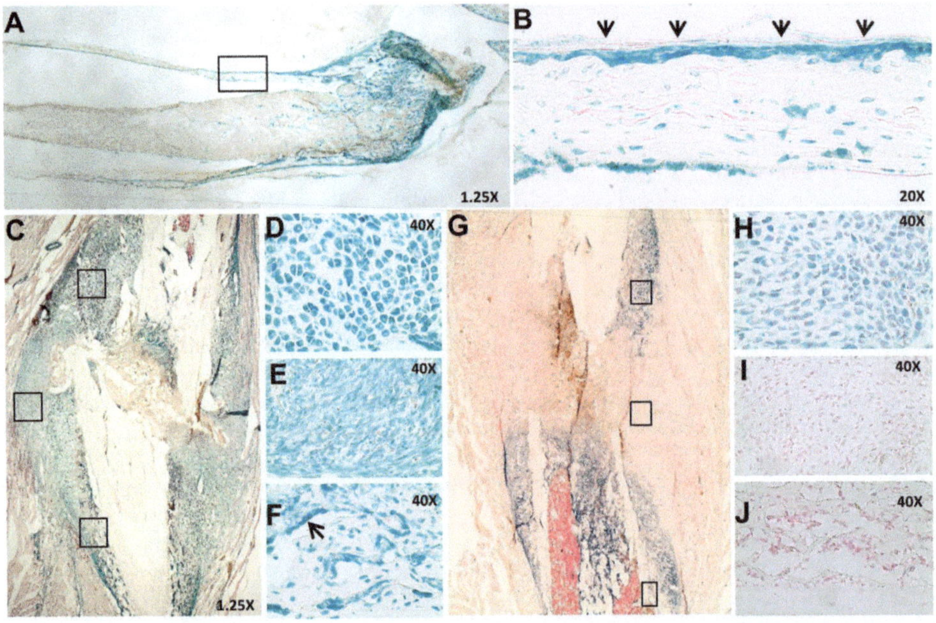

Figure 1. Efficient Prx1Cre- and Col2Cre-mediated targeted gene recombination in fracture callus. A tissue section from long bone of *Prx1Cre; RosaR* mice show intense LacZ staining in bone and cartilage, but not in bone marrow (A). The boxed region in A, shown at a higher magnification (20×), demonstrates LacZ staining in periosteum (arrows in B). Fracture callus at day 7 from *Prx1Cre; RosaR* shows intense LacZ staining throughout the callus region at the cortical bone junction (C). Boxed regions in C (from top to bottom), shown at a higher magnification (20×), illustrate effective gene recombination in chondrocytes (D), mesenchyme (E) and osteoblasts (arrows in F). *Col2Cre; RosaR* fracture callus at day 5 shows effective gene recombination in chondroprogenitors and chondrocytes, but not mesenchymal cells (G). Higher magnification images (20×) in the boxed region (from top to bottom) show positive LacZ staining in chondrocytes (H) but not in mesenchyme cells (I) or osteoblasts (J).

cartilage in the fracture callus, *Cox-2$^{f/f}$; Prx1Cre* mice had an average of 52% mesenchyme and 12% immature cartilage in the fracture callus (Fig. 2K, open bar, n = 10, $p<0.05$). As a result, the percentage of new bone formation in *Cox-2$^{f/f}$; Prx1Cre* mice was reduced by nearly 3-fold as compared to their Cre-negative controls. In *Cox-2$^{f/f}$; Col2Cre* callus, the percentage area of mesenchyme was increased to 25% of the total callus. However, unlike *Cox-2$^{f/f}$; Prx1Cre* callus, which was primarily occupied by mesenchyme and poorly differentiated cartilage, the *Cox-2$^{f/f}$; Col2Cre* callus had an average of 23% mature cartilage and 3% immature cartilage at the cortical bone junctions, leading to a 1.8-fold reduction of new bone formation in the fracture callus (Fig. 2K, gray bar, n = 10, $p<0.05$).

Cox-2 deficient periosteal progenitors exhibit impaired osteogenic and chondrogenic differentiation in cell culture

To further understand the role of Cox-2 in periosteum-mediated repair, PDMPCs were isolated from the periosteum of *Cox-2$^{f/f}$; Prx1Cre* mice and their Cre-negative littermate controls. Cox-2-deficient PDMPCs exhibited reduced ALP staining both at the basal level and following BMP-2 stimulation (Fig. 3A). Prx1Cre-mediated *Cox-2* gene deletion also markedly reduced *ALP*, *RUNX2*, *OSX* and *OCN* gene expression, both in untreated cultures and upon BMP-2 treatment (Fig. 3B). Western blot analyses demonstrated a modest, but statistically significant, induction of Cox-2 protein by BMP-2 treatment in control cells and the absence of Cox-2 protein in PDMPCs isolated from *Cox-2$^{f/f}$; Prx1Cre* mice (Fig. 3C). Quantification of Western blot data from three experiments demonstrates an average of ~1.5 fold induction of Cox-2 by BMP-2 in monolayer cultures from COX-2^{ff} (wild type) mice and ~95% reduction of Cox-2 protein in the Cox-2$^{f/f}$; Prx1Cre cells (Fig. 3D).

Chondrogenesis and chondrocyte differentiation were examined in PDMPC micromass cultures (Fig. 4). Two time points that reflect chondrogenesis onset (day 1) and chondrocyte maturation (day7) were examined [22,23], in the presence and absence of BMP-2 treatment (n = 3 per group). In contrast to monolayer culture, Western blot analyses demonstrated that Cox-2 protein was markedly induced by BMP-2 in the high-density micromass cultures (Fig. 4A), suggesting Cox-2 as a BMP-2 responsive gene in chondrogenic conditions. The induction of Cox-2 expression by BMP-2 was further confirmed by RT-PCR analyses (Fig. S2); these data demonstrate robust induction of *Cox-2* mRNA expression in both day 1 and day 7 BMP-2 treated cultures. Prx1Cre-mediated *Cox-2* gene deletion decreased chondrogenesis and chondrocyte differentiation induced by BMP-2, as evidenced by reduced Alcian Blue staining (Fig. 4B), suppressed *SOX-9* expression at day 1 and further reduced expression of a set of chondrocyte marker gene expression at day 7 (Fig. 4C). Of note is that *Cox-2* gene deletion reduced BMP-2-induced *Col2a1* expression by 50%, but blocked the expression of BMP-2-induced chondrocyte maturation genes, namely *Col10a1*, *Ihh*, *MMP13 and Col11a1* at day 7 (Fig. 3C), suggesting that mesenchymal cell-specific Cox-2 expression is required for both chondrogenesis and chondrocyte maturation and hypertrophy. Consistently, *ALP* and *OCN*, the bone marker genes associated with endochondral ossification, were similarly reduced in BMP-2-treated culture at day 7, demonstrating a key role of Cox-2 in mesenchymal differentiation.

To obtain a deeper understanding of the molecular regulation of osteogenic and chondrogenic differentiation of PDMPCs, gene expression microarray analyses were performed. These differential

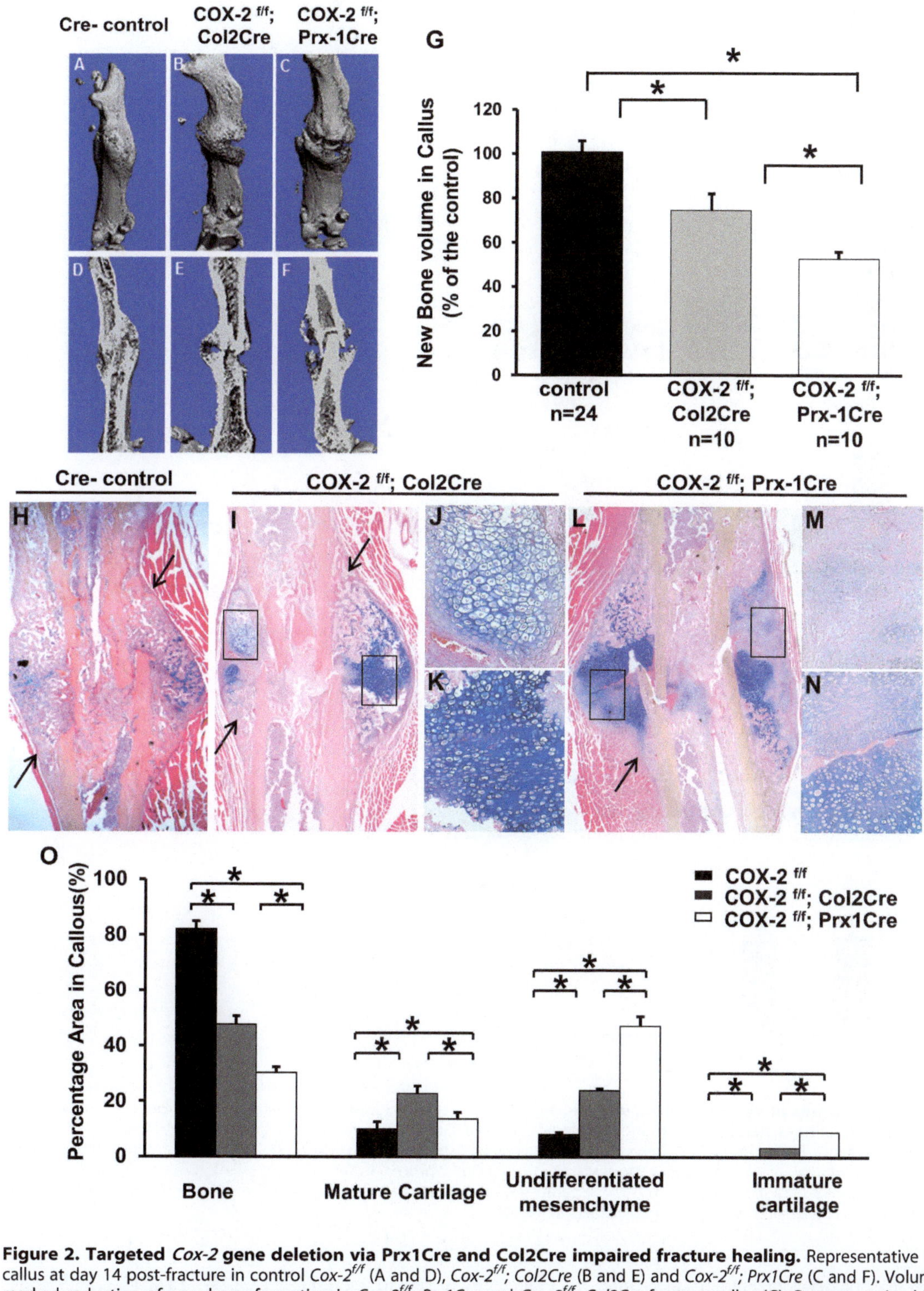

Figure 2. Targeted *Cox-2* gene deletion via Prx1Cre and Col2Cre impaired fracture healing. Representative micro-CT images of fracture callus at day 14 post-fracture in control *Cox-2$^{f/f}$* (A and D), *Cox-2$^{f/f}$; Col2Cre* (B and E) and *Cox-2$^{f/f}$; Prx1Cre* (C and F). Volumetric analyses demonstrate marked reduction of new bone formation in *Cox-2$^{f/f}$; Prx1Cre* and *Cox-2$^{f/f}$; Col2Cre* fracture callus (G). Representative histology sections of fracture callus at day 14 from control *Cox-2$^{f/f}$* (H), *Cox-2$^{f/f}$; Col2Cre* (I–K), and *Cox-2$^{f/f}$; Prx1Cre* (L–N) mice. Boxed regions in I show presence of mature (J) and under-differentiated chondrocytes (K) in *Cox-2$^{f/f}$; Col2Cre* fracture callus. Boxed regions in L show poorly differentiated mesenchyme (M) and immature cartilage (N) in *Cox-2$^{f/f}$; Prx1Cre* fracture callus. Arrows indicate regions of intramembraneous bone formation in H, I and L. Quantitative histomorphometric analyses show the composition of bone, cartilage and mesenchyme tissue in periosteal callus (K). Data are presented as means ± SEM, * $p<0.05$. n = 10.

gene profiling studies are directed at identifying Cox-2 mediated differences in gene expression in micromass cultures of *Cox-2$^{f/f}$; Prx1Cre* and *Cox-2$^{f/f}$* PDMPCs. In the absence of BMP-2 at day 1, 143 genes were found to be suppressed by 2-fold or more in the Cox-2 deficient cells as compared to the control PDMPCs. Biological GO enrichment analyses show functional cluster

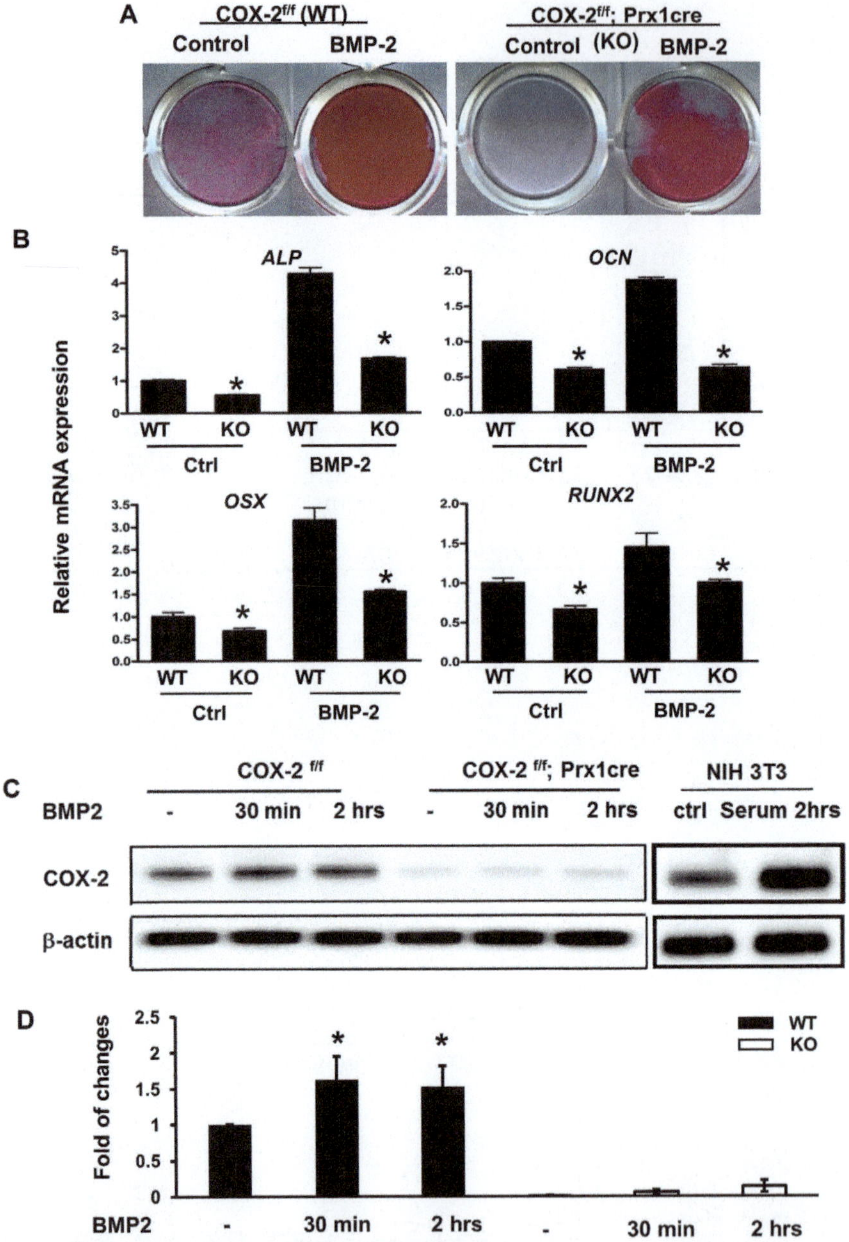

Figure 3. Osteogenic differentiation was impaired in Cox-2 deficient PDMPCs. Periosteal progenitors were isolated from *Cox-2^f/f^* (WT) and *Cox-2^f/f^; Prx1Cre* (KO) mice. Monolayer cultures demonstrate reduced differentiation of *Cox-2* deficient cells, both under basal conditions and in response to BMP-2 stimulation, as evidenced by reduced ALP staining (A) and decreased osteogenic gene expression at day 7 (B). * indicates p<0.05, as compared to the control. Western blot analyses demonstrate a modest induction of Cox-2 protein in WT cells and ablation of Cox-2 protein in Cox-2 deficient cells (C). Quantification of western blot analyses from three separate experiments shows induction of Cox-2 protein in WT cells and near absence of Cox-2 protein in the Prx-1Cre-mediated conditional KO cells (*, p<0.05).

categories of genes involved in bone development and ossification process (11 genes, p<4.0E-5), immune/inflammatory response (21 genes, p<8.2E-5), growth factor activity (7 genes, p<3.3E-4), Wnt pathway (6 genes, p<0.001) and morphogenesis of a branching structure (7 genes, p<0.005) (Table S1). Several known key regulators associated with bone/cartilage ossification and remodeling were significantly suppressed in the Cox-2 deficient cells, namely *Sox9* (2.7-fold), *Sp7 (OSX)* (2.2-fold), *MMP13* (4.5-fold), *MMP9* (4.8-fold), *RANKL (3.7-fold) and Vitamin D receptor (VDR)* (4.8-fold), suggesting reduced osteogenic/chondrogenic potential and bone/cartilage remodeling activity in Cox-2 deficient cells. Following micromass culture for 7 days, PDMPCs underwent spontaneous differentiation to induce a series of genes critical for bone formation, namely *SP7* (5.1-fold), *BMP4* (23.5-fold), and *FGFR3* (4.3-fold), and *Osteocalcin* (4-fold). Among the genes associated with bone/cartilage development and ossification, we identified 25 genes that were significantly suppressed at day 7 in the Cox-2 deficient cells (Fig. S3B), providing further evidence to show the disruption of bone morphogenetic pathway in micromass culture as a consequence of targeted *Cox-2* gene deletion in PDMPCs.

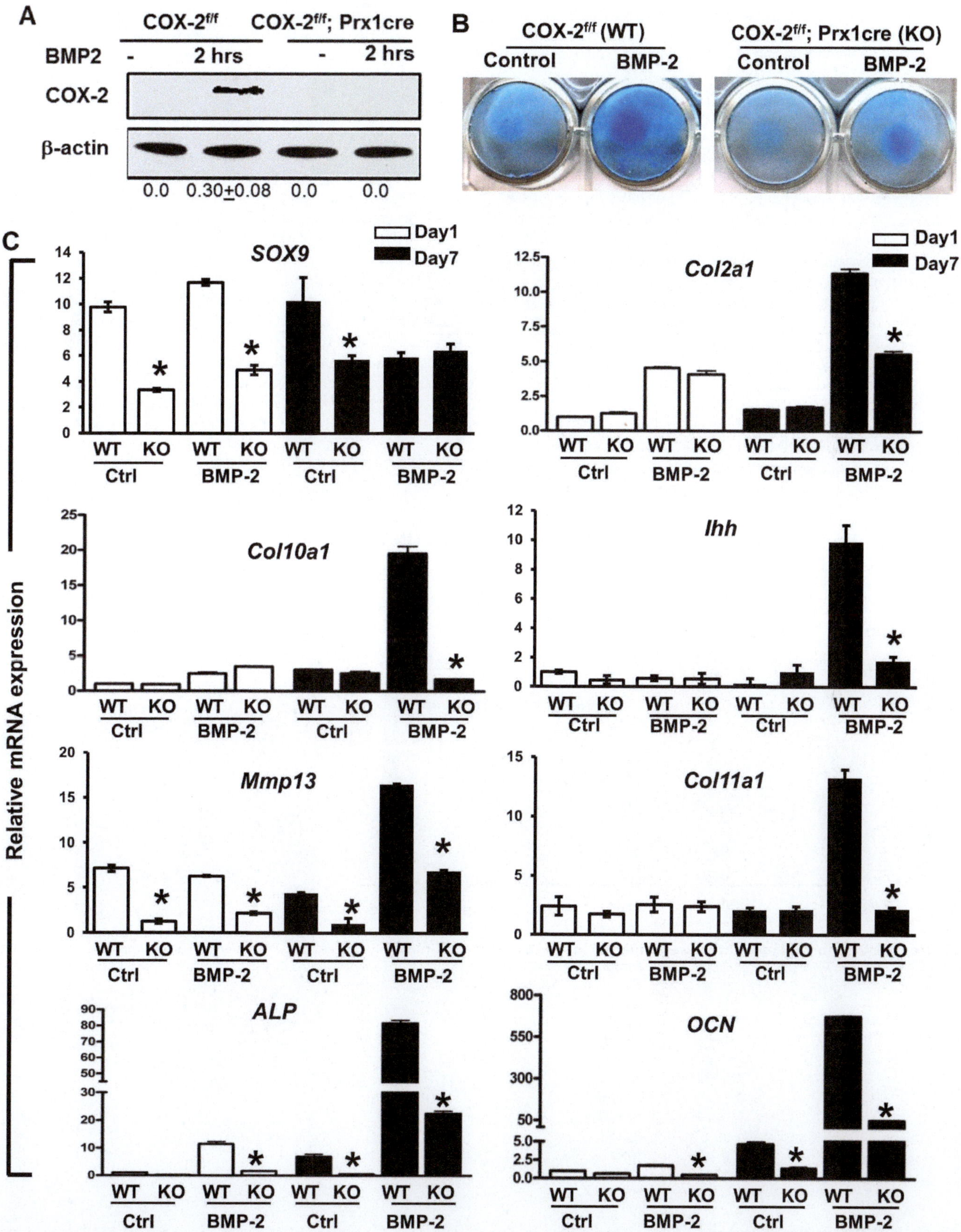

Figure 4. Chondrogenic differentiation was impaired in periosteal progenitors from mice with a targeted *Cox-2* gene deletion. Periosteal mesenchymal progenitors were isolated from *Cox-2*$^{f/f}$ (WT) and *Cox-2*$^{f/f}$*; Prx1Cre* (KO) periosteum. Western blot analyses demonstrated marked Cox-2 induction by BMP-2 in WT cells and absence of Cox-2 protein in Cox-2 deficient cells. Numbers at the bottom of the image show

normalized density ratio of each lane in western blot analyses (A). Micromass cultures demonstrate impaired chondrogenesis and chondrocyte differentiation in KO cells at day 1 and day 7, as indicated by Alcian Blue staining (B) and Real Time PCR analyses of genes associated with chondrocyte differentiation and bone formation (C). * $p<0.05$, as compared to the control.

To further identify BMP responsive genes whose expression is mediated by COX-2, we separately analyzed the gene profiling in control and Cox-2 deficient PDMPCs at day 1 and day 7 following BMP-2 treatment. At day 1, among 193 BMP-2-responsive genes whose expression were changed by 2-fold or more in control *Cox-2*$^{f/f}$ cells, 30 of these genes had significantly suppressed expression in Cox-2 deficient cells in response to BMP-2. These 30 genes are known to be involved in regulation of cellular proliferation and differentiation and in developmental process associated with bone/cartilage formation (Fig. 5A). Among genes that were markedly down-regulated by one day of exposure to BMP-2 in *Cox-2*$^{f/f}$ (WT) cells, 20 of those genes were less down-regulated by BMP-2 in *Cox-2* deficient cells (Fig. 5B). These genes were functionally mapped to annotation categories of immune process and response to stress.

Markedly differences in gene expression profiles were identified in samples treated with BMP-2 at day 7. In control *Cox-2*$^{f/f}$ cells, a total of 1183 unique genes were identified that exhibited a change of 2-fold or more following BMP-2 treatment (Fig. S4A). Among BMP-2 upregulated genes, 447 unique transcripts had significantly reduced expression in BMP-2-treated *Cox-2* deficient cells. Gene ontology (GO) enrichment analyses using DAVID and Partek-associated software annotated these 449 differentially expressed genes into several major categories, including bone/cartilage development and ossification ($p = 2.0E\text{-}8$), glycolysis/gluconeogenesis ($p = 7.1E\text{-}7$), extracellular matrix ($p = 3.0E\text{-}10$), angiogenesis and vessel development ($p<0.01$) (Table 1). Among genes down-regulated by BMP-2 in *Cox-2*$^{f/f}$ WT cells, 208 genes showed less suppressed expression by BMP-2 in *Cox-2* deficient cells. These genes were functionally mapped to annotation categories of immune system response, leukocytes and osteoclast differentiation, biological adhesion, and angiogenesis (Table 1). The marked differences in gene expression profile between Cox-2 deficient cells and control PDMPCs in response to BMP-2 strongly suggest Cox-2 as one of the important downstream mediators of BMP-2.

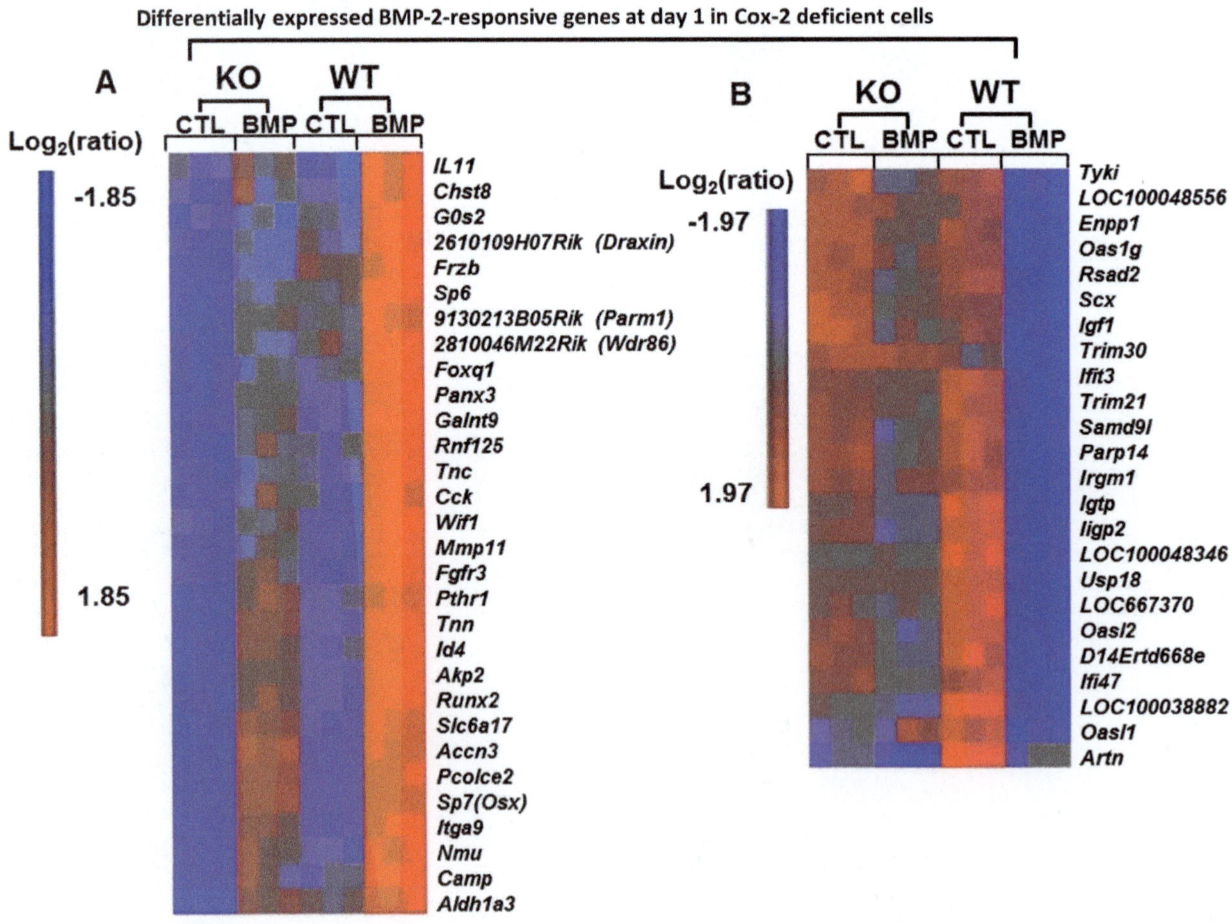

Figure 5. Differentially down- and up-regulated genes in *Cox-2*$^{f/f}$ and *Cox-2*$^{f/f}$; *Prx1Cre* PDMPCs in response to BMP-2. Heat map showing differential expression of 30 BMP-2-upregulated genes (A) and 24 BMP-2-downregulated genes (B) in Cox-2$^{f/f}$ (WT) in micromass cultures at day 1 and their corresponding expression levels in BMP-2 treated *Cox-2*$^{f/f}$; *Prx1Cre* (KO) micromass cultures. Each column shows the relative gene expression of a sample for the indicated pathway-associated genes. Gene up-regulation is presented in red and gene down-regulation is in blue.

Table 1. Go classification of the differentially expressed genes in Cox-2 deficient cells at day 7 in response to BMP-2.

Functional classification	Fisher exact p value	Genes included in the group
Upregulated by BMP-2 in WT, significantly suppressed in KO (447 genes)		
Bone/cartilage development process (ossification)	2.0E-8	39
Glycolysis/gluconeogenesis	7.1E-7	14
Extracellular matrix	3.0E-10	27
Angiogenesis and vessel development	<0.01	24
Down-regulated by BMP-2 in WT, significantly less regulated in KO (208 genes)		
Immune system response	3.0E-5	42
Leukocytes and osteoclasts differentiation	9.6E-4	13
Biological adhesion	6.3E-3	15
angiogenesis	<0.01	14

The table lists major functional categories enriched by DAVID using differentially expressed, BMP-2 up-regulated or down-regulated genes following seven days of culture in the presence or absence of BMP-2. Fisher exact P values for the gene-enrichment categories were generated by DAVID. "Genes included in the group" indicate the number of genes enriched for that category from the input gene list.

Enriched biological pathway analyses demonstrate dysregulation of the HIF1, PI3K-AKT and Wnt pathways in Cox-2 deficient PDMPCs

The genes differentially expressed in *Cox-2^f/f^ and Cox-2^f/f^; Prx1Cre* PDMPCs at day 1 and day 7 in the presence and absence of BMP-2 were further analyzed using the KEGG pathway database available in the Partek Genomic Suite. The main signaling pathways dysregulated by the absence of Cox-2 are the PI3K-AKT, HIF-1 and Wnt pathways. At day 1, genes annotated to the PI3K-AKT pathway, whose expression were suppressed in *Cox-2* deficient cells in the presence of BMP-2, include *FGFR2* (1.4-fold, $p<0.01$), *FGFR3* (2.6-fold, $p<0.01$), *Itga9 (1.6fold, p< 0.01), Tnc (2.4-fold, p<0.01), Tnn (2.2fold, p<0.01)*. At day 7, 34 of the annotated PI3K-AKT pathway genes had significantly altered expression in *Cox-2* deficient cells; eight of these genes were down-regulated, relative to wild-type cells, in the absence of any treatment and 26 of these genes were down-regulated, relative to wild type cells, following BMP-2 treatment (Fig. 6, top panel A).

Additional remarkable changes identified in Cox-2 deficient PDMPCs were the altered gene expressions annotated to the hypoxia inducible factor 1 (HIF-1) pathway. Among 41 HIF-1 pathway genes identified from control *Cox-2^f/f^* cells at day 7, 24 genes showed altered expression in the Cox-2 deficient cells (Fig. 6. top panel B). Real-time PCR analyses further confirmed the suppressed expression of several key genes of the HIF-1 pathway, namely *EGLN1, EGLN3, VEGFA, ANGPT4 and HIF-1a* in Cox-2 deficient cells day 7 (Fig. 6C). These data indicate strongly a key role for Cox-2 in modulating HIF-1 pathway activation in PDMPCs.

Wnt pathway genes were also enriched among the genes differentially expressed between *Cox-2^f/f^ and Cox-2^f/f^; Prx1Cre* PDMPCs at days 1 and 7. Several well-documented Wnt pathway inhibitory genes involved in bone metabolism were significantly suppressed at basal level in $Cox\text{-}2^{f/f}$; Prx1Cre PDMPCs at day 1 in micromass culture, including *Prickle1, Cdh2, Frzb, Sfrp1 and 2* (Fig. 7A). At day 7, 28 Wnt pathway-associated genes were suppressed in untreated cultures or following BMP-2 treatment. The altered genes included Wnt pathway receptors, as well as positive and negative regulators of the Wnt signaling pathway (Fig. 7B). Real-time PCR analyses further confirmed the altered expression of several key Wnt pathway associated genes in *Cox-2^f/f^; Prx1Cre* PDMPCs, namely, *Wif-1, N-cadherin, LRP4, FRZB, and TCF7* (Fig. 7C).

Discussion

During fracture healing mesenchymal progenitors residing in periosteum undergo osteogenic and chondrogenic differentiation to induce intramembranous and endochondral bone formation. To understand the spatiotemporal control of periosteal mesenchymal progenitor cell differentiation during repair and regeneration, we specifically deleted the *Cox2* gene in mesenchyme via Prx1cre or in cartilage via Col2Cre. Our studies show that Cox-2 acts at the early mesenchyme differentiation stage and mediates both osteogenic and chondrogenic differentiation of PDMPC during repair. Targeted *Cox-2* deletion via Prx1Cre in mesenchyme disrupted the entire differentiation program of mesenchyme progenitors, leading to reduction of bone formation and accretion of mesenchyme and immature cartilage in the callus (Figure 1). By contrast, targeted *Cox-2* deletion via *Col2Cre* expression in cartilage impaired fracture healing primarily by disrupting chondrocyte maturation, vascular invasion and endochondral bone formation. Consistent with the *in vivo* observation, cell differentiation and gene profiling analyses showed that *Prx1Cre*-mediated *Cox-2* deletion blunted osteogenic PDMPC differentiation, attenuated chondrogenesis and blocked BMP-2-induced chondrocyte maturation and terminal differentiation. Our data are consistent with the previous observation which demonstrates a marked induction of *Cox-2* mRNA at the onset of endochondral and intramembranous repair in early fracture callus [14,15], further providing direct evidence for a unique spatiotemporal role of Cox-2 in osteogenic and chondrogenic differentiation of periosteal progenitor cells in bone repair and regeneration.

To obtain mechanistic information underlying impaired fracture healing in Cox-2 deficient mice, we utilized a previously established method which allows isolation and *in vitro* analyses of mesenchymal progenitors derived from autografted periosteal callus (PDMPCs) [17,18,24]. This procedure permits robust isolation and recovery of otherwise limiting cell populations for biochemical and molecular analyses. By analyzing the differentiation potential and gene profiling of PDMPCs obtained directly from the healing site, we demonstrated that Cox-2 deficient cells exhibited decreased osteogenic and chondrogenic differentiation

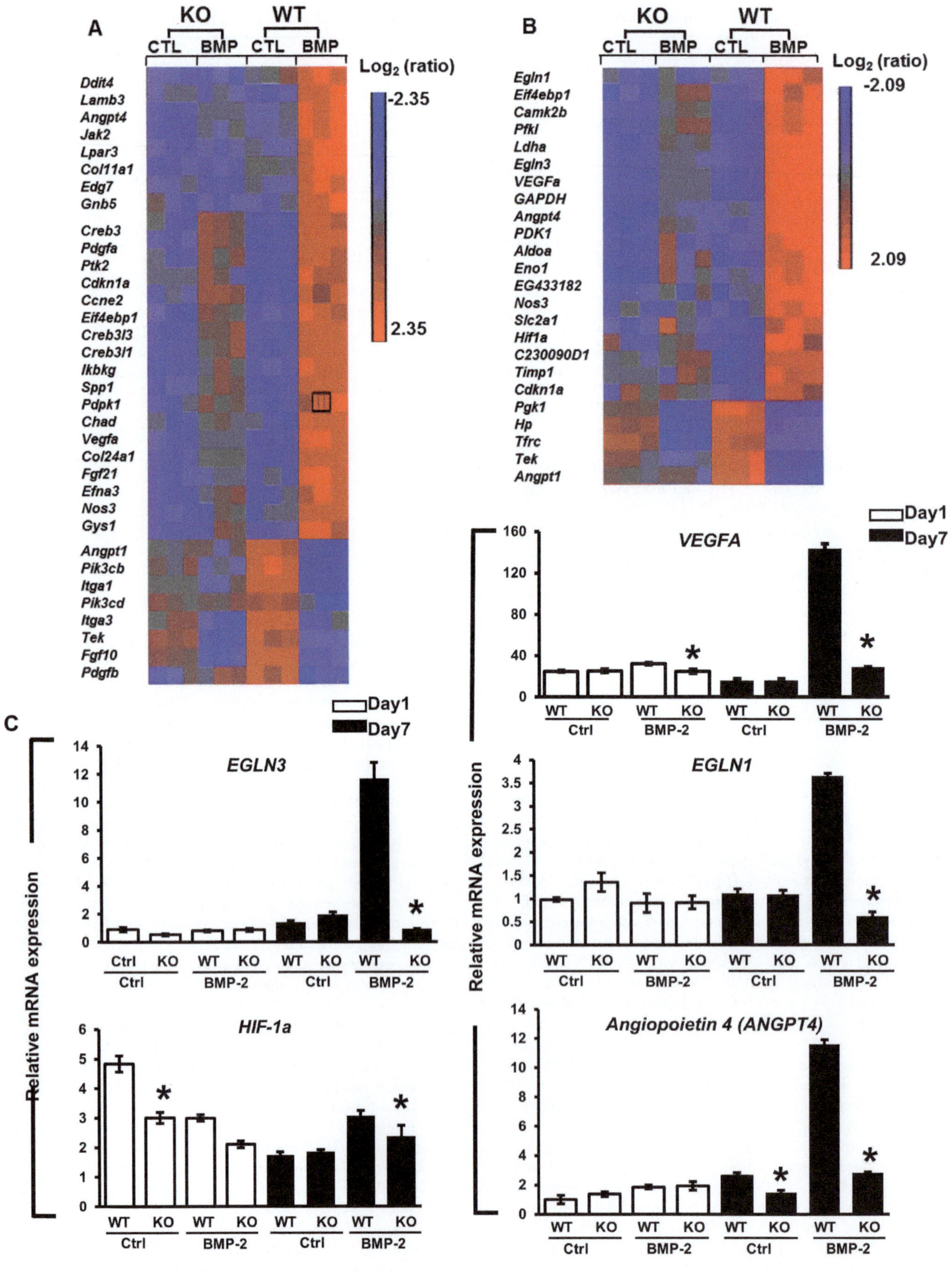
A
KO
WT
CTL
BMP
CTL
BMP
Log2 (ratio)
-2.35
2.35
Ddit4
Lamb3
Angpt4
Jak2
Lpar3
Col11a1
Edg7
Gnb5
Creb3
Pdgfa
Ptk2
Cdkn1a
Ccne2
Eif4ebp1
Creb3l3
Creb3l1
Ikbkg
Spp1
Pdpk1
Chad
Vegfa
Col24a1
Fgf21
Efna3
Nos3
Gys1
Angpt1
Pik3cb
Itga1
Pik3cd
Itga3
Tek
Fgf10
Pdgfb
B
KO
WT
CTL
BMP
CTL
BMP
Log2 (ratio)
-2.09
2.09
Egln1
Eif4ebp1
Camk2b
Pfkl
Ldha
Egln3
VEGFa
GAPDH
Angpt4
PDK1
Aldoa
Eno1
EG433182
Nos3
Slc2a1
Hif1a
C230090D1
Timp1
Cdkn1a
Pgk1
Hp
Tfrc
Tek
Angpt1
C
Day1
Day7
Relative mRNA expression
VEGFA
EGLN3
EGLN1
HIF-1a
Angiopoietin 4 (ANGPT4)
WT
KO
Ctrl
BMP-2
*

Figure 6. Dysregulation of the PI3K/AKT and HIF-1pathways in Cox-2 deficient PDMPCs. Heat maps showing differentially expressed genes associated with the PI3K/AKT (A) and the HIF-1 pathway (B) in micromass cultures in the presence and absence of BMP-2 for seven days. Each column shows the relative gene expression of a sample for the indicated pathway-associated genes. RT-PCR analyses further quantitate the values for the key genes in the HIF-1 pathway at day 1 (white bars) and day 7 (black bars) (C), namely *VEGFA, EGLN1, EGLN3, HIF-1a* and *ANGPT4*. * $p<0.05$, as compared to the control.

potential under basal culture conditions, for both monolayer and micromass culture. Gene profiling analyses revealed significant down-regulation in Cox-2 deficient cells of a set of key genes that control bone/cartilage ossification and remodeling as compared to the wild type controls; the genes *Sox9*, *Sp7 (OSX)*, *MMP13*, *MMP9*, *RANKL* and *VDR*. The reduced expression of this key set of genes in Cox-2 deficient mesenchymal progenitors is likely to explain the impaired bone formation and delayed cartilage remodeling observed in the Cox-2 mutant mice at the onset of fracture healing, indicating that the differentiation of the mesenchymal progenitors depends on Cox-2 expression during initiation of healing. The data are consistent with the anabolic effects of prostaglandins, e.g. prostaglandin E2 (PGE2) in stimulating bone formation and bone/cartilage remodeling in repair [15,25–27], underscoring a direct role of Cox-2 from cells of mesenchymal lineages in modulating expression of this key set of genes in repair and regeneration. In addition to the altered gene expression associated with bone formation, GO analyses also identified functional gene clusters (Table S1) that regulate immune and inflammatory responses, suggesting that Cox-2 deletion in mesenchymal progenitors could further modify immune response and change local inflammatory microenvironments at the onset of bone healing [28,29].

By analyzing PDMPC differentiation in response to BMP-2 treatment, our study demonstrated a key role of Cox-2 in BMP-2-induced mesenchymal differentiation. BMP-2 is known for its strong osteo-inductive and chondro-inductive actions on mesenchymal progenitors *in vivo* and *in vitro* [30]. Recent studies have further established BMP-2 as a critical gene in the initiation of bone fracture repair [31]. Similar to Cox-2, BMP-2 deletion via Prx1Cre produces minimal effects on embryonic long bone development (23). However, postnatal deletion of the BMP-2 gene in periosteum impairs chondrogenic and osteogenic differentiation of mesenchymal progenitor cells and impedes periosteum-mediated endochondral and intramembranous bone formation [17,32]. While we observed modest Cox-2 protein induction in monolayer cultures, both Cox-2 protein and mRNA were markedly induced by BMP-2 in micromass cultures, suggesting a key role of Cox-2 in BMP-2 mediated chondrogenic differentiation of PDMPCs. Prx1Cre-mediated *Cox-2* deletion further attenuated BMP-2-induced osteogenic differentiation in monolayer culture and completely blocked chondrocyte maturation and terminal differentiation in micromass culture. These data speak directly to the mechanism by which BMP-2 mediates bone differentiation, and establishes Cox-2 as a critical downstream mediator of BMP-2 action, demonstrating an important role of the BMP-2/Cox-2 axis in control of chondrogenic and osteogenic differentiation of mesenchymal progenitors in postnatal bone tissue repair.

By using GO pathway enrichment analyses, we identified the phosphoinositide 3-kinase/protein kinase B (PI3K/AKT), Hypoxia Inducible Factor-1 (HIF-1) and the Wnt pathway as key signaling pathways targeted by Cox-2 in BMP-2-induced PDMPC differentiation. The PI3K/AKT pathway crosstalks with a number of signaling pathways, including BMP/TGFβ signaling pathway, mTOR, NF-κb, JAK/STAT, MAPK, CREB, P53 and VEGF, which are known for their roles in stem/progenitor cell proliferation, osteoblast and chondrocyte differentiation, apoptosis and angiogenesis [33–35]. The PI3K/AKT pathway also plays a role in regulating glycolysis and gluconeogenesis processes [36,37], which are markedly affected by Cox-2 deletion (Table 1). A link between Cox-2 and the PI3K/AKT pathway has recently been reported in mouse and human osteoblasts [38]. Downregulation of COX-2 via gene silencing suppresses phosphorylation of AKT and PTEN. Interestingly, PGE2, one of the potential downstream products resulting from cyclooxygenase activity, failed to reverse COX-2-dependent AKT phosphorylation, suggesting a potential PGE2 independent mechanism(s) in BMP-2/COX-2/PI3K/AKT-mediated regulation of cell differentiation.

The HIF-1 pathway plays a central role in cellular response to hypoxic condition and is essential for bone/cartilage development and chondrocyte survival [39]. The HIF-1 pathway is also critically important in bone repair and regeneration [40,41]. While a direct link between HIF-1 pathway and Cox-2-mediated repair remains to be established, hypoxia regulates PGE2 release in osteoblasts [42,43] and COX-2/PGE2 signalling is involved in a hypoxia-induced angiogenic response in endothelial cells [44].The central player of HIF-1 pathway is HIF-1α, which is regulated at the post-transcriptional level by the HIF prolyl-hydroxylase domain enzymes (PHDs) (gene name: Egl nine homologs, Eglns). Eglns hydroxylate the α-subunit of HIF-1α, enabling binding of the von Hippel-Lindau (VHL) protein for poly-ubiquitination, which ultimately leads to proteolytic proteasomal degradation of HIF-1α [45,46]. In our current study, HIF-1α expression was only modest regulated during chondrogenic differentiation. However, the HIF prolyl-hydroxylase domain enzymes Egln1 and Egln3 were markedly induced by BMP-2 in PDMPCs at day 7, and this induction was abolished in the *Cox-2* deficient cells. The data suggest a requirement for Cox-2 expression in BMP-2 induction of *Egln1* and *3*, and their likely subsequent involvement in chondrocyte differentiation, vascular invasion and endochondral bone formation. In addition to *Egln1* and *Egln3*, a subset of genes associated with hypoxia, angiogenesis and vasculogenesis, namely *VEGFA* and *Angiopoietin 4* (*ANGPT4*), *Ddit4*, *Eif4ebp1*, *Camk2b*, *Pfkl*, *Ldha*, *Aldoa*, *PDK1*, *Slc2a1* were also markedly suppressed in *Cox-2* deficient PDMPCs (Fig. 6B). These data suggest a central role for Cox-2 from mesenchymal lineage in coordinating osteogenesis and angiogenesis in response to hypoxia during endochondral bone repair.

The Wnt pathway is known to play key roles in bone and cartilage development [47]. Canonical Wnt pathway activation favors osteoblastic differentiation, but inhibits chondrogenesis [48,49]. Activation of β-catenin signaling further stimulates chondrocyte hypertrophy and vascular invasion [50]. Although detailed molecular actions of the Wnt pathway on different phases of endochondral bone repair remain to be determined, genetic manipulation of Wnt signaling in mice demonstrates that inhibition of Wnt/β-catenin expression suppresses early chondrogenesis but favors osteogenesis, leading to accelerated but reduced fracture repair [51–53]. In our current study, we noted that Cox-2 inactivation in PDMPCs down regulated a group of genes that are classified as negative regulators of the canonical Wnt pathway; e.g., *N-cadherin*, *FRZB* and *Sfrps*, along with Sox9 at day 1 (Fig. 7A) Contrary to accelerated repair observed in a Wnt/β-catenin gain-of-function mouse model, Cox-2 deficiency is associated with a

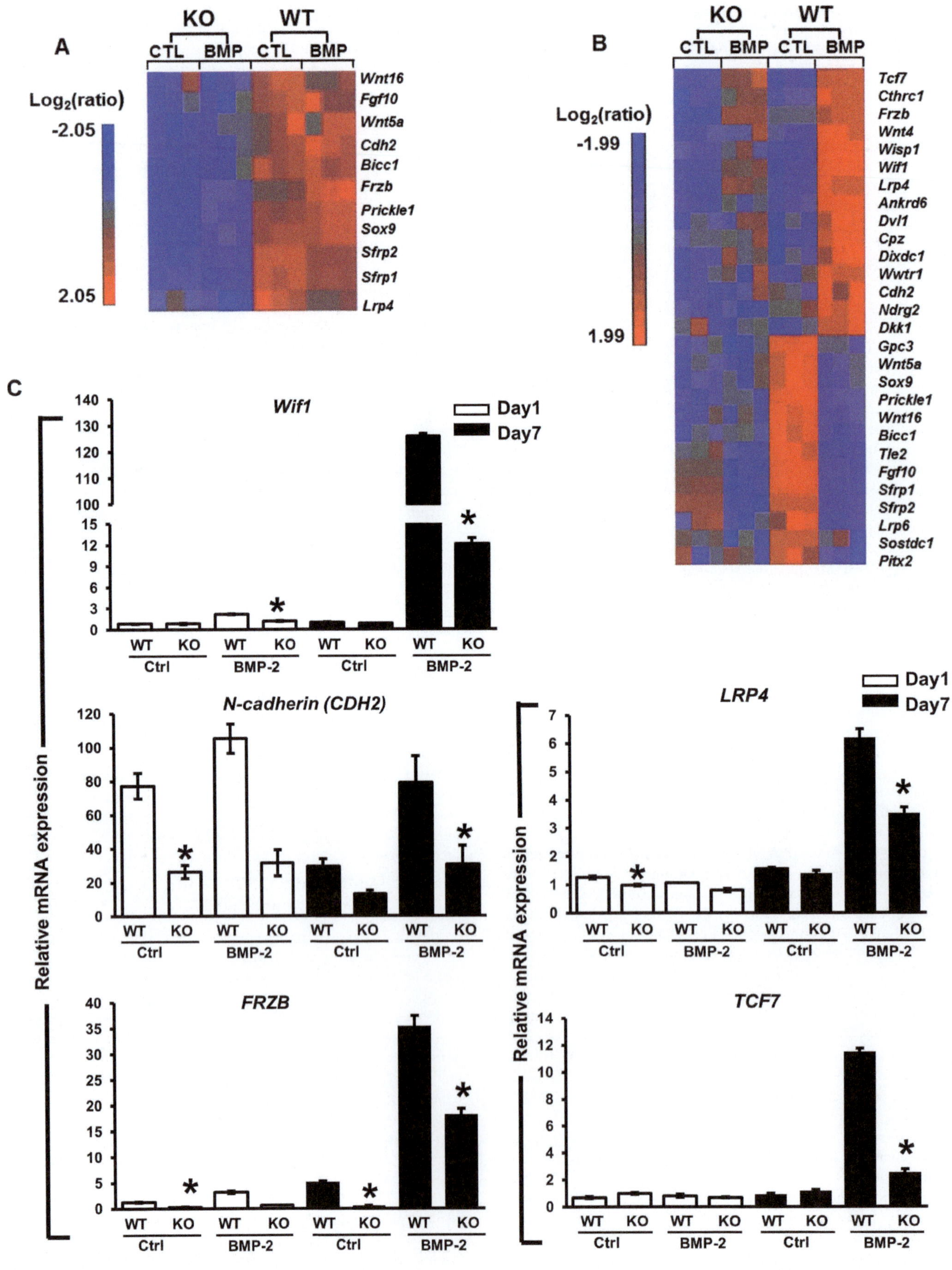
A
KO
WT
CTL
BMP
CTL
BMP
Log2(ratio)
-2.05
2.05
Wnt16
Fgf10
Wnt5a
Cdh2
Bicc1
Frzb
Prickle1
Sox9
Sfrp2
Sfrp1
Lrp4
B
KO
WT
CTL
BMP
CTL
BMP
Log2(ratio)
-1.99
1.99
Tcf7
Cthrc1
Frzb
Wnt4
Wisp1
Wif1
Lrp4
Ankrd6
Dvl1
Cpz
Dixdc1
Wwtr1
Cdh2
Ndrg2
Dkk1
Gpc3
Wnt5a
Sox9
Prickle1
Wnt16
Bicc1
Tle2
Fgf10
Sfrp1
Sfrp2
Lrp6
Sostdc1
Pitx2
C
Wif1
Day1
Day7
N-cadherin (CDH2)
LRP4
FRZB
TCF7
Relative mRNA expression
WT
KO
Ctrl
BMP-2

Figure 7. Deferentially expressed genes associated with the Wnt pathway in Cox-$2^{f/f}$ and Cox-$2^{f/f}$; Prx1Cre PDMPCs. Heat maps showing differentially expressed genes associated with the Wnt pathway at day 1 (A) and day 7 (B) micromass cultures. Each column shows the relative gene expression of a sample for the indicated Wnt pathway-associated genes. RT-PCR demonstrates expression of key genes in the Wnt pathway at day 1 (white bars) and day 7 (black bars) in cells with a targeted *Cox-2* gene deletion and in their littermate controls (C), namely *Wif1*, *N-cadherin (CDH2)*, *LRP4*, *FRZB*, and *TCF7*. * $p<0.05$, as compared to the control.

marked reduction of osteogenesis *in vitro* and *in vivo*, indicating that Cox-2 orchestrates a complex signaling interplay in conjunction with Wnt pathway regulators during repair and regeneration.

NSAIDs (non-steroidal anti-inflammatory drugs) which often inhibit both Cox-1 and Cox-2 are well known as having a negative effect on fracture healing in rat models [54,55]. Prolonged use of targeted Cox-2 inhibitors delays fracture healing in rats [13]. Transient inhibition of Cox-2 has small and reversible effects on fracture healing, suggesting that the adverse effect of Cox-2 inhibition may be both dosage and duration dependent [56,57]. Pharmacological inhibition of Cox-2 activity is also reported to have an inhibitory effect on differentiation of human and mouse mesenchymal stem cells [58,59]. Pharmacological studies are often confounded by dosing issue, specificity and the potential off-targeting effects of the drug. Using a gene targeting approach, our current study moves the field forward, we believe, by identifying cells that are likely to be the specific (or a specific) cell type in which COX-2 expression plays a modulatory role in fracture repair, and demonstrates the consequences of targeted Cox-2 gene deletion on fracture repair *in vivo*.

In summary, using cell-type specific *Cox-2* gene deletion, we demonstrate a spatial and temporal role for Cox-2 function in endochondral and intramembranous bone repair; targeted *Cox-2* gene deletion inhibits BMP-2-induced osteogenic, chondrogenic and angiogenic responses in periosteum-derived mesenchymal progenitors. Gene profiling analyses uncovered Cox-2-targeted pathways, e.g., the HIF-1, PI3K/AKT and Wnt pathways that modulate periosteal progenitor cell differentiation in bone fracture repair and regeneration. Identification of critical genes/targets in periosteal-derived mesenchymal progenitor cell differentiation could assist in identification of novel drug targets, facilitating development of new therapeutic solutions for bone repair and regeneration.

Supporting Information

Figure S1 Cox-$2^{f/f}$; Prx1cre mice have normal long bone length and cortical bone morphology. Quantitative measurements show identical length (A) and cortical thickness (B) in tibias of two-month-old Cox-$2^{f/f}$ and Cox-$2^{f/f}$; Prx1Cre mice. Data are presented as means ± SEM, n = 6.

Figure S2 *Cox-2* mRNA expression in day 1 and day 7 micromass cultures. Real Time PCR analyses show robust induction of Cox-2 gene expression by BMP-2 in micromass culture. Cox-2 mRNA was reduced by more than 95% in the Cox-$2^{f/f}$; Prx1Cre cells isolated from periosteal callus. * $p<0.05$, as compared to the control.

Figure S3 Comparison of Cox-$2^{f/f}$ (WT) and Cox-$2^{f/f}$; Prx1cre PDMPC gene expression profiles at day 1 vs. day 7 identified 1159 differentially expressed genes that exhibited a change of 2 fold or more. Hierarchical clustering analyses were used to generate the heat maps showing expression of these genes in Cox-$2^{f/f}$ (WT) and Cox-$2^{f/f}$; prx1cre (KO) cells at day 1 and 7 (A). Subsets of genes (111genes) associated with bone/cartilage formation and mineralization in Cox-$2^{f/f}$ and Cox-$2^{f/f}$; prx1cre cells at day 1 and 7 are further illustrated in the heat maps generated by hierarchical clustering analyses (B). The suppressed genes in Cox-$2^{f/f}$; prx1cre (KO) cells as compared to the Cox-$2^{f/f}$ (WT) cells at day 7 are listed in no particular order at the bottom. Gene up-regulation is presented in red and gene down-regulation is in blue.

Figure S4 Heat map showing expression of 1183 BMP-2 responsive genes in Cox-$2^{f/f}$ (WT) and Cox-$2^{f/f}$; prx1cre cells (KO) at day 7 (A). Among them, 181 unique probes associated with bone/cartilage formation and mineralization in Cox-$2^{f/f}$ (WT) and Cox-$2^{f/f}$; prx1cre (KO) cells were subjected to hierarchical clustering analyses to generate a heat map (B). Thirty-nine genes representing significantly suppressed genes in the KO cells at basal level or following BMP-2 treatment are listed at bottom without particular order. Gene up-regulation is presented in red and gene down-regulation is in blue.

Table S1 Go classification of the differentially expressed genes in Cox-2 deficient cells at day 1 without any treatment. Table S1 lists major functional categories enriched by DAVID using differentially expressed genes in Cox-2 deficient cells at day 1 without BMP-2 treatment. Genes suppressed or increased by 2 fold or more in the absence of Cox-2 were separately analyzed. Fisher exact P values for the gene-enrichment categories were generated from a reference gene list provided by Partek Genomic Suite software. "Genes included in the group" indicate the number of genes enriched for that category from the input gene list.

Table S2 Additional RT-PCR primers used for RT-PCR analyses in this study are listed.

Acknowledgments

We thank Ryan Tierry, Sarah Mack and Nehal for their assistance with histological work and Michael Thullen for microCT analyses.

Author Contributions

Conceived and designed the experiments: XPZ RJO. Performed the experiments: CH MX HC JJ. Analyzed the data: CH XPZ HRH. Contributed reagents/materials/analysis tools: HRH. Wrote the paper: XPZ HRH.

References

1. Eyre-Brook AL (1984) The periosteum: its function reassessed. Clin Orthop Relat Res: 300–307.
2. Malizos KN, Papatheodorou LK (2005) The healing potential of the periosteum molecular aspects. Injury 36 Suppl 3: S13–19.
3. McKibbin B (1978) The biology of fracture healing in long bones. J Bone Joint Surg Br 60-B: 150–162.

4. Colnot C, Zhang X, Knothe Tate ML (2012) Current insights on the regenerative potential of the periosteum: molecular, cellular, and endogenous engineering approaches. J Orthop Res 30: 1869–1878.
5. Barnes GL, Kostenuik PJ, Gerstenfeld LC, Einhorn TA (1999) Growth factor regulation of fracture repair. J Bone Miner Res 14: 1805–1815.
6. Gerstenfeld LC, Cullinane DM, Barnes GL, Graves DT, Einhorn TA (2003) Fracture healing as a post-natal developmental process: molecular, spatial, and temporal aspects of its regulation. J Cell Biochem 88: 873–884.
7. Zuscik MJ, Hilton MJ, Zhang X, Chen D, O'Keefe RJ (2008) Regulation of chondrogenesis and chondrocyte differentiation by stress. J Clin Invest 118: 429–438.
8. Smith WL, Langenbach R (2001) Why there are two cyclooxygenase isozymes. J Clin Invest 107: 1491–1495.
9. Agarwal S, Reddy GV, Reddanna P (2009) Eicosanoids in inflammation and cancer: the role of COX-2. Expert Rev Clin Immunol 5: 145–165.
10. Morham SG, Langenbach R, Loftin CD, Tiano HF, Vouloumanos N, et al. (1995) Prostaglandin synthase 2 gene disruption causes severe renal pathology in the mouse. Cell 83: 473–482.
11. Robertson G, Xie C, Chen D, Awad H, Schwarz EM, et al. (2006) Alteration of femoral bone morphology and density in COX-2−/− mice. Bone 39: 767–772.
12. Zhang X, Schwarz EM, Young DA, Puzas JE, Rosier RN, et al. (2002) Cyclooxygenase-2 regulates mesenchymal cell differentiation into the osteoblast lineage and is critically involved in bone repair. J Clin Invest 109: 1405–1415.
13. Simon AM, Manigrasso MB, O'Connor JP (2002) Cyclo-oxygenase 2 function is essential for bone fracture healing. J Bone Miner Res 17: 963–976.
14. Naik AA, Xie C, Zuscik MJ, Kingsley P, Schwarz EM, et al. (2009) Reduced COX-2 expression in aged mice is associated with impaired fracture healing. J Bone Miner Res 24: 251–264.
15. Xie C, Liang B, Xue M, Lin AS, Loiselle A, et al. (2009) Rescue of impaired fracture healing in COX-2−/− mice via activation of prostaglandin E2 receptor subtype 4. Am J Pathol 175: 772–785.
16. Lau KH, Kothari V, Das A, Zhang XB, Baylink DJ (2013) Cellular and molecular mechanisms of accelerated fracture healing by COX2 gene therapy: studies in a mouse model of multiple fractures. Bone 53: 369–381.
17. Wang Q, Huang C, Xue M, Zhang X (2011) Expression of endogenous BMP-2 in periosteal progenitor cells is essential for bone healing. Bone 48: 524–532.
18. Wang Q, Huang C, Zeng F, Xue M, Zhang X (2010) Activation of the Hh pathway in periosteum-derived mesenchymal stem cells induces bone formation in vivo: implication for postnatal bone repair. Am J Pathol 177: 3100–3111.
19. Ishikawa TO, Herschman HR (2006) Conditional knockout mouse for tissue-specific disruption of the cyclooxygenase-2 (Cox-2) gene. Genesis 44: 143–149.
20. Bonnarens F, Einhorn TA (1984) Production of a standard closed fracture in laboratory animal bone. J Orthop Res 2: 97–101.
21. Zhang X, Xie C, Lin AS, Ito H, Awad H, et al. (2005) Periosteal progenitor cell fate in segmental cortical bone graft transplantations: implications for functional tissue engineering. J Bone Miner Res 20: 2124–2137.
22. Wang Y, Belflower RM, Dong YF, Schwarz EM, O'Keefe RJ, et al. (2005) Runx1/AML1/Cbfa2 mediates onset of mesenchymal cell differentiation toward chondrogenesis. J Bone Miner Res 20: 1624–1636.
23. Zhang X, Ziran N, Goater JJ, Schwarz EM, Puzas JE, et al. (2004) Primary murine limb bud mesenchymal cells in long-term culture complete chondrocyte differentiation: TGF-beta delays hypertrophy and PGE2 inhibits terminal differentiation. Bone 34: 809–817.
24. Huang C, Tang M, Yehling E, Zhang X (2013) Overexpressing Sonic Hedgehog Peptide Restores Periosteal Bone Formation in a Murine Bone Allograft Transplantation Model. Mol Ther.
25. Paralkar VM, Borovecki F, Ke HZ, Cameron KO, Lefker B, et al. (2003) An EP2 receptor-selective prostaglandin E2 agonist induces bone healing. Proc Natl Acad Sci U S A 100: 6736–6740.
26. Ninomiya T, Hosoya A, Hiraga T, Koide M, Yamaguchi K, et al. (2011) Prostaglandin E(2) receptor EP(4)-selective agonist (ONO-4819) increases bone formation by modulating mesenchymal cell differentiation. Eur J Pharmacol 650: 396–402.
27. Li X, Pilbeam CC, Pan L, Breyer RM, Raisz LG (2002) Effects of prostaglandin E2 on gene expression in primary osteoblastic cells from prostaglandin receptor knockout mice. Bone 30: 567–573.
28. Zhang Q, Shi S, Liu Y, Uyanne J, Shi Y, et al. (2009) Mesenchymal stem cells derived from human gingiva are capable of immunomodulatory functions and ameliorate inflammation-related tissue destruction in experimental colitis. J Immunol 183: 7787–7798.
29. Yaqub S, Tasken K (2008) Role for the cAMP-protein kinase A signaling pathway in suppression of antitumor immune responses by regulatory T cells. Crit Rev Oncog 14: 57–77.
30. Riley EH, Lane JM, Urist MR, Lyons KM, Lieberman JR (1996) Bone morphogenetic protein-2: biology and applications. Clin Orthop: 39–46.
31. Tsuji K, Bandyopadhyay A, Harfe BD, Cox K, Kakar S, et al. (2006) BMP2 activity, although dispensable for bone formation, is required for the initiation of fracture healing. Nat Genet 38: 1424–1429.
32. Chappuis V, Gamer L, Cox K, Lowery JW, Bosshardt DD, et al. (2012) Periosteal BMP2 activity drives bone graft healing. Bone 51: 800–809.
33. Manning BD, Cantley LC (2007) AKT/PKB signaling: navigating downstream. Cell 129: 1261–1274.
34. Mukherjee A, Rotwein P (2009) Akt promotes BMP2-mediated osteoblast differentiation and bone development. J Cell Sci 122: 716–726.
35. Mukherjee A, Wilson EM, Rotwein P (2010) Selective signaling by Akt2 promotes bone morphogenetic protein 2-mediated osteoblast differentiation. Mol Cell Biol 30: 1018–1027.
36. DeBerardinis RJ, Lum JJ, Hatzivassiliou G, Thompson CB (2008) The biology of cancer: metabolic reprogramming fuels cell growth and proliferation. Cell Metab 7: 11–20.
37. Wallace DC (2005) Mitochondria and cancer: Warburg addressed. Cold Spring Harb Symp Quant Biol 70: 363–374.
38. Li CJ, Chang JK, Wang GJ, Ho ML (2011) Constitutively expressed COX-2 in osteoblasts positively regulates Akt signal transduction via suppression of PTEN activity. Bone 48: 286–297.
39. Schipani E, Ryan HE, Didrickson S, Kobayashi T, Knight M, et al. (2001) Hypoxia in cartilage: HIF-1alpha is essential for chondrocyte growth arrest and survival. Genes Dev 15: 2865–2876.
40. Wan C, Gilbert SR, Wang Y, Cao X, Shen X, et al. (2008) Activation of the hypoxia-inducible factor-1alpha pathway accelerates bone regeneration. Proc Natl Acad Sci U S A 105: 686–691.
41. Zou D, Zhang Z, Ye D, Tang A, Deng L, et al. (2011) Repair of critical-sized rat calvarial defects using genetically engineered bone marrow-derived mesenchymal stem cells overexpressing hypoxia-inducible factor-1alpha. Stem Cells 29: 1380–1390.
42. Lee CM, Genetos DC, Wong A, Yellowley CE (2010) Prostaglandin expression profile in hypoxic osteoblastic cells. J Bone Miner Metab 28: 8–16.
43. Lee CM, Genetos DC, You Z, Yellowley CE (2007) Hypoxia regulates PGE(2) release and EP1 receptor expression in osteoblastic cells. J Cell Physiol 212: 182–188.
44. Zhao L, Wu Y, Xu Z, Wang H, Zhao Z, et al. (2012) Involvement of COX-2/PGE2 signalling in hypoxia-induced angiogenic response in endothelial cells. J Cell Mol Med 16: 1840–1855.
45. Jaakkola P, Mole DR, Tian YM, Wilson MI, Gielbert J, et al. (2001) Targeting of HIF-alpha to the von Hippel-Lindau ubiquitylation complex by O2-regulated prolyl hydroxylation. Science 292: 468–472.
46. Ivan M, Haberberger T, Gervasi DC, Michelson KS, Gunzler V, et al. (2002) Biochemical purification and pharmacological inhibition of a mammalian prolyl hydroxylase acting on hypoxia-inducible factor. Proc Natl Acad Sci U S A 99: 13459–13464.
47. Regard JB, Zhong Z, Williams BO, Yang Y (2012) Wnt signaling in bone development and disease: making stronger bone with Wnts. Cold Spring Harb Perspect Biol 4.
48. Akiyama H, Lyons JP, Mori-Akiyama Y, Yang X, Zhang R, et al. (2004) Interactions between Sox9 and beta-catenin control chondrocyte differentiation. Genes Dev 18: 1072–1087.
49. Day TF, Guo X, Garrett-Beal L, Yang Y (2005) Wnt/beta-catenin signaling in mesenchymal progenitors controls osteoblast and chondrocyte differentiation during vertebrate skeletogenesis. Dev Cell 8: 739–750.
50. Dao DY, Jonason JH, Zhang Y, Hsu W, Chen D, et al. (2012) Cartilage-specific beta-catenin signaling regulates chondrocyte maturation, generation of ossification centers, and perichondrial bone formation during skeletal development. J Bone Miner Res 27: 1680–1694.
51. Chen Y, Alman BA (2009) Wnt pathway, an essential role in bone regeneration. J Cell Biochem 106: 353–362.
52. Chen Y, Whetstone HC, Lin AC, Nadesan P, Wei Q, et al. (2007) Beta-catenin signaling plays a disparate role in different phases of fracture repair: implications for therapy to improve bone healing. PLoS Med 4: e249.
53. Gaur T, Wixted JJ, Hussain S, O'Connell SL, Morgan EF, et al. (2009) Secreted frizzled related protein 1 is a target to improve fracture healing. J Cell Physiol 220: 174–181.
54. Altman RD, Latta LL, Keer R, Renfree K, Hornicek FJ, et al. (1995) Effect of nonsteroidal antiinflammatory drugs on fracture healing: a laboratory study in rats. J Orthop Trauma 9: 392–400.
55. Allen HL, Wase A, Bear WT (1980) Indomethacin and aspirin: effect of nonsteroidal anti-inflammatory agents on the rate of fracture repair in the rat. Acta Orthop Scand 51: 595–600.
56. Gerstenfeld LC, Einhorn TA (2004) COX inhibitors and their effects on bone healing. Expert Opin Drug Saf 3: 131–136.
57. Gerstenfeld LC, Thiede M, Seibert K, Mielke C, Phippard D, et al. (2003) Differential inhibition of fracture healing by non-selective and cyclooxygenase-2 selective non-steroidal anti-inflammatory drugs. J Orthop Res 21: 670–675.
58. Kellinsalmi M, Parikka V, Risteli J, Hentunen T, Leskela HV, et al. (2007) Inhibition of cyclooxygenase-2 down-regulates osteoclast and osteoblast differentiation and favours adipocyte formation in vitro. Eur J Pharmacol 572: 102–110.
59. Wang JH, Liu YZ, Yin LJ, Chen L, Huang J, et al. (2013) BMP9 and COX-2 form an important regulatory loop in BMP9-induced osteogenic differentiation of mesenchymal stem cells. Bone 57: 311–321.

2

Microstructural Parameters of Bone Evaluated Using HR-pQCT Correlate with the DXA-Derived Cortical Index and the Trabecular Bone Score in a Cohort of Randomly Selected Premenopausal Women

Albrecht W. Popp[1]*, Helene Buffat[1], Ursula Eberli[2], Kurt Lippuner[1], Manuela Ernst[2], R. Geoff Richards[2], Vincent A. Stadelmann[2], Markus Windolf[2]

1 Department of Osteoporosis, Inselspital, Berne University Hospital and University of Berne, Berne, Switzerland, **2** AO Research Institute Davos, Davos, Switzerland

Abstract

Background: Areal bone mineral density is predictive for fracture risk. Microstructural bone parameters evaluated at the appendicular skeleton by high-resolution peripheral quantitative computed tomography (HR-pQCT) display differences between healthy patients and fracture patients. With the simple geometry of the cortex at the distal tibial diaphysis, a cortical index of the tibia combining material and mechanical properties correlated highly with bone strength ex vivo. The trabecular bone score derived from the scan of the lumbar spine by dual-energy X-ray absorptiometry (DXA) correlated ex vivo with the micro architectural parameters. It is unknown if these microstructural correlations could be made in healthy premenopausal women.

Methods: Randomly selected women between 20–40 years of age were examined by DXA and HR-pQCT at the standard regions of interest and at customized sub regions to focus on cortical and trabecular parameters of strength separately. For cortical strength, at the distal tibia the volumetric cortical index was calculated directly from HR-pQCT and the areal cortical index was derived from the DXA scan using a Canny threshold-based tool. For trabecular strength, the trabecular bone score was calculated based on the DXA scan of the lumbar spine and was compared with the corresponding parameters derived from the HR-pQCT measurements at radius and tibia.

Results: Seventy-two healthy women were included (average age 33.8 years, average BMI 23.2 kg/m^2). The areal cortical index correlated highly with the volumetric cortical index at the distal tibia ($R = 0.798$). The trabecular bone score correlated moderately with the microstructural parameters of the trabecular bone.

Conclusion: This study in randomly selected premenopausal women demonstrated that microstructural parameters of the bone evaluated by HR-pQCT correlated with the DXA derived parameters of skeletal regions containing predominantly cortical or cancellous bone. Whether these indexes are suitable for better predictions of the fracture risk deserves further investigation.

Editor: Dominique Heymann, Faculté de médecine de Nantes, France

Funding: This study was funded by the AO Research program. The funders had no role in study design, data collection and analysis, decision to publish, or preparation of the manuscript.

Competing Interests: The authors have declared that no competing interests exist.

* E-mail: albrecht.popp@insel.ch

Introduction

In addition to low bone mass, osteoporosis was characterized in the WHO Technical Report of 1994 [1] by the micro architectural deterioration of bone tissue. Predominantly driven by sex steroid hormone levels changing with aging, the structures of the long bones are altered by enhanced endosteal resorption and are only in part compensated by periosteal apposition [2]. This change translates into altered micro architecture of the trabecular and cortical bone in vivo as assessed by high resolution imaging techniques, such as high-resolution peripheral quantitative computed tomography (HR-pQCT) [3]. For the cortex, trabecularization of the cortical bone with aging has been suggested [4]. Accordingly, ex-vivo micrographs of the femoral cortex demonstrated increasing porosity and thinning of the cortex by coalescence of the intracortical pores [5].

Different studies have demonstrated the direct relationship between the mechanical properties of specific anatomical regions and their architecture ex vivo [6,7] and in silico [8–10]. Even if the differences in the areal bone mineral density (aBMD) measurements by dual-energy X-ray absorptiometry (DXA) at the standardized sites were inexistent or mild, these structural parameters could distinguish between individuals with or without prevalent low velocity fractures [11,12]. The standard regions of interest (ROI) used in the clinically applied HR-pQCT measurements at the distal radius and tibia were formerly focused on the trabecular bone [13], but meanwhile the quantification of the cortical bone derived indices, including the cortical porosity (Ct.Po) based on automated segmentation from HR-pQCT images, has been implemented [14].

A low aBMD is predictive of the individual fracture risk in postmenopausal women when measured at the hip, lumbar spine, or radius [15,16]. The best predictive ability was observed when the measurements were performed at the same skeletal sites that sustained a fracture later. Whereas the tibial epiphysis (T-EPI) consists predominantly of trabecular bone, the tibial diaphysis (T-DIA) is predominantly composed of cortical bone. The authors previously showed that, in a cohort of randomly selected postmenopausal women, aBMD measured by DXA at both tibial subregions was predictive for non-vertebral fracture risk [17]. T-scores were generally higher at the T-DIA than at the T-EPI suggesting that the T-DIA might be suitable for identifying other contributors of an individual's fracture risk, including parameters related to the shape and size.

Because of the growing share of cortex from distal to proximal the ratio of trabecular and cortical bone is highly variable at the tibial metaphysis [18]. A more proximal region of interest with thicker and more homogeneous cortices, such as the T-DIA, has a simple geometric structure, similar to a hollow cylinder. The combination of the aBMD at the T-DIA and the structural parameters derived from DXA scans and confirmed by HR-pQCT can improve the prediction of local bone strength ex vivo [19]. It is unknown whether this combination of material and structural competence can be confirmed by both of the techniques in a standardized procedure in vivo.

The trabecular bone score (TBS) is a DXA-derived parameter that focuses on the cancellous architecture. This score quantifies the gray-level texture out of the DXA scan of the lumbar spine [20]. TBS was shown not to correlate or to correlate weakly with the aBMD in postmenopausal women ranging from 0.2 to 0.58 [21–23]. In epidemiological studies, TBS was significantly lower in the women with incidental fractures compared to the controls [24]. Even improvements in the TBS could be observed in postmenopausal women under antiresorptive treatment in a randomized controlled trial [22]. While the correlation of this texture parameter to the parameters of microarchitecture, e.g., the degree of connectivity, the trabecular number and separation, was performed ex vivo by micro-computed tomography [25], little is known if these correlations can be confirmed by the HR-pQCT measurement of these parameters at the appendicular skeleton in vivo.

The aim of this study was to evaluate whether and to what extent the DXA-derived cortical and trabecular structural parameters correlate with the bone microstructural parameters assessed using HR-pQCT in premenopausal women.

Materials and Methods

Study participants

In December 2012, study invitations were mailed to a total of 485 women selected from commercially available address listings categorized by sex, age, and the region of Davos, Switzerland. Mobile, non-institutionalized, not pregnant (confirmed by a negative pregnancy test) randomly selected women between 20–40 years old were eligible. The exclusion criteria were a known bone disease or immobilization (relative or absolute immobilization was defined as unable to stand or walk at least one hour per day). In total, 72 women were included in this study, sixty-nine of these women were white. The left upper and lower extremities were examined or the nonfractured contralateral extremity in cases of prior fracture on the left side (Fig. 1). All of the measurements occurred at the AO Research Institute Davos, Switzerland.

Ethical Statement

The study was approved by the local ethics committee for medical sciences (Ethics Committee of the Canton of Zurich, Switzerland, registration number 2012-0464). All of the participants provided prior written informed consent and were monetarily compensated for their efforts.

DXA Measurements

DXA densitometer measurements (Hologic Discovery C^{TM}, Hologic, Bedford, MA, USA) were performed with a mobile device provided by the Department of Osteoporosis, University Hospital Berne, Switzerland. aBMD was measured at the lumbar spine (L1-4; LS), the femoral neck (FN) and total hip (TH), the distal radius (Rad 1/3), and at the two customized subregions of the distal tibia (T-EPI, T-DIA). The detailed standardized procedures for the tibial BMD measurements by DXA were previously published [26]. The ROI is defined as the 120 mm height and 129 mm width area that starts 10 mm above the top of the ankle joint space. T-EPI corresponds to the distal 40 mm of the ROI, and T-DIA corresponds to the proximal 40 mm of the ROI (Fig. 2). aBMD is expressed in grams of hydroxyapatite (HA) per square centimeter of the projected area. The obtained aBMD values of the femoral neck were expressed as the standard deviation (SD) of the mean value of the young healthy population (T-scores) derived from the National Health and Nutrition Examination Survey in the United States of America (NHANES III) [27]. The scans were performed according to the manufacturer's guidelines, and the analyses were conducted according to the recommendations of the International Society of Clinical Densitometry. Spine phantom scanning was routinely performed on a daily basis for quality control. A least significant change at the 95% confidence level of 0.020 g/cm^2 for the aBMD at the total hip was achieved as the reproducibility index for the technician involved.

DXA-Derived Parameters of Cortical and Trabecular Bone

Assuming a hollow cylindrical shape of the T-DIA, the DXA-derived cortical thickness (Ct.Th) was calculated using the DICOM images of the DXA scan at the distal tibia. DXA gray-scale images were imported into Matlab^{TM} programming environment (MATLAB^{TM}, MathWorks Inc., Natick, MA, USA). The region of interest was automatically extracted for all data sets. Image data was segmented using an edge detection filter based on the algorithm proposed by Canny [28]. Canny threshold was kept constant at 0.05 resulting in a binary image showing the inner and outer borders of the cortex. A Butterworth filter was applied for smoothing the edges (Fig. 3). Cortex diameter (DIA) was defined as mean pixel distance between the outermost edges. Ct.Th was calculated as mean distance between outer and inner edges of the medial cortex projection, because the individual variation of Ct.Th is wider at the medial cortex than at the lateral cortex, i.e., the cortex closer to the fibula (own observation, unpublished data). Values were transformed to millimeter by isometric scaling (2.0 pixels/mm). Estimating the bony cross section as ideal tube the polar moment of inertia (pMOI) was computed according to formula I.

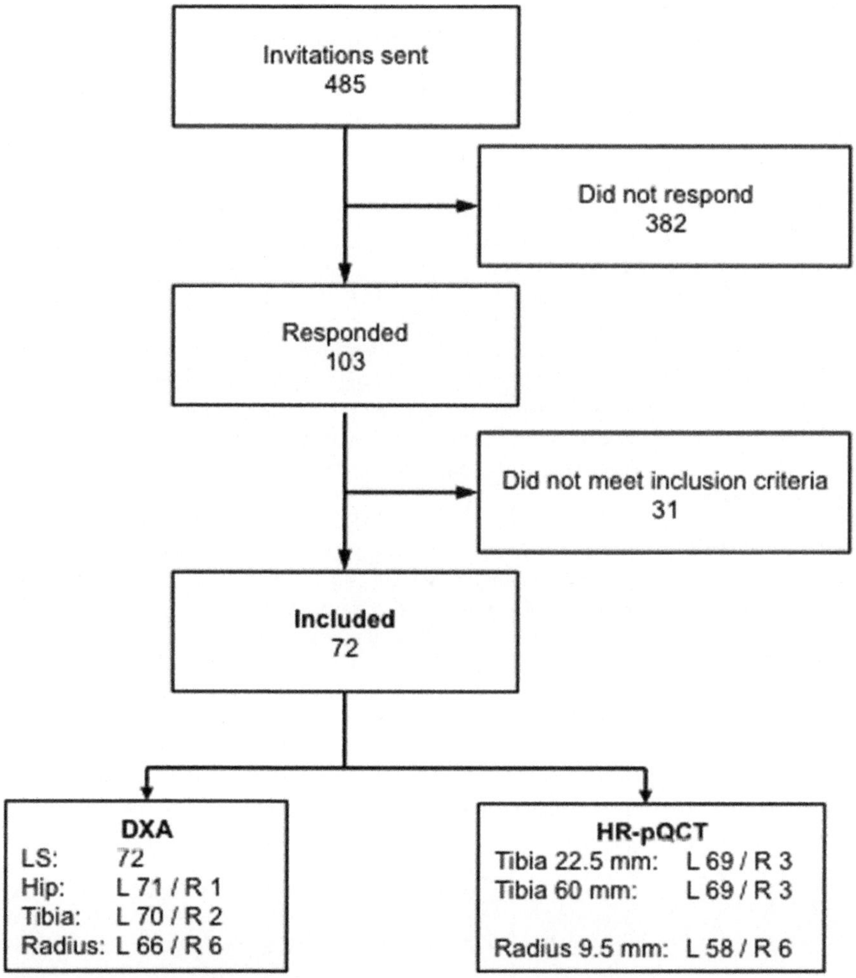

Figure 1. Consort flow diagram.

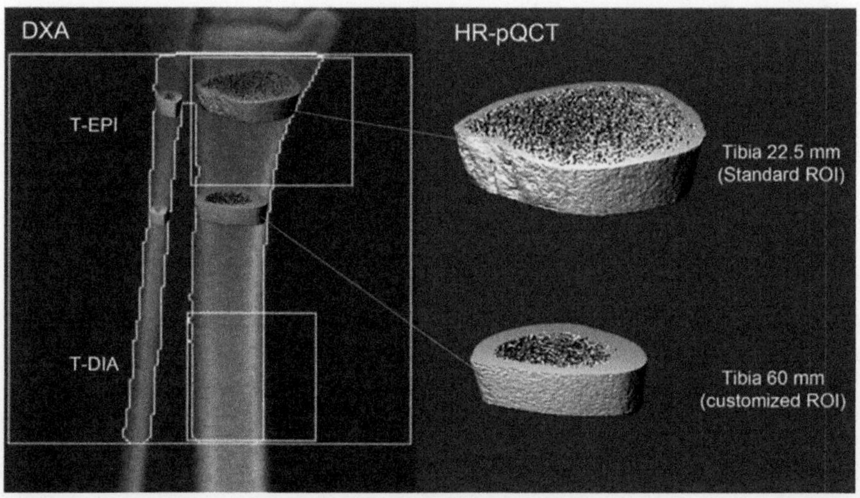

Figure 2. Regions of interest at the left distal tibia by DXA (left) and the volumes of interest as 3D reconstructions by HR-pQCT (right).

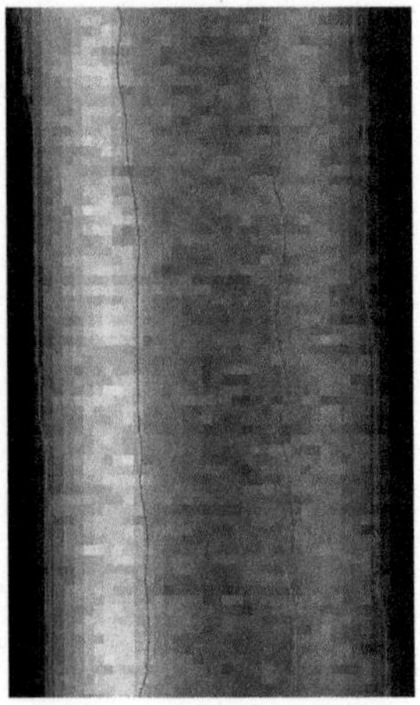

Figure 3. ROI of a representative DXA data set of the tibial diaphysis. The cortex edges as derived from image filtering are depicted as blue (outer diameter) and red lines (intramedullary channel).

$$\mathrm{pMOI} = \frac{\pi}{4}\left[\left(\frac{\mathrm{DIA}}{2}\right)^4 - \left(\frac{\mathrm{DIA}}{2} - \mathrm{Ct.Th}\right)^4\right] \quad \text{(I)}$$

A new parameter was introduced as cortical index for diaphyseal bone strength (CI), defined as product of a material (aBMD) and a structural component (pMOI). Because this CI is calculated from the two-dimensional DXA data, it is called the areal CI (aCI) in formula II.

$$\mathrm{aCI} = \mathrm{aBMD} * \mathrm{pMOI} \quad \text{(II)}$$

TBS was evaluated in the identical ROI as those used for the LS BMD. The dimensionless TBS values were calculated as the mean of the individual measurements for vertebrae L1-L4 from the DXA using TBS iNsight® Software (version 1.8.2; Med-Imaps, Bordeaux, France).

HR-pQCT Measurements

HR-pQCT (XtremeCT, Scanco Medical AG, Brüttisellen, Switzerland) measurements were performed by immobilizing the left forearm and the left distal tibia in a carbon fiber shell and scanning as previously described [29–31]. In addition to the standard ROI at the radius (radius 9.5 mm) and at the tibia (tibia 22.5 mm), a third customized ROI was scanned starting at the distal tibia 60 mm above the endplate (tibia 60 mm) to increase the amount of cortex measured (Fig. 2). A stack of 110 parallel CT slices was acquired at the distal starting points of all of the sites in the proximal direction using 60 kVp and a 126 mm field of view reconstructed across an image matrix size of 1536×1536, with a voxel size of 82 μm. These provided a 3D image of 9.02 mm in the axial direction. The attenuation data were converted to the equivalent hydroxyapatite (HA) densities. The manufacturer's phantom was scanned daily for quality control.

The bone morphological parameters were evaluated using the standard protocols provided by the manufacturer. The parameters of interest were the total volumetric bone mineral density (vBMD), the bone volume fraction (BV/TV), the trabecular bone density (Tb. BMD), the trabecular thickness (Tb.Th), the trabecular number (Tb.N), the trabecular separation (Tb.Sp), the inhomogeneity of the trabecular network, defined as Tb.1/N.SD, and connectivity density of the trabecular network (Conn.D), the cortical bone density (Ct.BMD) and the cortical thickness (Ct.Th). The cortical porosity (Ct.Po) and the polar moment of inertia (pMOI), as a structural index of resistance to torsion, were calculated using an automated image processing chain [14,32]. As an analogue to the calculation from DXA, the vBMD at both ROI of the tibia multiplied by the pMOI leads to the volumetric cortical index (vCI) as a potential parameter of cortical strength. Scans with severe movement artifacts, such as a blurry trabecular area or skewed or discontinued cortical faces, were excluded. Based on the categories (1 = best, 5 = worst), seven forearm scans of grade 3 and higher were excluded [33]. Additionally, a single forearm measurement by HR-pQCT was lost for technical reasons.

Table 1. Baseline characteristics.

n = 72	mean	SD
Age (years)	33.8	5.5
Height (cm)	167.6	6.2
Weight (kg)	65.2	12.1
BMI (kg/m2)	23.2	4.1
Calcium intake (mg per day)	816.0	402
	n	%
Nulliparas	42	58.3
Smoker total	19	26.4
former	10	13.9
current	9	12.5
Family history for osteoporosis	22	30.6
BMI < 18.5 kg/m^2	3	4.2
Ever glucocorticoid use	6	8.3

Table 2. Areal BMD and the structural derivates by DXA.

DXA		mean	SD
aBMD			
FN	g/cm^2	0.853	0.119
TH	g/cm^2	0.952	0.116
LS	g/cm^2	1.039	0.138
Rad 1/3	g/cm^2	0.712	0.046
T-DIA	g/cm^2	1.362	0.108
T-EPI	g/cm^2	0.750	0.096
Structural derivates			
Ct.Th (T-DIA)	mm	3.8	0.58
pMOI (T-DIA)	mm^4	1.9298	0.64
aCI	g*cm^2	2.62	0.856
TBS	-	1.399	0.087

Table 3. Volumetric BMD and the structural parameters by HR-pQCT.

HR-pQCT		radius 9.5 mm		tibia 22.5 mm		tibia 60 mm	
	Unit	*mean*	*SD*	*mean*	*SD*	*mean*	*SD*
total vBMD	mgHA/cm^3	307.6	53.3	303.2	50.1	550.3	79.3
BV/TV	%	13.7	2.8	14.1	2.9	7.6	2.6
Cortical parameters							
Ct.BMD	mgHA/cm^3	846.2	44.7	874.8	33.2	997.9	20.9
Ct.Th	mm	0.760	0.151	1.229	0.221	2.521	0.267
pMOI	mm^4	7694	2228	41104	11140	20031	4967
Ct.Po	%	2.8	1.0	4.3	1.2	1.2	0.5
vCI	gHA*cm	0.234	0.072	1.231	0.352	1.079	0.222
Trabecular parameters							
Tb.BMD	mgHA/cm^3	164.4	34.2	169.7	34.5	91.2	31.2
Tb.N	1/mm	1.944	0.246	1.912	0.312	1.476	0.424
Tb.Th	mm	0.070	0.009	0.074	0.011	0.052	0.011
Tb.Sp	mm	0.453	0.073	0.464	0.094	0.690	0.247
Inhomogeneity	mm	0.187	0.038	0.209	0.053	0.373	0.177
Conn.D	mm^{-3}	3.300	0.816	3.39	1.01	1.020	0.570

Statistical Analysis

The analyses were conducted with PASW statistical software (version 21.0; SPSS™, Chicago, IL). The two-sided p values <0.05 were considered to indicate statistical significance. The descriptive data were presented as the mean ± standard deviation (SD). After checking the variables of interest for normality (Kolmogorov-Smirnov test), the correlations between the structural parameters were expressed as R Pearson's coefficient. To compare correlations, Fisher's transformation was applied.

Results

Baseline Characteristics

Seventy-two healthy premenopausal women were included in the study. The anthropometric baseline characteristics are shown

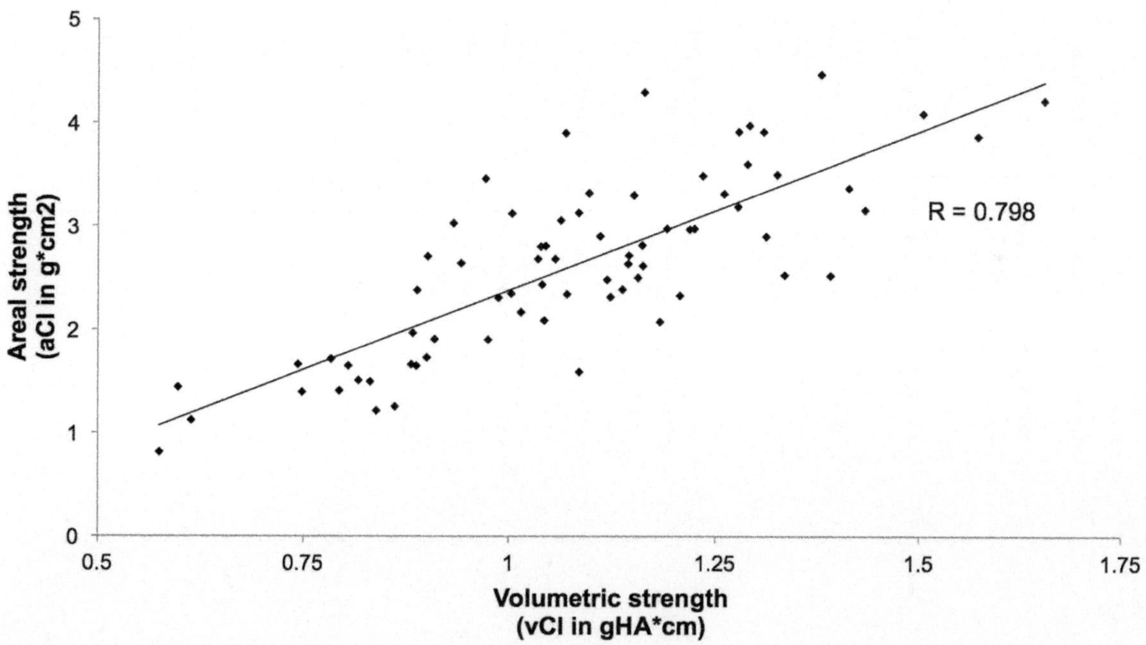

Figure 4. Correlation between the aCI (DXA) and the vCI (HR-pQCT) at the distal tibia.

Table 4. Correlations between the parameters derived from DXA and HR-pQCT.

	DXA									
HR-pQCT radius tibia 22.5 mm tibia 60 mm	**aBMD FN**	**aBMD TH**	**aBMD LS**	**aBMD Rad 1/3**	**aBMD T-DIA**	**aBMD T-EPI**	**Ct.Th T-DIA**	**pMOI T-DIA**	**aCI T-DIA**	**TBS**
total vBMD	**0.501 0.532** *0.295*	**0.586 0.603 0.307**	**0.334** *0.275* 0.020	**0.521 0.496 0.429**	**0.459 0.570 0.601**	**0.564 0.748 0.467**	*0.259* **0.586 0.566**	**−0.440 −0.333 −0.600**	*−0.337* −0.177 **−0.433**	0.242 *0.254* 0.029
BV/TV	**0.544 0.659 0.594**	**0.707 0.736 0.644**	**0.608 0.631 0.680**	**0.363 0.407** 0.227	**0.457 0.558 0.442**	**0.736 0.889 0.664**	**0.374 0.521** *0.247*	−0.117 0.075 0.169	0.015 0.220 *0.290*	**0.494 0.508 0.572**
Ct.BMD	*0.300* 0.196 −0.101	*0.288* 0.210 −0.113	0.045 −0.117 *−0.293*	**0.465 0.377** *0.257*	0.241 0.183 0.073	0.209 0.184 −0.068	0.065 0.119 −0.007	**−0.492 −0.436 −0.525**	**−0.417 −0.370 −0.494**	0.008 −0.017 *−0.295*
Ct.Th	**0.441 0.399 0.382**	**0.506 0.492 0.440**	*0.288* 0.163 0.186	**0.525 0.446 0.471**	**0.422 0.542 0.791**	**0.506 0.650 0.665**	0.230 **0.612 0.755**	**−0.326** *−0.285 −0.242*	−0.212 −0.134 −0.029	0.154 0.185 0.167
pMOI	0.115 0.205 0.149	*0.295* **0.302** *0.234*	**0.479 0.514 0.412**	−0.003 −0.030 −0.063	0.135 0.118 0.073	**0.448 0.368 0.466**	0.245 0.105 −0.002	**0.704 0.829 0.892**	**0.748 0.821 0.897**	*0.276* **0.351 0.315**
vCI	**0.411 0.542 0.452**	**0.640 0.680 0.564**	**0.684 0.708 0.588**	**0.324** *0.284 0.267*	**0.408 0.477 0.585**	**0.764 0.820 0.714**	**0.384 0.461 0.450**	**0.417 0.599 0.645**	**0.542 0.729 0.798**	**0.408 0.512 0.447**
Ct.Po	0.016 0.135 0.271	0.109 0.200 0.259	0.289 **0.415** *0.298*	−0.166 −0.122 −0.024	0.128 0.208 *0.301*	0.236 **0.308** *0.300*	0.110 *0.252* **0.308**	0.171 **0.338** 0.131	0.196 **0.392** 0.208	0.227 0.155 *0.247*
Tb.BMD	**0.544 0.659 0.593**	**0.707 0.735 0.643**	**0.608 0.630 0.681**	**0.363 0.408** 0.227	**0.458 0.559 0.442**	**0.737 0.889 0.665**	**0.373 0.522** *0.248*	−0.118 0.073 0.167	0.014 0.221 *0.288*	**0.493 0.508 0.570**
Tb.N	**0.467 0.525 0.604**	**0.532 0.565 0.611**	**0.517 0.645 0.565**	*0.307 0.268 0.274*	**0.400 0.420 0.552**	**0.589 0.627 0.636**	0.230 *0.260* **0.321**	−0.058 *0.253* 0.189	0.056 **0.358 0.330**	**0.432 0.527 0.497**
Tb.Th	**0.432 0.353** 0.115	**0.624 0.411** 0.167	**0.455** 0.136 *0.287*	*0.296 0.280* −0.082	**0.363** *0.293* −0.098	**0.608 0.533** 0.167	**0.389 0.437** −0.035	−0.152 −0.195 −0.002	−0.046 −0.011 −0.015	**0.373** 0.109 0.188
Tb.Sp	**−0.452 −0.517 −0.546**	**−0.551 −0.570 −0.582**	**−0.528 −0.672 −0.592**	**−0.322** *−0.280 −0.301*	**−0.415 −0.422 −0.526**	**−0.614 −0.656 −0.610**	*−0.272 −0.287 −0.295*	0.079 *−0.257* −0.208	–−0.040 **−0.360 −0.337**	**−0.428 −0.572 −0.570**
Inhomogeneity	**−0.475 −0.482 −0.571**	**−0.531 −0.503 −0.584**	**−0.487 −0.634 −0.536**	*−0.306 −0.233* **−0.355**	*−0.394 −0.322* **−0.550**	**−0.547 −0.563 −0.595**	−0.222 −0.183 **−0.306**	0.071 *−0.264* −0.100	−0.043 **−0.344** *−0.243*	**−0.408 −0.498 −0.510**
Conn.D	**0.425 0.432 0.466**	**0.496 0.464 0.473**	**0.499 0.596 0.575**	0.188 0.142 0.092	**0.377 0.346** *0.279*	**0.558 0.497 0.449**	0.228 0.155 0.040	0.061 **0.310 0.376**	0.172 **0.397 0.450**	**0.416 0.461 0.428**

$p<0.05$ (italic); **$p<0.01$ (bold).**

in Table 1. The mean age was 33.8 years; the mean height and BMI were 167.6 cm and 23.2 kg/m^2, respectively. Forty-two women were nulliparas, and 9 of 72 women were current smokers. The mean calcium intake was 816 mg per day. Thirty-eight females had prevalent fractures, mainly in the forearms (18), phalanges (14) and ankle (6). Twenty-two women or 30.6 % reported a potentially positive family history for osteoporosis, i.e. any self-reported major osteoporotic fracture (clinical spine, forearm, hip or shoulder fracture) among first-/second-grade relatives. As shown in Table 2, the femoral neck BMD was 0.853 g/cm^2, corresponding to a mean NHANES T-score of 0.04 (±1.08) SD. All of the areal and volumetric density parameters at all of the ROI were normally distributed (Tables 2 and 3). While the magnitude of extent of the vBMD was similar at the standard ROI of the radius 9.5 mm and the tibia 22.5 mm, the one at the tibia 60 mm was higher because of the higher portion of the cortical compartment. The Ct.Po was lower at the tibia 60 mm compared to the tibia 22.5 mm (1.2±0.5 % vs. 4.3±1.2 %).

Correlation Analysis Between the Cortical Parameters

For the cortex at the distal tibia, a significant correlation ($R = 0.74$, $p<0.01$, Table 4) was found between the CI measured at the tibia 22.5 mm by DXA and HR-pQCT, indicating that the bone strengths assessed by both techniques were predictive of each other. The correlation coefficient was even higher at the tibia 60 mm (Fig. 4), where the portion of cortical bone is more substantial, but without reaching statistical significance ($p = 0.3$).

Correlation Analysis Between the DXA-derived and HR-pQCT Parameters of the Trabecular Bone

The TBS of L1-4 correlated significantly ($p<0.01$) with the following parameters at the radius 9.5 mm and the tibia 22.5 mm: positively with the Tb.BMD, BV/TV, Tb.N, Conn.D, and negatively with the TbSp, inhomogeneity (Table 4). Correlations between the TBS and the Tb.Th, the total vBMD, the Ct.BMD, the Ct.Th or the Ct.Po were absent or inconsistent between the different skeletal sites. Among these healthy women, the TBS correlated with the aBMD at the lumbar spine and femoral neck ($R = 0.660$ and 0.532).

Discussion

The CI and TBS represent DXA derived parameters of the cortical and cancellous bone. This study showed for the first time that the corresponding structural parameters of the bone evaluated by HR-pQCT correlate with these DXA derived parameters in a cohort of randomly selected premenopausal women. In clinical practice, the aBMD is the only bone-specific parameter currently used to assess the fracture risk. By integrating the cortical and cancellous bone of a defined skeletal area, DXA scans provide bone mass of the projected area as expressed as the aBMD. If specific skeletal sites revealed a substantial amount of cortical or cancellous bone, these structural parameters could be quantified. The distal tibial diaphysis offers simple geometry similar to a hollow cylinder and a high percentage of cortical bone. Ex vivo material and structural characteristics of the bone at the T-DIA were previously shown to be predictive of the bone strength assessed by biomechanical testing [19]. As shown in the present study, the determination of the pMOI on a DXA scan of the tibia allowed for calculation of the CI by integrating the potential bone material (BMD) and the mechanical properties (pMOI). This index correlated highly with the index obtained by applying HR-pQCT. The correlation between those cortical parameters is stepwise, increasing from the radius 9 mm to the tibia 22.5 mm to the tibia 60 mm, which may reflect that a higher cortex portion better predicts its quantity, even if it is enhanced by considering two subregions of the same tibia. Interestingly, the cortical porosity at the distal tibia decreases the more proximal it is measured, which might reflect less transition from trabecular to cortical bone in the tibial diaphysis. Further studies are needed to confirm if this standardized quantification of the cortex in individuals at risk is predictive for the incidences of fractures.

By focusing on the cancellous bone contained in the lumbar spine, this ROI is predestinated for the assessment of the trabecular structure. TBS is a texture parameter that evaluates the pixel gray-level variations in DXA images of the lumbar spine. Ex vivo, these variations reflect the altered micro architecture of the trabecular bone such as the Conn.D, Tb.Sp or Tb.N assessed by high-resolution micro computed tomography [20,25]. In our cohort of healthy young women, the TBS correlated highly with these parameters of the microstructures, although the resolution of HR-pQCT is lower compared to that used ex vivo. Similar correlations were described recently in a pooled cohort of pre- and postmenopausal Chinese American and white women with exception that the strongest association has been found between TBS and vBMD [34]. In postmenopausal women with osteoporosis, the TBS did not correlate or correlated weakly with the aBMD of the lumbar spine [22]. In contrast to that, R was highly significant between aBMD at the LS and TBS in this study in healthy controls indicating that normal bone mass and not altered, homogeneous texture correlate highly with each other.

This study has some limitations. All of the measurements were performed in healthy premenopausal women and will not necessarily translate into findings of other cohorts, e.g., postmenopausal women or men. The sample might be selective (e.g., the subjects were from rural mountain areas; the regional calcium rich dietary habits of the subjects may have had an effect). For both of the bone structures, only one skeletal region was considered, and the findings may differ when applying a similar methodology to other sites of the skeleton. Whether the CI reflects more than regional bone strength is speculative. The strengths of the study included the number of randomly selected healthy women and the consistency of the study results of the hip aBMD to the data obtained by the NHANES III, which demonstrates the balance of the sample.

In this cohort of randomly selected healthy women, microstructural parameters of bone assessed by the 3D technique were predictable through information deducted from regular 2D DXA scans. This approach may add information to improve the prediction of individual fracture risks in a clinical setting.

Author Contributions

Conceived and designed the experiments: AP MW. Performed the experiments: HB VS UE ME AP. Analyzed the data: HB UE ME MW VS AP. Contributed reagents/materials/analysis tools: RGR MW VS KL. Wrote the paper: AP MW HB. Revised the manuscript content: MW RGR VS KL AP. Takes responsibility for the integrity of the data analysis: MW AP.

References

1. WHO Study Group - no authors listed (1994) Assessment of fracture risk and its application to screening for postmenopausal osteoporosis. Report of a WHO Study Group. World Health Organ Tech Rep Ser 843: 1–129.
2. Seeman E (2003) Invited Review: Pathogenesis of osteoporosis. J Appl Physiol 95: 2142–2151.

3. Khosla S, Riggs BL, Atkinson EJ, Oberg AL, McDaniel LJ, et al. (2006) Effects of sex and age on bone microstructure at the ultradistal radius: a population-based noninvasive in vivo assessment. J Bone Miner Res 21: 124–131.
4. Seeman E, Delmas PD (2006) Bone quality—the material and structural basis of bone strength and fragility. N Engl J Med 354: 2250–2261.
5. Zebaze RM, Ghasem-Zadeh A, Bohte A, Iuliano-Burns S, Mirams M, et al. (2010) Intracortical remodelling and porosity in the distal radius and post-mortem femurs of women: a cross-sectional study. Lancet 375: 1729–1736.
6. Cordey J, Schneider M, Belendez C, Ziegler WJ, Rahn BA, et al. (1992) Effect of bone size, not density, on the stiffness of the proximal part of normal and osteoporotic human femora. J Bone Miner Res 7 Suppl 2: S437–444.
7. Holzer G, von Skrbensky G, Holzer LA, Pichl W (2009) Hip fractures and the contribution of cortical versus trabecular bone to femoral neck strength. J Bone Miner Res 24: 468–474.
8. Hernandez CJ, Gupta A, Keaveny TM (2006) A biomechanical analysis of the effects of resorption cavities on cancellous bone strength. J Bone Miner Res 21: 1248–1255.
9. Liu XS, Zhang XH, Sekhon KK, Adams MF, McMahon DJ, et al. (2010) High-resolution peripheral quantitative computed tomography can assess microstructural and mechanical properties of human distal tibial bone. J Bone Miner Res 25: 746–756.
10. Nishiyama KK, Macdonald HM, Hanley DA, Boyd SK (2012) Women with previous fragility fractures can be classified based on bone microarchitecture and finite element analysis measured with HR-pQCT. Osteoporos Int.
11. Stein EM, Liu XS, Nickolas TL, Cohen A, Thomas V, et al. (2010) Abnormal microarchitecture and reduced stiffness at the radius and tibia in postmenopausal women with fractures. J Bone Miner Res 25: 2572–2581.
12. Vico L, Zouch M, Amirouche A, Frere D, Laroche N, et al. (2008) High-resolution pQCT analysis at the distal radius and tibia discriminates patients with recent wrist and femoral neck fractures. J Bone Miner Res 23: 1741–1750.
13. Laib A, Ruegsegger P (1999) Calibration of trabecular bone structure measurements of in vivo three-dimensional peripheral quantitative computed tomography with 28-microm-resolution microcomputed tomography. Bone 24: 35–39.
14. Burghardt AJ, Buie HR, Laib A, Majumdar S, Boyd SK (2010) Reproducibility of direct quantitative measures of cortical bone microarchitecture of the distal radius and tibia by HR-pQCT. Bone 47: 519–528.
15. Black DM, Cummings SR, Genant HK, Nevitt MC, Palermo L, et al. (1992) Axial and appendicular bone density predict fractures in older women. J Bone Miner Res 7: 633–638.
16. Marshall D, Johnell O, Wedel H (1996) Meta-analysis of how well measures of bone mineral density predict occurrence of osteoporotic fractures. BMJ 312: 1254–1259.
17. Popp AW, Senn C, Franta O, Krieg MA, Perrelet R, et al. (2009) Tibial or hip BMD predict clinical fracture risk equally well: results from a prospective study in 700 elderly Swiss women. Osteoporos Int 20: 1393–1399.
18. Sode M, Burghardt AJ, Kazakia GJ, Link TM, Majumdar S (2010) Regional variations of gender-specific and age-related differences in trabecular bone structure of the distal radius and tibia. Bone 46: 1652–1660.
19. Popp AW, Windolf M, Senn C, Tami A, Richards RG, et al. (2012) Prediction of bone strength at the distal tibia by HR-pQCT and DXA. Bone 50: 296–300.
20. Pothuaud L, Carceller P, Hans D (2008) Correlations between grey-level variations in 2D projection images (TBS) and 3D microarchitecture: applications in the study of human trabecular bone microarchitecture. Bone 42: 775–787.
21. Hans D, Goertzen AL, Krieg MA, Leslie WD (2011) Bone microarchitecture assessed by TBS predicts osteoporotic fractures independent of bone density: the Manitoba study. J Bone Miner Res 26: 2762–2769.
22. Popp AW, Guler S, Lamy O, Senn C, Buffat H, et al. (2013) Effects of zoledronate versus placebo on spine bone mineral density and microarchitecture assessed by the trabecular bone score in postmenopausal women with osteoporosis: A three-year study. J Bone Miner Res 28: 449–454.
23. Silva BC, Boutroy S, Zhang C, McMahon DJ, Zhou B, et al. (2013) Trabecular bone score (TBS)--a novel method to evaluate bone microarchitectural texture in patients with primary hyperparathyroidism. J Clin Endocrinol Metab 98: 1963–1970.
24. Boutroy S, Hans D, Sornay-Rendu E, Vilayphiou N, Winzenrieth R, et al. (2012) Trabecular bone score improves fracture risk prediction in non-osteoporotic women: the OFELY study. Osteoporos Int.
25. Hans D, Barthe N, Boutroy S, Pothuaud L, Winzenrieth R, et al. (2011) Correlations between trabecular bone score, measured using anteroposterior dual-energy X-ray absorptiometry acquisition, and 3-dimensional parameters of bone microarchitecture: an experimental study on human cadaver vertebrae. J Clin Densitom 14: 302–312.
26. Casez JP, Troendle A, Lippuner K, Jaeger P (1994) Bone mineral density at distal tibia using dual-energy X-ray absorptiometry in normal women and in patients with vertebral osteoporosis or primary hyperparathyroidism. J Bone Miner Res 9: 1851–1857.
27. Looker AC, Wahner HW, Dunn WL, Calvo MS, Harris TB, et al. (1998) Updated data on proximal femur bone mineral levels of US adults. Osteoporos Int 8: 468–489.
28. Canny J (1986) A computational approach to edge detection. IEEE Trans Pattern Anal Mach Intell 8: 679–698.
29. Boutroy S, Bouxsein ML, Munoz F, Delmas PD (2005) In vivo assessment of trabecular bone microarchitecture by high-resolution peripheral quantitative computed tomography. J Clin Endocrinol Metab 90: 6508–6515.
30. Cohen A, Liu XS, Stein EM, McMahon DJ, Rogers HF, et al. (2009) Bone microarchitecture and stiffness in premenopausal women with idiopathic osteoporosis. J Clin Endocrinol Metab 94: 4351–4360.
31. Sornay-Rendu E, Boutroy S, Munoz F, Delmas PD (2007) Alterations of cortical and trabecular architecture are associated with fractures in postmenopausal women, partially independent of decreased BMD measured by DXA: the OFELY study. J Bone Miner Res 22: 425–433.
32. Nishiyama KK, Macdonald HM, Buie HR, Hanley DA, Boyd SK (2010) Postmenopausal women with osteopenia have higher cortical porosity and thinner cortices at the distal radius and tibia than women with normal aBMD: an in vivo HR-pQCT study. J Bone Miner Res 25: 882–890.
33. Sode M, Burghardt AJ, Pialat JB, Link TM, Majumdar S (2011) Quantitative characterization of subject motion in HR-pQCT images of the distal radius and tibia. Bone 48: 1291–1297.
34. Silva BC, Walker MD, Abraham A, Boutroy S, Zhang C, et al. (2013) Trabecular Bone Score Is Associated With Volumetric Bone Density and Microarchitecture as Assessed by Central QCT and HRpQCT in Chinese American and White Women. J Clin Densitom 16: 554–561.

3

Calcitonin Inhibits SDCP-Induced Osteoclast Apoptosis and Increases Its Efficacy in a Rat Model of Osteoporosis

Yi-Jie Kuo[1,2], Fon-Yih Tsuang[3], Jui-Sheng Sun[4,5], Chi-Hung Lin[6], Chia-Hsien Chen[6], Jia-Ying Li[7], Yi-Chian Huang[8], Wei-Yu Chen[7], Chin-Bin Yeh[9], Jia-Fwu Shyu[7,9]*

1 Department of Orthopaedic, Taipei Medical University Hospital, Taipei, Taiwan, Republic of China, **2** Institute of Clinical Medicine, National Yang Ming University, Taipei, Taiwan, Republic of China, **3** Division of Neurosurgery, Department of Surgery, National Taiwan University Hospital, Taipei, Taiwan, Republic of China, **4** Department of Orthopaedic Surgery, National Taiwan University Hospital-Hsin Chu, Hsin-Chu, Taiwan, Republic of China, **5** Graduate Institute of Clinical Medicine, College of Medicine, Taipei Medical University, Taipei, Taiwan, Republic of China, **6** Institute of Microbiology and Immunology, National Yang Ming University, Taipei, Taiwan, Republic of China, **7** Department of Biology and Anatomy, National Defense Medical Center, Taipei, Taiwan, Republic of China, **8** Institute of Anatomy and Cell Biology National Yang Ming University, Taipei, Taiwan, Republic of China, **9** Department of Psychiatry, Tri-Service General Hospital, Taipei, Taiwan, Republic of China

Abstract

Introduction: Treatment for osteoporosis commonly includes the use of bisphosphonates. Serious side effects of these drugs are caused by the inhibition of bone resorption as a result of osteoclast apoptosis. Treatment using calcitonin along with bisphosphonates overcomes these side-effects in some patients. Calcitonin is known to inhibit bone resorption without reducing the number of osteoclasts and is thought to prolong osteoclast survival through the inhibition of apoptosis. Further understanding of how calcitonin inhibits apoptosis could prove useful to the development of alternative treatment regimens for osteoporosis. This study aimed to analyze the mechanism by which calcitonin influences osteoclast apoptosis induced by a bisphosphate analog, sintered dicalcium pyrophosphate (SDCP), and to determine the effects of co-treatment with calcitonin and SDCP on apoptotic signaling in osteoclasts.

Methods: Isolated osteoclasts were treated with CT, SDCP or both for 48 h. Osteoclast apoptosis assays, pit formation assays, and tartrate-resistant acid phosphatase (TRAP) staining were performed. Using an osteoporosis rat model, ovariectomized (OVX) rats received calcitonin, SDCP, or calcitonin + SDCP. The microarchitecture of the fifth lumbar trabecular bone was investigated, and histomorphometric and biochemical analyses were performed.

Results: Calcitonin inhibited SDCP-induced apoptosis in primary osteoclast cultures, increased Bcl-2 and Erk activity, and decreased Mcl-1 activity. Calcitonin prevented decreased osteoclast survival but not resorption induced by SDCP. Histomorphometric analysis of the tibia revealed increased bone formation, and microcomputed tomography of the fifth lumbar vertebrate showed an additive effect of calcitonin and SDCP on bone volume. Finally, analysis of the serum bone markers CTX-I and P1NP suggests that the increased bone volume induced by co-treatment with calcitonin and SDCP may be due to decreased bone resorption and increased bone formation.

Conclusions: Calcitonin reduces SDCP-induced osteoclast apoptosis and increases its efficacy in an in vivo model of osteoporosis.

Editor: Agustin Guerrero-Hernandez, Cinvestav-IPN, Mexico

Funding: This work was funded by National Defense Medical Center of Medical Research Grants (DOD-100-C-11-02) and Tri-Service General Hospital of Medical Research Grants (TSGH-C99-011-12-S03). The funders had no role in study design, data collection and analysis, decision to publish, or preparation of the manuscript.

Competing Interests: The authors have declared that no competing interests exist.

* E-mail: jiafwu.shyu@msa.hinet.net

Introduction

Bisphosphonates are the most commonly prescribed first line medication for osteoporosis despite causing side effects, including low bone turnover, hypocalcemia, and osteonecrosis of the jaw due to decreased bone formation as well as increased bone fracture due to reduced bone resorption [1,2]. Although the molecular mechanisms by which they inhibit bone resorption vary among the bisphosphonates, they collectively induce osteoclast apoptosis. Specifically, simple bisphosphonates are incorporated into non-hydrolysable adenosine triphosphate analogues, inducing osteoclast apoptosis [3]. The more potent nitrogen-containing bisphosphonates inhibit farnesyl pyrophosphate synthase, a key enzyme of the mevalonate pathway, which is essential for protein prenylation in osteoclasts [3,4]. Thus, bisphosphonates inhibit bone resorption by disrupting osteoclast function and survival.

Calcitonin has also been used as a therapy for osteoporosis, hypercalcemia, and Paget's disease. This 32-amino-acid peptide hormone induces hypocalcemia by inhibiting osteoclast-induced bone resorption. Although it has been used for nearly 30 years, it is less widely used than bisphosphonates and estrogen [5–7]. In addition, the physiological role of calcitonin in calcium homeostasis and bone remodeling as well as its effects on bone cells remains unclear. For example, studies using calcitonin-null mice indicate that it may be involved in protecting the skeleton during periods of "calcium stress", such as growth, pregnancy, and lactation [8]. However, in the basal state, only modest effects on regulating bone remodeling and calcium homeostasis were observed [9]. Furthermore, calcitonin primarily inhibits bone resorption [10,11] without reducing the number of osteoclasts [12]. Although the apoptotic signaling pathways regulated by calcitonin in osteoclasts remain to be fully elucidated, the phosphokinase A (PKA) pathway is likely involved [13]. In addition, calcitonin protects osteoclasts from the effects of a nitric oxide-releasing compound, a highly effective apoptotic stimulus [14]. Downregulation of Cox activity by calcitonin inhibits the function, but not survival of osteoclasts [15]. However, it may also interfere with bone remodeling by inhibiting bone formation [16,17] although not markedly in humans [1]. Combined use of calcitonin and anti-resorptive agents with different modes of action may overcome the side-effects experienced by some patients taking bisphosphonates.

Sintered dicalcium pyrophosphate (SDCP) is a pyrophosphate analog developed by Lin et al. [18]. It was proven biocompatible with bone in an in vivo animal model [18] and in vitro cell culture model [19]. Furthermore, in ovariectomized rats, SDCP increased bone mass [20] by inducing osteoclast apoptosis [21]. Moreover, the effects of SDCP were comparable to those observed for alendronate, a bisphosphonate commonly used clinically [20]. However, further studies are necessary to fully elucidate its mechanism of action.

Because calcitonin may prolong osteoclast survival through inhibition of apoptosis, this study aimed to analyze its influence on osteoclast apoptosis induced by a bisphosphate analog, SDCP. Specifically, the effects of calcitonin and SDCP co-treatment on osteoclast apoptosis and survival were assessed. In addition, the mechanism by which calcitonin influences SDCP-induced apoptosis of osteoclasts was determined. Finally, this study aimed to investigate the potential synergistic effects of calcitonin and SDCP co-treatment in ovariectomized rats by assessing bone volume, trabecular number, thickness, and separation as well as bone formation. Because the present osteoporosis treatments, including bisphosphonates, have side effects, the investigation of such potential alternative treatments is warranted. The examination of the effects of co-treatment with calcitonin and SDCP on osteoclast apoptotic signaling may help elucidate the mechanism by which calcitonin exerts its antiapoptotic effect in osteoclasts.

Results

Effects of Calcitonin and SDCP on Osteoclast Apoptosis

As shown in Fig. 1, osteoclast apoptosis was assessed using the TUNEL assay. Confocal analysis of osteoclasts cultured in control medium for 48 h revealed approximately 5% of TUNEL stain-positive cells (Fig. 1A and B). SDCP induced a time-dependent increase in TUNEL stain-positive cells, which became apparent after 12 hours and reached a maximum level at 48 hours of treatment. Both DNase and SDCP treatment increased TUNEL stain-positive cells to 100.0±0% and 72.8±11.6%, respectively (Fig. 1B). As compared to control and SCDP-treated cells, addition of calcitonin significantly decreased the number of TUNEL-positive osteoclasts (2.0±0.9 vs. 5.2±2.3% and 27.0±11.1 vs. 72.8±11.6%, respectively; Fig. 1B).

Apoptosis was also assessed using annexin-V staining (Fig. 2). In osteoclasts cultured for 18 h, treatment with TGF-β1, the positive control, and SDCP increased annexin-V-positive cells by

A

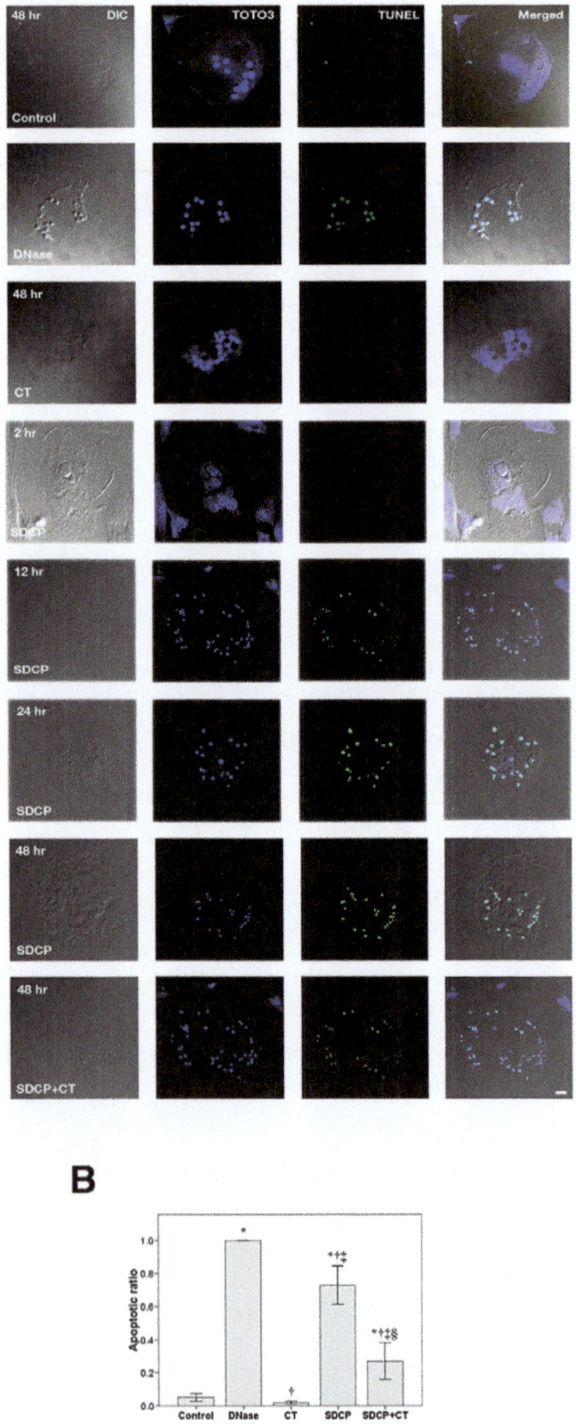

Figure 1. Detection of osteoclast apoptosis using TUNEL analysis. (A) Osteoclasts were treated with CT (10 nM), SDCP (10 μM), or both for the times indicated. Osteoclasts treated with DNase I (3 U/mL) were included as positive controls. Green nuclear labeling indicates apoptotic cells. Nuclei were counterstained using TOTO-3 (blue). Difference interference contrast (DIC) images show morphology of the cells. Bar = 20 μm. (B) Quantitative results of the experiment shown in panel A. *P*<0.05 compared to *control group, †DNase group, ‡CT group, and §SDCP group after Bonferroni adjustment, mean ± SD, n = 6 in each group.

24.9±4.6% and 14.6±4.0%, respectively. Upon cotreatment with calcitonin and SDCP, a significant decrease in annexin-V-positive cells was observed as compared with those cells treated with SDCP alone (6.7±0.6 vs. 14.6±0.4%; Fig. 2A and B). Because these data demonstrate that SDCP induced osteoclast apoptosis, the TGF-β1 treatment group was eliminated from subsequent experiments.

Calcitonin Inhibits SDCP-induced Expression of Cleaved Caspase 3 in Osteoclasts

To determine the effects of SDCP and calcitonin on caspase-3 cleavage, Western blot analysis was employed (Fig. 3). Exposure of osteoclasts to 0.1, 1 and 10 nM calcitonin for 18 h induced a dose-dependent decrease of cleaved caspase-3 (Fig. 3A). In addition, exposure of osteoclasts to 10 μM SDCP induced an increase in cleaved caspase-3, which was inhibited with the addition of 10 nM calcitonin (Fig. 3A). Cleaved caspase-3 was also assessed using confocal analysis of immunofluorescent-labeled cells; decreased cleaved caspase-3 labeling was observed in osteoclasts treated with calcitonin and SDCP as compared to those treated with SDCP alone (13.4±1.5 vs. 32.9±3.2%; Fig. 3B and C).

Regulation of Apoptosis-related Protein Expression and Activation by Calcitonin and SDCP

The effects of calcitonin and SDCP on Bcl-2 and Mcl-1 expression as well as caspase cleavage were assessed using Western blot analysis (Fig. 4). Calcitonin alone and with SDCP increased Bcl-2 expression in osteoclasts; SDCP only slightly increased Bcl-2 expression (Fig. 4A). However, SDCP decreased Mcl-1 expression, which was partially reversed by the addition of calcitonin with the SDCP (Fig. 4A); calcitonin alone only slightly reduced Mcl-1 expression (Fig. 4A). FasL, the positive control, increased caspase-8 cleavage whereas both calcitonin and SDCP induced little activation of caspase-8 in osteoclasts (Fig. 4B). Calcitonin decreased and SDCP increased caspase-9 cleavage in osteoclasts, which was inhibited by calcitonin co-treatment (Fig. 4B). Because this data indicates that SDCP induces apoptosis through a pathway distinct from FasL, the FasL treatment group was eliminated from subsequent experiments.

Calcitonin Inhibits Osteoclast Apoptosis through Bcl-2 and Erk Signaling Pathway

As shown in Fig. 5, the effects of calcitonin and SDCP treatment on apoptosis-related signaling pathways were determined by Western blot analysis. Pretreatment of osteoclasts with HA14-1, a Bcl-2 inhibitor, blocked the reduction in cleaved caspase-3 and -9 induced by calcitonin treatment (Fig. 5A). In addition, pre-treatment of osteoclasts with PD98059, an Erk1/2 inhibitor, blocked the calcitonin-induced increase of Bcl-2 and SDCP-induced decrease of Mcl-1 (Fig. 5B). The SDCP-induced increase of cleaved caspase-9 was also blocked by PD98059 pre-treatment, but the calcitonin-induced decrease was not. Finally, the decreased cleaved caspase-9 by cotreatment with calcitonin and SDCP as well as the calcitonin-induced decrease of cleaved caspase-3 were sensitive to PD98059 pretreatment (Fig. 5B).

Calcitonin Reduces the Inhibitory Effect of SDCP on Osteoclast Survival but not Activity

The effects of calcitonin and SDCP cotreatment on osteoclast number, size and bone resorption were determined (Fig. 6). In osteoclasts treated with calcitonin, TRAP staining revealed a significant decrease in cell number and size as compared to those cells in control medium, which was further decreased with SDCP treatment alone. However, combined treatment of calcitonin and SDCP alleviated the SDCP-induced decrease in osteoclast number and size (Fig. 6A). A similar inhibitory effect on pit number and area was observed on dentine discs in the calcitonin and SDCP alone groups. Combined treatment of calcitonin and SDCP induced a further decrease in pit number (Fig. 6B).

Calcitonin Increases the Therapeutic Efficacy of SDCP in an in vivo Osteoporosis Model

The influence of calcitonin-SDCP cotreatment on bone deposition was determined in an in vivo model of osteoporosis (Fig. 7). Ovariectomy or sham operation was performed in 3-month-old female Sprague Dawley rats. After four weeks, ovariectomized rats received normal saline, calcitonin, SDCP, or calcitonin plus SDCP treatment for four additional weeks after which micro-computed tomography analysis of the fifth lumbar vertebrates and histomorphometric analysis of the tibia were

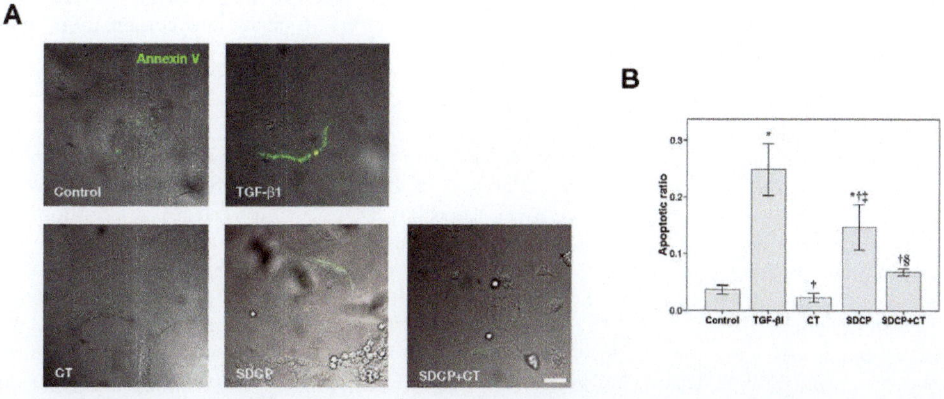

Figure 2. Detection of apoptosis by annexin V labeling in osteoclasts. (A) Osteoclasts were treated with CT (10 nM), SDCP (10 μM), or both for 18 h. Osteoclasts treated with TGF-βI (10 ng/mL) were included as positive controls. Green cellular membrane labeling indicates apoptotic cells. Only cells without propidium iodide (red) labeling were considered to be apoptotic. DIC images and nucleus stain were performed as described in Fig. 1. Bar = 10 μm. (B) Quantitative results of the experiment shown in panel A. The measurement of apoptosis was calculated as the percentage of positive annexin V labeling cells in a total of at least 500 osteoclasts. $P<0.05$ compared to *control group, †TGF-β1 group, ‡CT group; and §SDCP group after Bonferroni adjustment, mean ± SD, n = 6 in each group.

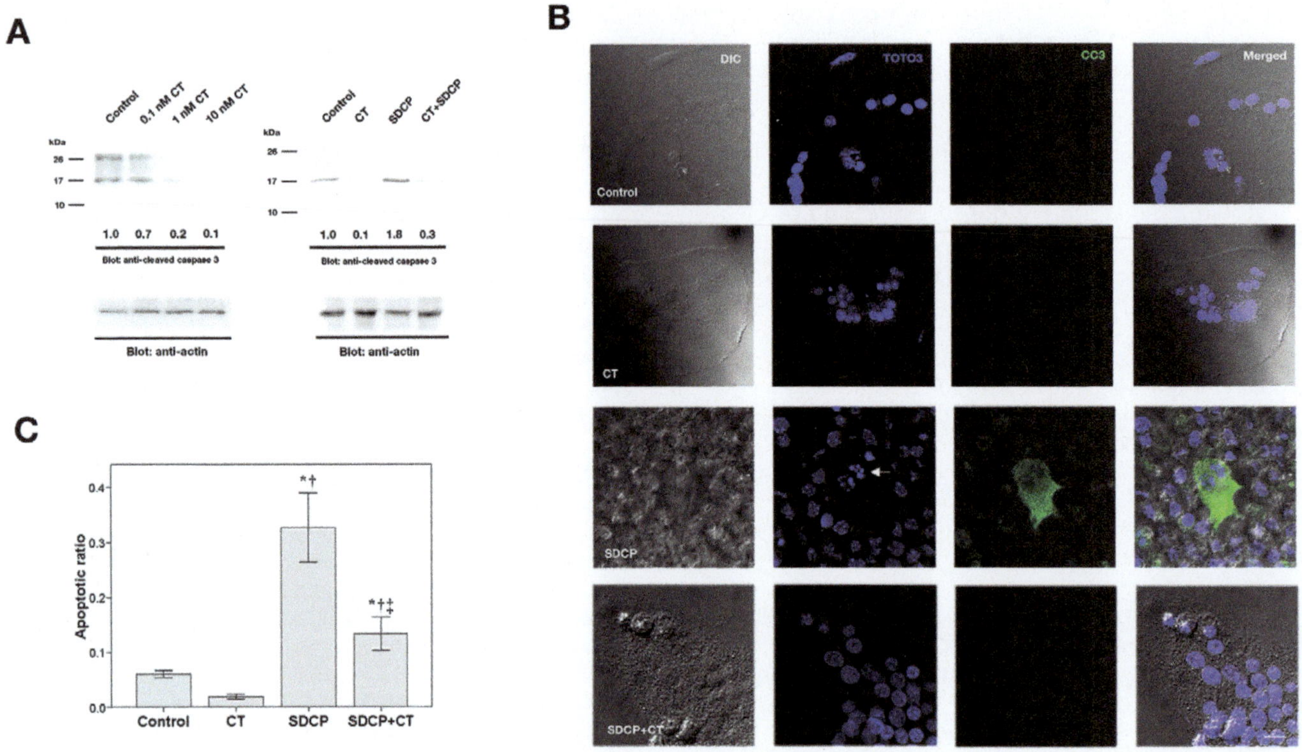

Figure 3. Calcitonin inhibits SDCP-induced expression of cleaved caspase 3 in osteoclasts. (A) Western blot analysis of cleaved caspase 3 expression in osteoclasts treated with CT (10 nM), SDCP (10 μM), or both. Protein levels were quantified by densitometry, corrected for the sample load based on actin expression, and expressed as fold-increase or decrease relative to the control lane. Each blot is representative of at least three replicate experiments. (B) Confocal analysis of immunofluorescent labeling of cleaved caspase 3 in calcitonin- or SDCP-treated osteoclast. Green intracellular cleaved caspase 3 labeling and blue TOTO3-labeled nuclear chromatin condensation (white arrow) indicate cells that underwent apoptosis. Bar = 10 μm. (C) Quantitative results of the experiment shown in panel B. The measurement of apoptosis was calculated as a percentage of positive cleaved caspase-3–labelled cells in a total of at least 500 osteoclasts. $P<0.05$ compared to *control group, † CT group, and ‡SDCP group after Bonferroni adjustment, mean ± SD, n = 6 in each group.

undertaken on the five-month-old rats. Although the 2D images also included cortical bone, regions of interest containing trabecular bone were selected for subsequent quantification. Significant increases in bone loss were observed in ovariectomized rats as compared to those of the sham controls (Fig. 7A and B). As compared to untreated ovariectomized rats, calcitonin treatment significantly increased percent bone volume and trabecular number. Compared to calcitonin treatment, SDCP induced further but not significant changes in these bone parameters; however, cotreatment with calcitonin and SDCP significantly increased percent bone volume and trabecular number in ovariectomized rats (Fig. 7A and 7B). No additional benefits in trabecular separation and thickness were observed upon cotreatment with calcitonin and SDCP. As shown in Figure 7C, a significant increase in bone formation was observed in ovariectomized rats, which was further increased upon calcitonin treatment. SDCP treatment in ovariectomized rats decreased bone formation, which was reversed by cotreatment with calcitonin (Fig. 7C).

Analysis of bone resorption and formation markers was next carried out after various treatments with calcitonin and SDCP (Fig. 7D). Analysis of a serum bone resorption marker, CTX-I, revealed increased bone resorption in ovariectomized rats as compared to those receiving the sham operation (Fig. 7D). Significant decreases in CTX-I were found in the calcitonin treatment group as compared to the untreated group. In both SDCP treatment and cotreatment groups, a further reduction in CTX-I was observed. Increases in the serum bone formation marker, P1NP, were observed in ovariectomized rats as compared to those receiving the sham operation (Fig. 7D). Further increases in P1NP levels were observed in ovariectomized rats receiving calcitonin. Although decreased P1NP levels were observed in the SDCP treatment group as compared to the calcitonin and vehicle groups, a significant increase was found in ovariectomized rats receiving the combination treatment of calcitonin and SDCP.

Discussion

[LOSSEST]Because calcitonin may prolong osteoclast survival through inhibition of apoptosis, this study aimed to analyze its influence on osteoclast apoptosis induced by a bisphosphate analog, SDCP. Cotreatment of calcitonin and SDCP was chosen because the in vivo therapeutic effects of SDCP were comparable to those observed for alendronate, a conventional bisphosphonate [20]. In addition, the efficacy of cotreatment with these agents was explored in ovariectomized rats. In primary osteoclast cultures, calcitonin inhibited SDCP-induced apoptosis, resulting in increased osteoclast number and size. However, the SDCP-induced reduction in bone resorption was not affected by calcitonin. Furthermore, an additive effect of calcitonin and SDCP on increased bone formation, increasing bone volume, was observed in ovariectomized rats.

In contrast to most other antiresorptive agents, calcitonin treatment inhibits the function but not the survival of osteoclasts

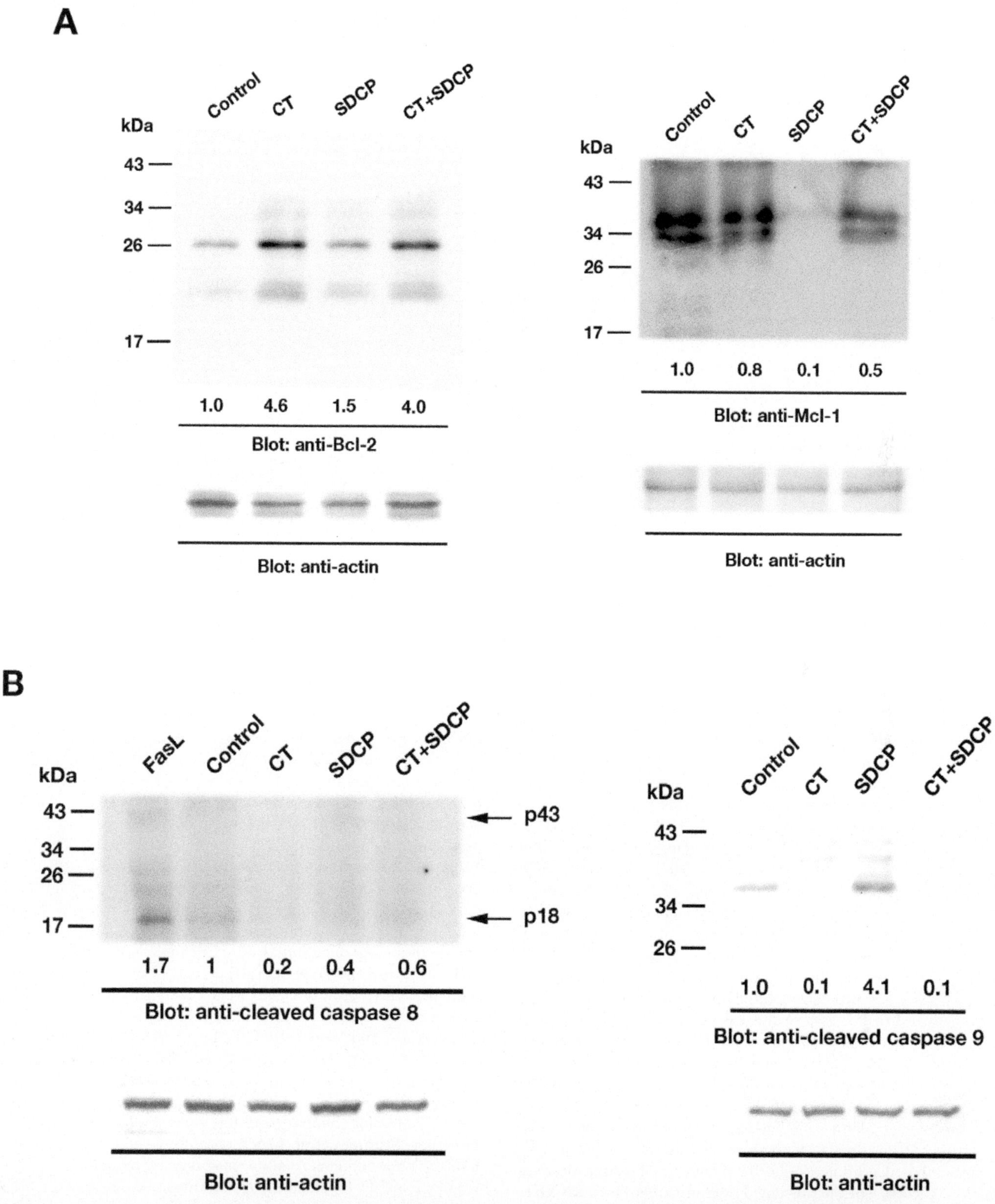

Figure 4. Regulation of apoptotic signaling by calcitonin and SDCP. (A) Western blot analysis of Bcl-2 and Mcl-1 expression in osteoclasts treated with CT (10 nM), SDCP (10 μM), or both. (B) Caspase 8 and 9 activation in response to CT (10 nM) or SDCP (10 μM) stimulation. Western blot analysis revealed the presence of two fragments (p43 and p18), corresponding to the cleaved caspase 8 under the treatment of FasL (10 ng/mL). Western blot analysis of cleaved caspase 9 was shown in the right panel. Protein levels were quantified by densitometry, corrected for the sample load based on actin expression, and expressed as fold-increase or decrease relative to the control lane. Each blot is representative of at least three replicate experiments.

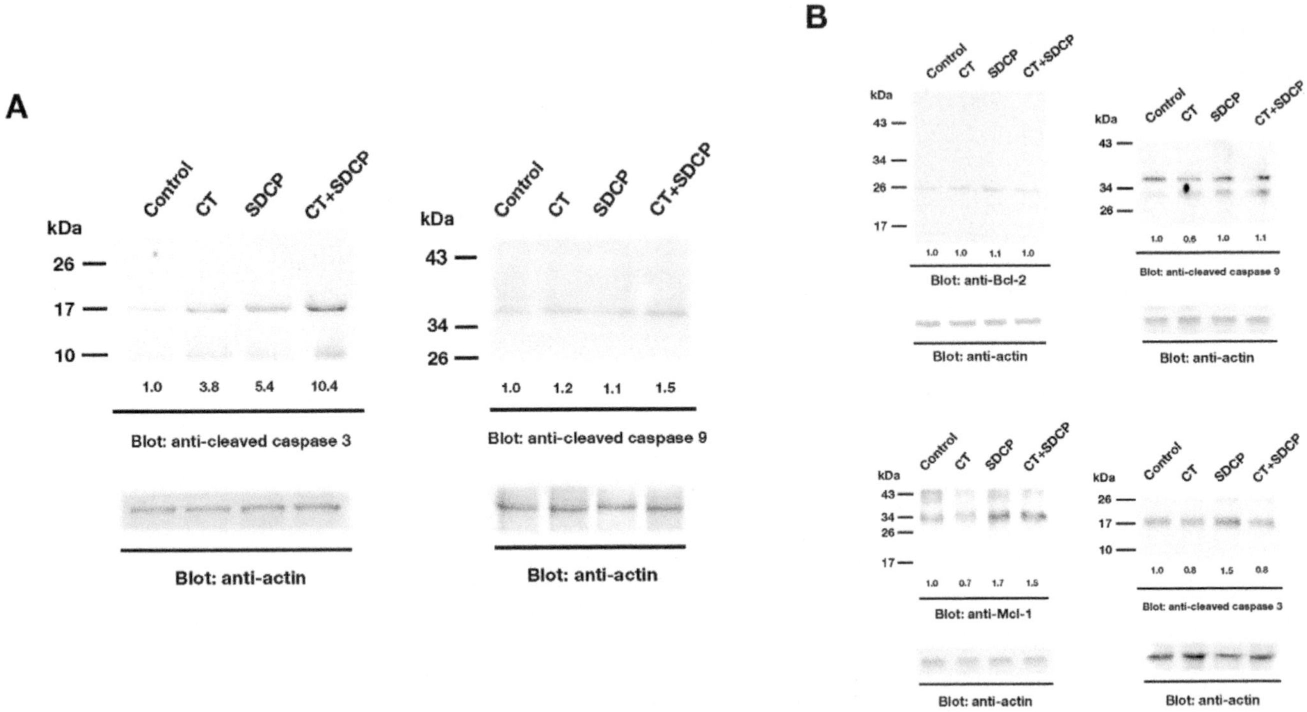

Figure 5. Calcitonin inhibits osteoclast apoptosis through Bcl-2 and Erk signaling. (A) Western blot analysis of expression of caspase 3 and 9. Osteoclasts were first treated with HA14-1 (50 μM) for 2 h and then CT (10 nM), SDCP (10 μM), or both were added to the culture medium. (B) Examination of apoptotic signaling regulated by calcitonin and SDCP in the presence of an Erk inhibitor. Osteoclasts were first treated with PD98059 (5 μM) for 2 h and then CT (10 nM), SDCP (10 μM), or both were added to the culture medium. Protein levels were quantified by densitometry, corrected for the sample load based on actin expression, and expressed as fold-increase or decrease relative to the control lane. Each blot is representative of at least three replicate experiments.

[22]. Indeed, calcitonin may play an important role in osteoclast survival by preventing apoptosis [10,13–15]. To decrease bone resorption by osteoclasts, calcitonin induces cytoskeletal changes [23], causing cell detachment [11], decreasing mobility [24], and interaction with integrin-related signaling [10]. As in osteoclasts cultured on glass or bone [13], the present study showed that calcitonin promoted osteoclast survival in cells treated with SDCP by reducing apoptosis as observed by reduced chromatin condensation and DNA degradation, annexin-V staining, and caspase-3 cleavage. However, little activation of caspase 8 was observed in osteoclasts treat with calcitonin or SDCP, indicating that calcitonin and SDCP may not function through the extrinsic apoptotic pathway. This notion is corroborated by the effect of these agents on Bcl-2 family proteins. Specifically, calcitonin alone and combined with SDCP increased Bcl-2 expression in osteoclasts. In addition, SDCP reduced Mcl-1 expression, which was partially reversed with calcitonin cotreatment. These results indicate that calcitonin inhibits osteoclast apoptosis at least in part by increasing Bcl-2 expression, whereas SDCP treatment induces apoptosis by decreasing Mcl-1 expression. Consistent with these results, Sutherland et al. [25] reported that alendronate induced osteoclast apoptosis by decreasing Mcl-1 levels, which is prevented by co-treatment with RANKL. Further studies will be undertaken to elucidate the mechanism by which SDCP reduces Mcl-1 expression.

The antiapoptotic proteins Mcl-1, Bcl-2, and Bcl-xL differentially inhibit activator BH3-only proteins Bim, Bid, and Puma, which can directly activate Bak and Bax [26]. In the present study, the BH3-mimetic molecule, HA14-1, blocked the calcitonin-mediated reduction in caspase-3 and -9 activation. Thus, upregulation of Bcl-2 by calcitonin is likely the mechanism by which calcitonin prevents SDCP-induced osteoclast apoptosis.

Calcitonin receptor couples to multiple G proteins and activates multiple signaling pathways [27]. In osteoclasts, calcitonin activates Erk1/2 [15], mediating osteoclast survival [28]. Erk promotes cell survival by direct phosphorylation and inhibition of caspase-9 during development and tissue homeostasis [29]. In the present study, calcitonin-induced Bcl-2 expression, and inhibition of caspase-3 and -9 activation were sensitive to the Erk1/2 inhibitor, PD98059, confirming that Erk1/2 is involved in the antiapoptotic signaling induced by calcitonin in osteoclasts.

To achieve more powerful therapeutic effects, a combination of multiple anti-resorption agents might be needed for osteoporosis patients. Ogawa et al. [30] showed an additive effect on trabecular architecture and bone strength in ovariectomized rats after cotreatment with calcitonin and alendronate. In addition, a combined therapy of calcitonin and alendronate in patients with rheumatoid arthritis for 12 months had additive effects, significantly increasing lumbar and hip bone mineral density [31]. However, Iwamoto et al. [32] reported no significant changes in lumbar bone mineral density in postmenopausal osteoporotic women treated with alendronate and calcitonin compared to those receiving alendronate alone. This may be due to the short treatment period (6 months) [32]. In the present study, both calcitonin and SDCP increased the percent bone volume and trabecular number and thickness, and decreased trabecular separation in ovariectomized rats although not all these parameters reached significance. Calcitonin-SDCP cotreatment further increased percent bone volume, illustrating an additive effect by the combined treatment for osteoporosis. Further studies are

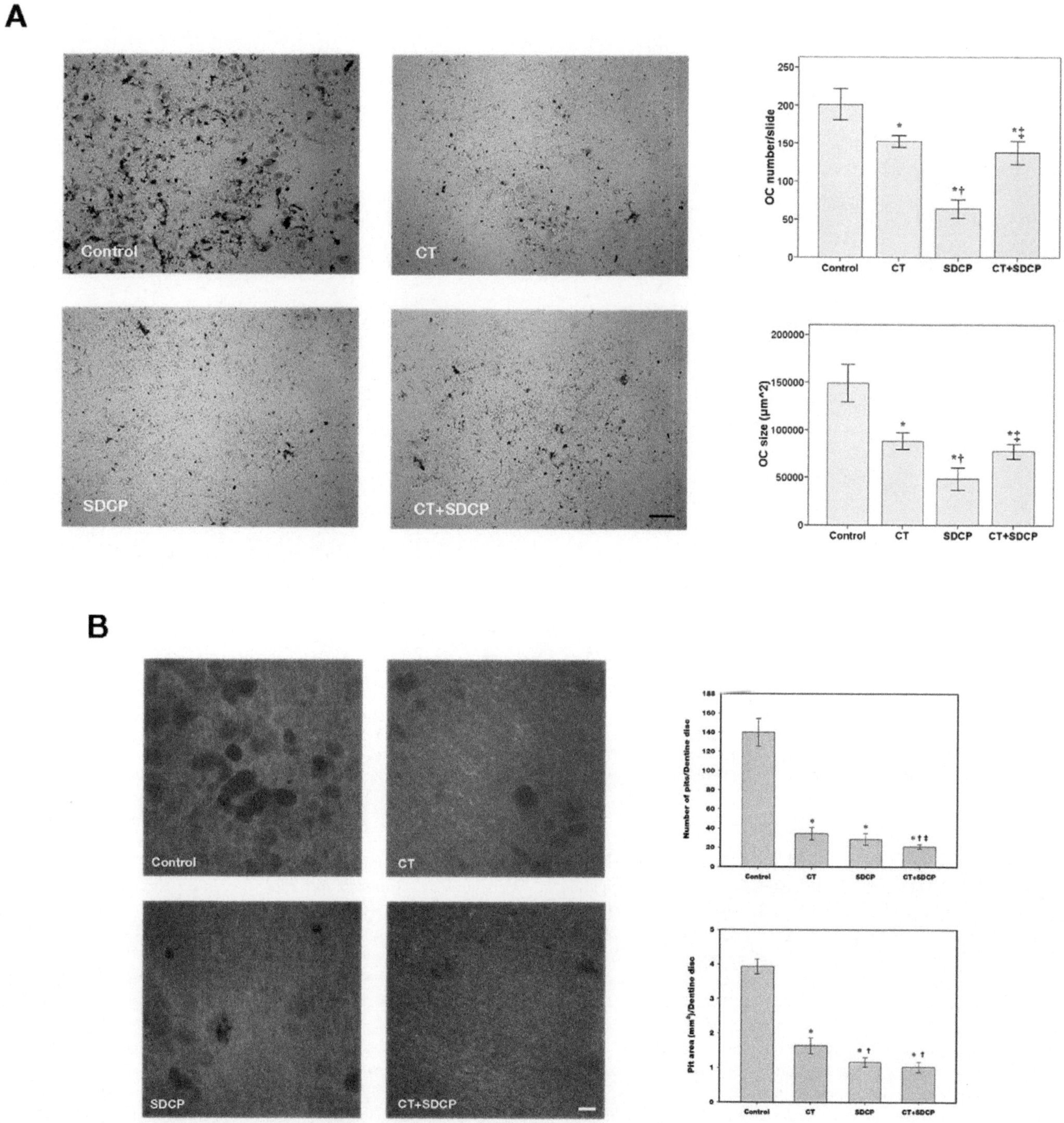

Figure 6. Calcitonin reduces inhibitory effect of SDCP on osteoclast survival but not activity. (A) TRAP stain of osteoclasts treated with CT (10 nM), SDCP (10 μM), or both. Red intracellular stain with multiple nuclei indicates positive labeling. Quantitative results of cell number and size were shown in right panel. Bar = 500 μm. (B) Pit formation assay. Osteoclasts were cultured on dentine discs and treated with CT (10 nM), SDCP (10 μM), or both. Quantitative results of the number and area of resorption pits were shown in right panel. Bar = 50 mm. $P<0.05$ compared to *control group, † CT group, and ‡SDCP group after Bonferroni adjustment, mean ± SD, n = 6 in each group.

necessary to determine whether combined therapy of pyrophosphate analog and calcitonin may represent a new strategy for osteoporosis treatment.

A balance between osteoblast and osteoclast activity is required for normal bone formation and maintenance. A coupling mechanism has been described in which resorption products and osteoclast-derived factors stimulate bone formation by osteoblast lineage cells [33]. Similarly, osteoblast lineage cells regulate osteoclast formation and activity [33]. Therefore, because of the coupled nature of remodeling, most of the anti-resorptive agents available also reduce bone formation directly or indirectly, limiting their effect on bone mass. Drugs that uncouple bone resorption from bone formation (e.g. inhibitors of chloride channels, cathepsin K, vacuolar H+ATPase and Src) may have a greater

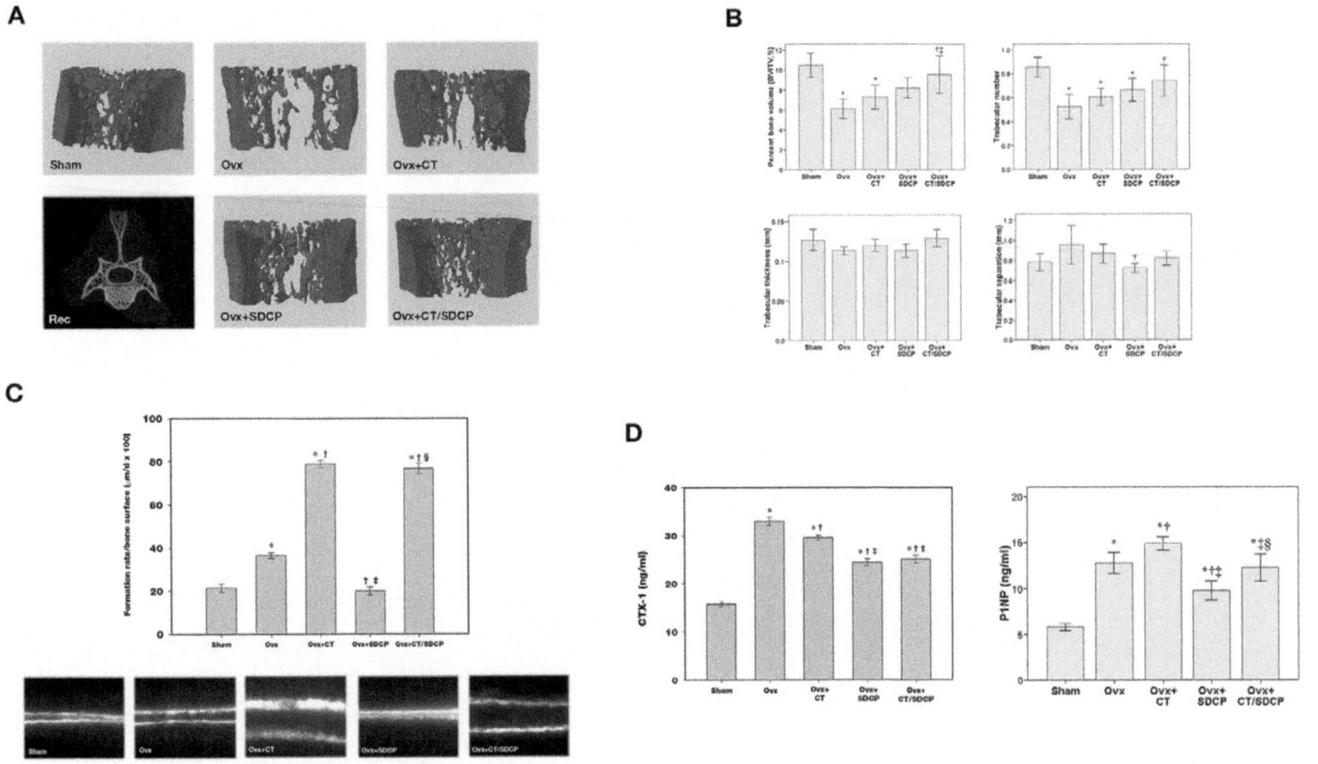

Figure 7. Calcitonin increases therapeutic efficacy of SDCP to treat osteoporotic rats. (A) Micro-computed tomography analysis of 5th lumbar vertebrate in ovariectomized (OVX) rats treated with CT (5 IU/kg/day), SDCP (1 mg/kg/day), or both. Figures are representative 3D reconstruction images from each treatment groups except lower left panel which is 2D reconstruction image shows the contouring method used to delineate the trabecular bone region. (B) Quantitative results of the experiment shown in panel A. (C) Calcein double-labeling in OVX rats. Representative fluorescent micrographs show that the distance between the two labeled mineralization fronts. The quantification of the bone formation rate per bone surface is shown in the right panel. (D) Serum bone resorption marker (CTX-1) and bone formation marker (P1NP) were determined by ELISA. $P<0.05$ compared to *sham group, †Ovx group, ‡Ovx+CT group, and §Ovx+SDCP group after Bonferroni adjustment, mean ± SD, n = 6 in each group.

effect in terms of increasing bone mass. In the present study, combined therapy of calcitonin and SDCP had less of an effect on inhibiting bone resorption and induced more bone formation as compared to SDCP treatment alone as observed by pit formation assay, CTX-1 and P1NP expression, and calcein double labeling. Consistent with these results, calcitonin increased bone formation in ovariectomized rats [34,35] and anabolic effect was observed in glucocorticoid-induced osteopenia [36]. Though results from calcitonin and calcitonin receptor-null mice suggest that it is a physiologic inhibitor of bone formation, the mechanism of how calcitonin regulates bone formation remains unknown [37]. The results from the present study suggest that calcitonin-induced inhibition of osteoclast apoptosis may be an important factor in this process.

There are some study limitations that warrant further discussion. For example, this study analyzes the effect of combination therapy using the bisphosphonate analog, SDCP, without comparing them with a conventional bisphosphonate, such as alendronate. In addition, the effects of SDCP alone or with calcitonin on osteoblasts were not assessed in the present study. However, Sun et al. [38] reported that SDCP inhibited osteoblast proliferation, which was mediated by the promotion of osteoblast differentiation and the increased synthesis of prostaglandin E2. Also, the effect of calcitonin and SDCP on apoptosis was only addressed in vitro without further studies seeding the osteoclasts on bone. Because this study will permit a correlation of anti-resorptive effects versus apoptosis, it will be carried out in future studies. Furthermore, 3-month old rats were used for the *in vivo* study. Because their skeletons are immature, the effect of bone growth cannot be separated from the effect of calcitonin or SDCP treatment to the rat skeleton. However, by the end of the study, the rats were five months of age. In conclusion, this study confirmed that calcitonin inhibits osteoclast apoptosis; it inhibited SDCP-induced apoptosis in primary osteoclast cultures. In addition, calcitonin-SDCP combination therapy inhibited bone resorption to a lesser extent and induced more bone formation as compared to SDCP alone. The benefits of combination therapy for osteoporosis warrant further investigation as a possible treatment for postmenopausal osteoporosis.

Materials and Methods

Reagents

Salmon calcitonin was purchased from Sigma-Aldrich (St. Louis, MO, USA). SDCP was purchased from Purzer Pharmaceutical Co., Taipei, Taiwan. TGF-βI was obtained from Peprotech (Rockey Hill, NJ, USA). HA14-1, a Bcl-2 inhibitor, was purchased from Enzo Life Science (Plymouth Meeting, PA, USA). PD98059, a MEK1 inhibitor, was purchased from Cell Signaling Technology (Danvers, MA, USA). Fas ligand (FasL) was purchased from R&D System (Minneapolis, MN, USA).

Isolation and Treatment of Rabbit Osteoclasts

New Zealand white rabbits approximately 7-day-old (90–120 g) were used as the source of bone cells for purification of osteoclasts as previously described [11]. For subsequent imaging analyses, unpurified cultures were employed; however, purified cultures (>90% purity) were used for the molecular analysis. Purification of the cultures was performed using 0.02% EDTA and 0.001% pronase E for 5 min at 37°C. The experiment was performed with the approval of the Laboratory Animal Center of the National Defense Medical Center in Taipei, Taiwan. Purified osteoclasts were cultured in alpha-minimum essential medium (α-MEM, Sigma-Aldrich), pH 6.9, supplemented with 26 mM sodium bicarbonate, 10 mM HEPES, 1% penicillin/streptomycin, and 5% fetal bovine serum (FBS, HyClone, Logan, Utah, USA). Unless otherwise indicated, osteoclasts were treated with CT (10 nM), SDCP (10 μM), or both for 18 h for short-term changes including analysis of signaling molecules to 48 h for TUNEL and TRAP analysis.

Confocal Microscopic Analysis of Osteoclast Apoptosis

1.5×10^4 osteoclasts were cultured on 22×22 mm glass coverslips for 18 h after which they were treated with CT (10 nM), SDCP (10 μM) or both for 48 h. After the cells were washed with phosphate buffered saline (PBS), they were fixed in 4% paraformaldehyde for 10 min and permeabilized with 0.1% Triton X-100 in PBS for 5 min. The cells were subsequently incubated in 1% bovine serum albumin (BSA) in PBS for 1 h. Apoptosis was determined using an In Situ Cell Death Kit (Roche Applied Science, Mannheim, Germany) based on the TdT-mediated fluorescein dUTP nick-end labeling (TUNEL) method, according to the recommendations of the manufacturer. Negative controls included omission of TdT, and positive controls included DNase I treatments. Nuclei were counterstained using TOTO-3 diluted 1:5000 (Molecular Probes, Inc., Eugene, OR, USA). For each treatment, at least 500 osteoclasts in three glass coverslips were counted. Measurement of apoptosis was calculated as a percentage of apoptotic nuclei versus total nuclei [39].

Apoptosis of cells was also determined by analysis of Annexin Vas well as cleaved caspase staining. 1.5×10^4 osteoclasts were cultured on 22×22 mm glass coverslips for 18 h after which they were treated with CT (10 nM), SDCP (10 μM) or both for 18 h. For Annexin V staining, an Annexin V-FITC Apoptosis Detection kit (BioVision, Mountain View, CA, USA) was used, according to the recommendation of the manufacturer. Propidium iodide (50 μg/ml) was added to the binding buffer to detect necrosis. For analysis of cleaved caspase-3, cells were incubated with anticleaved caspase-3 polyclonal antibody (Cell Signaling Technology) in 1% BSA PBS at 4°C for 16 h, and then with Cy-3-conjugated anti-rabbit IgG antibody (Jackson Immunoresearch Laboratories, West Grove, PA, USA) in PBS for 1 h. Microscopy was performed using a confocal microscope equipped with difference interference contrast light path (LSM 510, Zeiss, Göttingen, Germany). Annexin V- and active caspase-3–positive osteoclasts were counted manually as stated above, and the apoptosis rate was statistically analyzed. Multi-nucleated cells were considered osteoclasts if they had more than three nuclei.

Tartrate-resistant Acid Phosphatase (TRAP) Staining

1.5×10^4 osteoclasts were cultured on 22×22 mm glass coverslips for 18 h after which they were treated with CT (10 nM), SDCP (10 μM) or both for 72 h. They were then stained for TRAP using a kit that uses 50 mM tartrate and following the manufacturer's instructions (Sigma-Aldrich). For each treatment, at least 500 osteoclasts in three glass coverslips were counted. Osteoclasts were defined as cells with more than three nuclei. The number of $TRAP^+$ cells per coverslip was determined by light microscope (Axio Imager A2, Zeiss).

Pit Formation Assay

In the Pit formation assay, 1×10^3 osteoclasts were cultured on dentine discs (Immunodiagnostic Systems Inc, Fountain Hills, AR) in a 96-well plate for 18 h after which they were treated with CT (10 nM), SDCP (10 μM),or both for 72 h. For most groups, there were 4 dentine discs per group. To measure the areas containing resorption lacunae, cells were removed, and the dentine discs were incubated in 0.25 M ammonium hydroxide, washed with distilled water, and then stained with 0.5% (wt/vol) toluidine blue. The images of the resorbed areas were measured using a reflective optical microscope (LSM 510, Zeiss), and the results were expressed as the number of resorption pits and total area resorbed per dentine disc.

Western Blot Analysis

Purified osteoclasts ($1.5 \pm 0.5 \times 10^5$/10 cm dish) were cultured in α-MEM for 18 h after which they were treated with CT (10 nM), SDCP (10 μM), or both for 18 h. They were then washed twice with PBS, and lysed with cold lysis buffer (150 mM NaCl, 50 mM Tris, pH 7.5, 0.25% sodium deoxycholate, 0.1% Nonidet P-40, 1 mM sodium orthovanadate, 1 mM sodium fluoride, 1 mM phenylmethylsulfonyl fluoride, 10 μg/mL aprotinin, and 10 μg/mL leupeptin). The cell lysate was obtained by centrifugation at 16,000×g at 4°C for 30 min. The protein concentration was measured with a Bicinconinic acid kit (Pierce, Rockford, IL, USA), and 30 μg of total protein was separated on a 12% SDS-polyacrylamide gel. After the proteins were transferred to nitrocellulose membranes (Whatman, Dassel, Germany), the membranes were blocked with 5% skim milk in TBS-T (20 mM Tris, pH 7.6, 137 mM NaCl, and 0.1% Tween-20) and incubated with antibodies specific for cleaved caspase-3, 8, and 9 (Cell Signaling Technology) or anti-Bcl-2 and anti-Mcl-1(Santa Cruz, CA, USA). Proteins were visualized using the appropriate secondary antibody conjugated to horseradish peroxidase (HRP; Santa Cruz), followed by the application of ECL reagents (Amersham, Buckinghamshire, UK). The bands were quantified by densitometry (ProXPRESS Proteomic Imaging System, Perkin Elmer, Melbourne, VIC, Australia), and normalized to the loading control, actin. The influence of various treatments was expressed as fold-increase or decrease relative to the control lane. Each analysis was carried out in at least three independent experiments.

In vivo Osteoporosis Model

Fifty 3-month-old female Sprague–Dawley rats were purchased from the Laboratory Animal Center, National Defense Medical Center (Taipei, Taiwan) and acclimated under standard laboratory conditions at 22±2°C and 50±10% humidity. Food and water were available ad libitum during the acclimatization period. A sham-operation (n = 10) or ovariectomy (OVX, n = 40) was performed. Four weeks after the surgery, OVX rats were divided into four groups: vehicle, calcitonin (50 IU/ml, subcutaneous injection of 5 IU/kg/day), SDCP (2.5 mg/ml, oral administration of 1 mg/kg/day), and calcitonin+SDCP (n = 10 for each group). Rats were treated five times per week for four weeks. The sham and OVX vehicle groups received the vehicle, an isotonic sodium chloride solution, orally. SDCP was administered orally by catheter at 1.0 mg/kg/day five times per week as previously described [20]. Salmon calcitonin (Miacalcic by Novartis-Pharma) was administered by subcutaneously injection at 5 IU/kg/day five times per week. The vehicle and drug were given on the same days, and the treatment period lasted 4 weeks. The animal study was carried out in accordance with ethical guidelines for animal care, and the experimental protocols were approved by the animal care committee of National Defense Medical Center.

Whole blood samples were obtained with plastic syringes via intracardiac puncture immediately following sacrifice at five months of age (8 weeks after surgery). The blood samples were allowed to clot at room temperature after which the serum was separated by centrifugation, divided into 500-μL aliquots, and stored at −80°C until further analysis. The lumbar vertebrae were also removed and stored at −80°C for subsequent assessment of trabecular microstructure.

Micro-computed Tomography

Microarchitecture of the fifth lumbar trabecular bone was investigated using a microcomputed tomography (Skyscan 1174; Skyscan, Aartselaar, Belgium) as previously described [40]. The X-ray source was set at 50 kV, with a pixel size at 11 μm. Four hundred projections were acquired over an angular range of 180° (angular step of 0.45°). The image slices were reconstructed using the cone-beam reconstruction software version 2.6 based on the Feldkamp algorithm (Skyscan). The registered data sets were segmented into binary images. Simple global thresholding methods were used due to the low noise and relatively good resolution of the data sets. The trabecular bone was extracted by drawing ellipsoid contours with the CT analyzer software (Skyscan). Trabecular bone volume (BV/TV; percentage), trabecular number, and trabecular separation were calculated by the mean intercept length method. Trabecular thickness was calculated according to the method of Hildebrand and Ruegsegger [41].

Histomorphometric Analysis

Eight weeks after ovariectomy, the rats received an intraperitoneal injection of calcein (30 mg/kg) and another injection 8 days later. Two days later they were sacrificed [42]. The proximal tibia were dehydrated in graded ethanol, defatted in acetone, and embedded undecalcified in London resin (London Resin Co., London, United Kingdom) after staining with Villanueva bone stain (Polyscience Ltd, Warrington, PA, USA). Frontal sections of the tibiae (7 μm thick) were prepared. Measurements were performed on the entire marrow region within the cortical shell of the proximal tibia metaphysis from 1–4 mm distal to the growth plate-metaphyseal junction using an Image Analysis System (Osteomeasure, Inc., Atlanta, GA, USA). Bone area, perimeter, single- and double-labeling surface were measured, and trabecular number, thickness, and separation as well as the bone formation rate/bone surface (BFR/BS) were calculated.

Biochemical Analyses

Serum type 1 carboxyterminal collagen fragments (CTX-1) were measured using the RatLaps enzyme immunoassay (EIA; Immunodiagnostic Systems, UK), and the amino-terminal propeptide of type 1 procollagen (P1NP) was measured using the Rat PINP EIA (Immunodiagnostic Systems), according to the manufacturer's instructions.

Statistical Analysis

Means and standard deviations (SDs) were calculated for each group. Comparisons were performed using ANOVA with post-hoc comparison adjusted by the Bonferroni method. Data were analyzed with SAS 9.0 (SAS Institute Inc., Cary, NC), and a P value <0.05 was considered statistically significant.

Acknowledgments

We would like to thank Tzu-Hui Chu for her expert technical assistance.

Author Contributions

Conceived and designed the experiments: J-FS Y-JK J-SS C-HL. Performed the experiments: J-FS Y-JK F-YT C-HC J-YL Y-CH W-YC C-BY. Analyzed the data: J-FS Y-JK C-HL C-HC J-YL Y-CH W-YC C-BY. Contributed reagents/materials/analysis tools: J-FS Y-JK F-YT J-SS C-HL. Wrote the paper: J-FS Y-JK.

References

1. Rogers MJ, Frith JC, Luckman SP, Coxon FP, Benford HL, et al. (1999) Molecular mechanisms of action of bisphosphonates. Bone 24: 73S–79S.
2. Drake MT, Clarke BL, Khosla S (2008) Bisphosphonates: mechanism of action and role in clincal practice. Mayo Clin Proc 83: 1032–1045.
3. Rogers MJ, Crockett JC, Coxon FP, Mönkkönen J (2011) Biochemical and molecular mechanisms of action of bisphosphonates. Bone 49: 34–41.
4. Luckman SP, Hughes DE, Coxon FP, Graham R, Russell G, et al. (1998) Nitrogen-containing bisphosphonates inhibit the mevalonate pathway and prevent post-translational prenylation of GTP-binding proteins, including Ras. J Bone Miner Res 13: 581–589.
5. Karsdal MA, Henriksen K, Arnold M, Christiansen C (2008) Calcitonin: a drug of the past or for the future? Physiologic inhibition of bone resorption while sustaining osteoclast numbers improves bone quality. BioDrugs 22: 137–144.
6. de Paula FJ, Rosen CJ (2010) Back to the future: revisiting parathyroid hormone and calcitonin control of bone remodeling. Horm Metab Res 42: 299–306.
7. Gallagher JC, Sai AJ (2010) Molecular biology of bone remodeling: implications for new therapeutic targets for osteoporosis. Maturitas 65: 301–307.
8. Woodrow JP, Sharpe CJ, Fudge NJ, Hoff AO, Gagel RF, et al. (2006) Calcitonin plays a critical role in regulating skeletal mineral metabolism during lactation. Endocrinology 147: 4010–4021.
9. Davey RA, Turner AG, McManus JF, Chiu WS, Tjahyono F, et al. (2008) Calcitonin receptor plays a physiological role to protect against hypercalcemia in mice. J Bone Miner Res 23: 1182–1193.
10. Marzia M, Chiusaroli R, Neff L, Kim NY, Chishti AH, et al. (2006) Calpain is required for normal osteoclast function and is down-regulated by calcitonin. J Biol Chem 281: 9745–9754.
11. Shyu JF, Shih C, Tseng CY, Lin CH, Sun DT, et al. (2007) Calcitonin induces podosome disassembly and detachment of osteoclasts by modulating Pyk2 and Src activities. Bone 40: 1329–1342.
12. Stern PH (2007) Antiresorptive agents and osteoclast apoptosis. J Cell Biochem 101: 1087–1096.
13. Selander KS, Härkönen PL, Valve E, Mönkkönen J, Hannuniemi R, et al. (1996) Calcitonin promotes osteoclast survival in vitro. Mol Cell Endocrinol 122: 119–129.
14. Kanaoka K, Kobayashi Y, Hashimoto F, Nakashima T, Shibata M, et al. (2000) A common downstream signaling activity of osteoclast survival factors that prevent nitric oxide-promoted osteoclast apoptosis. Endocrinology 141: 2995–3005.
15. Miyazaki T, Neff L, Tanaka S, Horne WC, Baron R (2003) Regulation of cytochrome c oxidase activity by c-Src in osteoclasts. J Cell Biol 160: 709–718.
16. Hoff AO, Catala-Lehnen P, Thomas PM, Priemel M, Rueger JM, et al. (2002) Increased bone mass is an unexpected phenotype associated with deletion of the calcitonin gene. J Clin Invest 110: 1849–1857.
17. Huebner AK, Schinke T, Priemel M, Schilling S, Schilling AF, et al. (2006) Calcitonin deficiency in mice progressively results in high bone turnover. J Bone Miner Res 2006; 21: 1924–1934.
18. Lin FH, Lin CC, Lu CM, Liu HC, Sun JS, et al. (1995) Mechanical properties and histological evaluation of sintered beta-Ca2P2O7 with Na4P2O7.10H2O addition. Biomaterials 16: 793–802.
19. Sun JS, Tsuang YH, Liao CJ, Liu HC, Hang YS, et al. (1997) The effects of calcium phosphate particles on the growth of osteoblasts. J Biomed Mater Res 37: 324–334.
20. Sun JS, Huang YC, Tsuang YH, Chen LT, Lin FH (2002) Sintered dicalcium pyrophosphate increases bone mass in ovariectomized rats. J Biomed Mater Res59: 246–253.
21. Sun JS, Huang YC, Lin FH, Chen LT (2003) The effect of sintered dicalcium pyrophosphate on osteoclast metabolism: an ultrastructural study. J Biomed Mater Res A 64: 616–621.
22. Karsdal MA, Henriksen K, Arnold M, Christiansen C (2008) Calcitonin- A drug of the Past or for the Future? BioDrugs 22: 137–144.
23. Chambers TJ, Athanasou NA, Fuller K (1984) Effect of parathyroid hormone and calcitonin on the cytoplasmic spreading of isolated osteoclasts. J Endocrinol 102: 281–286.

24. Zaidi M, Chambers TJ, Moonga BS, Oldoni T, Passarella E, et al. (1990) A new approach for calcitonin determination based on target cell responsiveness. J Endocrinol Invest 13: 119–126.
25. Sutherland KA, Rogers HL, Tosh D, Rogers MJ (2009) RANKL increases the level of Mcl-1 in osteoclasts and reduces bisphosphonate-induced osteoclast apoptosis in vitro. Arthritis Res Ther 11: R58.
26. Tanaka S, Wakeyama H, Akiyama T, Takahashi K, Amano H, et al. (2010) Regulation of osteoclast apoptosis by bcl-2 family protein bim and caspase-3. Adv Exp Med Biol 658: 111–116.
27. Horne WC, Sanjay A, Baron R (2008) Regulating Bone Resorption: Targeting Integrins, Calcitonin Receptor, and Cathepsin K, in: J.P. Bilezikian, T.J. Martin (Eds.) Principles of Bone Biology 3rd ed., Academic Press, New York, NY, USA, 221–236.
28. Miyazaki T, Katagiri H, Kanegae Y, Takayanagi H, Sawada Y, et al. (2000) Reciprocal role of ERK and NF-kappaB pathways in survival and activation of osteoclasts. J Cell Biol 148: 333–342.
29. Allan LA, Morrice N, Brady S, Magee G, Pathak S, et al. (2003) Inhibition of caspase-9 through phosphorylation at Thr 125 by ERK MAPK. Nat Cell Biol 5: 647–654.
30. Ogawa K, Hori M, Takao R, Sakurada T (2005) Effects of combined elcatonin and alendronate treatment on the architecture and strength of bone in ovariectomized rats. J Bone Miner Metab 23: 351–358.
31. Ozoran K, Yildirim M, ÖNDER M, Sivas F, Inanir A (2007) The bone mineral density effects of calcitonin and alendronate combined therapy in patients with rheumatoid arthritis. APLAR J Rheumatol 10: 17–22.
32. Iwamoto J, Uzawa M, Sato Y, Takeda T, Matsumoto H. (2009) Effects of short-term combined treatment with alendronate and elcatonin on bone mineral density and bone turnover in postmenopausal women with osteoporosis. Ther Clin Risk Manag 5: 499–505.
33. Martin T, Gooi JH, Sims NA. (2009) Molecular mechanisms in coupling of bone formation to resorption. Crit Rev Eukaryot Gene Expr 19: 73–88.
34. Mochizuki K, Inoue T. (2000) Effect of salmon calcitonin on experimental osteoporosis induced by ovariectomy and low-calcium diet in the rat. J Bone Miner Metab 18: 194–207.
35. Davey RA, Morris HA. (2005) The effects of salmon calcitonin-induced hypocalcemia on bone metabolism in ovariectomized rats. J Bone Miner Metab 23: 359–365.
36. Furuichi H, Fukuyama R, Izumo N, Fujita T, Kohno T, et al. (2000) Bone-anabolic effect of salmon calcitonin on glucocorticoid-induced osteopenia in rats. Biol Pharm Bull 23: 946–951.
37. Huebner AK, Keller J, Catala-Lehnen P, Perkovic S, Streichert T, et al. (2008) The role of calcitonin and alpha-calcitonin gene-related peptide in bone formation. Arch Biochem Biophys 473: 210–217.
38. Sun JS, Tsuang YH, Liao CJ, Liu HC, Hang YS, et al. (1999) The effect of sintered beta-dicalcium pyrophosphate particle size on newborn Wistar rat osteoblasts. Artif Organs 23: 331–338.
39. Penolazzi L, Lampronti I, Borgatti M, Khan MT, Zennaro M, et al. (2008) Induction of apoptosis of human primary osteoclasts treated with extracts from the medicinal plant Emblica officinalis. BMC Complement Altern Med 8: 59.
40. Bouxsein ML, Boyd SK, Christiansen BA, Guldberg RE, Jepsen KJ, et al. (2010) Guidelines for assessment of bone microstructure in rodents using micro-computed tomography. J Bone Miner Res 25: 1468–1486.
41. Hildebrand T, Ruegsegger P. (1997) Quantification of Bone Microarchitecture with the Structure Model Index. Comput Methods Biomech Biomed Engin 1: 15–23.
42. Lin C, Moniz C, Chambers TJ, Chow JWM (1996) Colitis causes bone loss in rats through suppression of bone formation. Gastroenterol; 11: 1263–1271.

4

Zoledronate Effects on Systemic and Jaw Osteopenias in Ovariectomized Periostin-Deficient Mice

Nicolas Bonnet[1]*, Philippe Lesclous[2,3], Jean Louis Saffar[2], Serge Ferrari[1]

1 Division of Bone Diseases, Department of Internal Medicine Specialties, Geneva University Hospital, Geneva, Switzerland, **2** Laboratoire Pathologies, Imagerie et Biothérapie de l'organe dentaire EA 2496, Université Paris-Descartes, Faculté de Chirurgie Dentaire, Paris, France, **3** INSERM-UMRS 791, LIOAD: Laboratoire d'Ingénierie Ostéo-Articulaire et Dentaire, STEP: Skeletal Tissue Engineering and Physiopathology group, Nantes University, School of Dentistry, Hôtel Dieu Hospital, LUNAM Université, Nantes, France

Abstract

Osteoporosis and periodontal disease (PD) are frequently associated in the elderly, both concurring to the loss of jaw alveolar bone and finally of teeth. Bisphosphonates improve alveolar bone loss but have also been associated with osteonecrosis of the jaw (ONJ), particularly using oncological doses of zoledronate. The effects and therapeutic margin of zoledronate on jaw bone therefore remain uncertain. We reappraised the efficacy and safety of Zoledronate (Zol) in ovariectomized (OVX) periostin (Postn)-deficient mice, a unique genetic model of systemic and jaw osteopenia. Compared to vehicle, Zol 1M (100 µg/kg/month) and Zol 1W (100 µg/kg/week) for 3 months both significantly improved femur BMD, trabecular bone volume on tissue volume (BV/TV) and cortical bone volume in both OVX Postn$^{+/+}$ and Postn$^{-/-}$ (all $p<0.01$). Zol 1M and Zol 1W also improved jaw alveolar and basal BV/TV, although the highest dose (Zol 1W) was less efficient, particularly in Postn$^{-/-}$. Zol decreased osteoclast number and bone formation indices, i.e. MAR, MPm/BPm and BFR, independently in Postn$^{-/-}$ and Postn$^{+/+}$, both in the long bones and in deep jaw alveolar bone, without differences between Zol doses. Zol 1M and Zol 1W did not reactivate inflammation nor increase fibrous tissue in the bone marrow of the jaw, whereas the distance between the root and the enamel of the incisor (DRI) remained high in Postn$^{-/-}$ vs Postn$^{+/+}$ confirming latent inflammation and lack of crestal alveolar bone. Zol 1W and Zol 1M decreased osteocyte numbers in Postn$^{-/-}$ and Postn$^{+/+}$ mandible, and Zol 1W increased the number of empty lacunae in Postn$^{-/-}$, however no areas of necrotic bone were observed. These results demonstrate that zoledronate improves jaw osteopenia and suggest that in Postn$^{-/-}$ mice, zoledronate is not sufficient to induce bone necrosis.

Editor: Carlos M. Isales, Georgia Health Sciences University, United States of America

Funding: These studies were supported by a Swiss National Science Foundation grant No. 3100A0-116633/1 and EC 201099-TALOS (to S.F). The funders had no role in study design, data collection and analysis, decision to publish, or preparation of the manuscript.

Competing Interests: The authors have the following interests: Co-author Serge Ferrari has declared a conflict of interest since he serves as an expert in trials about ONJ cases in the US involving Novartis; however, he is not an employee of this company nor is he directly remunerated by the company for this expertise. There are no patents, products in development or marketed products to declare.

* E-mail: nicolas.bonnet@unige.ch

Introduction

Periodontal disease (PD) is a common problem as it is estimated that 48.2% of the US population aged more than 30 years is affected, with up to 20% of subjects showing severe tooth attachment loss in the NHANES III survey [1]. Moreover, PD seems to be frequently associated with osteoporosis [2], which could further aggravates the risk of tooth loosening [3,4]. Periodontal disease, especially measured by alveolar bone loss, is a strong predictor for incident of tooth loss in postmenopausal women, approximately one-third of adults age 65 and older losses one or more tooth [5]. Bisphosphonates, particularly alendronate and risedronate, have been shown to exert favorable effects on PD [6,7]. Clinical studies demonstrated a reduction of radiological and/or clinical signs of PD, including alveolar bone loss, gingival index and bleeding [8], [9], [10], [11], [12]. These beneficial effect of bisphosphonates on mandibular bone loss have also been demonstrated in animal models of PD such as the rice rat [13,14], and/or as induced by elastic rings [15,16], tooth ligature [7,17], and bacterial inoculations [18,19].

On another side, the occurrence of osteonecrosis of the jaw (ONJ) in some patients receiving bisphosphonates, particularly high-dose zoledronate for the prevention of skeletal complications of malignancy, has raised important questions regarding the role of these drugs in the development of ONJ [20,21]. Tooth extraction is commonly considered as a precipitating factor for bisphosphonates-related osteonecrosis of the jaw (BRONJ) [22,23]. However apparently spontaneous BRONJ, i.e. without any surgical traumatism of alveolar bone, also occurs. Nethertheless, it seems that PD is a crucial factor in the development of ONJ in patients receiving bisphosphonates. Indeed, oral preventive measures avoiding tooth mobility, periodontal diseases, presence of root fragments, decays, granulomas, edentulism and periapical conditions [24] decrease ONJ incidence [25,26]. Consistent with these clinical observations, lesions reminiscent of ONJ have been observed following administration of high-dose zoledronate in rats with severe PD [27,28]. Hence tooth ligature and cumulative high doses of zoledronate in rats (66 µg/kg, i.e equivalent to 4 mg/60 kg in humans, three times per week for 3 weeks) led to the appearance of necrotic bone in the mandible [27], arguing that both the presence of infectious/inflammatory sockets and lack of bone remodeling due to bisphosphonates concur to the development of ONJ-like lesions, despite a significant reduction of alveolar bone loss [27]. Similarly, in the rice rat model (Oryzomys Palustris) with periodontitis, high dose zoledronate (80 μg/kg I.V, once monthly during 18 and 24 weeks) induced ONJ-like lesions characterized by areas of exposed necrotic alveolar bone, increased osteocyte apoptosis and presence of bacterial colonies [28]. Whether the start of the necrosis process is secondary to PD [27] or is primarily an aseptic process [29], however remains questionable.

Several drug-related mechanisms have been suggested to eventually explain the contribution of bisphosphonates to the development of ONJ, all so far unproven, including an impairment of soft tissue and/or bone vascularization; a direct toxicity on the gingival epithelium; a direct toxicity on bone cells, particularly osteocytes; and of course the suppression of bone turnover [30]. Experimental models of aggressive PD (above) however do not allow to clarify the potential pathophysiological role of bisphosphonates in the development of ONJ beyond the absence of removal of necrotic bone fragments induced inflammation/infection. Whether bisphosphonates can actually cause jaw bone necrosis in absence of injury/inflammation, as observed in some patients without tooth extraction or severe PD, therefore remains debatable.

Periostin deficient mice (*Postn*$^{-/-}$) represent a unique opportunity to reappraise the effects of bisphosphonates on the jaw. Periostin is a matricellular protein synthesized by osteoblast/osteocytes, that is linked to type I collagen in the periodontal ligament, where it regulates fibrillogenesis [31], [32]. Periostin-deficient mice show severe alterations in tooth eruption, resulting from a failure to digest collagen fibers in the shear zone of the periodontal ligament [33]. As a consequence, the enamel and dentin of the incisors are compressed and disorganized, and these mice develop inflammatory infiltrates (particularly neutrophils) in the periodontal ligament, loss of crestal (superficial) alveolar bone and alveolar bone loss underneath. The severity of PD can be moderated by feeding the mice a soft diet, indicating that the trigger of the inflammatory infiltrate in the periodontal ligament is traumatic mastication [33]. On a soft diet, *Postn*$^{-/-}$ mice do not have overt PD with inflammation, however they still present alveolar and systemic osteopenia [34]. Accordingly, we used old *Postn*$^{-/-}$ mice kept on a soft diet to reappraise the intrinsic effects of high dose zoledronate on the jaw. Here we hypothesize that zoledronate will improve jaw and systemic osteopenia, without causing necrosis of alveolar bone in absence of overt PD. Our results indicate that zoledronate improves jaw and systemic osteopenia without causing alveolar bone necrosis in absence of overt PD, despite a decrease in osteocyte number.

Materials and Methods

Animals

Postn Lac Z knock-in mice (*Postn*$^{-/-}$) were generated as reported previously [33]. *Postn*$^{-/-}$ mice were subsequently bred with C57BL/6J mice, and DNA analyzed by PCR was used to identify Postn heterozygous mice. We interbred mice that were heterozygous carriers of this mutation and obtained wild-type (*Postn*$^{+/+}$) and homozygous mutant (*Postn*$^{-/-}$) offspring with the expected Mendelian distribution. They were subsequently backcrossed for 10 generations, resulting in a genome of 99% C57BL/6J. Mice were housed five per cage, maintained under standard non barriers conditions and had access to water and a soft diet ad libitum (Harlan Teklad 2019,SDS, England). Under those experimental conditions, the malnutrition that is otherwise observed in the *Postn*$^{-/-}$ mice under a standard (hard) diet that causes the enamel and dentin defects of the incisors and molars [33], is partially prevented. This dietary adaptation also reduces the severity of PD [33], i.e. inflammation. All mice received the same diet during the experiment. Ten month-old female *Postn*$^{-/-}$ and *Postn*$^{+/+}$ mice were OVX (8/gr) or Sham-operated (6/gr) and administered directly after the surgery subcutaneous Zol either once weekly (Zol 1W, 100 μg/kg/week), or once monthly (Zol 1M, 100 μg/kg/month), or vehicle (Veh) for 3 months, corresponding to a cumulative dose of 16 mg/60 kg/month (ZOL 1W) or 4 mg/60 kg/month (ZOL 1M), respectively. These drug exposures correspond to 4 times, and 1 time respectively, of the monthly dose of zoledronate prescribed for the prevention of skeletal-related events in cancer patients [27,35]. The duration of treatment has been chosen based on previous study describing the structural effects of Zol in rodents [36–38]. Lumbar spine, femurs and mandible were excised and stored in ethanol for micro-computed tomography analysis & histomorphometry and kept at −20°C for biomechanical analysis. All surgical procedures were performed under ketamin/xylasin, and OVX animals received Buprenorphin (0.05 mg/kg) just after surgery and every 12 h for 2days. Ethics Statement: animal procedures were approved by the University Of Geneva School Of Medecine Ethical Committee and the State of Geneva Veterinarian Office.

In vivo measurement of bone mineral density

Total body, femoral and spinal bone mineral density (BMD, g/cm^2) were measured *in vivo* at 10, 11.5 and 13 months of age by dual-energy X-ray absorptiometry (PIXImus2, GE lunar, Madison WI) [39].

Ex vivo measurement of morphology and microarchitecture

Micro-computed tomography (microCT UCT40, Scanco Medical AG, Basserdorf Switzerland) was used to assess trabecular bone volume fraction and microarchitecture in the excised 5th lumbar spine body and distal femur, and cortical bone geometry at the midshaft femoral diaphysis as previously described [40]. Briefly, trabecular and cortical bone regions were evaluated using isotropic 12 μm voxels.

For the vertebral trabecular region, we evaluated 250 transverse CT slices between the cranial and caudal end plates, excluding 100 μm near each endplate. For the femoral and tibial trabecular region, to eliminate the primary spongiosa, we analyzed one hundred slices from the 50 slices under the distal growth plate.

Femoral cortical geometry was assessed using 50 continuous CT slides (600 μm) located at the femoral midshaft. Images were segmented using an adaptative-iterative thresholding approach rather than a fixed threshold. Morphometric variables were computed from binarized images using direct, three-dimensional techniques that do not rely on prior assumptions about the underlying structure [41]. For the trabecular bone regions, we assessed the bone volume fraction (BV/TV, %), trabecular thickness (TbTh, μm), trabecular number (TbN, mm^{-1}), trabecular connectivity density (Tb Conn Density, mm^{-3}) and structural model index (SMI). The structure model index was measured to determine the prevalence of plate-like or rod-like trabecular structures, where 0 represents 'plates' and 3 'rods' [41]. For cortical bone at the femoral and tibial midshaft, we measured the cortical tissue volume (CtTV, mm^3), bone volume (CtBV, mm^3), the marrow volume (BMaV, mm^3) and the average cortical width (CtTh, μm).

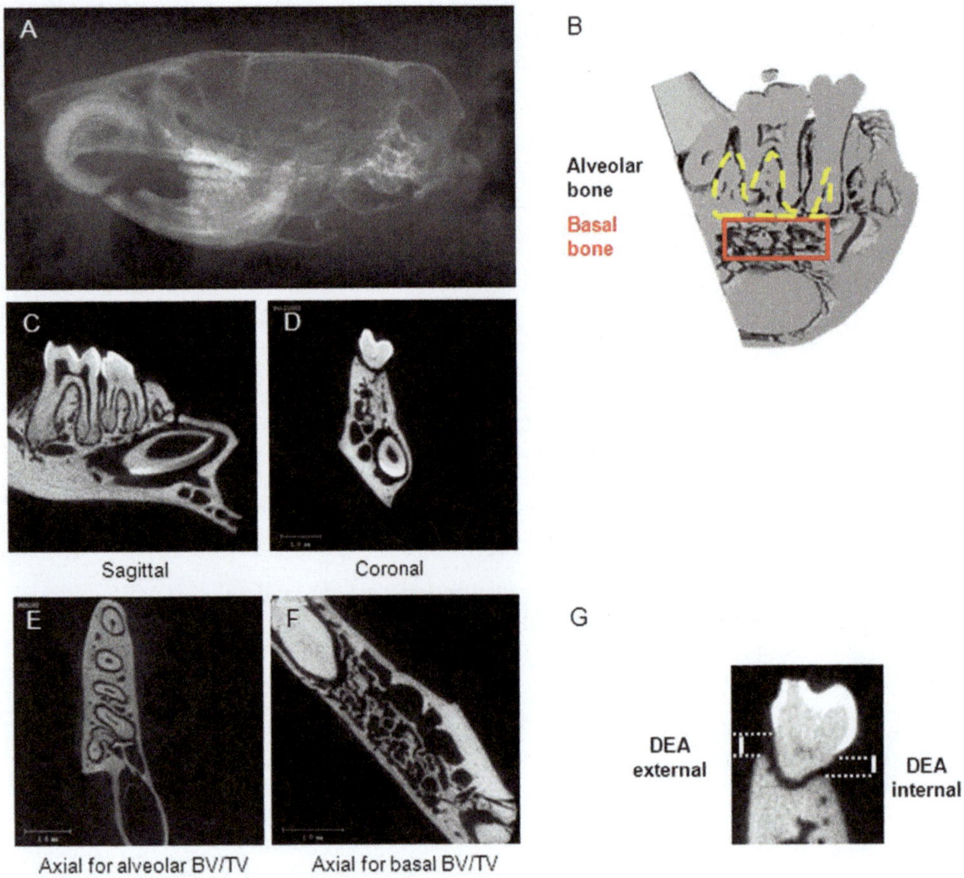

Figure 1. 2D and 3D images of microcomputed tomography. (A) Scout view of the *Postn*$^{-/-}$ mice showing alteration of the enamel (*) that affects the incisor from the apex to the incisor edge. (B) 3D reconstruction of our region of interest for the alveolar and basal bone compartment. (C) Sagittal slice (D) coronal slice (E) Axial slice at the alveolar bone compartment (F) Axial slice at the basal bone compartment. (G) Illustration of the external and internal Distance between cement-Enamel junction and Alveolar bone (DEA), an index of exposed bone in the oral cavity.

For mandible alveolar and basal bone volume fraction (BV/TV) analysis, the head of the mice was oriented with the nasal cavity floor parallel to the horizontal plane and the midpalatal suture parallel to the midsagital plane to obtain axial CT slides (Fig. 1).

The Distance between cementum-Enamel junction and Alveolar bone (DEA), an index of alveolar bone loss, was measured at the mesial root of M1 on coronal CT slides, which represents the mean of external and internal DEA (Fig. 1).

Histomorphometry

To measure dynamic indices of bone formation, mice received subcutaneous injections of calcein (20 mg/kg, Sigma, Buchs, Switzerland) 9 and 2 days before euthanasia.

Femur were embedded in methyl-methacrylate (Merck, Darmstadt, Germany) as previously described [42] [34], and 20-µm-thick transversal sections of the midshaft were cut with a saw (FinOcut, Metkon, Instruments LTD) than sanded to 10-µm-thick and mounted unstained for evaluation of fluorescence. Five-8 µm thick sagital sections were cut with a Leica Corp. Polycut E microtome (Leica Corp. Microsystems AG, Glattburg, Switzerland) and stained with modified Goldner's trichrome, and histomorphometric measurements were performed on the secondary spongiosa of the distal femur metaphysis and on the endocortical and periosteal bone surfaces in the middle of the femur, using a Leica Corp. Q image analyser at 40× magnification. All parameters were calculated and expressed according to standard formulas and nomenclatures [43] : mineral apposition rate (MAR, µm/day), single labeled surface (sLS/BPm, %), and double-labeled surface (dLS/BPm, %). Mineralizing surface per bone surface (MS/BPm, %) was calculated by adding dLS/BPm and one-half sLS/BPm. Bone formation rate (BFR/BPm, $\mu m^3/\mu m^2$/day) was calculated as the product of MS/BPm and MAR. Three slides per sample were analyzed for the bone formation indices. Osteocyte number and lacunae per bone area were counted on two toluidine blue stained slides of the midshaft cross-sectionnal femur per sample.

The right mandible was removed and fixed in cold (4°C) 70% ethanol. After dehydratation, the bone samples were embedded without demineralization in methylmethacrylate and polymerized at – 20° for 48 h [44]. Longitudinal sections (4 µm thick) were cut with a polycut E microtome (Leica, Wetzlar, Germany). They were stained with toluidine blue (pH 3.8) or Sirius red or hematoxylin-eosin or processed for tartrate-resistant acid phosphatase (TRAP) revelation. Two sections for each stained sample were quantified per animal. Toluidine blue staining was used to visualize osteocytes and their lacunae (expressed in number per square millimeter of trabecular bone surface) in the zone of interest, i.e the trabecular bone segment comprised between the end of the M1 root and the underlying incisor. Empty osteocyte lacunae were evaluated and necrotic bone defined as a loss of more than five contiguous osteocytes with confluent areas of empty

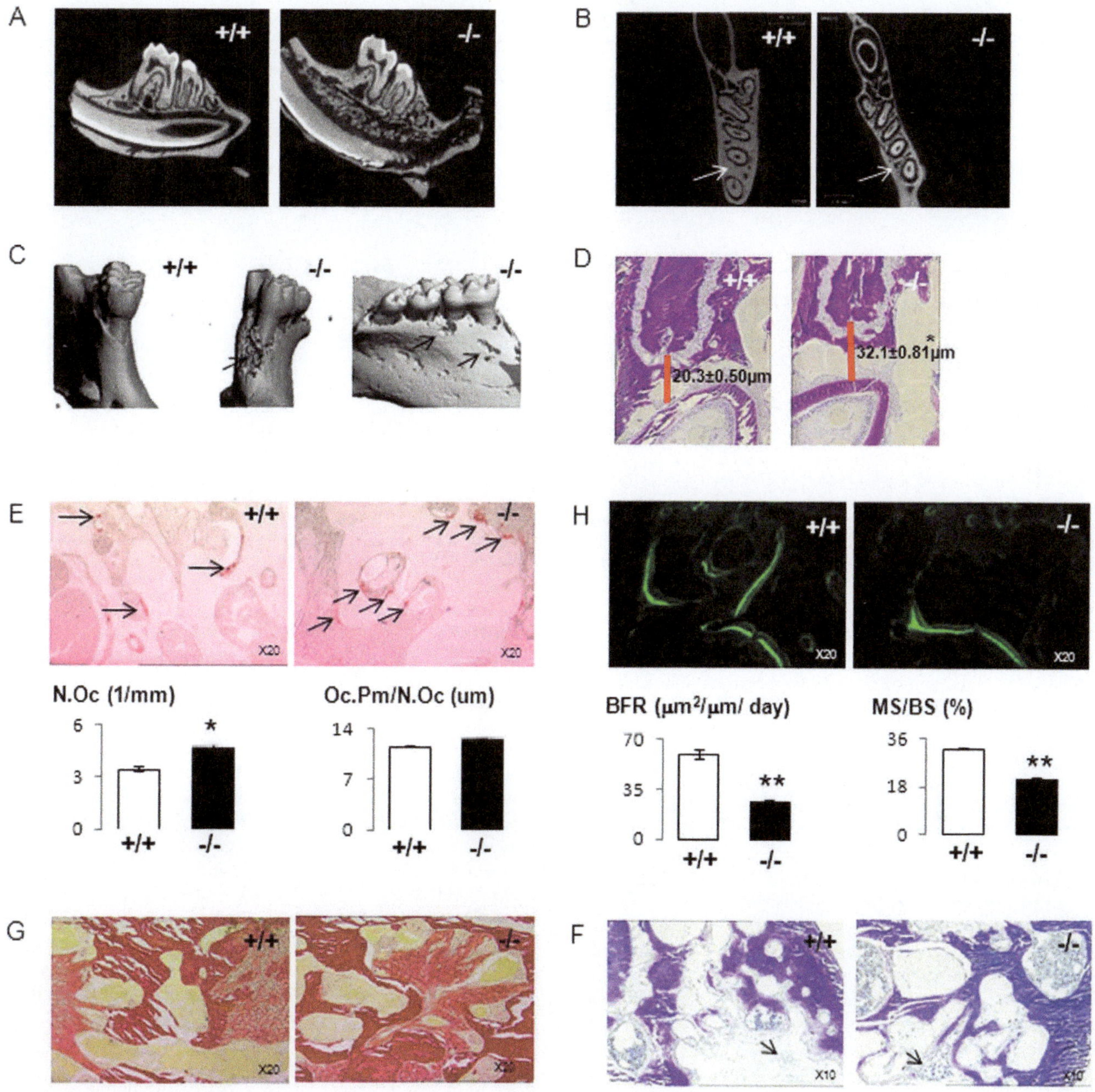

Figure 2. Periodontal disease disturbance and mandibule osteopenia in *Postn*$^{-/-}$ mice aged of 13 months. (A,B) Sagital and axial 2D image, arrows indicate alteration of the alveolar bone between roots in *Postn*$^{-/-}$ vs *Postn*$^{+/+}$. (C) 3D reconstruction of the mandible, arrows shows loss of the alveolar bone and therefore tooth exhibition in *Postn*$^{-/-}$ vs *Postn*$^{+/+}$. (D) Toluidine blue staining, red bar shows a lower distance between the root and the enamel of the incisor in *Postn*$^{-/-}$ vs *Postn*$^{+/+}$. (E) TRAP staining, arrow indicate higher osteoclast in *Postn*$^{-/-}$ vs *Postn*$^{+/+}$ mice, Number of Osteoclast (N.Oc), activity of the osteoclast illustrated by the ratio Osteoclast Perimeter on Osteoclast Number (Oc.Pm/N.Oc), * $p<0.05$. (H) Fluorescent calcein labels on alveolar surfaces, Bone Formation Rate (BFR), Mineralizing Surface per Bone Surface (MS/BS). (G) Sirius red staining. (F) Toluidine blue staining, no sign of active inflammation are noted, arrows indicate residual inflammation around the periodontal incisive ligament.

lacunae [27]. Sirius red staining, specific for tissue collagen, was used to visualize the fibrous network in the bone marrow area. Hematoxilin-eosin was used to characterize inflammatory cells and further quantify areas of osteonecrosis. Distance between the Root and the enamel of the Incisor (DRI) was also evaluated on the hematoxilin-eosin stained sections.

TRAP was detected by using hexazotized pararosanilin (Sigma, St Louis, MO) and naphtol ASTR phosphate (Sigma, St Louis, MO) to reveal osteoclasts, ; non-osteoclastic acid phosphatase was inhibited by adding 100 mMol/L L(+)-tartric acid (Sigma, St Louis, MO) to the substrate solution. The following parameters were recorded: the number of TRAP+ osteoclasts in contact with trabeculae (N.Oc/TBPm ; expressed in cells per millimeter of trabecular bone surface) ; the resorption surface (OcS/BS ; expressed in %) ; the average length of the zone of contact per osteoclast (Oc.Pm/N.Oc ; given in microns) considered as a sensitive indicator of osteoclast activity [45]. Dynamic indices of bone formation were evaluated as described above for the femur.

Table 1. Influence of zoledronate on bone turnover/remodelling indices in femur and jaw.

	Parameters	*SH Postn*$^{+/+}$	Veh	*OVX Postn*$^{+/+}$ Zol1M	Zol1W	*SH Postn*$^{-/-}$	Veh	*OVX Postn*$^{-/-}$ Zol1M	Zol1W
FEMUR	Ps MAR (μm/day)	0.49±0.04*	0.26±0.09	0.37±0.07	0.18±0.05	0.29±0.09$^{\#}$	0.23±0.11	0.17±0.05$^{\#}$	0±0$^{\#}$
Periosteal	Ps BFR/BPm (μm²/μm/ day)	0.10±0.02	0.04±0.03	0.05±0.02	0.01±.002	0.02±0.01$^{\#}$	0.04±0.03	0.01±0.004	0±0
	Ps MPm/BPm (%)	0.20±0.03**	0.06±0.02	0.13±0.04	0.05±0.02	0.08±0.02$^{\#}$	0.10±0.05	0.07±0.02	0.009±0.002
Endocortical	Ec MAR (μm/day)	0.77±0.05	0.63±0.07	0.02±0.02****	0±0****	0.41±0.09$^{\#}$	0.48±0.04$^{\#}$	0.29±0.04****	0±0****
	Ec BFR/BPm (μm²/μm/ day)	0.24±0.03	0.16±0.03	0.001±0.001****	0±0****	0.11±0.03$^{\#}$	0.15±0.03	0.002±0.002***	0±0****
	Ec MPm/BPm (%)	0.32±0.04*	0.27±0.04	0.06±0.01****	0.02±0.003****	0.22±0.04	0.30±0.04	0.10±0.01***	0.03±0.006****
JAW									
Alveolar	Tb MAR (μm/day)	1.87±0.21	1.43±0.12	1.07±0.14****	1.03±0.1****	1.27±0.06$^{\#\#\#}$	1.18±0.08$^{\#\#\#}$	0.99±0.03***	0.94±0.04****
	Tb BFR/BS (μm²/μm³/ day)	59.11±3.35	25.16±1.03	15.01±1.60****	14.08±1.55****	20.66±1.50$^{\#\#\#}$	18.33±2.23$^{\#\#}$	14.41±1.82***	13.33±1.75***
	Tb MS/BS (%)	32.33±2.1	36.36±2.52	16.13±0.97**	14.31±0.95***	26.29±1.48$^{\#}$	21.65±1.16$^{\# \#}$	14.22±0.58****	12.43±1.63****

$^{*}p<0.05$, $^{**}p<0.01$, $^{***}p<0.001$, $^{****}p<0.0001$ vs OVXvehicle of the respective genotype. $^{\#}p<0.05$ vs *Postn*$^{+/+}$ of the respective treatments. Means ± SEM. Ps: periosteum, Ec: endocortical, Tb: trabecular. mineral apposition rate (MAR), mineralisation perimeter (MPm), mineralisation surface (MS), Bone formation rate (BFR), bone perimeter (BPm), bone surface (BS). Ovariectomitzed mice (OVX n = 8/gr) or Sham-operated (SH n = 6/gr).

Testing of mechanical resistance

The night before mechanical testing, bones were thawed slowly at 7°C and then maintained at room temperature. The length of the femur (distance from intermalleolar to intercondylar region) was measured using callipers with an integrated electronic digital display and the midpoint of the shaft was determined. The femur then was placed on the material testing machine on two supports separated by a distance of 9.9 mm and load was applied to the midpoint of the shaft, thus creating a three-point bending test. Between each preparation step, the specimens were kept immersed in physiological solution. The mechanical resistance to failure was tested using a servo-controlled electromechanical system (Instron 1114, Instron corp., High Wycombe, UK) with actuator displaced at 2 mm/minute. Both displacement and load were recorded. All tested samples (n = 8 per group) have been included in the analysis. Ultimate force (maximal load, measured in Newtons [N]), stiffness (slope of the linear part of the curve, representing the elastic deformation, N/mm), and energy (surface under the curve, N*mm) were calculated. Ultimate stress (N/mm^2) and Young's modulus (MPa) were determined by the equations previously described by Turner and Burr [46]. Reproducibility was 3.3% for midshaft femur as previously described elsewhere [47].

Data analysis

The power calculation to perform our study was based on our primary criteria, the improvement of bone alterations by Zol. We first tested the effects of Zol within groups (*Postn*$^{-/-}$ and *Postn*$^{+/+}$) by unpaired t-tests. To compare the effects of genotype and the response to treatments Zol, we used a two way ANOVA. As appropriate, post hoc testing was performed using Fisher's protected Least Squares Difference (PLSD). Differences were considered significant at $p<0.05$. Data were presented as mean ± SEM.

Results

Jaw bone alterations in *Postn*$^{-/-}$ mice

Postn$^{-/-}$ mice fed a hard diet develop severe PD, with bone and teeth alterations [33]. To assess the severity of these alterations in *Postn*$^{-/-}$ mice receiving a soft diet, dissected mandibles of 13-months-old intact mice were imaged by histological sections and microCT. 2D and 3D microCT images illustrate alterations of the crestal alveolar bone as well as the deeper alveolar bone and cementum-enamel junction, particularly around the proximal root of the first molar (Fig. 2A–C). Quantitatively, *Postn*$^{-/-}$ present lower basal and alveolar BV/TV (−31.6% and −21.4% vs *Postn*$^{+/+}$, $p<0.01$). The alteration of alveolar bone was confirmed histologically by the higher distance between the molar root and the enamel of the underlying incisor, 'DRI' (Fig. 2D). In this bone area, *Postn*$^{-/-}$ mice presented a higher osteoclast number (4.67±0.34, 1/mm vs 3.42±0.14, 1/mm in *Postn*$^{+/+}$ mice, $p<0.01$) and lower bone formation indices (Fig. 2E–H, table 1). Sirius red staining indicated large medullar spaces filled by fibrous tissue in almost all *Postn*$^{-/-}$ mice, whereas no fibrous tissue was detectable in *Postn*$^{+/+}$ mice (Fig. 2G), suggesting that an inflammatory episode had previously occurred in the mandible of *Postn*$^{-/-}$ mice. Consistent with previous descriptions [33], *Postn*$^{-/-}$ mice showed some inflammatory infiltrates around the periodontal ligament (Fig. 2F). In contrast, and likely due to the effects of a soft diet, no signs of active inflammation were noted in gingival, periradicular and jaw bone compartments at 13 months of age (Fig. 2F). These observations indicate that *Postn*$^{-/-}$ mice fed a soft diet present alveolar and systemic osteopenia without overt PD.

Effects of zoledronate

Bone structure. As previously described in male *Postn*$^{-/-}$ mice [34], both intact and OVX female *Postn*$^{-/-}$ mice had lower femur BMD, trabecular bone microarchitecture (BV/TV) and

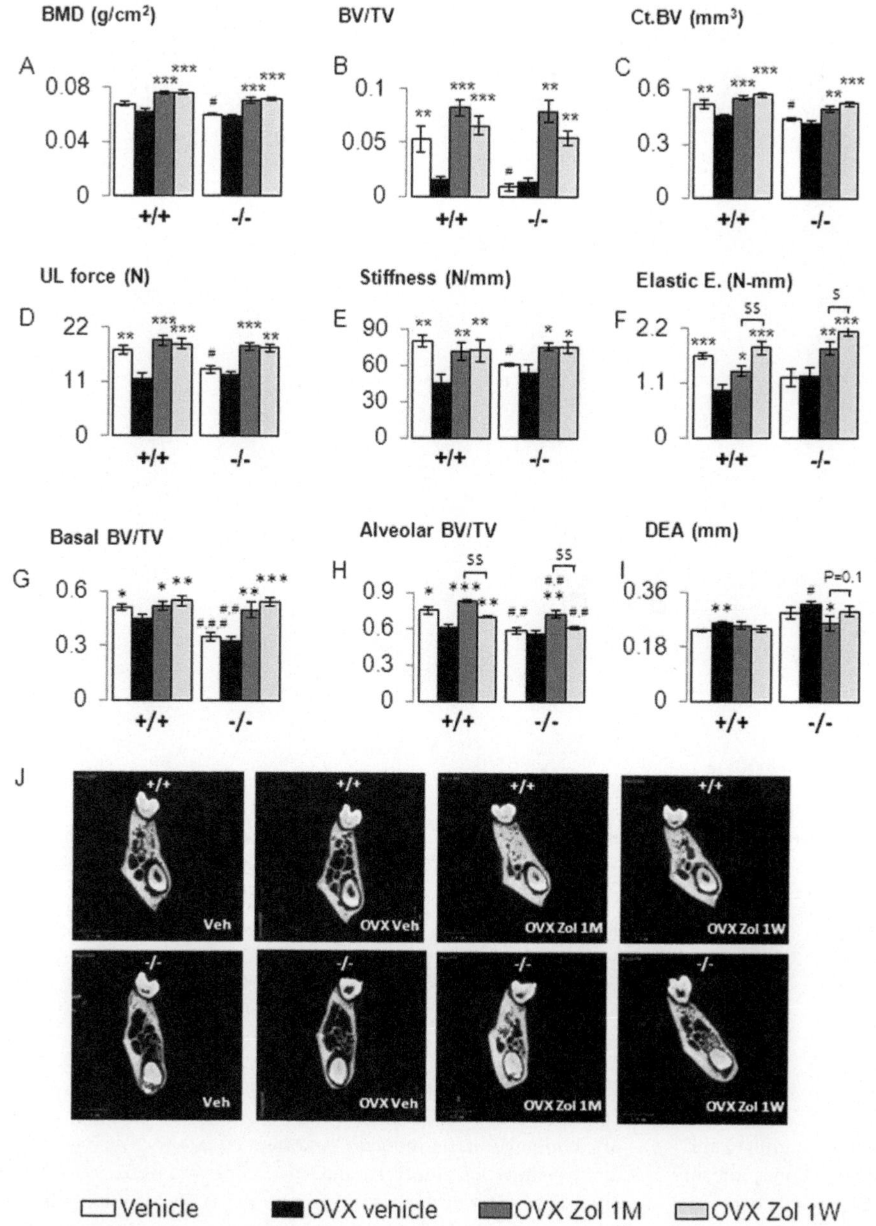

Figure 3. Zoledronate effect on the femur and mandible site in *Postn*$^{+/+}$ and *Postn*$^{-/-}$ mice. (A) Femur Bone Mineral Density (BMD). (B) Trabecular bone volume on tissue volume (BV/TV) of the distal femur. (C) Cortical Bone Volume (CtBV). (D, E, F) Biomechanical parameters obtain by three points bending test, (ultimate, UL; energy, E). (G, H) Basal bone volume fraction and alveolar bone volume fraction respectively obtains by microcomputed-tomography. (I) Mean of the internal and external Distance between cement-Enamel junction and Alveolar bone (DEA). (J) 2D coronal illustration of the effect of zoledronate one injection per month (Zol 1M) and one injection per week (Zol 1W) in ovariectomized (OVX) *Postn*$^{+/+}$ and *Postn*$^{-/-}$ mice. * $p<0.05$, ** $p<0.01$, *** $p<0.001$ vs OVX vehicle in the respective genotype of *Postn*$^{+/+}$ and *Postn*$^{-/-}$. # $p<0.05$, ## $p<0.01$, ### $p<0.001$ vs *Postn*$^{+/+}$ in the respective treatment. \$ $p<0.05$, \$\$ $p<0.01$ significant differences between OVX Zol 1M and OVX Zol 1W. Bars show means (± sem).

cortical bone volume (CtBV) compared to *Postn*$^{+/+}$ (−13.8%, −83.0% and −15.4% respectively, all $p<0.01$, Table 1). Bone formation indices were also decreased in the femur and mandible of *Postn*$^{-/-}$ mice (Table 1).

Compared to vehicle, Zol 1M (100 µg/kg/month) and Zol 1W (100 µg/kg/week) significantly improved BMD, femur BV/TV and CtBV in both OVX Postn$^{+/+}$ and Postn$^{-/-}$ mice (Fig. 3A–C, all $p<0.01$). Accordingly, biomechanical properties of the femur were improved by Zol in both genotypes (Fig. 3D–F).

In the mandible, Zol 1W and 1M also improved basal BV/TV both in Postn$^{-/-}$ and Postn$^{+/+}$ mice ($p<0.01$) (Fig. 3G). As a consequence the distance between the molar root and the enamel of the underlying incisor (DRI) decreased in response to Zol in both Postn$^{-/-}$ and Postn$^{+/+}$ (Fig 4H). Zol 1M also significantly increased alveolar BV/TV vs Veh in Postn$^{-/-}$ (+27%, $p<0.01$) and in Postn$^{+/+}$ (+35%, $p<0.001$) (Fig. 3H & 3J). However, Postn$^{-/-}$ and Postn$^{+/+}$ mice treated with Zol 1W had significantly lower alveolar BV/TV vs Zol 1M (all $p<0.01$). Moreover, Zol 1M decreased vs Veh the Distance between cement-Enamel junction

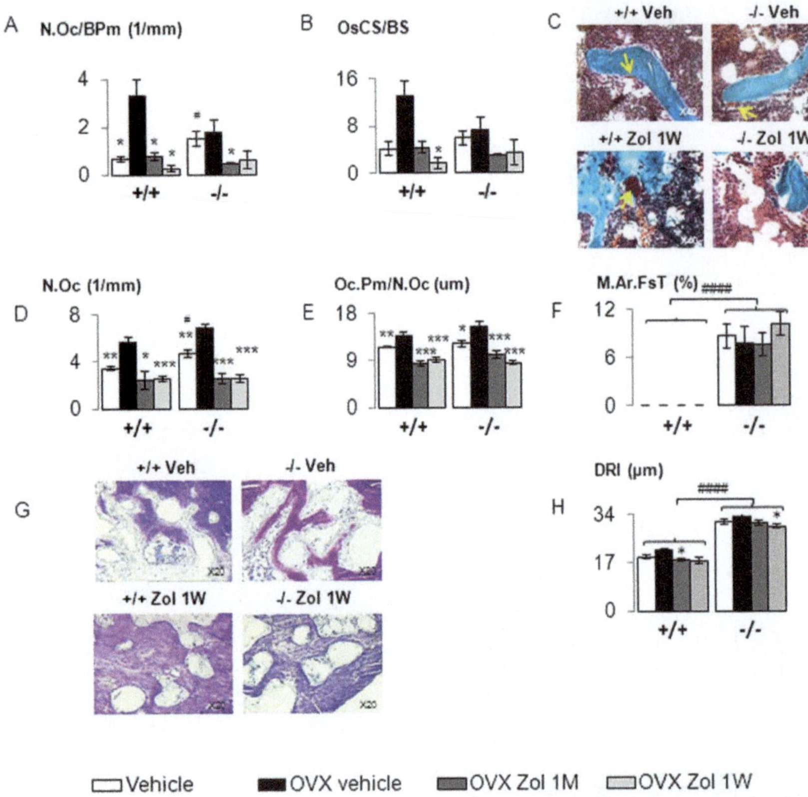

Figure 4. Zoledronate effect on bone resorption and sign of inflammation in *Postn*$^{+/+}$ and *Postn*$^{-/-}$ mice. (A–C) Histomorphometry parameter and images perform on the femur. (A) Number of Osteoclast on Bone Perimeter (N.Oc/BPm), (B) Osteoclast Surface on Bone Surface (OcS/BS), (C) Goldner staining, yellow arrows indicate normal size of osteoclast in vehicle groups and shows giant osteoclast under zoledronate treatment either in *Postn*$^{+/+}$ and *Postn*$^{-/-}$ mice. (D–H) Histomorphometry parameter and images perform on the mandible. (D) Osteoclast Number (N.Oc), (E) Osteoclast Perimeter on Osteoclast Number (Oc.Pm/N.Oc). (F) Medullary area filled by fibrous tissue (M.Ar.FsT). (G) Toluidine blue staining, note that Zol1W do not active inflammation. (H) Distance between the Root and the enamel of the Incisor (DRI). * $p<0.05$, ** $p<0.01$, *** $p<0.001$ vs OVX vehicle in the respective genotype of *Postn*$^{+/+}$ and *Postn*$^{-/-}$. # $p<0.05$, ## $p<0.01$, #### $p<0.0001$ vs *Postn*$^{+/+}$ in the respective treatment. Bars show means (± sem).

and Alveolar bone (DEA) in Postn$^{-/-}$ ($p<0.05$, Fig. 3I), whereas Zol 1W did not.

Bone remodelling. Zol decreased osteoclast number and surface in Postn$^{-/-}$ and Postn$^{+/+}$, both in the long bones and in deep jaw alveolar bone (Fig. 4A–E), without differences between Zol doses. As previously described, we confirmed the presence of giant osteoclasts with Zol in both Postn$^{-/-}$ and Postn$^{+/+}$ (Fig. 4C). Zol did not affect bone formation indices at the periosteum either in Postn$^{-/-}$ nor Postn$^{+/+}$ mice (Table 1). In contrast Zol at both doses significantly decreased bone formation indices, i.e. MAR, MPm/BPm and BFR, at the endocortical and alveolar compartments in Postn$^{-/-}$ and Postn$^{+/+}$ mice (Table 1).

Alveolar bone histopathology. Clinical and histological examination revealed no osteonecrotic area in the mandible of either group. Zol did not influence the size of medullar area filled by fibrous tissue (Fig. 4H). There was also no evidence of inflammatory infiltrates in any area of the mandible in relation to Zol treatment (Fig 4G). However, Zol decreased the number of osteocytes in deep bone area in both Postn$^{+/+}$ (−17% and −11% vs veh, respectively in Zol1M and Zol1W, $p<0.05$) and Postn$^{-/-}$ mice (−26% and −27% vs veh, respectively in Zol1M and Zol1W, $p<0.05$, Fig. 5A). In Postn$^{-/-}$, but not Postn$^{+/+}$ mice, Zol 1W also increased the percentage of empty lacunae (+33.9% in Zol1W vs veh, $p<0.05$). However, we did not observe areas of adjacent empty lacunae that define necrotic bone tissue [27] (Fig. 5C–D).

By comparison, no reduction in osteocyte number or increase in the percentage of empty lacunae with Zol was observed in long bones (Fig. 5B). On the contrary, in OVX Postn$^{+/+}$ mice, Zol 1M and 1W significantly decreased the percentage of empty lacunae vs veh (Fig. 5B).

Discussion

Despite the prominent benefits of bisphosphonates on preventing osteoporotic fractures and the improvement of alveolar bone and tooth loss in PD with these drugs, the occurrence of ONJ, particularly with oncological doses of i.v. zoledronate, has raised new concerns about their therapeutic margin, -i.e. the difference between the optimal effective dose and the dose at which unacceptable adverse effects occur-. Our results indicate that in absence of cancer, injury and/or severe inflammation, zoledronate at up to 4 fold the human oncological dose is safe and effective in improving jaw (and systemic) bone loss in rodents. They further indicate that suppressed bone turnover together with alterations of bone mass and quality, as observed in *Postn*$^{-/-}$ mice, is not sufficient to induce jaw bone necrosis. Periodontal disease and particularly periodontitis is characterized by inflammation of the periodontal tissues (gingival tissue, alveolar bone and periodontal

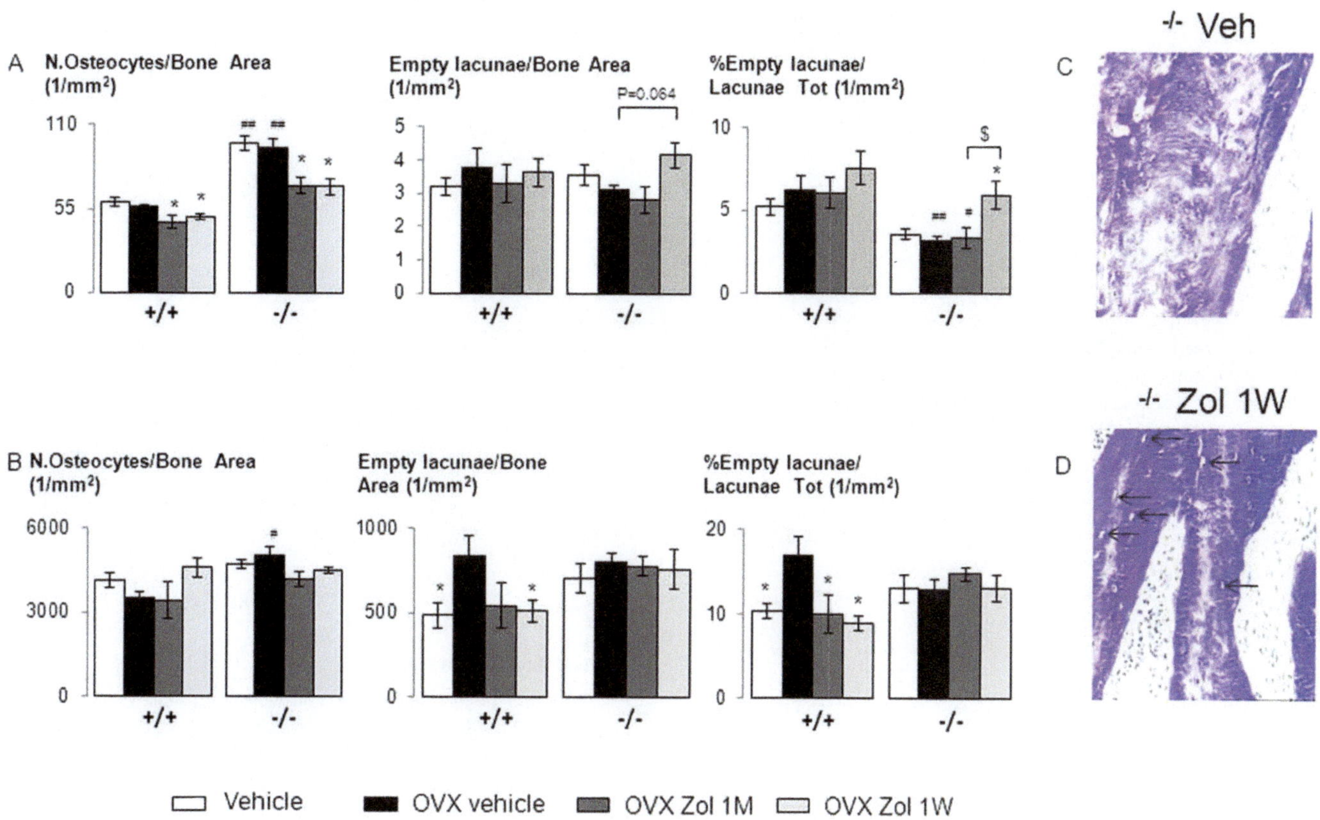

Figure 5. Zoledronate effect on osteocyte number and empty lacunae in jaw and femur site of *Postn*$^{+/+}$ and *Postn*$^{-/-}$ mice. Osteocyte number and empty lacunae in the jaw (A) and the mid-shaft femur (B), (C–D) Toluidine blue, (C) Full of osteocyte lacunae with osteocyte in vehicle (Veh) *Postn*$^{-/-}$, (D) Less osteocyte and more empty lacunae (arrow) in zoledronate one injection per week (Zol 1W) vs vehicle in *Postn*$^{-/-}$ mice. * $p<0.05$ vs OVX vehicle in the respective genotype of *Postn*$^{+/+}$ and *Postn*$^{-/-}$. # $p<0.05$, ## $p<0.01$ vs *Postn*$^{+/+}$ in the respective treatment. $ $p<0.05$ OVX Zol 1M. Bars show means (± sem).

ligament) caused by pathogenic microflora, loss of connective tissue and crestal alveolar bone [48]. Periostin-deficient mice fed a soft diet represent a unique genetic model of systemic and jaw bone alterations. In these conditions, crestal alveolar bone is affected as DEA increased, and the periodontal ligament appeared enlarged. Basal bone, which does not belong to the periodontal tissue, was also affected as BV/TV and fibrous areas were increased. This is sustained by an imbalance of bone remodeling secondary to a decrease of bone formation and an increase of bone resorption. However no prominent inflammatory infiltrates were observed in periodontal tissues, mucosa and bone, nor were periodontal pockets present, indicating the absence of overt PD.

In this model, even supra-pharmacological exposure to Zol, i.e 4 folds the human oncological dose, did not reactivate inflammation and/or worsen the DRI. Although, Zol decreased osteoclast and osteocyte number, and increased the percentage of empty lacunae in *Postn*$^{-/-}$, no area of necrotic bone was observed. Hence, in absence of active inflammation, suppression of bone turnover (by BPs) together with alterations of alveolar bone mass and bone quality, i.e collagen fibers as in *Postn*$^{-/-}$ [34], is not sufficient to induce bone necrosis. Our results markedly differ from previous observations in which zoledronate was administered at various doses in animal models subjected to severe surgical procedure (ligature [27] or extraction [49,50]), induction of PD by high sucrose diet [28], metastatic processes, bacteria inoculation [51] and/or cytotoxic drugs (dexamethasone, docetaxel…) [52]. In these models, in addition to cellular infiltration, lesions reminiscent of ONJ have sometimes been observed. Taken together these experiments suggest that injury/inflammation is an pre-requisite for the development of necrosis.

In wild-type OVX mice, Zol 1W still improved trabecular and compact bone in the femur and basal bone in the jaw, i.e similar to the oncologic dose (Zol 1M), as previously described [36]. However, in the jaw alveolar compartment, BV/TV remained lower with weekly Zol administration. The concomitant decrease of osteocytes, osteoclasts and bone remodeling (i.e low BFR) in the jaw, could suggest a lower cell viability and / or replacement rate with frequently dosed Zol, i.e low remodeling levels. In contrast, we did not observe a significant reduction of osteocyte number in the femur. Toxic effects of BPs on fibroblasts and epithelial cells have been reported in-vitro and at high concentrations [53], [54], [55], and suggested on osteocytes in vivo [56–57]. However despite many studies, direct effects of BPs on bone osteoblasts/ osteocytes have been difficult to demonstrate in vivo using clinically relevant doses [58]. The site-specific effects of BPs on osteocytes observed in our study could be explained by some differences in the biology of jaw vs peripheral osteoblasts, which have various embryonic origins: in the long bones the osteoblast lineage derives from the trunk lateral plate mesoderm, whereas in the mandible it derives from the paraxial mesoderm [59]. It could also be explained by the different remodeling rate between these skeletal sites, which is higher in the jaw [60], potentially facilitating the accumulation of BPs in the bone matrix [61], [62]. However, after a single infusion of Zol in dogs, drug concentration in jaw and teeth was not higher than in tibia and actually lower than in pelvis or vertebrae [63]. Repeated administration of ibandronate in rats also showed the absence of preferential intake in the jaw [64].

It has been shown that the decrease of bone turnover by Zoledronate does not affect serum periostin levels or periostin immunostaining in mice [65,66]. In contrast, in absence of periostin, high dose Zol was the least effective on the jaw BV/TV. Hence, *Postn*$^{-/-}$ mice receiving Zol 1W maintained a lower alveolar BV/TV compared to mice receiving Zol 1M, and its absolute value did not differ from placebo. Moreover, in these mice, Zol 1W increased the number of empty osteocytic lacunae. Basal bone turnover is lower in *Postn*$^{-/-}$, however the decrease of bone formation indices in response to Zol was not more pronounced in absence of periostin. Hence, it is unlikely that the poor gain of alveolar BV/TV under Zol in *Postn*$^{-/-}$ mice could be explained by an over-suppression of bone turnover.

In a model of fibrosis [67], interleukin-4, -13, two anti-inflammatory cytokines, induced periostin expression, whereas during periodontal inflammation periostin staining is down-regulated [68]. On another side, *Postn*$^{-/-}$ mice have latent PD, and inflammatory cells produce cytokines that decrease osteoblast functions. However, *Postn*$^{-/-}$ mice did not present an increased infiltration of jaw bone by inflammatory cells in response to Zol. We previously reported that loading and PTH increases periostin expression in osteocytes [34], and that periostin decreases the expression of apoptotic molecules such as caspase 3 [47], potentially through direct binding to intergrin $\alpha V\beta 5$ which activate downstream FAK and Akt pathways. In others tissues, increased periostin expression have also been suggested to represent an adaptative cell response to maintain cell survivals against an environmental stress [69], [70], [71]. Therefore, it is possible that absence of periostin promoted BPs pro-apoptotic effects on osteocytes [61–62], which together with low bone turnover would explain the persistence and accumulation of empty osteocytic lacunae. We cannot exclude that with a higher number of animals and a longer duration of treatment the accumulation of empty osteocytic lacunae would have led to the detection of bone necrosis.

To conclude, zoledronate improved systemic and alveolar bone alterations in OVX *Postn*$^{-/-}$ mice, without producing jaw bone necrosis.

Acknowledgments

We thank Dr. Conway (Program in Developmental Biology and Neonatal Medicine, Wells Center for Pediatric Research, Indiana University School of Medicine, Indianapolis, USA) for providing the periostin deficient mice. We thank Pr Rizzoli for providing assistance in designing these experiments and for his constructive feedback throughout the experience. We thank Ms Madeleine Lachize (1), Juliette Cicchini (1), Anne-Laure Bonnet (2) and Annie Llorens (2) for her technical assistance.

Author Contributions

Conceived and designed the experiments: NB PL SF. Performed the experiments: NB PL. Analyzed the data: NB PL JLS SF. Contributed reagents/materials/analysis tools: NB PL JLS SF. Wrote the paper: NB PL SF.

References

1. Albandar JM, Kingman A (1999) Gingival recession, gingival bleeding, and dental calculus in adults 30 years of age and older in the United States, 1988–1994. J Periodontol 70: 30–43.
2. Lerner UH (2006) Inflammation-induced bone remodeling in periodontal disease and the influence of post-menopausal osteoporosis. J Dent Res 85: 596–607.
3. Koduganti RR, Gorthi C, Reddy PV, Sandeep N (2009) Osteoporosis: 'A risk factor for periodontitis'. J Indian Soc Periodontol 13: 90–96.
4. Wactawski-Wende J (2001) Periodontal diseases and osteoporosis: association and mechanisms. Ann Periodontol 6: 197–208.
5. Tezal M, Wactawski-Wende J, Grossi SG, Dmochowski J, Genco RJ (2005) Periodontal disease and the incidence of tooth loss in postmenopausal women. J Periodontol 76: 1123–1128.
6. Wactawski-Wende J, Grossi SG, Trevisan M, Genco RJ, Tezal M, et al. (1996) The role of osteopenia in oral bone loss and periodontal disease. J Periodontol 67: 1076–1084.
7. Duarte PM, de Assis DR, Casati MZ, Sallum AW, Sallum EA, et al. (2004) Alendronate may protect against increased periodontitis-related bone loss in estrogen-deficient rats. J Periodontol 75: 1196–1202.
8. El-Shinnawi UM, El-Tantawy SI (2003) The effect of alendronate sodium on alveolar bone loss in periodontitis (clinical trial). J Int Acad Periodontol 5: 5–10.
9. Lane N, Armitage GC, Loomer P, Hsieh S, Majumdar S, et al. (2005) Bisphosphonate therapy improves the outcome of conventional periodontal treatment: results of a 12-month, randomized, placebo-controlled study. J Periodontol 76: 1113–1122.
10. Jeffcoat MK, Cizza G, Shih WJ, Genco R, Lombardi A (2007) Efficacy of bisphosphonates for the control of alveolar bone loss in periodontitis. J Int Acad Periodontol 9: 70–76.
11. Rocha ML, Malacara JM, Sánchez-Marin FJ, Vazquez de la Torre CJ, Fajardo ME (2004) Effect of alendronate on periodontal disease in postmenopausal women: a randomized placebo-controlled trial. J Periodontol 75: 1579–1585.
12. Rocha M, Nava LE, Vázquez de la Torre C, Sánchez-Márin F, Garay-Sevilla ME, et al. (2001) Clinical and radiological improvement of periodontal disease in patients with type 2 diabetes mellitus treated with alendronate: a randomized, placebo-controlled trial. J Periodontol 72: 204–209.
13. Leonard EP, Reese WV, Mandel EJ (1979) Comparison of the effects of ethane-1-hydroxy-1,1-diphosphonate and dichloromethylene diphosphonate upon periodontal bone resorption in rice rats (Oryzomys palustris). Arch Oral Biol 24: 707–708.
14. Gotcher JE, Jee WS (1981) The progress of the periodontal syndrome in the rice rat. I. Morphometric and autoradiographic studies. J Periodontal Res 16: 275–291.
15. Shoji K, Horiuchi H, Shinoda H (1995) Inhibitory effects of a bisphosphonate (risedronate) on experimental periodontitis in rats. J Periodontal Res 30: 277–284.
16. Mitsuta T, Horiuchi H, Shinoda H (2002) Effects of topical administration of clodronate on alveolar bone resorption in rats with experimental periodontitis. J Periodontol 73: 479–486.
17. Alencar VB, Bezerra MM, Lima V, Abreu AL, Brito GA, et al. (2002) Disodium chlodronate prevents bone resorption in experimental periodontitis in rats. J Periodontol ;(): 73: 251–256.
18. Tani-Ishii N, Minamida G, Saitoh D, Chieda K, Omuro H, et al. (2003) Inhibitory effects of incadronate on the progression of rat experimental periodontitis by porphyromonas gingivalis infection. J Periodontol 74: 603–609.
19. Weinreb M, Quartuccio H, Seedor JG, Aufdemorte TB, Brunsvold M, et al. (1994) Histomorphometrical analysis of the effects of the bisphosphonate alendronate on bone loss caused by experimental periodontitis in monkeys. J Periodontal Res 29: 35–40.
20. Bilezikian JP (2006) Osteonecrosis of the jaw--do bisphosphonates pose a risk? N Engl J Med 355: 2278–2281.
21. Rizzoli R, Burlet N, Cahall D, Delmas PD, Eriksen EF, et al. (2008) Osteonecrosis of the jaw and bisphosphonate treatment for osteoporosis. Bone 42: 841–847.
22. Khosla S, Burr D, Cauley J, Dempster DW, Ebeling PR, et al. (2007) Bisphosphonate-associated osteonecrosis of the jaw: report of a task force of the American Society for Bone and Mineral Research. J Bone Miner Res 22: 1479–1491.
23. Hoff AO, Toth BB, Altuntag K, Johnson MM, Warnecke CL, et al. (2008) Frequency and risk factors associated with osteonecrosis of the jaw in cancer patients treated with intravenous bisphosphonates. J Bone Miner Res 23: 826–836.
24. Dental management of patients receiving oral bisphosphonate therapy: expert
25. panel recommendations. (2006) J Am Dent Assoc 137: 1144–1150.
26. Dimopoulos MA, Kastritis E, Bamia C, Melakopoulos I, Gika D, et al. (2009) Reduction of osteonecrosis of the jaw (ONJ) after implementation of preventive measures in patients with multiple myeloma treated with zoledronic acid. Ann Oncol 20: 117–120.
27. Ripamonti CI, Maniezzo M, Campa T, Fagnoni E, Brunelli C, et al. (2009) Decreased occurrence of osteonecrosis of the jaw after implementation of dental preventive measures in solid tumour patients with bone metastases treated with bisphosphonates. Ann Oncol 20: 137–145.
28. Aghaloo TL, Kang B, Sung EC, Shoff M, Ronconi M, et al. (2011) Periodontal disease and bisphosphonates induce osteonecrosis of the jaws in the rat. J Bone Miner Res 26: 1871–1882.

29. Aguirre JI, Akhter MP, Kimmel DB, Pingel JE, Williams A, et al. (2012) Oncologic doses of Zoledronic acid induce osteonecrosis of the jaw-like lesions in rice rats (oryzomys palustris) with periodontitis. J Bone Miner Res in press.
30. Lesclous P, Abi Najm S, Carrel JP, Baroukh B, Lombardi T, et al. (2009) Bisphosphonate-associated osteonecrosis of the jaw: a key role of inflammation? Bone 45: 843–852.
31. Reid IR, Cornish J (2011) Epidemiology and pathogenesis of osteonecrosis of the jaw. Nat Rev Rheumatol 8: 90–96.
32. Norris RA, Damon B, Mironov V, Kasyanov V, Ramamurthi A, et al. (2007) Periostin regulates collagen fibrillogenesis and the biomechanical properties of connective tissues. J Cell Biochem 101: 695–711.
33. Rani S, Barbe MF, Barr AE, Litvin J (2009) Periostin-like-factor and Periostin in an animal model of work-related musculoskeletal disorder. Bone 44: 502–512.
34. Rios H, Koushik SV, Wang H, Wang J, Zhou HM, et al. (2005) periostin null mice exhibit dwarfism, incisor enamel defects, and an early-onset periodontal disease-like phenotype. Mol Cell Biol 25: 11131–11144.
35. Bonnet N, Standley KN, Bianchi EN, Stadelmann V, Foti M, et al. (2009) The matricellular protein Periostin is required for Sclerostin inhibition and the anabolic response to mechanical loading and physical activity. J Biol Chem 284: 35939–35950.
36. Van Poznak CH, Von Roenn JH, Temin S (2011) American society of clinical oncology clinical practice guideline update: recommendations on the role of bone-modifying agents in metastatic breast cancer. J Oncol Pract 7: 117–121.
37. Gasser JA, Ingold P, Venturiere A, Shen V, Green JR (2008) Long-term protective effects of zoledronic acid on cancellous and cortical bone in the ovariectomized rat. J Bone Miner Res 23: 544–551.
38. Sheng ZF, Xu K, Ma YL, Liu JH, Dai RC, et al. (2009) Zoledronate reverses mandibular bone loss in osteoprotegerin-deficient mice. Osteoporos Int 20: 151–159.
39. Huja SS, Fernandez SA, Phillips C, Li Y (2009) Zoledronic acid decreases bone formation without causing osteocyte death in mice. Arch Oral Biol 54: 851–856.
40. Iida-Klein A, Lu SS, Yokoyama K, Dempster DW, Nieves JW, et al. (2003) Precision, accuracy, and reproducibility of dual X-ray absorptiometry measurements in mice in vivo. J Clin Densitom 6: 25–33.
41. Bouxsein ML, Pierroz DD, Glatt V, Goddard DS, Cavat F, et al. (2005) beta-Arrestin2 regulates the differential response of cortical and trabecular bone to intermittent PTH in female mice. J Bone Miner Res 20: 635–643.
42. Hildebrand T, Ruegsegger P (1997) A new method for the model-independent assessment of thickness in the three-dimensional images. Journal of Microscopy 185: 67–75.
43. Chappard D, Palle S, Alexandre C, Vico L, Riffat G (1987) Bone embedding in pure methyl methacrylate at low temperature preserves enzyme activities. Acta Histochem 81: 183–190.
44. Parfitt AM, Drezner MK, Glorieux FH, Kanis JA, Malluche H, et al. (1987) Bone histomorphometry: standardization of nomenclature, symbols, and units. Report of the ASBMR Histomorphometry Nomenclature Committee. J Bone Miner Res 2: 595–610.
45. Lasfargues JJ, Saffar JL (1993) Inhibition of prostanoid synthesis depresses alveolar bone resorption but enhances root resorption in the rat. Anat Rec 237: 458–465.
46. McMillan PJ, Dewri RA, Joseph EE, Schultz RL, Deftos LJ (1989) Rapid changes of light microscopic indices of osteoclast-bone relationships correlated with electron microscopy. Calcif Tissue Int 44: 399–405.
47. Turner CH, Burr DB (1993) Basic biomechanical measurements of bone: a tutorial. Bone 14: 595–608.
48. Bonnet N, Conway SJ, Ferrari SL (2012) Regulation of beta catenin signaling and parathyroid hormone anabolic effects in bone by the matricellular protein periostin. Proc Natl Acad Sci U S A 109: 15048–15053.
49. Pihlstrom BL, Michalowicz BS, Johnson NW (2005) Periodontal diseases. Lancet 366: 1809–1820.
50. Allen MR, Kubek DJ, Burr DB, Ruggiero SL, Chu TM (2011) Compromised osseous healing of dental extraction sites in zoledronic acid-treated dogs. Osteoporos Int 22: 693–702.
51. Abtahi J, Agholme F, Sandberg O, Aspenberg P (2012) Bisphosphonate-induced osteonecrosis of the jaw in a rat model arises first after the bone has become exposed. No primary necrosis in unexposed bone. J Oral Pathol Med In press.
52. Sonis ST, Watkins BA, Lyng GD, Lerman MA, Anderson KC (2009) Bony changes in the jaws of rats treated with zoledronic acid and dexamethasone before dental extractions mimic bisphosphonate-related osteonecrosis in cancer patients. Oral Oncol 45: 164–172.
53. Allen MR, Ruggiero SL (2011) Osteonecrosis of the Jaw: Recent Clinical and Preclinical Advances. IBMS BoneKEy 8: 141–153.
54. Ravosa MJ, Ning J, Liu Y, Stack MS (2011) Bisphosphonate effects on the behaviour of oral epithelial cells and oral fibroblasts. Arch Oral Biol 56: 491–498.
55. Scheper MA, Badros A, Chaisuparat R, Cullen KJ, Meiller TF (2009) Effect of zoledronic acid on oral fibroblasts and epithelial cells: a potential mechanism of bisphosphonate-associated osteonecrosis. Br J Haematol 144: 667–676.
56. Cornish J, Bava U, Callon KE, Bai J, Naot D, et al. (2011) Bone-bound bisphosphonate inhibits growth of adjacent non-bone cells. Bone 49: 710–716.
57. Hansen T, Kunkel M, Weber A, James Kirkpatrick C (2006) Osteonecrosis of the jaws in patients treated with bisphosphonates - histomorphologic analysis in comparison with infected osteoradionecrosis. J Oral Pathol Med 35: 155–160.
58. Roelofs AJ, Coxon FP, Ebetino FH, Lundy MW, Henneman ZJ, et al. (2010) Fluorescent risedronate analogues reveal bisphosphonate uptake by bone marrow monocytes and localization around osteocytes in vivo. J Bone Miner Res 25: 606–616.
59. Russell RG, Watts NB, Ebetino FH, Rogers MJ (2008) Mechanisms of action of bisphosphonates: similarities and differences and their potential influence on clinical efficacy. Osteoporos Int 19: 733–759.
60. Yu YY, Lieu S, Hu D, Miclau T, Colnot C (2012) Site Specific Effects of Zoledronic Acid during Tibial and Mandibular Fracture Repair. PLoS One 7: e31771.
61. Mavropoulos A, Rizzoli R, Ammann P (2007) Different responsiveness of alveolar and tibial bone to bone loss stimuli. J Bone Miner Res 22: 403–410.
62. Masarachia P, WeinrebM, Balena R, Rodan GA (1996) Comparison of the distribution of 3Halendronate and 3H-etidronate in rat and mouse bones. Bone 19: 281–290.
63. Cremers S, Papapoulos S (2011) Pharmacology of bisphosphonates. Bone 49: 42–49.
64. Weiss HM, Pfaar U, Schweitzer A, Wiegand H, Skerjanec A, et al. (2008) Biodistribution and plasma protein binding of zoledronic acid. Drug Metab Dispos 36: 2043–2049.
65. Bauss F, Pfister T, Papapoulos S (2008) Ibandronate uptake in the jaw is similar to long bones and vertebrae in the rat. J Bone Miner Metab 26: 406–408.
66. Contié S, Voorzanger-Rousselot N, Litvin J, Bonnet N, Ferrari S, et al. (2010) Development of a New ELISA for Serum Periostin: Evaluation of Growth-Related Changes and Bisphosphonate Treatment in Mice. Calcif Tissue Int 87: 341–350.
67. Merle B, Garnero P (2012) The multiple facets of periostin in bone metabolism. Osteoporos Int In press.
68. Takayama G, Arima K, Kanaji T, Toda S, Tanaka H, et al. (2006) Periostin: a novel component of subepithelial fibrosis of bronchial asthma downstream of IL-4 and IL-13 signals. J Allergy Clin Immunol 118: 98–104.
69. Padial-Molina M, Volk SL, Taut AD, Giannobile WV, Rios HF (2012) Periostin is Down-regulated during Periodontal Inflammation. J Dent Res In press.
70. Rios HF, Ma D, Xie Y, Giannobile WV, Bonewald LF, et al. (2008) Periostin Is Essential for the Integrity and Function of the Periodontal Ligament During Occlusal Loading in Mice. J Periodontol 79: 1480–1490.
71. Ma D, Lu H, Xu L, Xu X, Xiao W (2009) Mechanical loading promotes Lewis lung cancer cell growth through periostin. In Vitro Cell Dev Biol Anim 45: 467–472.
72. Ouyang G, Liu M, Ruan K, Song G, Mao Y, et al. (2009) Upregulated expression of periostin by hypoxia in non-small-cell lung cancer cells promotes cell survival via the Akt/PKB pathway. Cancer Lett 281: 213–219.

5

Differential Roles of MAPK Kinases MKK3 and MKK6 in Osteoclastogenesis and Bone Loss

David L. Boyle[1], Deepa Hammaker[1]*, Meghan Edgar[1], Mario M. Zaiss[2], Stefan Teufel[3], Jean Pierre David[3], Georg Schett[4], Gary S. Firestein[1]

1 Medicine, University of California San Diego, La Jolla, California, United States of America, **2** Global Health Institute, École Polytechnique Fédèrale de Lausanne, Switzerland, **3** Institute of Osteology and Biomechanics, University Medical Center Hamburg-Eppendorf, Hamburg, Germany, **4** Department of Internal Medicine 3, University of Erlangen-Nuremberg, Friedrich Alexander University, Erlangen, Germany

Abstract

Bone mass is maintained by osteoclasts that resorb bone and osteoblasts that promote matrix deposition and mineralization. Bone homeostasis is altered in chronic inflammation as well as in post-menopausal loss of estrogen, which favors osteoclast activity that leads to osteoporosis. The MAPK p38α is a key regulator of bone loss and p38 inhibitors preserve bone mass by inhibiting osteoclastogenesis. p38 function is regulated by two upstream MAPK kinases, namely MKK3 and MKK6. The goal of this study was to assess the effect of MKK3- or MKK6-deficiency on osteoclastogenesis in vitro and on bone loss in ovariectomy-induced osteoporosis in mice. We demonstrated that MKK3 but not MKK6, regulates osteoclast differentiation from bone marrow cells in vitro. Expression of NFATc1, a master transcription factor in osteoclastogenesis, is decreased in cells lacking MKK3 but not MKK6. Expression of osteoclast-specific genes Cathepsin K, osteoclast-associated receptor and MMP9, was inhibited in MKK3−/− cells. The effect of MKK-deficiency on ovariectomy-induced bone loss was then evaluated in female WT, MKK3−/− and MKK6−/− mice by micro-CT analysis. Bone loss was partially inhibited in MKK3−/− as well as MKK6−/− mice, despite normal osteoclastogenesis in MKK6−/− cells. This correlated with the lower osteoclast numbers in the MKK-deficient ovariectomized mice. These studies suggest that MKK3 and MKK6 differentially regulate bone loss due to estrogen withdrawal. MKK3 directly mediates osteoclastogenesis while MKK6 likely contributes to pro-inflammatory cytokine production that promotes osteoclast formation.

Editor: Dominique Heymann, Faculté de médecine de Nantes, France

Funding: Supported by the NIH grants AI-070555 and AI-067752. The funders had no role in study design, data collection and analysis, decision to publish, or preparation of the manuscript.

Competing Interests: The authors have declared that no competing interests exist.

* E-mail: dhammaker@ucsd.edu

Introduction

Homeostatic maintenance of bone mass and strength requires the concerted actions of bone-forming osteoblasts and bone-resorbing osteoclasts [1]. Imbalances in bone remodeling that favor osteoclast differentiation, survival and activation occur in chronic inflammatory diseases such as rheumatoid arthritis (RA) as well as in post-menopausal osteoporosis [2,3]. Pro-inflammatory cytokines such as IL-1, TNF, and IL-6 in chronic inflammation or the loss of estrogen in menopause regulate bone resorption by increasing the expression of Receptor Activator of NF-κB ligand (RANKL) on osteoblasts and stromal cells or by amplifying RANKL-mediated differentiation of monocytes to osteoclasts [4–7]. The interaction of RANKL with its cognate receptor RANK, expressed on osteoclasts, initiates signaling that enhances osteoclast activity, leading to accelerated bone loss and fractures [8].

RANK and RANKL belong to the TNF receptor superfamily [9,10]. The binding of RANKL to RANK recruits the adapter protein TNF receptor associated factor-6 (TRAF6) to the plasma membrane [11]. RANK, RANKL, and TRAF6 are essential for osteoclastogenesis as mice lacking these molecules have profound defects in bone resorption [11]. The RANK/TRAF6 complex activates several pathways including NF-κB and the MAPKs, JNK and p38, which induce the expression of NFATc1, considered one of the master transcription factors of osteoclastogenesis [12,13]. NFATc1, in conjunction with the transcription factors AP-1, PU.1 and micropthalmia transcription factor (MITF), is required for the expression of osteoclast specific genes such as tartrate-resistant acid phosphatase (TRAP) and Cathepsin K that promote bone resorption and demineralization [14,15].

The p38 family of MAPKs, most notably p38α, is an essential regulator of RANKL-mediated osteoclastogenesis, which makes it a potential therapeutic target for osteoporosis [16]. Several studies have shown that p38 inhibitors prevented inflammatory bone destruction in animal models and in some cases, reversed the existing disease [17–19]. MAPK kinases, MKK3 and MKK6, are two upstream enzymes that differentially regulate p38 function [20]. Our previous studies have shown that MKK3 is required for optimal p38α activation while MKK6 regulates pro-inflammatory cytokine production in response to LPS and TNF [21]. In addition, either MKK3- or MKK6-deficiency reduces arthritis severity and joint destruction in passive serum transfer K/BxN arthritis or collagen-induced arthritis [21–23]. The goal of this study was to assess the role of MKK3 and MKK6 in p38-regulated bone resorption. Therefore, we evaluated the effect of MKK3- and MKK6-deficiency on osteoclastogenesis in vitro and on bone

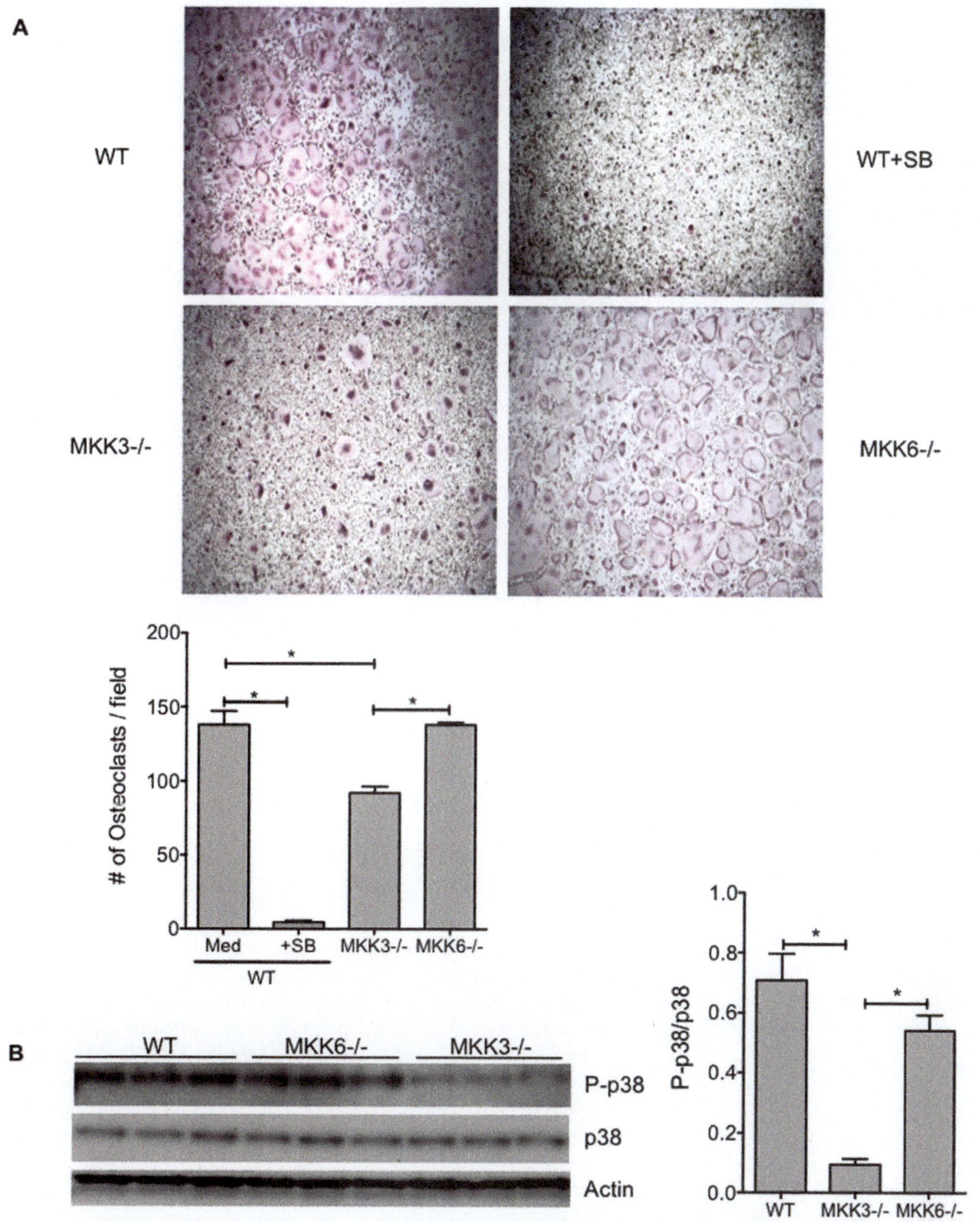

Figure 1. Effect of MKK-deficiency in osteoclastogenesis in vitro. (A) WT, MKK3−/− and MKK6−/− bone marrow cells were cultured to induce osteoclastogenesis and analyzed by TRAP staining (n = 3/group). The number of osteoclasts were counted in 5 pre-defined locations per well and the data are represented as mean ± SEM. Numbers of osteoclasts were reduced in SB-treated WT and MKK3−/− cells compared with WT. Osteoclastogenesis in MKK6−/− group were comparable to WT cells. *p<0.05 (B) Phosphorylation of p38 in MKK-deficient osteoclasts. Western blot analysis showed that P-p38 levels were significantly lower in MKK3−/− but not in MKK6−/− compared with WT group. *p<0.05.

preservation in vivo using an ovariectomy model of osteoporosis. These studies show that blocking either MKK3 or MKK6 has beneficial effects on bone preservation by differentially regulating osteoclastogenesis or function.

Materials and Methods

Mice

Female wildtype (WT) C57Bl/6 mice (6–8 weeks old) were purchased from Charles River Laboratories (Wilmington, MA). Female MKK3−/− and MKK6−/− mice (C57Bl/6 background) were obtained from Dr. Richard Flavell (Yale University, CT).

Ethics Statement

All experimental animal protocols were reviewed and approved by the University of California San Diego Institutional Animal Care and Use Committee. This study was carried out in strict accordance with the recommendations in the Guide for the Care

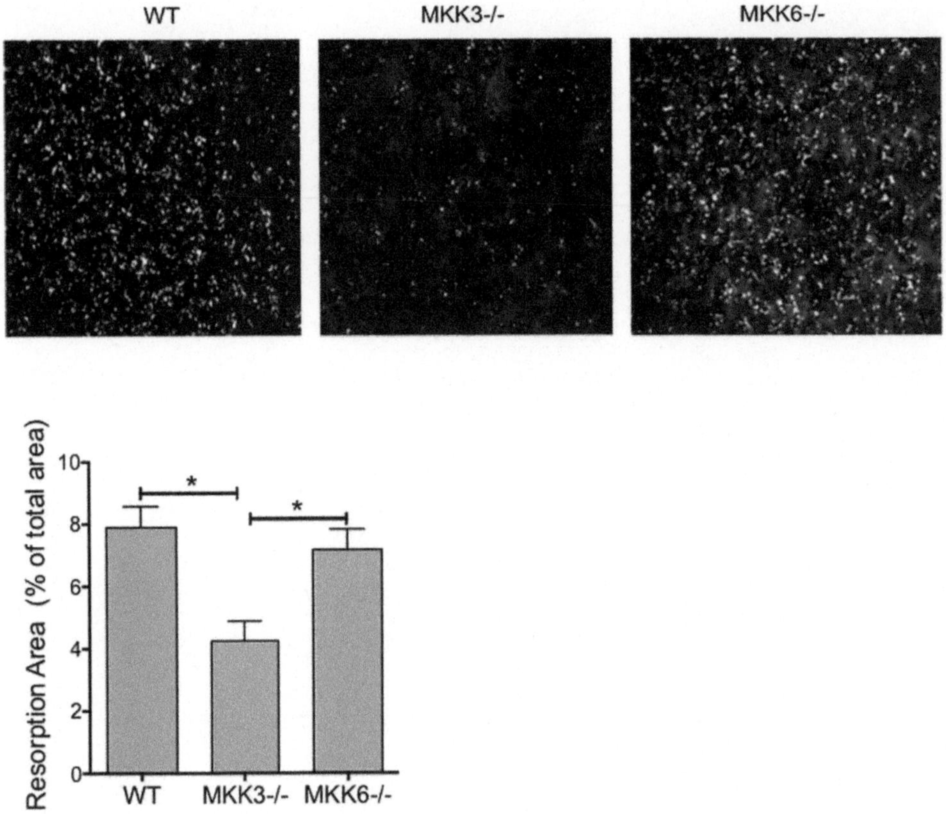

Figure 2. Bone resorption by MKK3- and MKK6-deficient osteoclasts. WT, MKK3−/− and MKK6−/− bone marrow cells were differentiated into osteoclasts on a calcium matrix and subjected to Von Kossa staining to determine resorption activity. The resorption pit area was calculated in eight areas/well and data are shown as percent resorbed area/total area. Resorption activity was significantly reduced in MKK3−/− but not MKK6−/− osteoclasts compared with WT. n = 3/group, *p<0.05.

and Use of Laboratory Animals of the National Institutes of Health. All surgeries were performed under isoflurane vaporizer, and all efforts were made to minimize suffering. Mice were housed using standard housing conditions and allowed access to food and water ad libitum.

Generation of Osteoclasts

Bone marrow was isolated from WT, MKK3−/−, and MKK6−/− femora and tibias. The red blood cells were lysed and the remaining cells were counted and seeded in T75 flasks at 1×10^6 cells/ml. The cells were cultured for 24 h in αMEM (1X) containing GlutaMAX (Invitrogen, Carlsbad, CA) supplemented with 10% FBS, 5% penicillin-streptomycin, and 30 ng/ml of recombinant murine M-CSF (Peprotech, Rocky Hill, NJ). After 24 hours, the non-adherent cells were seeded in 24-well plates (1×10^6 cells/ml) with 30 ng/ml of M-CSF and 50 ng/ml of receptor activator of NF-κB ligand (RANKL) (R&D, Minneapolis, MN). The culture medium was replaced every 72 h and supplemented with M-CSF and RANKL for 5–8 days until multinucleated osteoclasts were observed. In some experiments, cells were cultured for 5 days with 3 μM SB203580 (p38 inhibitor) or DMSO (EMD Chemicals, Gibbstown, NJ).

Osteoclast Differentiation and Activity

Tartrate-resistant acid phosphatase (TRAP) staining: Differentiated cells were stained using the Acid Phosphatase, Leukocyte (TRAP) kit (Sigma-Aldrich, St. Louis, MO). Osteoclasts were defined as multinucleated (≥3 nuclei), TRAP positive cells and were counted in 5 pre-defined locations in each well. The data are represented as average count in each well.

Bone resorption assay: Bone marrow monocytes (BMM) were seeded at 3×10^5 cells/well for 8 days on an Osteologic™ Bone Cell Culture System (BD Biocoat™, Bedford, MA) (4). The cell culture system was then subjected to von Kossa staining. Eight defined areas of each well were imaged and the resorption pits were quantified using Image Pro Plus software (Media Cybernetics, Bethesda, MD). The average resorption was calculated per area for each well and the data are expressed as a percentage of resorbed area/total area.

Ovariectomy

At 16 weeks of age, female WT, MKK3−/−, and MKK6−/− mice were subjected to ovariectomy or sham-surgery and allowed to recover for 6 weeks. To confirm ovariectomy, leutinizing hormone (LH) was measured in serum by sandwich ELISA (Ligand assay and analysis core lab at the University of Virginia).

Micro-Computed Tomography (micro-CT) and Bone Histomorphometry

Micro-CT images of the tibias were acquired as described previously [13]. Briefly, the tibias were harvested, fixed in 10% neutral buffered formalin for 24 h and stored in 70% ethanol. All quantifications were performed with digital image analysis (OsteoMeasure; Osteometrics, Atlanta, GA). The following parameters were measured: fraction of bone volume of the total

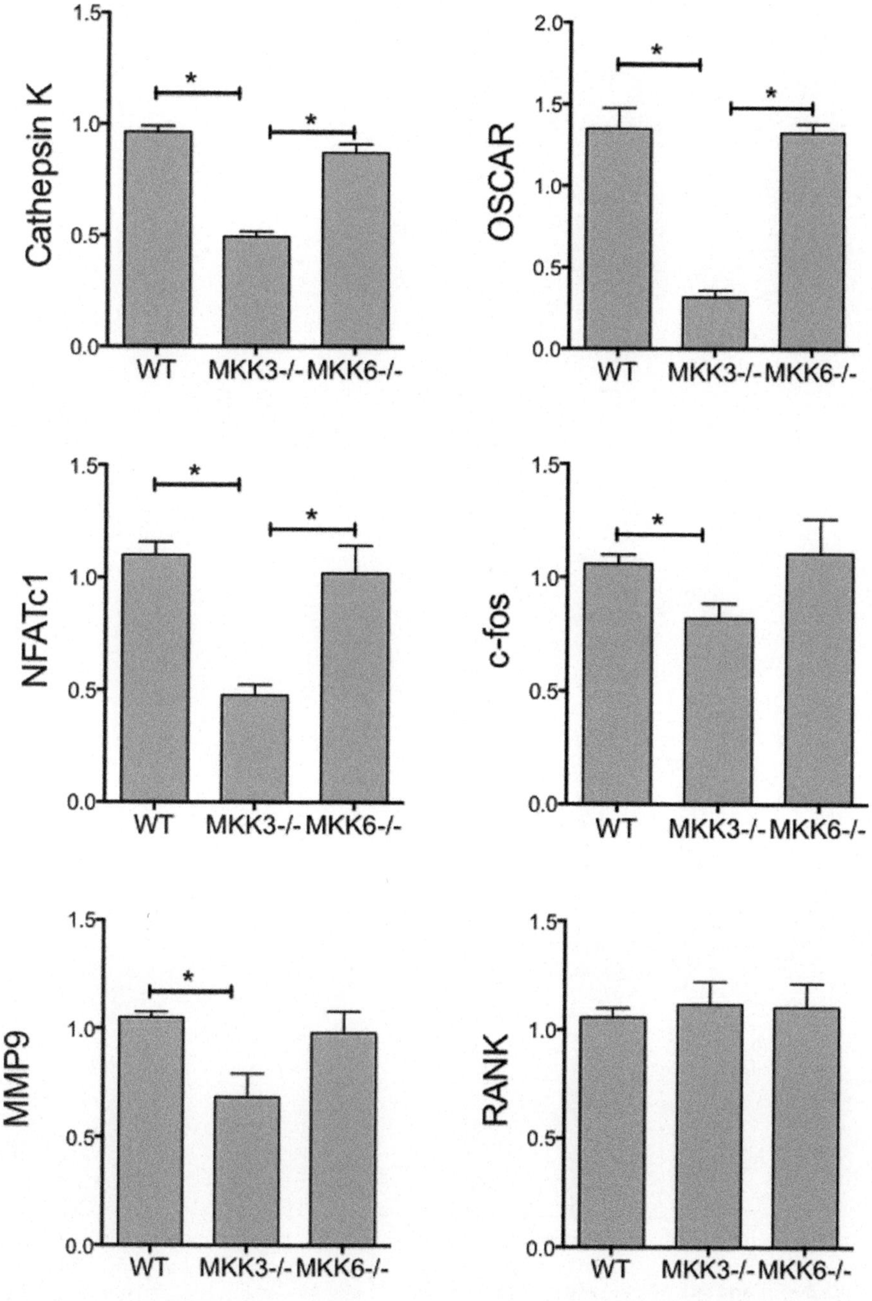

Figure 3. Gene expression in MKK3−/− and MKK6−/− osteoclasts. WT, MKK3−/− and MKK6−/− osteoclast RNA was isolated and subjected to qPCR using gene-specific primer probe sets (n = 3/group). Expression of NFATc1, cFos, Cathepsin K, OSCAR and MMP9 was significantly lower in MKK3−/− but not MKK6−/− cells, compared with WT. RANK expression was comparable in WT, MKK3−/− and MKK6−/− groups. *$p<0.05$.

sample volume (bone volume/tissue volume (BV/TV)), trabecular number (Tb.N), trabecular thickness (Tb.Th), and trabecular separation (Tb.Sp).

Histomorphometric analysis was performed on methacrylate-embedded undecalcified plastic sections of bone and were stained using von Kossa's stain and TRAP stain. To measure bone formation rate (BFR), all mice were injected with calcein green solution (30 mg/kg, Sigma, MO) at 10 days and 2 days prior to harvesting. The tibias were prepared as described above and the measurements were performed using an image analysis system (OsteoMeasure) and the bone formation rate was calculated and the data are shown as $\mu m^3/\mu m^2$/year.

Gene Expression Analysis

Total RNA was isolated from cells and 500 ng RNA was used for first-strand cDNA synthesis (Life Technologies, NY). Quantitative real-time PCR was performed using Taqman gene expression assay primer/probe sets and GeneAmp 7300 system (Applied Biosystems, Foster City, CA) [24]. Ct values were normalized to hypoxanthine-guanine phosphoribosyl transferase 1 (Hprt1) using the ΔΔCt method.

Western Blot Analysis

Osteoclasts were lysed using a lysis buffer containing 50 mM HEPES (pH 7.4), 150 mM NaCl, 25 mM $MgCl_2$, 1 mM EDTA

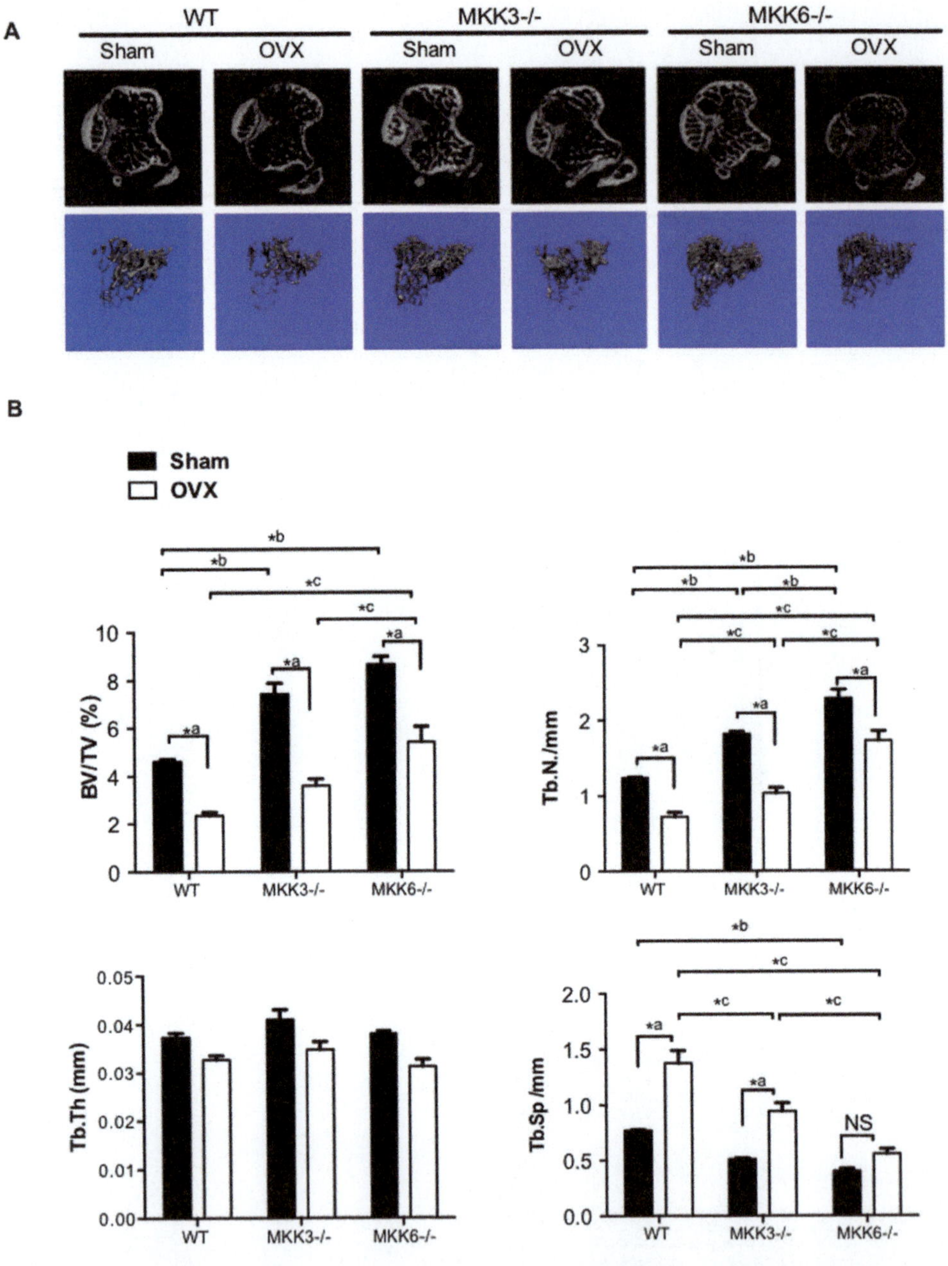

Figure 4. Ovariectomy-induced bone loss in MKK3−/− and MKK6−/− mice. (A) WT, MKK3−/− and MKK6−/− mice were subjected to ovariectomy and bone loss was calculated using micro-CT analysis (n = 5/group). Representative images are shown. Significant bone loss was observed in all three groups. (B) Bone volume and trabecular number were elevated in MKK3−/− and MKK6−/− sham-treated or OVX mice compared with respective WT controls. Trabecular thickness was similar in sham-treated and OVX mice. Trabecular separation was significantly higher in WT and MKK3−/− mice after OVX. MKK3- and MKK6-deficient mice had high bone mass phenotype compared with WT in sham-treated or OVX groups.

(pH8.0), 10% glycerol, 1% Triton X-100, 20 mM ß-glycerophosphate, 10 mM NaF, 1 mM Na_2VO_4, 0.4% cocktail protease inhibitor (Roche, Indianapolis, IN). Protein was quantified using a Micro BCA protein assay kit (Thermo Scientific, Waltham, MA) and separated using a Nupage® Bis-Tris 4–12% polyacrylamide gel (Invitrogen) and transferred onto a PVDF membrane. The membrane was probed with antibodies specific for mouse phospho-p38 (Sigma), total p38 (Cell Signaling Technology, Danvers, MA), and Actin (Sigma, MO). Western blots were developed using the Immun-star™ Western C Kit and images were analyzed using the Versadoc Imaging System and Quantity One software (Bio-Rad Laboratories, Hercules, CA).

Statistical Analysis

Comparisons between WT, MKK3−/−, and MKK6−/− cells were analyzed by one-way ANOVA and Tukey's or Kruskal-Wallis multiple comparison tests, unless otherwise stated. Ovariectomy data were analyzed by two-way ANOVA and Tukey's multiple comparison test. Data were analyzed using GraphPad

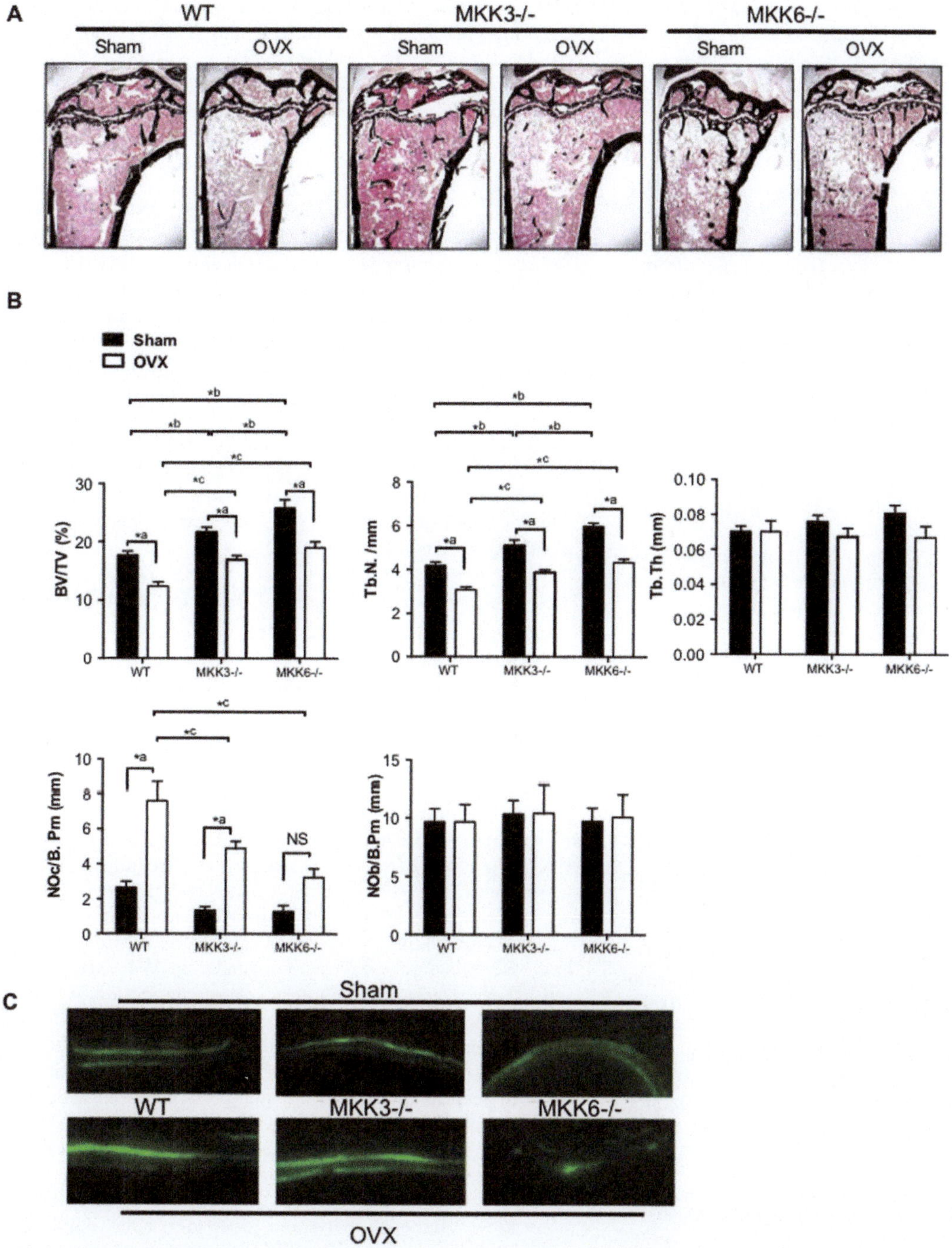

Figure 5. Histomorphometric analysis of bone in ovariectomized MKK3−/− and MKK6−/− mice. (A) Tibial bone sections from sham and OVX-treated mice were stained and representative figures are shown (n = 5/group) (B) Histomorphometric analysis showed that bone volume and trabecular number were elevated in MKK6−/− mice compared with WT after sham surgery or OVX. Trabecular thickness was unaltered after OVX in the three groups. TRAP-staining showed lower osteoclast numbers (NOc/B.Pm) after OVX in MKK3−/− and MKK6−/− compared with WT mice. Osteoblast numbers were unaltered after OVX in the three groups. (C) Bone formation rate was evaluated by injecting mice with calcein green solution at 10 days and 2 days prior to harvesting. The tibias were evaluated for bone formation rate (n = 3/group). Bone formation rate was unaltered by MKK-deficiency in sham- or OVX-treated mice compared with WT controls. *$p<0.05$.

Prism 6.0 and the comparisons were considered statistically significant if $p<0.05$.

Results

Effect of MKK3- and MKK6-deficiency on Osteoclastogenesis in vitro

To evaluate the role of MKK3 and MKK6 in osteoclast differentiation, we cultured WT and MKK3- and MKK6-

deficient bone marrow cells in the presence of M-CSF and RANKL. WT cells were cultured in the presence or absence of the p38 inhibitor SB203580 (SB). Osteoclastogenesis was significantly decreased in MKK3−/− ($p = 0.0012$) and SB-treated WT group ($p<0.0001$) compared with WT control (Figure 1A, n = 3 mice/group). MKK3−/− osteoclast numbers were also significantly lower than MKK6−/− cells ($p = 0.0012$). Surprisingly, osteoclast numbers in MKK6−/− group were comparable to the WT control. We next determined the level of phosphorylation of p38 (P-p38) in cultured WT, MKK3−/− and MKK6−/− osteoclasts by Western blot analysis. MKK3−/− cells had significantly reduced P-p38 levels compared with WT or MKK6−/− (Figure 1B, $p = 0.0009$ and $p = 0.005$, respectively). These data show that MKK3, but not MKK6, is an important regulator of osteoclast differentiation in vitro.

Bone Resorption Activity in MKK3- and MKK6-deficient Osteoclasts

Bone resorption of MKK-deficient osteoclasts was then determined by their ability to demineralize matrix and form resorption pits. Resorption was visualized using Von Kossa staining (Figure 2). MKK3−/− osteoclasts had a significantly lower number of resorptive pits than WT ($p = 0.0061$) or MKK6−/− cells ($p = 0.027$, Kruskal-Wallis test), suggesting that MKK3 is a key regulator of osteoclast differentiation in vitro.

Gene Expression in MKK3−/− and MKK6−/− Osteoclasts

Osteoclast differentiation requires the expression of a number of well-characterized markers such as NFATc1 and Cathepsin K, which regulate osteoclast function. To determine the effect of MKK-deficiency on these markers, we compared gene expression in WT, MKK3−/−, and MKK6−/− osteoclasts by qPCR (Figure 3). Expression of Cathepsin K and osteoclast-associated receptor (OSCAR) was significantly reduced in MKK3−/− osteoclasts compared with WT ($p<0.001$, respectively) or MKK6−/− cells ($p<0.001$, respectively). Similarly, NFATc1 expression was significantly reduced in MKK3−/− cells compared with WT ($p = 0.004$) or MKK6−/− osteoclasts ($p = 0.009$). Expression of c-fos and MMP9 (gelatinase B) was inhibited only in MKK3−/− cells ($p = 0.037$ and $p = 0.031$, respectively, t-test) compared with WT. In contrast, RANK expression was not decreased in MKK-deficient cells. These data show that in vitro expression of osteoclast-specific markers is inhibited in the absence of MKK3.

Ovariectomy-induced Bone Loss in MKK3- and MKK6-deficient Mice

Loss of estrogen in ovariectomized (OVX) mice is associated with increased bone turnover with bone resorption exceeding formation, leading to a net bone loss. Thus far, our data have shown that MKK3-deficiency decreases osteoclastogenesis and bone resorption in vitro, suggesting that a lack of MKK3 might preserve bone in vivo. We therefore examined the effect of MKK-deficiency on bone preservation after ovariectomy. The efficiency of the surgery was confirmed by showing increased levels of luteinizing hormone (LH) in post-surgical sera (Figure S1). Trabecular bone density at the proximal tibia was evaluated in OVX or sham control mice using micro-CT (Figure 4A, n = 5/group).

Micro-CT analysis showed significantly higher bone volume (BV/TV) and trabecular number (Tb.N.) in sham MKK3−/− mice compared with WT sham control (Figure 4B, BV: $p = 0.003$, Tb.N: $p = 0.006$). Surprisingly, sham MKK6−/− mice had a significantly elevated bone volume and Tb.N. compared with sham WT control (BV: $p<0.0001$, Tb.N: $p<0.0001$). Together, these data suggest that both MKK3 and MKK6 play a role in physiological bone homeostasis. While a significant bone loss was observed after OVX in all three genotypes, bone volume and Tb.N were modestly elevated in OVX MKK3−/− and significantly increased in MKK6−/− mice compared to the OVX WT control. These results suggest that MKK6−/− mice were partially protected from OVX-mediated bone loss, maintaining a bone volume similar to sham-treated WT controls. Trabecular thickness was virtually unchanged in OVX or sham control WT and MKK−/− mice. In contrast, trabecular separation (Tb. Sp) was significantly higher after OVX in WT ($p = 0.002$) and MKK3−/− ($p = 0.005$) but not in MKK6−/−, compared with their respective sham controls. Trabecular separation was significantly lower in OVX MKK3−/− ($p = 0.003$) and MKK6−/− ($p<0.0001$) compared with OVX WT mice, indicating a higher bone mass in MKK-deficient mice. Together, the in vivo data demonstrate that MKK3- and MKK6-deficiency are associated with a high bone mass phenotype, which is partially maintained after OVX.

Histomorphometric Analysis of Bone in Ovariectomized MKK3- and MKK6-deficient Mice

To further evaluate the effect of MKK3- and MKK6-deficiency in estrogen-deficient mice, undecalcified tibial bone sections from OVX and sham control mice were stained and subjected to histomorphometric analysis (Figure 5A, B). Consistent with the micro-CT data, bone volume (%BV/TV) was significantly higher in sham- and OVX-treated MKK3−/− ($p<0.05$ for each) and MKK6−/− mice compared to respective WT controls ($p<0.001$, for each). OVX led to a reduction of bone volume in the WT, MKK3−/− and MKK6−/− groups (n = 5/treatment, $p<0.001$, respectively). Nonetheless, bone volume and trabecular number were at least partially maintained in MKK-mutants, indicating a similar bone volume after OVX as sham-treated WT mice. Trabecular thickness (Tb.Th) was similar in WT, MKK3−/−, and MKK6−/− mice, both after sham-treatment and OVX.

TRAP staining showed higher osteoclast numbers (NOc/bone perimeter) in OVX WT mice compared with sham-treated WT mice ($p<0.001$). However, MKK3- and MKK6-deficient mice had significantly lower osteoclast numbers compared with sham-treated or OVX WT mice (MKK3−/−: $p<0.01$, MKK6−/−: $p<0.001$). Interestingly, the number of osteoblasts (NOb) and bone formation rate was not altered in MKK3 and MKK6 mutants. These results suggest that MKK-deficiency inhibits osteoclast formation in vivo but does not alter numbers of osteoblasts or bone formation (Figure 5C). Together, these data show that MKK-deficiency induced high bone mass by lowering osteoclast numbers in vivo.

Discussion

Osteoclast differentiation and activation is regulated by p38 MAPK, at least in part by mediating the effects of pro-inflammatory cytokines [25,26]. Several studies have shown that p38 inhibitors protect against bone resorption in inflammation, possibly through the direct effects on osteoclasts as well as through inhibition of p38-induced cytokine expression. For instance, p38α activation is essential for TNF-mediated inflammatory bone loss, and a selective p38α inhibitor prevented trabecular bone loss and increased cortical bone area in ovariectomized rats [13,27]. Our previous studies demonstrated clinical benefits of MKK3- and

MKK6-deficiency in acute and chronic models of arthritis [21–23]. Inflammation-induced bone loss in the joints was markedly reduced in the absence of MKK3 or MKK6, with a corresponding decrease in serum IL-6 and synovial MMP [22]. In the present study, we extend our observations on bone protection by evaluating the effect of MKK3- and MKK6-deficiency on osteoclastogenesis and bone loss due to estrogen withdrawal in ovariectomized mice.

Our data show that MKK3 and MKK6 differentially regulate osteoclastogenesis. MKK3 is required for optimal osteoclastogenesis and function. MKK6 was unable to effectively compensate for the absence of MKK3 in the osteoclasts. MKK6-deficiency, on the other hand, did not affect osteoclastogenesis in vitro. Consistent with our previous studies, P-p38 levels were markedly reduced in MKK3−/− but normal in MKK6−/− osteoclasts [21]. Osteoclast numbers and resorption activity correlated with p38 activation in MKK3−/− and MKK6−/− cells and are in agreement with previous studies [16]. Expression of NFATc1 and c-fos were reduced in MKK3−/− osteoclasts, indicating that p38 function is necessary for the induction of these transcription factors that are involved in osteoclast differentiation [28]. Cathepsin K, OSCAR, and matrix metalloproteinase 9 (MMP9) expression was reduced in MKK3-deficient osteoclasts. This is consistent with the requirement of NFATc1 in the transcription of these osteoclast-specific markers [15,29,30]. Together, these results indicate that MKK3, rather than MKK6, is a principal regulator of RANKL-induced signaling in osteoclastogenesis in vitro. These data are in accordance with other studies showing that p38 regulates the early phases of osteoclast differentiation [31,32]. However, those studies suggested that MKK6, but not MKK3, is necessary for osteoclastogenesis in vitro, where it enhances cell survival but not bone resorption. The differences might be partly due to differences in the methodology, such as the efficiency of inhibiting MKK3 and MKK6 using viral transduction of dominant-negative MKK3 and MKK6 constructs compared with using bone marrow-derived osteoclasts of MKK3−/− and MKK6−/− mice.

Osteoclastogenesis in vivo is regulated by a number of factors such as vitamin D, parathyroid hormone, prostaglandins and most notably, estrogen [33–36]. Estrogen is a key modulator of both the immune system and bone homeostasis [37]. It regulates bone remodeling by decreasing osteoclast life span by promoting apoptosis [38,39]. Estrogen inhibits expression of RANKL on osteoblasts, stromal cells, and lymphocytes, and increases production of osteoprotegerin (OPG), an inhibitor of RANK signaling [1]. In menopause, the loss of estrogen is associated with elevated levels of IL-1, IL-6, TNF, and M-CSF, which support bone resorption [40,41]. Estrogen deficiency also triggers the differentiation of Th17 cells that produce the pro-inflammatory cytokine IL-17 [42]. IL-17 induces osteoblast and stromal cell production of IL-6, and TNF, which induce RANKL expression, accelerate osteoclastogenesis and lead to osteoporosis [43].

In this study, we showed that both MKK3- and MKK6-deficiency is associated with high bone mass and at least partially inhibited bone loss after ovariectomy, even though our in vitro studies did not show major effects of MKK6 on in vitro osteoclastogenesis. Histomorphometric data demonstrated that high bone mass in MKK3 and MKK6-deficiency correlates with reduced osteoclast numbers. The decrease in osteoclast numbers in MKK6-deficient mice could be due to decreased p38-regulated cytokine production, such as IL-6, since a direct effect on osteoclasts was not observed. The bone protection is consistent with our previous studies showing reduced inflammation and joint destruction in MKK3−/− and MKK6−/− mice, where a direct effect on osteoclasts for MKK3 and an indirect effect by blocking cytokines for MKK6 were found [22].

The study also found no major effect on osteoblast number and bone formation rate in MKK3- and MKK6- deficient mice. The regulation of bone homeostasis and skeletal formation was recently evaluated in MKK3- and MKK6-deficient mice [44]. That study showed that both MKK3−/− and MKK6−/− mice had reduced bone mass resulting from defective osteoblast differentiation. The reason for the discrepancy is unclear but might be partly due to strain variations in mice and the different ages of the mice used, 5 weeks compared with 20 weeks for our study.

In conclusion, MKK3 and MKK6 affect bone mass through regulation of osteoclast numbers in vivo. MKK6 and to a lesser extent MKK3 mitigate bone loss in conjunction with estrogen deficiency. While MKK3 likely mediates direct effects on osteoclasts through RANKL signaling, MKK6 likely contributes to the production of pro-inflammatory cytokines such as IL-6 and IL-17 that increase RANKL expression. Targeting upstream p38 kinases, such as MKK3 and MKK6 might modulate bone loss during inflammation and estrogen deficiency.

Supporting Information

Figure S1 Serum leutinizing hormone (LH) in ovariectomized mice. The efficiency of the ovariectomy was evaluated by measuring LH in sera. LH levels were significantly elevated in ovariectomized WT, MKK3−/−, and MKK6−/− sera compared with sham-treated sera (n = 8/group, *$p<0.05$).

Acknowledgments

The authors thank Dr. Pamela Mellon and Dr. Christine Glidewell-Kenney for advice on ovariectomy surgeries and on the LH confirmations.

Author Contributions

Conceived and designed the experiments: DLB GS GSF. Performed the experiments: ME MMZ ST. Analyzed the data: DLB DH ME JD GS GSF. Contributed reagents/materials/analysis tools: MMZ ST JD GS. Wrote the paper: DH DLB JD GS GSF.

References

1. Khosla S (2001) Minireview: the OPG/RANKL/RANK system. Endocrinology 142: 5050–5055.
2. Kimble RB, Srivastava S, Ross FP, Matayoshi A, Pacifici R (1996) Estrogen deficiency increases the ability of stromal cells to support murine osteoclastogenesis via an interleukin-1and tumor necrosis factor-mediated stimulation of macrophage colony-stimulating factor production. J Biol Chem 271: 28890–28897.
3. Manolagas SC (1995) Role of cytokines in bone resorption. Bone 17: 63S–67S.
4. Wei S, Kitaura H, Zhou P, Ross FP, Teitelbaum SL (2005) IL-1 mediates TNF-induced osteoclastogenesis. J Clin Invest 115: 282–290.
5. Kim JH, Jin HM, Kim K, Song I, Youn BU, et al. (2009) The mechanism of osteoclast differentiation induced by IL-1. J Immunol 183: 1862–1870.
6. Faienza MF, Ventura A, Marzano F, Cavallo L (2013) Postmenopausal osteoporosis: the role of immune system cells. Clin Dev Immunol 2013: 575936.
7. David JP, Schett G (2010) TNF and bone. Curr Dir Autoimmun 11: 135–144.
8. Feng X (2005) RANKing intracellular signaling in osteoclasts. IUBMB Life 57: 389–395.
9. Raggatt LJ, Partridge NC (2010) Cellular and molecular mechanisms of bone remodeling. J Biol Chem 285: 25103–25108.
10. Boyle WJ, Simonet WS, Lacey DL (2003) Osteoclast differentiation and activation. Nature 423: 337–342.
11. Asagiri M, Takayanagi H (2007) The molecular understanding of osteoclast differentiation. Bone 40: 251–264.

12. Strait K, Li Y, Dillehay DL, Weitzmann MN (2008) Suppression of NF-kappaB activation blocks osteoclastic bone resorption during estrogen deficiency. Int J Mol Med 21: 521–525.
13. Zwerina J, Hayer S, Redlich K, Bobacz K, Kollias G, et al. (2006) Activation of p38 MAPK is a key step in tumor necrosis factor-mediated inflammatory bone destruction. Arthritis Rheum 54: 463–472.
14. Sharma SM, Bronisz A, Hu R, Patel K, Mansky KC, et al. (2007) MITF and PU.1 recruit p38 MAPK and NFATc1 to target genes during osteoclast differentiation. J Biol Chem 282: 15921–15929.
15. Troen BR (2006) The regulation of cathepsin K gene expression. Ann N Y Acad Sci 1068: 165–172.
16. Bohm C, Hayer S, Kilian A, Zaiss MM, Finger S, et al. (2009) The alpha-isoform of p38 MAPK specifically regulates arthritic bone loss. J Immunol 183: 5938–5947.
17. Hill RJ, Dabbagh K, Phippard D, Li C, Suttmann RT, et al. (2008) Pamapimod, a novel p38 mitogen-activated protein kinase inhibitor: preclinical analysis of efficacy and selectivity. J Pharmacol Exp Ther 327: 610–619.
18. Caverzasio J, Higgins L, Ammann P (2008) Prevention of trabecular bone loss induced by estrogen deficiency by a selective ααalpha inhibitor. J Bone Miner Res 23: 1389–1397.
19. Medicherla S, Ma JY, Mangadu R, Jiang Y, Zhao JJ, et al. (2006) A selective p38 alpha mitogen-activated protein kinase inhibitor reverses cartilage and bone destruction in mice with collagen-induced arthritis. J Pharmacol Exp Ther 318: 132–141.
20. Inoue T, Hammaker D, Boyle DL, Firestein GS (2005) Regulation of p38 MAPK by MAPK kinases 3 and 6 in fibroblast-like synoviocytes. J Immunol 174: 4301–4306.
21. Yoshizawa T, Hammaker D, Boyle DL, Corr M, Flavell R, et al. (2009) Role of MAPK kinase 6 in arthritis: distinct mechanism of action in inflammation and cytokine expression. J Immunol 183: 1360–1367.
22. Hammaker D, Topolewski K, Edgar M, Yoshizawa T, Fukushima A, et al. (2012) Decreased collagen-induced arthritis severity and adaptive immunity in MKK-6-deficient mice. Arthritis Rheum 64: 678–687.
23. Inoue T, Boyle DL, Corr M, Hammaker D, Davis RJ, et al. (2006) Mitogen-activated protein kinase kinase 3 is a pivotal pathway regulating p38 activation in inflammatory arthritis. Proc Natl Acad Sci U S A 103: 5484–5489.
24. Boyle DL, Rosengren S, Bugbee W, Kavanaugh A, Firestein GS (2003) Quantitative biomarker analysis of synovial gene expression by real-time PCR. Arthritis Res Ther 5: R352–360.
25. Matsumoto M, Sudo T, Saito T, Osada H, Tsujimoto M (2000) Involvement of p38 mitogen-activated protein kinase signaling pathway in osteoclastogenesis mediated by receptor activator of NF-kappa B ligand (RANKL). J Biol Chem 275: 31155–31161.
26. Mbalaviele G, Anderson G, Jones A, De Ciechi P, Settle S, et al. (2006) Inhibition of p38 mitogen-activated protein kinase prevents inflammatory bone destruction. J Pharmacol Exp Ther 317: 1044–1053.
27. Matsumoto M, Sudo T, Maruyama M, Osada H, Tsujimoto M (2000) Activation of p38 mitogen-activated protein kinase is crucial in osteoclastogenesis induced by tumor necrosis factor. Febs Lett 486: 23–28.
28. Huang H, Chang EJ, Ryu J, Lee ZH, Lee Y, et al. (2006) Induction of c-Fos and NFATc1 during RANKL-stimulated osteoclast differentiation is mediated by the p38 signaling pathway. Biochem Biophys Res Commun 351: 99–105.
29. So H, Rho J, Jeong D, Park R, Fisher DE, et al. (2003) Microphthalmia transcription factor and PU.1 synergistically induce the leukocyte receptor osteoclast-associated receptor gene expression. J Biol Chem 278: 24209–24216.
30. Sundaram K, Nishimura R, Senn J, Youssef RF, London SD, et al. (2007) RANK ligand signaling modulates the matrix metalloproteinase-9 gene expression during osteoclast differentiation. Exp Cell Res 313: 168–178.
31. Yamashita T, Kobayashi Y, Mizoguchi T, Yamaki M, Miura T, et al. (2008) MKK6-p38 MAPK signaling pathway enhances survival but not bone-resorbing activity of osteoclasts. Biochem Biophys Res Commun 365: 252–257.
32. Huang H, Ryu J, Ha J, Chang EJ, Kim HJ, et al. (2006) Osteoclast differentiation requires TAK1 and MKK6 for NFATc1 induction and NF-kappaB transactivation by RANKL. Cell Death Differ 13: 1879–1891.
33. Khosla S, Oursler MJ, Monroe DG (2012) Estrogen and the skeleton. Trends Endocrinol Metab 23: 576–581.
34. Armas LA, Recker RR (2012) Pathophysiology of osteoporosis: new mechanistic insights. Endocrinol Metab Clin North Am 41: 475–486.
35. Shibata T, Shira-Ishi A, Sato T, Masaki T, Masuda A, et al. (2002) Vitamin D hormone inhibits osteoclastogenesis in vivo by decreasing the pool of osteoclast precursors in bone marrow. J Bone Miner Res 17: 622–629.
36. Bolon B, Carter C, Daris M, Morony S, Capparelli C, et al. (2001) Adenoviral delivery of osteoprotegerin ameliorates bone resorption in a mouse ovariectomy model of osteoporosis. Mol Ther 3: 197–205.
37. Krum SA, Brown M (2008) Unraveling estrogen action in osteoporosis. Cell Cycle 7: 1348–1352.
38. Krum SA, Miranda-Carboni GA, Hauschka PV, Carroll JS, Lane TF, et al. (2008) Estrogen protects bone by inducing Fas ligand in osteoblasts to regulate osteoclast survival. EMBO J 27: 535–545.
39. Nakamura T, Imai Y, Matsumoto T, Sato S, Takeuchi K, et al. (2007) Estrogen prevents bone loss via estrogen receptor alpha and induction of Fas ligand in osteoclasts. Cell 130: 811–823.
40. Passeri G, Girasole G, Jilka RL, Manolagas SC (1993) Increased interleukin-6 production by murine bone marrow and bone cells after estrogen withdrawal. Endocrinology 133: 822–828.
41. Srivastava S, Weitzmann MN, Kimble RB, Rizzo M, Zahner M, et al. (1998) Estrogen blocks M-CSF gene expression and osteoclast formation by regulating phosphorylation of Egr-1 and its interaction with Sp-1. J Clin Invest 102: 1850–1859.
42. Tyagi AM, Srivastava K, Mansoori MN, Trivedi R, Chattopadhyay N, et al. (2012) Estrogen deficiency induces the differentiation of IL-17 secreting Th17 cells: a new candidate in the pathogenesis of osteoporosis. PLoS One 7: e44552.
43. Tokuda H, Kanno Y, Ishisaki A, Takenaka M, Harada A, et al. (2004) Interleukin (IL)-17 enhances tumor necrosis factor-alpha-stimulated IL-6 synthesis via p38 mitogen-activated protein kinase in osteoblasts. J Cell Biochem 91: 1053–1061.
44. Greenblatt MB, Shim JH, Zou W, Sitara D, Schweitzer M, et al. (2010) The p38 MAPK pathway is essential for skeletogenesis and bone homeostasis in mice. J Clin Invest 120: 2457–2473.

6

The Haploinsufficient Hematopoietic Microenvironment Is Critical to the Pathological Fracture Repair in Murine Models of Neurofibromatosis Type 1

Xiaohua Wu[1,2], Shi Chen[1,2], Yongzheng He[1,2], Steven D. Rhodes[2,3], Khalid S. Mohammad[5], Xiaohong Li[1,2], Xianlin Yang[1,2], Li Jiang[1,2], Grzegorz Nalepa[1,2,4], Paige Snider[1,2], Alexander G. Robling[3], D. Wade Clapp[1,2], Simon J. Conway[1,2,3], Theresa A. Guise[5], Feng-Chun Yang[1,2,3]*

1 Department of Pediatrics, Indiana University School of Medicine, Indianapolis, Indiana, United States of America, 2 Herman B Wells Center for Pediatric Research, Indiana University School of Medicine, Indianapolis, Indiana, United States of America, 3 Anatomy and Cell Biology, Indiana University School of Medicine, Indianapolis, Indiana, United States of America, 4 Pediatric Hematology-Oncology, Indiana University School of Medicine, Indianapolis, Indiana, United States of America, 5 Endocrinology and Metabolism, Department of Internal Medicine, Indiana University School of Medicine, Indianapolis, Indiana, United States of America

Abstract

Germline mutations in the *NF1* tumor suppressor gene cause neurofibromatosis type 1 (NF1), a complex genetic disorder with a high predisposition of numerous skeletal dysplasias including short stature, osteoporosis, kyphoscoliosis, and fracture non-union (pseudoarthrosis). We have developed murine models that phenocopy many of the skeletal dysplasias observed in NF1 patients, including reduced bone mass and fracture non-union. We also show that the development of these skeletal manifestations requires an *Nf1* haploinsufficient background in addition to nullizygous loss of *Nf1* in mesenchymal stem/progenitor cells (MSCs) and/or their progenies. This is replicated in two animal models of NF1, *PeriCre*$^{+}$*;Nf1*$^{flox/-}$ and *Col2.3Cre*$^{+}$*;Nf1*$^{flox/-}$ mice. Adoptive transfer experiments demonstrate a critical role of the *Nf1+/−* marrow microenvironment in the impaired fracture healing in both models and adoptive transfer of WT bone marrow cells improves fracture healing in these mice. To our knowledge, this is the first demonstration of a non-cell autonomous mechanism in non-malignant NF1 manifestations. Collectively, these data provide evidence of a combinatory effect between nullizygous loss of *Nf1* in osteoblast progenitors and haploinsufficiency in hematopoietic cells in the development of non-malignant NF1 manifestations.

Editor: Pranela Rameshwar, University of Medicine and Dentistry of New Jersey, United States of America

Funding: This work was supported in part by the Department of Defense (DOD) grant no. NF043032 to FCY and grant no. NF073112 to FCY; March of Dimes grant no. YF08-246 to FCY; National Institute of Neurological Disorders and Stroke grant no. NS052606 to WC, SJC and FCY; and the Indiana Clinical and Translational Sciences Institute. The funders had no role in study design, data collection and analysis, decision to publish, or preparation of the manuscript.

Competing Interests: The authors have declared that no competing interests exist.

* E-mail: fyang@iupui.edu

Introduction

Bone integrity is maintained by the balance between osteoclasts originated from hematopoietic stem cells and mesenchymal-derived osteoblasts. Osteoclasts are multinucleated cells specialized in bone resorption, whereas osteoblasts are bone forming cells derived from the mesenchymal stem cells. The development of the osteoblast and osteoclast lineages is tightly coupled [1]. Imbalances in coupling of the two lineages leads to defective skeletal development [2] as well as abnormal hematopoiesis [3,4].

Mutations in the *NF1* tumor suppressor gene cause neurofibromatosis type 1 (NF1), a common chronic debilitating disorder that affects 1 in 3,000 individuals [5,6,7,8,9]. Neurofibromin, the protein encoded by *NF1*, functions at least in part as a GTPase activating protein (GAP) for Ras. Loss of heterozygosity of the tumorigenic cell is required for genesis of tumors in individuals with NF1 [10,11]. However, recent studies have also identified a key role of the microenvironment in tumor progression in both plexiform neurofibromas [12] and optic gliomas [13,14] in NF1. Despite advances in understanding the cell-cell interactions in cancers affecting NF1 patients, little information of the molecular and cellular signaling of the microenvironment of the prevalent nonmalignant manifestations of NF1 exists, particularly those impacting the skeletal system that are prevalent in ~50% of NF1 patients [6,7,8,9,15,16,17,18,19,20]. Clinical studies have found that individuals with NF1 are at significant risk for generalized loss of bone mass (osteopenia and osteoporosis) [21,22,23,24,25,26] as well as focal skeletal abnormalities [25,27,28,29]. One focal skeletal abnormality, non-union of spontaneous fractures, also called pseudoarthrosis, is particularly debilitating and frequently affects the distal tibia. Despite a range of orthopedic procedures attempting to facilitate fracture healing, the typical clinical outcome is non-union of the fracture and ultimately amputation of the affected limbs.

Skeletal development and remodeling depends on the balance of interactions between osteoblasts-mesenchymal stem cell derived cells, and osteoclasts-specialized macrophages derived from hematopoietic stem cells that govern skeletal remodeling and bone resorption [30]. We have previously shown that NF1 patients and *Nf1* haploinsufficient mice have elevated osteoclast activity

[31]. However, the increase in lytic activity of osteoclasts alone is not sufficient to explain some of the osseous manifestations observed in the NF1 patients. Kolanczyk and colleagues observed bowing of the tibia and diminished growth in *Nf1*$^{flox/flox}$ mice that express Prx1Cre, which is expressed in undifferentiated mesenchymal cells in the limb bud. While those studies were informative concerning limb manifestations of the disease, the axial skeletal (e.g. kyphosis) are not modeled well due to a lack of expression of PrxCre in the vertebrae [32]. Elefteriou and colleagues utilized a genetic approach to delete *Nf1* in the osteoblast lineage by intercrossing *Nf1*$^{flox/flox}$ mice with *α1(I)* Collagen *Cre* transgenic mice and found that *Nf1* inactivation in osteoblasts affects osteoclast differentiation in addition to bone formation [33,34].

In the present study, we utilized two novel murine models and established that the hematopoietic microenvironment plays a critical role in fracture healing in the NF1 murine models. Our study provides strong evidence of a non-cell autonomous mechanism for the skeletal manifestations of NF1 and demonstrates that the hematopoietic microenvironment is instrumental for bone loss and impaired fracture healing process.

Results

Detection of periostin expression in MSCs, osteoblasts, and generation of *PeriCre*$^{+}$;*Nf1*$^{flox/-}$ mice

Endogenous full-length Periostin is expressed in primitive MSCs and epithelial cells [35,36]. To confirm 3.9 kb Periostin fragment promoter mediated Cre expression in adult MSCs and skeletal tissues, *PeriCre*$^{+}$ mice were intercrossed with transgenic reporter mice that have LacZ sequence knocked into the Rosa26 locus. The skeletal tissues of the intercrossed progeny were then subjected to β-gal staining. LacZ expression was abundant in the peripheral nervous system as expected [37] but was also detected in osteoblasts within the cartilaginous ribs as they begin the process of ossification, the long bone, and vertebrae cartilage of adult *PeriCre*$^{+}$;Rosa26$^{flox/flox}$ mice (data not shown). However, LacZ staining was not observed in *PeriCre*$^{-}$;Rosa26$^{flox/flox}$ littermates (Figure S1A, c, d). The expression of LacZ in bone tissue was confirmed following LacZ staining and hematoxylin/eosin (H&E) counterstaining (Figure S1A). Interestingly, LacZ expression within MSCs and skeletal tissues was detected only in mice 4 weeks of age or older, as *PeriCre* activity is initially restricted to the *in utero* heart valves, fetal and neonatal cardiac fibroblasts [38], and peripheral nervous system (Snider & Conway, unpublished data). Significantly, like the endogenous Periostin protein, *Peri*-Cre reporter expression is robustly localized to both the postnatal and adult outer periosteum, which gives rise to the bone collar covering all skeletal elements, including cancellous bone, and within the inner endosteal osteoblasts that secrete the vascularized bone-specific matrix [39]. LacZ expression was also examined in adult primary calvarial osteoblasts and MSCs *in vitro* following culture in specialized medium that selectively promotes the growth of these lineages. LacZ was strongly expressed in cultured adult calvarial osteoblasts and ~15% of the cultured MSCs were LacZ positive (Figure S1B, a, b).

PeriCre^{+} mice were then intercrossed with mice bearing either systemic or conditional genetic targeting of the *Nf1* allele (*Nf1*+/− and *Nf1*$^{flox/flox}$, respectively) to generate four experimental genotypes: *PeriCre*$^{-}$;*Nf1*$^{flox/flox}$ (control, referred to as WT mice), *PeriCre*$^{-}$;*Nf1*$^{flox/-}$ (referred to as *Nf1*+/−), *PeriCre*$^{+}$;*Nf1*$^{flox/flox}$ mice (*Nf1* null in MSCs and osteoblasts, otherwise systemically WT), and *PeriCre*$^{+}$;*Nf1*$^{flox/-}$ mice (*Nf1* null in MSCs and osteoblasts, otherwise systemically *Nf1* heterozygous). The offspring were genotyped by PCR (Figure S2). The postnatal deletion of neurofibromin protein was confirmed by western blot. A clear gene dose-dependent reduction of neurofibromin was detected in *Nf1*+/− MSCs and osteoblasts as compared to their WT counterparts and no neurofibromin was detected in adult *Nf1*−/− MSCs and osteoblasts (Figure S1C).

PeriCre^{+};*Nf1*$^{flox/-}$ mice have reduced bone mineral density (BMD) and bone volume

To evaluate whether the *PeriCre*$^{+}$;*Nf1*$^{flox/-}$ mouse model recapitulates the bone manifestations of NF1 patients, we measured skeletal mass and density in the four experimental genotypes. *PeriCre*$^{+}$;*Nf1*$^{flox/-}$ mice and *PeriCre*$^{+}$;*Nf1*$^{flox/flox}$ mice were born at the expected Mendelian ratio. Interestingly, syngeneic adult *PeriCre*$^{+}$;*Nf1*$^{flox/-}$ mice were smaller than the other three groups of mice (Figure S3A). Furthermore, *PeriCre*$^{+}$;*Nf1*$^{flox/-}$ mice had reduced body weight and length as compared to WT, *Nf1*+/−, or *PeriCre*$^{+}$;*Nf1*$^{flox/flox}$ mice (Figure S3B, C).

To investigate these skeletal phenotypes in more detail, a series of radiographic analyses were conducted to measure BMD and bone architecture. *PeriCre*$^{+}$;*Nf1*$^{flox/-}$ mice were shown to have reduced whole body BMD as compared to *PeriCre*$^{+}$;*Nf1*$^{flox/flox}$, WT, or *Nf1*+/− mice (Figure 1A) measured by peripheral Dual-Energy X-Ray Absorptiometry (pDEXA). When trabecular bone of 16-week old mice were evaluated using micro-computed tomography (μCT), the bone volume (BV/TV) was similar in WT, *Nf1*+/−, and *PeriCre*$^{+}$*Nf1*$^{flox/flox}$ mice, while *PeriCre*$^{+}$*Nf1*$^{flox/-}$ mice exhibited an ~23% reduction as compared to the other three genotypes (Figure 1B–C).

PeriCre^{+};*Nf1*$^{flox/-}$ mice have increased osteoclasts, reduced osteoblast formation, and altered bone turnover *in vivo*

Biochemical markers of bone turnover are indicative of the overall bone metabolism and provide additional information besides the measurement of BMD [40]. Therefore, we evaluated the osteoclast activity in the trabecular bone of the four genotypes of mice by tartrate-resistant acid phosphatase (TRACP) staining and scoring the TRACP^{+} osteoclasts surface (OcS) in the tibial trabeculae over trabecular bone surface (BS). A significantly greater OcS/BS ratio in the trabecular bone was observed in *Nf1*+/− and *PeriCre*$^{+}$;*Nf1*$^{flox/-}$ mice than WT and *PeriCre*$^{+}$;*Nf1*$^{flox/flox}$ mice as shown qualitatively and quantitatively in Figure 2A and Figure 2B, respectively. Furthermore, *PeriCre*$^{+}$;*Nf1*$^{flox/-}$ mice had significantly higher serum levels of TRACP5b compared to WT mice (1.26 unit±0.06 vs. 1.82unit±0.10, respectively, $p<0.005$) as measured by ELISA, suggesting an increased osteoclast development *in vivo*. In addition, a significantly lower number of osteoblasts was observed in *Nf1*+/−, *PeriCre*$^{+}$;*Nf1*$^{flox/flox}$ and *PeriCre*$^{+}$;*Nf1*$^{flox/-}$ mice compared to WT mice, as evaluated by counting osteoblasts in tibial trabecular bone on MacNeal's stained sections (Figure 2C–D). Interestingly, *PeriCre*$^{+}$;*Nf1*$^{flox/-}$ mice had reduced osteoblast numbers in comparison to *PeriCre*$^{+}$;*Nf1*$^{flox/flox}$ mice given that both genotypes of mice had a similar genetic background in mesenchymal-osteoblast lineage. This suggests an additional effect of the haploinsufficient hematopoietic microenvironment on the skeletal deficits in *PeriCre*$^{+}$;*Nf1*$^{flox/-}$ mice *in vivo*.

Labeling bones with fluorochrome markers provides a means to study the dynamic changes of bone formation [41]. Thus, we examined bone remodeling in the four genotypes of mice using fluorescent labeling. There was a 30% reduction in mineralizing surface (MS/BS), a 20% reduction in mineral apposition rate (MAR), and a 50% reduction in bone formation rate (BFR/BS) in

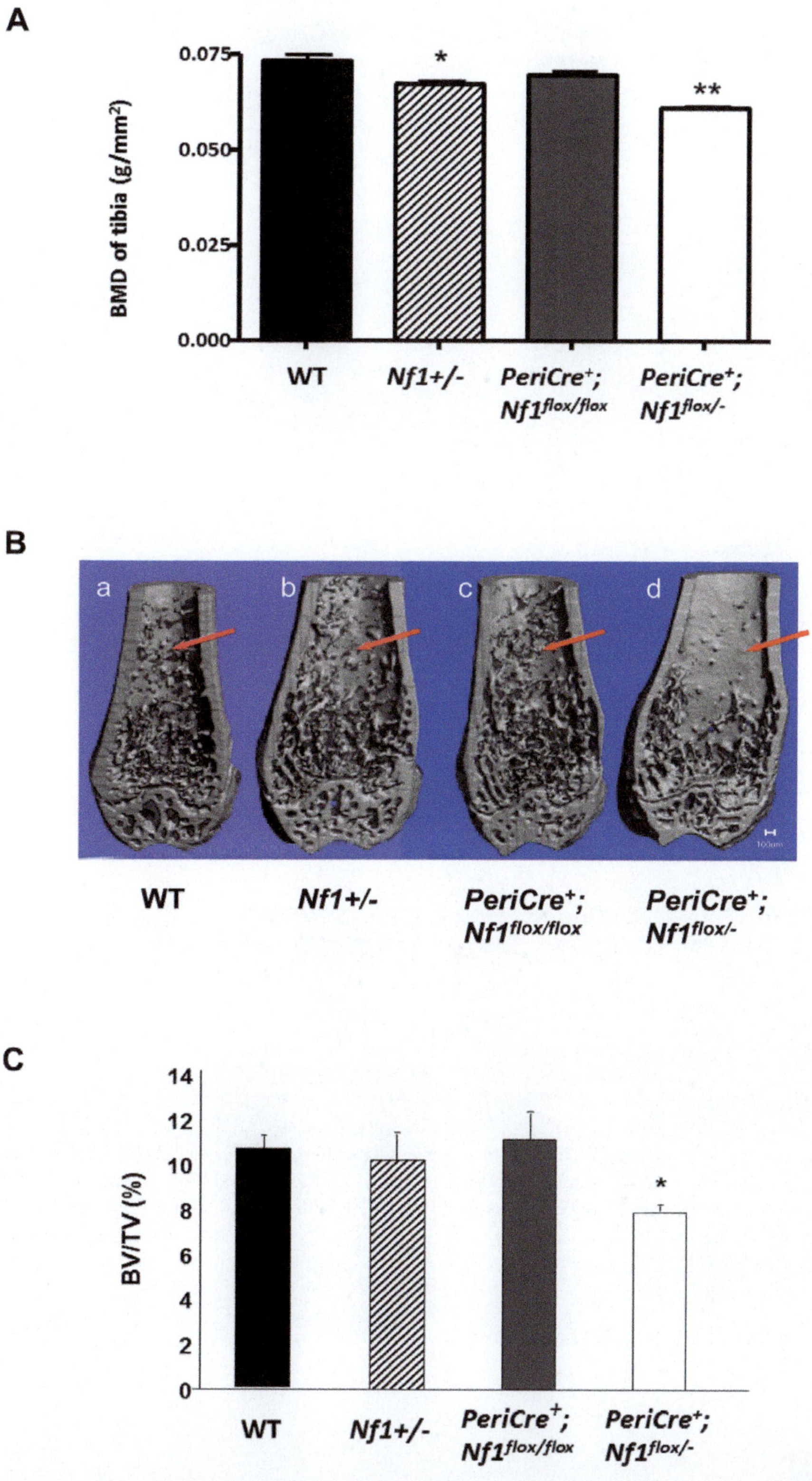

Figure 1. Loss of *Nf1* results in reduced bone mineral density (BMD), volume (BV), and trabecular architecture *in vivo*. (**A**) pDEXA scans on 4–6-month-old mice revealed a 22% reduction of whole body BMD in *PeriCre*$^{+}$;*Nf1*$^{flox/-}$ mice as compared to the other 3 genotypes of mice ($n \geq 9$/group, * and ** $P<0.05$). (**B**) µCT scans through the distal femur of 16-wk old mice revealed a significant reduction of trabecular bone volume in the *PeriCre*$^{+}$;*Nf1*$^{flox/-}$ mice. The anterior portion of each femur had been removed for the metaphyseal architecture analysis. Red arrows indicate the deficiency in the trabecular network in the *PeriCre*$^{+}$;*Nf1*$^{flox/-}$ mice vs. controls. (**C**) Quantitation of the trabecular bone volume reveals an ~22% reduction of bone volume per unit total volume (BV/TV) in the distal femoral metaphysis of *PeriCre*$^{+}$;*Nf1*$^{flox/-}$ mice as compared to the other genotypes ($n = 4$–6/group, * and ** $P<0.05$).

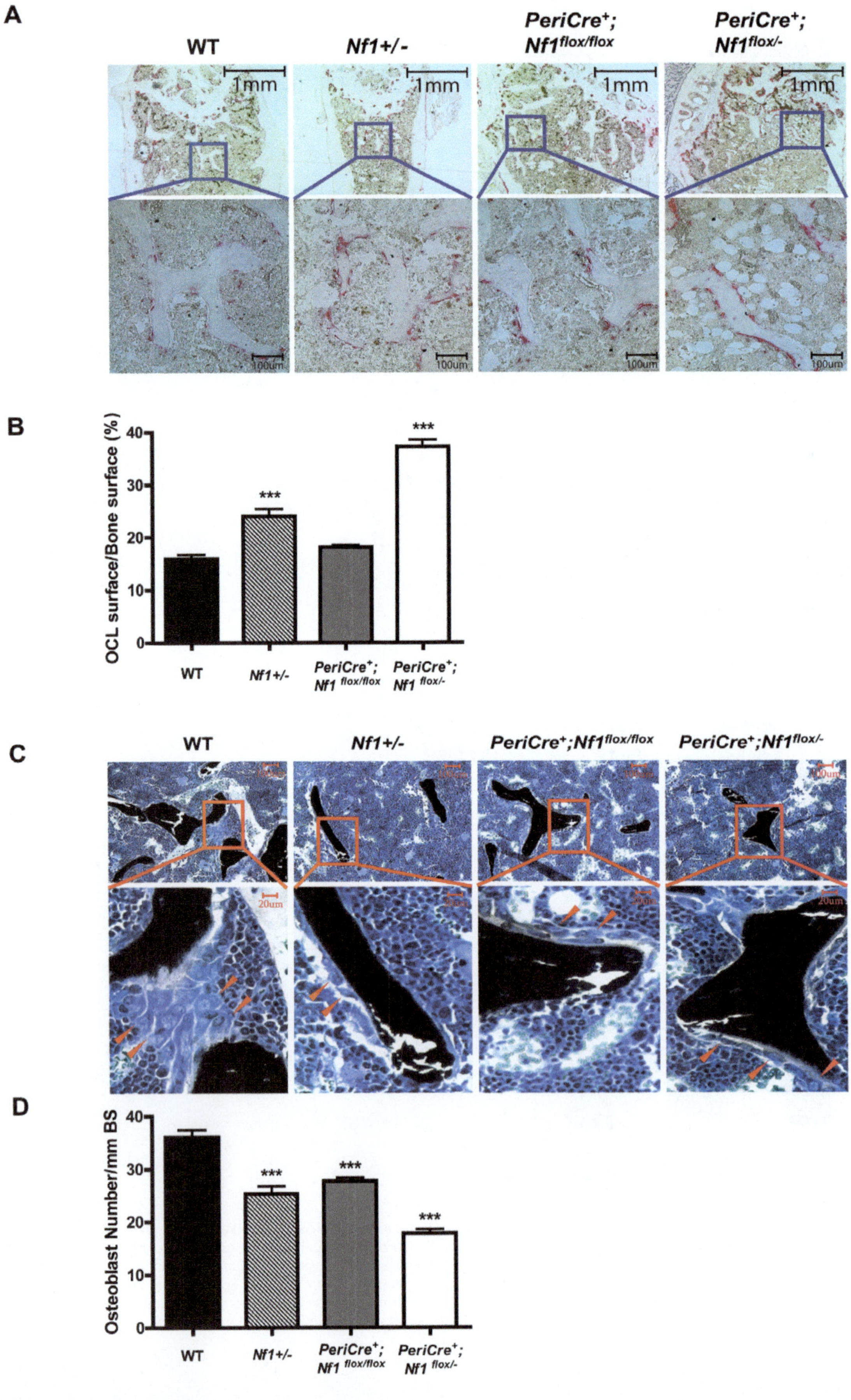
A
WT
Nf1+/-
PeriCre+; Nf1flox/flox
PeriCre+; Nf1flox/-
1mm
100um
B
OCL surface/Bone surface (%)
0
10
20
30
40
***
***
WT
Nf1+/-
PeriCre+; Nf1 flox/flox
PeriCre+; Nf1 flox/-
C
WT
Nf1+/-
PeriCre+;Nf1flox/flox
PeriCre+;Nf1flox/-
20um
D
Osteoblast Number/mm BS
0
10
20
30
40
***
***
***
WT
Nf1+/-
PeriCre+; Nf1 flox/flox
PeriCre+; Nf1 flox/-

Figure 2. *PeriCre$^+$;Nf1$^{flox/-}$* mice have increased osteoclasts and decreased osteoblasts *in vivo*. (**A**) TRACP staining revealed a significant increase of osteoclasts in *PeriCre$^+$;Nf1$^{flox/-}$* mice. Representative photomicrographs shows TRACP+ osteoclasts in tibia of each mouse genotype (Red staining are TRACP positive osteoclasts). (**B**) Quantitative data showing the change of surfaces/BS ratio. ***P<0.001 for *Nf1+/−* and *PeriCre$^+$; Nf1$^{flox/-}$* VS WT controls. (**C**) Representative photomicrograph showing MacNeal staining of the tibia of each mouse genotype (Red arrow heads are pointing to osteoblasts). (**D**) Quantitative data showing the osteoblast number in trabecular bone/ mm BS. ***P<0.001 for . WT control vs *PeriCre$^+$;Nf1$^{flox/-}$*, *Nf1+/−* and *PeriCre$^+$;Nf1$^{flox/flox}$* mice.

PeriCre$^+$;Nf1$^{flox/-}$ mice in comparison to control mice (Figure 3A–D). Together, these data suggest that *PeriCre$^+$;Nf1$^{flox/-}$* mice had a significant reduction in bone turnover in comparison to WT, *Nf1+/−*, or *PeriCre$^+$;Nf1$^{flox/flox}$* mice. The observation that skeletal phenotypes manifest in adult *PeriCre$^+$;Nf1$^{flox/-}$* mice, but not *PeriCre$^+$;Nf1$^{flox/flox}$* or *Nf1+/−* mice, suggests that the development of skeletal defects requires nullizygous loss of *Nf1* in MSCs/ osteoblasts and haploinsufficient loss of *Nf1* in other cell lineages.

PeriCre$^+$;Nf1$^{flox/-}$ mice have delayed fracture healing

Approximately 3% of young children with NF1 acquire pseudoarthrosis [42]. To assess whether the fracture healing process is altered in *PeriCre$^+$;Nf1$^{flox/-}$* mice, we induced three point bending fractures in the control and experimental mice. WT mice healed 28 days after the fracture as evaluated by X-ray (data not shown) and histological analysis following H&E, Masson Trichrome, McNeal staining and TRACP/Von Kossa staining (Figure 4 A, B). In contrast, only 15% of *PeriCre$^+$;Nf1$^{flox/-}$* mice had healed fractures after 28 days. While WT mice had a normal architecture in the fractured tibia, *Nf1+/−* and *PeriCre$^+$;Nf1$^{flox/-}$* tibias showed deficient trabecular and cortical bone formation and increased osteoclasts in the callus site and impairment was most severe in *Peri^{Cre+};Nf1$^{flox/-}$* mice (Figure 4A, B). These data are summarized in Figure 4C. To evaluate whether the fractures in *PeriCre$^+$;Nf1$^{flox/-}$* mice are delayed in healing or non-union, the fracture healing time was extended to 8 weeks after the fractures. As shown in Figure 4C, 33% of the *PeriCre$^+$;Nf1$^{flox/-}$* mice withstood the non-unioned fractures at the end of 8-weeks.

Col2.3Cre$^+$;Nf1$^{flox/-}$ mice have reduced bone mineral density (BMD) and reduced bone volume

Since the expression of periostin Cre is in both MSCs and osteoblasts, we sought to establish whether *Nf1* deficiency, specifically in the osteoblast lineage, would result in similar phenotypic skeletal manifestations. Conditional bi-allelic deletion of *Nf1* in osteoblasts was achieved by genetic intercross of *Nf1$^{flox/flox}$* mice with *Col2.3Cre+* mice, placing the *Cre* gene under the control of the 2.3-kb proximal fragment of the α1(I)-collagen promoter, which is specifically expressed in osteoblasts [33,43]. All genotypes of mice, including WT, *Nf1+/−*, *Col2.3Cre$^+$;Nf1$^{flox/flox}$*, and *Col2.3Cre$^+$;Nf1$^{flox/-}$* mice, were born at the expected Mendelian ratio. Similar to *PeriCre$^+$;Nf1$^{flox/-}$* mice, syngeneic adult *Col2.3-Cre$^+$;Nf1$^{flox/-}$* mice displayed an ~20% reduction in body weight and a 10% reduction in body length as compared to WT, *Nf1+/−*, or *Col2.3Cre$^+$;Nf1$^{flox/flox}$* mice (data not shown). To investigate these skeletal phenotypes in more detail, a series of radiographic analyses were conducted to measure BMD and bone architecture. At 8 weeks of age, *Col2.3Cre$^+$;Nf1$^{flox/-}$* mice had an ~10% reduction in tibial BMD as compared to WT, *Nf1+/−*, or *Col2.3Cre$^+$;Nf1$^{flox/flox}$* mice (Figure 5A) as measured by pDEXA. At 24 weeks of age, *Nf1+/−* tibiae showed a 13% reduction in BMD as compared to WT control mice. Yet, an even greater reduction of 22% in BMD was observed in tibiae of *Col2.3Cre$^+$;Nf1$^{flox/-}$* mice compared to WT mice (Figure 5B). However, no significant reduction of tibial BMD was found in *Col2.3Cre$^+$;Nf1$^{flox/flox}$* mice as compared to WT controls.

To compare the trabecular bone volume and architecture of long bone between the four mouse genotypes, micro-computed tomography (μCT) analysis was performed. *Col2.3Cre$^+$;Nf1$^{flox/-}$* mice exhibited an ~23% reduction in bone volume fraction (BV/TV) as compared to the WT and *Col2.3Cre$^+$; Nf1$^{flox/flox}$* mice (Figure 5C–D). *Nf1+/−* mice exhibited an ~16% reduction in BV/TV as compared to WT and *Col2.3Cre$^+$; Nf1$^{flox/flox}$* mice. This reduced bone volume in *Col2.3Cre$^+$; Nf1$^{flox/-}$* and *Nf1+/−* mice is consistent with the reduction of BMD in these mice.

Col2.3Cre$^+$;Nf1$^{flox/-}$ mice have increased osteoclast formation and reduced osteoblast number *in vivo*

We next identified osteoclasts in the distal femoral metaphysis by TRACP staining and scored the ratio of osteoclast surface over trabecular surface of each femur as a measure of osteoclast activity. Interestingly, a significantly greater CS/BS ratio in the trabecular bone was observed in *Nf1+/−* and *Col2.3Cre$^+$;Nf1$^{flox/-}$* mice as compared to WT and *Col2.3Cre$^+$;Nf1$^{flox/flox}$* mice (Figure 5E–F). The significant difference in CS/BS ratio was even more dramatic in *Col2.3Cre$^+$;Nf1$^{flox/-}$* mice. In addition, a significantly lower osteoblast number per millimeter trabecular bone surface was observed in *Nf1+/−*, *Col2.3Cre$^+$;Nf1$^{flox/flox}$* and *Col2.3Cre$^+$;Nf1$^{flox/-}$* mice as compared to WT mice (Figure 5G–H). Interestingly, *Col2.3Cre$^+$;Nf1$^{flox/-}$* mice had lower osteoblast number than *Col2.3Cre$^+$;Nf1$^{flox/flox}$* mice, even though both genotypes had identical *Nf1* alleles in the osteoblast lineage, suggesting the potential of an additional effect of the haploinsufficient hematopoietic microenvironment on bone formation *in vivo*.

Nf1+/− bone marrow transplantation impairs fracture healing in *Nf1$^{flox/flox}$;PeriCre+* mice

To formally test the hypothesis that the hematopoietic microenvironment has a key role in fracture healing in *PeriCreNf1$^{flox/flox}$* mice, bone marrow mononuclear cells (BMMNCs) from either WT or *Nf1+/−* donor mice, that also express an EGFP transgene, were transplanted into *PeriCre$^+$;Nf1$^{flox/-}$*, *PeriCre;Nf1 $^{flox/flox}$* recipient mice that had been previously treated with ionizing radiation [31]. The hematopoietic reconstitution was verified with flow cytometric analysis demonstrating that the reconstituted mice had >95% EGFP positive donor bone marrow cells and clonogenic myeloid progenitors (Figure S4). To clarify whether the donor mesenchymal stem cells were reconstituted in the recipient bone marrow, we cultured CFU-F using the recipient bone marrow cells. Two weeks later, we scored the CFU-F under the fluorescent microscope. All the CFU-Fs were negative in GFP, suggesting the mesenchymal stem cells were originated from recipients, but not the donor cells. This data indicated that the donor hematopoietic cells are key for the skeletal changes in the recipient mice.

To determine whether the transplantation of *Nf1+/−* bone marrow cells to *PeriCre$^+$;Nf1$^{flox/flox}$* mice alters fracture healing, all the recipient mice underwent 3-point bending fracture and the fracture healing process was investigated. Reconstitution with *Nf1+/−* BMMNCs resulted in a significant reduction in BV/TV as assessed by μCT (Figure 6 B–C). In addition, the fracture healing in *PeriCre;Nf1$^{flox/flox}$* mice transplanted with *Nf1+/−*

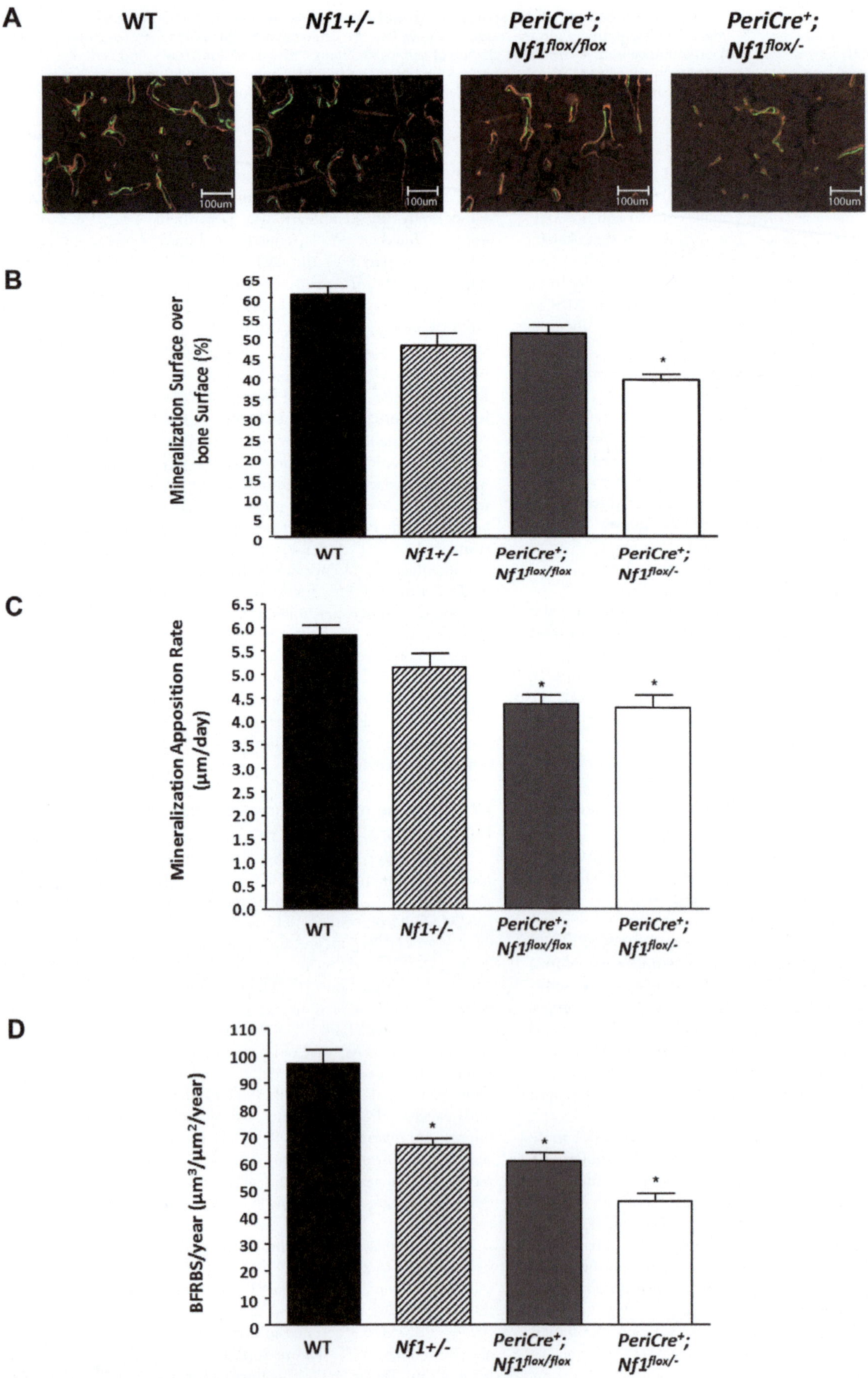
A
WT
Nf1+/-
PeriCre+; Nf1flox/flox
PeriCre+; Nf1flox/-
100um
100um
100um
100um
B
Mineralization Surface over bone Surface (%)
65
60
55
50
45
40
35
30
25
20
15
10
5
0
*
WT
Nf1+/-
PeriCre+; Nf1flox/flox
PeriCre+; Nf1flox/-
C
Mineralization Apposition Rate (µm/day)
6.5
6.0
5.5
5.0
4.5
4.0
3.5
3.0
2.5
2.0
1.5
1.0
0.5
0.0
*
*
WT
Nf1+/-
PeriCre+; Nf1flox/flox
PeriCre+; Nf1flox/-
D
BFRBS/year (µm3/µm2/year)
110
100
90
80
70
60
50
40
30
20
10
0
*
*
*
WT
Nf1+/-
PeriCre+; Nf1flox/flox
PeriCre+; Nf1flox/-

Figure 3. Loss of *Nf1* results in reduced bone turnover *in vivo*. (**A**) Representative photomicrographs showing the uptake of calcein and alizarin fluorochromes into newly mineralizing bone. (**B**) Quantification of the proportion of the total trabecular surface that was actively engaged in bone mineralization (MS/BS). (**C**) The radial rate of bone deposition at active sites (MAR) is shown. (**D**) The total rate of newly forming bone (BFRBS/year) was calculated and shown.

marrow was significantly impaired relative to those receiving WT bone marrow cells. This impaired fracture healing was confirmed by histological analysis (Figure 6D), which revealed that transplantation of *Nf1*+/−, but not WT BMMNCs, led to impaired fracture healing (Figure D). Similar results were obtained in a parallel study using *Nf1*+/− BMMNCs transplanted into *Nf1$^{flox/lfox}$;Col2.3Cre*+ recipients (Figure 6E). Most importantly, transplantation of WT BMMNCs restored the fracture healing of *Nf1$^{flox/l-}$;PeriCre*+ recipients (Figure 6 A–D) and *Nf1$^{flox/-}$;Col2.3Cre*+ recipients (Figure 6E). Collectively, these data indicate that the haploinsufficient bone marrow microenvironment plays an essential role in the skeletal manifestations of NF1, particularly in fracture non-union.

Discussion

Although skeletal manifestations collectively affect up to 50% of NF1 patients [44,45,46,47], the cellular mechanism(s) underlying the development of skeletal defects in NF1 patients are incompletely characterized. Previous attempts using other murine models have identified single lineage and phenotypic alterations that do not fully recapitulate the pathological phenotypes observed in individuals with NF1 [32,33,48,49]. The genetic intercrosses conducted in the present study provide novel murine models (*PeriCre$^+$;Nf1$^{flox/-}$* mice and *Col2.3Cre$^+$;Nf1$^{flox/-}$* mice) that closely recapitulate multiple skeletal phenotypes observed in NF1 patients, particularly the pathological non-union of fractures affecting young children.

In the present study, we generated two novel murine models using Cre-mediated recombination under the direction of either the MSC/osteoblast-selective periostin fragment promoter or the osteoblast-specific Col2.3 Cre promoter. In these mice, one *Nf1* allele was systemically deleted from all tissues (global knockout), while the remaining allele was conditionally deleted in mesenchymal stem/progenitor cells and/or osteoblasts. The two models allow us to compare the impact of the deficiency of *Nf1* at different stages during MSC and osteoblast development of the skeletal deficits. *PeriCre$^+$;Nf1$^{flox/-}$* mice and *Col2.3Cre$^+$;Nf1$^{flox/-}$* mice show increased osteoclast development compared to control mice *in vivo*. In addition, these mice display reduced bone mineral density (BMD) and impaired fracture healing compared to control mice.

Recent studies have begun to elucidate the interactions between haploinsufficient and nullizygous *Nf1* cells within the slow growing tumors found in individuals with NF1. Consistent with *Nf1* being a tumor suppressor gene, Zhu, et al have shown that nullizygosity of *Nf1* in the tumorigenic Schwann cell is required for plexiform neurofibroma progression [15]. However, in this model which results in a small fraction of *Nf1*−/− Schwann cells that likely appear analogous to the human situation, haploinsufficiency in non-tumorigenic lineages is also required [15]. Furthermore, Daginakatte, et al. have shown a similar phenomenon in optic gliomas in the NF1 murine model [13,14]. Recently, we reported that haploinsufficiency of *Nf1* in the hematopoietic microenvironment specifically has a critical role in plexiform neurofibroma formation [12]. Thus, while there is a structural framework that explains the development of slow growing tumors in NF1 patients, no such pathogenic framework to explain the genesis of non-malignant conditions exists. In the present study, we showed that the full development of skeletal manifestations in the NF1 murine model requires both the loss of *Nf1* in osteoblast precursors/osteoblasts and the haploinsufficiency of *Nf1* in the hematopoietic microenvironment. This data is consistent with a single case report by Stevenson and colleagues who found that localized nullizygous loss of NF1 in pseudarthrosis tissue is acquired by micro-dissection and NF1 haploinsufficiency in peripheral blood [29].

Given that our adoptive transfer study indicates that the *Nf1* haploinsufficient bone marrow cells are important for non-union to occur and WT bone marrow cells restores fracture healing, these observations lead to opportunities of clinical and therapeutic significance. Here, we show that *PeriCre$^+$;Nf1$^{flox/-}$* mice transplanted with *Nf1*+/−, but not WT bone marrow, exhibit impaired fracture healing. Most importantly, WT transplantation of bone marrow restored fracture healing of *PeriCre$^+$;Nf1$^{flox/-}$* and *Col2.3Cre$^+$;Nf1$^{flox/-}$* mice. We previously reported a key role for *Nf1* haploinsufficiency in the elevated bone resorptive activity in both murine and human NF1 osteoclasts [31]. This lineage is likely the key effector of the microenvironment. To our knowledge, this study provides the first evidence of a non-cell autonomous mechanism for the pathologic development of non-malignant NF1 pathologic manifestations. As such, these models provide an excellent platform to further study the cellular and molecular mechanism(s) underlying skeletal manifestations in NF1 patients. Future research investigating the specific lineage and molecular targets in the microenvironment that are critical for the non-union fracture healing in NF1 is necessary.

Collectively, these data demonstrate a critical role of the hematopoietic microenvironment in fracture healing in the NF1 population. Our study provides strong evidence of a non-cell autonomous mechanism for the skeletal manifestations of NF1 and demonstrates that the hematopoietic microenvironment is instrumental for bone loss and impaired fracture healing process.

Methods

Ethics statement

Animal care and experiments were conducted according to the guidelines established by the Indiana University Animal Care and Use Committee (IACUC). This study was approved by IACUC via Protocol Number 0000003401 originally approved on 6/19/09.

Animals

Nf1+/− mice were obtained from Dr. Tyler Jacks at the Massachusetts Institute of Technology (Cambridge, MA) [50]. *Nf1$^{flox/flox}$* mice were provided by Dr. Luis Parada at the University of Texas Southwestern Medical Center [15]. *3.9kb$^{peri-EGFP/Cre}$* (*PeriCre*) transgenic mice were generated as described elsewhere [38,51]. To examine the lineage distribution of Cre-Mediated recombination, adult *PeriCre* transgenic mice were crossed with ROSA26 reporter mice. *Col2.3Cre* transgenic mice were generated as described elsewhere [52]. All studies were approved by the Institutional Animal Care and Use Committee.

Histochemical detection of β-gal activity

To examine the Cre recombinase expression pattern in MSC and skeletal tissues, LacZ expression was determined as described previously [52]. Histochemical detection of β-gal activity was

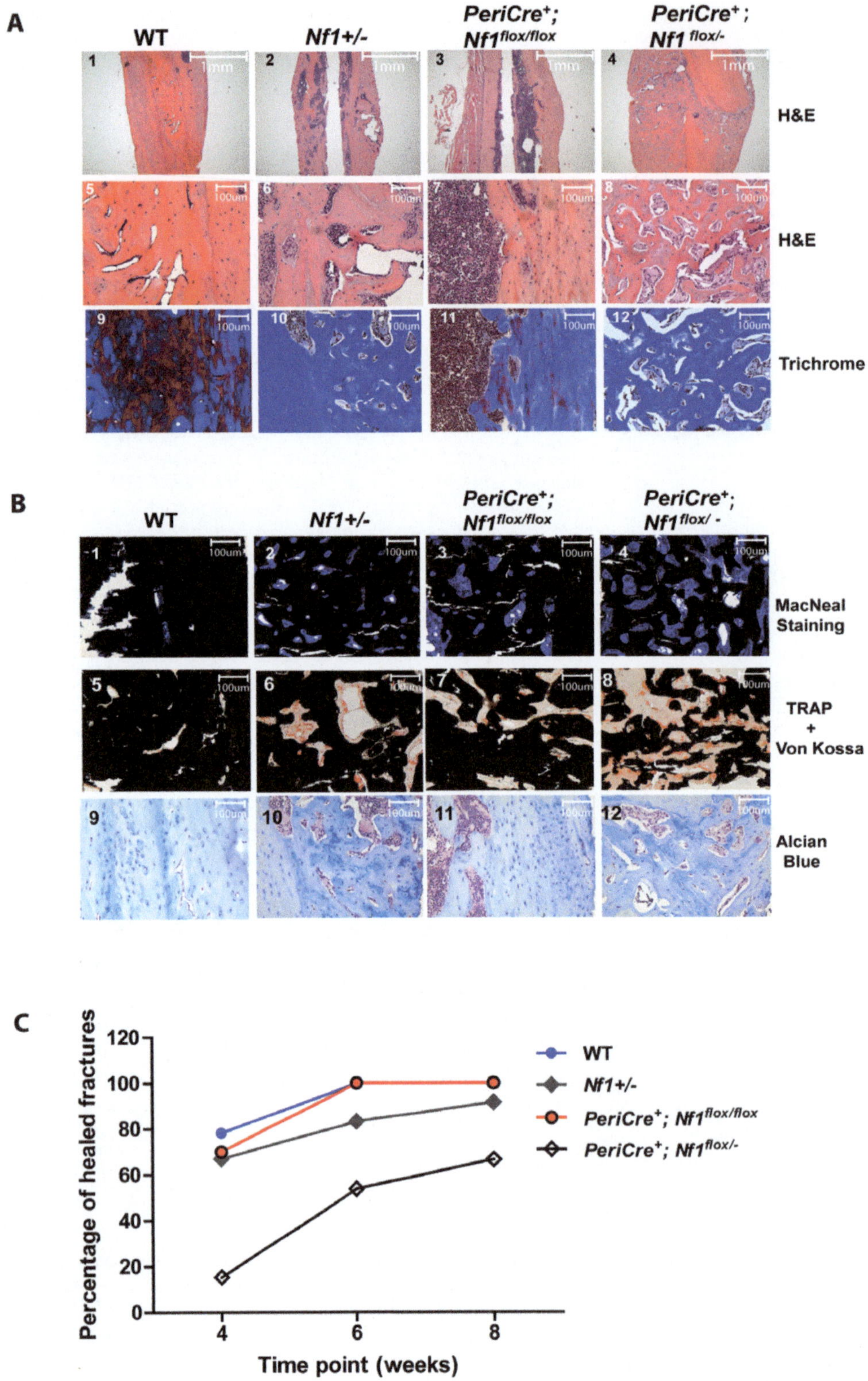

Figure 4. ***PeriCre*$^{+}$*;Nf1*$^{flox/-}$ mice have a delayed fracture healing process.** (**A**) H&E staining (upper and middle panels 1–4, 5–8) and Masson Trichrome staining (lower panels10–12). (**B**) McNeal/von Kossa staining (upper panels1–4), TRACP/Von Kossa (middle panels 5–8), and Alcian blue staining (lower panels 9–12) of the tibia 4 weeks after the fracture. (**C**) Percent of healed fractures at a series of time points.

performed on adult MSCs; cultured osteoblasts; calvaria, femur, and tibiae of *PeriCre*$^{+}$*;Nf1*$^{flox/-}$*;Rosa*$^{flox/flox}$ mice and *PeriCre*$^{-}$*; Nf1*$^{flox/-}$*;Rosa*$^{flox/flox}$ mice. Tissues/cells were fixed for 3 hours in a 0.1 M sodium phosphate buffer (PBS, pH 7.3) containing 0.2% gluteraldehyde, 5 mM EGTA, and 2 mM magnesium chloride. Following 3 wash cycles with a buffer containing 0.1 M PBS,

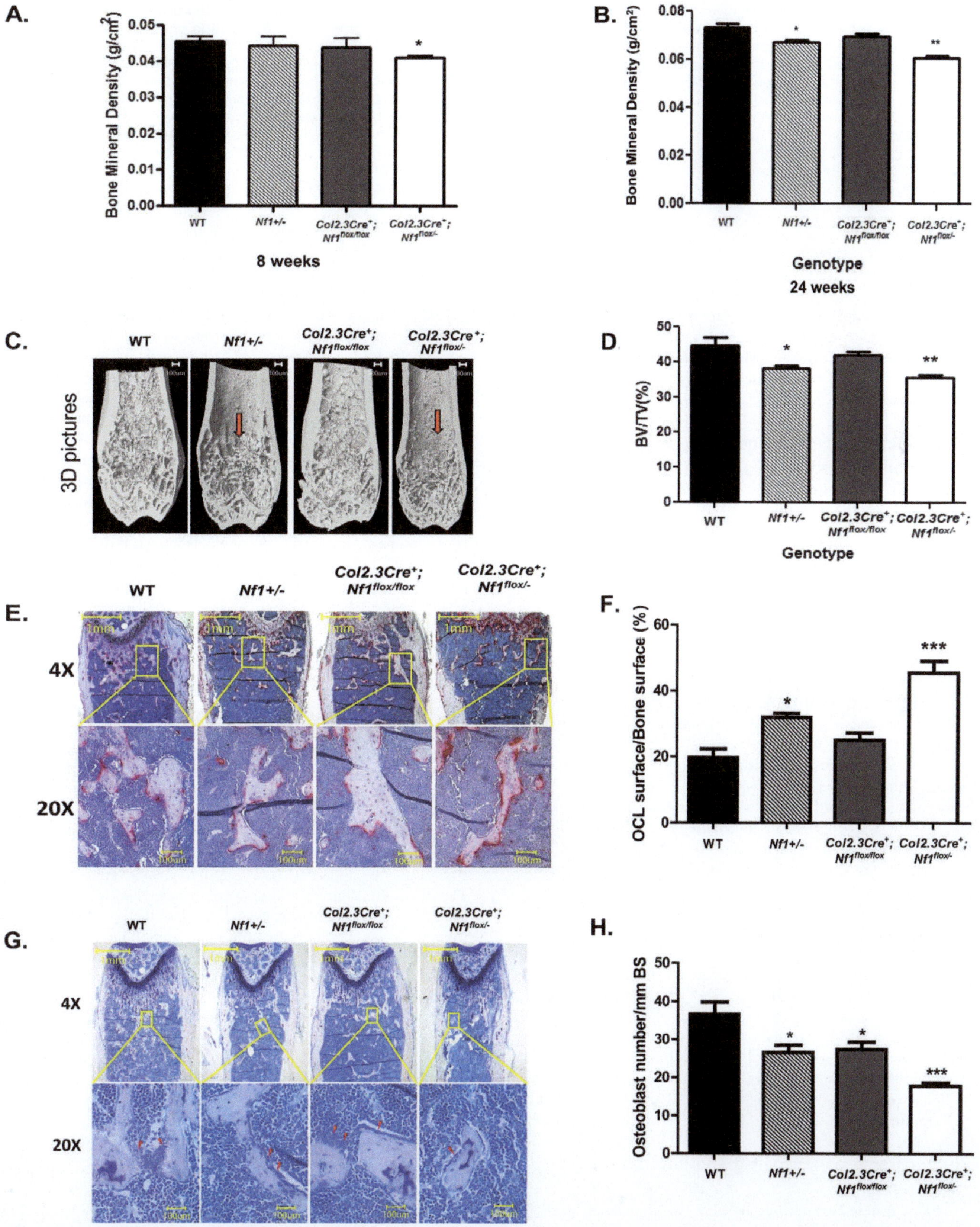

Figure 5. Loss of *Nf1* results in reduced bone mineral density (BMD), volume (BV), and trabecular architecture in *Col2.3Cre⁺;Nf1^flox/−^* mice *in vivo*. BMD was measured with pDEXA scans at 8 weeks (**A**) (*$p<0.05$) and 24 weeks (**B**) (*$p<0.05$, **$p<0.01$). WT (n = 12), *Nf1+/−* (n = 10), *Col2.3Cre⁺;Nf1^flox/flox^* (n = 12), and *Col2.3Cre⁺;Nf1^flox/−^* (n = 11). (**C**) Micro-CT (μCT) scans were performed on the distal femurs of 4 month old WT (n = 5), *Nf1+/−* (n = 5), *Col2.3Cre⁺;Nf1^flox/flox^* (n = 5) and *Col2.3Cre⁺;Nf1^flox/−^* (n = 5) mice. Representative reconstructed 3D pictures are shown. The anterior

portion of each femur has been removed for the metaphyseal architecture analysis. Deficiencies in the trabecular network are indicated by the red arrows. **(D)** Quantitation of 3D reconstruction and BV/TV ratio analysis. Trabecular bone formation is decreased in both *Nf1+/−* (*p<0.05) and *Col2.3Cre⁺;Nf1^flox/−^* (**p<0.01) mice as compared to WT and *Col2.3Cre⁺;Nf1^flox/flox^* mice. Four month old WT (n = 5), *Nf1+/−* (n = 5), *Col2.3Cre⁺;Nf1^flox/flox^* (n = 5), and *Col2.3Cre⁺; Nf1^flox/−^* (n = 5) mouse femur samples were processed for analysis. TRACP staining (**E, F**) and MacNeals' staining (**G, H**) were performed. **(E)** Representative photographs of the trabecular bone following TRACP staining (upper panel 4× and lower panel 20×) are shown. The red stained area indicates osteoclasts. **(F)** Quantitative analysis showing the change of osteoclast surface per bone surface. ***p<0.0001 as analyzed by ANOVA and Bonferroni's Multiple Comparison Test. **(G)** Representative photomicrographs (upper panel 4× and lower panel 20×) are shown. Light pink staining represents bony tissue (trabecular spicules). Blue staining represents the marrow cavity and includes bone marrow cells. Red arrow head are pointing to osteoblasts. **(H)** Quantitative data of osteoblast number over bone surface. One-way ANOVA analysis and Bonferroni's Multiple Comparison Test were used to evaluate statistical significance of the results. ***p<0.0001.

2 mM magnesium chloride, 0.01% deoxycholate, and 0.02% NonidetP40, tissues/cells were incubated for 4 hours at 37°C with β -gal staining solution containing 50 mg β -gal (Sigma Chemical Company, St. Louis, MO, USA), 0.106 g potassium ferrocyanide, and 0.082 g potassium ferricyanide in 50 ml wash buffer. After the staining, tissues/cells were washed 3 times with PBS and placed overnight in 10% formalin. The samples were then decalcified with 14% EDTA and embedded in paraffin. 6 μm thick sections were stained for LacZ with a hematoxylin counterstain.

Longitudinal *in vivo* peripheral dual-energy X-ray absorptiometry (pDEXA)

To evaluate the bone mass in each genotype of mice, bone mineral density (BMD) of the tibial diaphysis was evaluated *in vivo* using pDEXA (PIXImus II; GE-Lunar Corp., Madison, WI) [48]. Adult mice were anesthetized via inhalation of 2.5% isoflurane (IsoFlo; Abbott Laboratories, North Chicago, IL) mixed with O_2 (1.5 liter/min). The mice were placed in a prone position on the specimen tray and scanned. The head was excluded from total body scans. The region of interest included the central 50% of the whole tibia.

Micro (μ) computed tomography

Bone volume and microarchitecture in the distal femoral metaphysis were evaluated using a high-resolution desktop microcomputed tomography imaging system (μCT-20; Scanco Medical AG, Basserdorf, Switzerland). For evaluation of the trabecular envelope at the distal femoral metaphysis, each specimen was scanned with a slice increment of 9 μm. CT images were reconstructed, filtered (σ = 0.8 and support = 1.0), and thresholded (22% of maximum possible gray scale value) as previously described [53]. Scanning for the femur was started at 15% of the total femur length measured from the tip of the femoral condyle and extended proximally for 200 slices. The area for trabecular analysis was outlined within the trabecular compartment, excluding the cortical and subcortical bone. Every 10 sections were outlined manually, and the intermediate sections were interpolated with the contouring algorithm to create a volume of interest. Parameters of microarchitecture for both skeletal sites included bone volume (BV, mm^3) and bone volume fraction (BV/TV, %), as well as trabecular number (Tb.N, mm^{-1}), trabecular thickness (Tb.Th, μm), and trabecular separation (Tb.Sp, μm).

Fluorochrome bone labeling and histomorphometric measurements

Fluorochrome labeling of the bones was performed in 8 week-old mice by intraperitoneal injections of calcein (20 mg/kg, Sigma Chemical, St. Louis, MO, USA) and alizarin (20 mg/kg, Sigma) 8 and 3 days before sacrifice, as previously described [54]. After sacrifice, femurs were fixed in 10% neutral buffered formalin for 48 hours, dehydrated in graded ethanols, and embedded undecalcified in methylmethacrylate. Frontal sections (4 μm thick) were cut from the distal femur using a motorized microtome equipped with a tungsten-carbide knife (Leica Inc, Deerfield Il). The sections were reacted with tartrate-resistant acid phosphatase (TRACP) for identifying and measuring the osteoclast surface or mounted unstained for fluorochrome-derived bone formation parameters. One section per tibia was viewed at 160× magnification on a Leitz DMRXE microscope (Leica Mikroskopie und System GmbH, Wetzlar, Germany) and the image captured using a SPOT digital camera (Diagnostic Instruments, Inc., Sterling Heights, MI). The measurement area for the distal femoral metaphysis was determined by a region beginning 0.5 mm proximal to the midpoint of the growth plate, non-inclusive of cortical bone, and extending proximally for a total area of approximately 2.8 mm^2. Trabecular bone turnover was assessed by measuring the extent of single label (sL.Pm), double label (dL.Pm) and the area of bone (dL.Ar) between the calcein and alizarin labels using Image Pro Plus version 4.1 software (Media Cybernetics, Silver Spring, MD). Derived histomorphometric parameters included mineralizing surface (MS/BS, %), a measure of active bone-forming surface, calculated as follows: the [½ sL.Pm+dL.Pm]/Tt.Pm * 100; mineral apposition rate (MAR, μm/day), a measure of the rate of radial expansion of new bone, calculated as follows: dL.Ar/dL.Pm/4 dy; and bone formation rate, an overall measure of bone formation that combines MS/BS and MAR, calculated as follows: MS/BS * MAR * 3.65.

For histological analysis of cell populations, after sacrifice, tibiae were dissected from the mice and were fixed in 10% neutral buffered formalin for 48 hours, dehydrated in graded ethanols, and embedded undecalcified in methylmethacrylate. Frontal sections (4 μm thick) were cut from the tibiae using a motorized microtome equipped with a tungsten-carbide knife (Leica Inc, Deerfield Il). The sections were reacted with TRACP for identification and measuring of osteoclast surface. MacNeal and /or von Kossa staining were utilized for identifying osteoblasts and calcified bones. The sections were viewed at 200× magnification on a Leitz DMRXE microscope (Leica Mikroskopie und System GmbH, Wetzlar, Germany) and the images were captured using a SPOT digital camera (Diagnostic Instruments, Inc., Sterling Heights, MI). The quantification of osteoblast cell number and osteoclast surface were normalized to the bone surface in millimeters (mm), to control for the total amount of trabecular bone surface within each histological section.

Generation of fracture and X-ray scan

A single tibial fracture was induced as described previously [55,56,57]. With the animal lying supine on the operating table, an intramedullary rod (a 30-G needle) was surgically inserted via the proximal end of the tibiae into the medullary canal of the tibia, so as to stabilize the bone post-fracture and permit load-bearing. A 200-gram weight was dropped from a height of 30-cm to fracture the tibia between the middle to lower 1/3 of the bone. Mice were X-rayed following the fracture to verify standardization of the

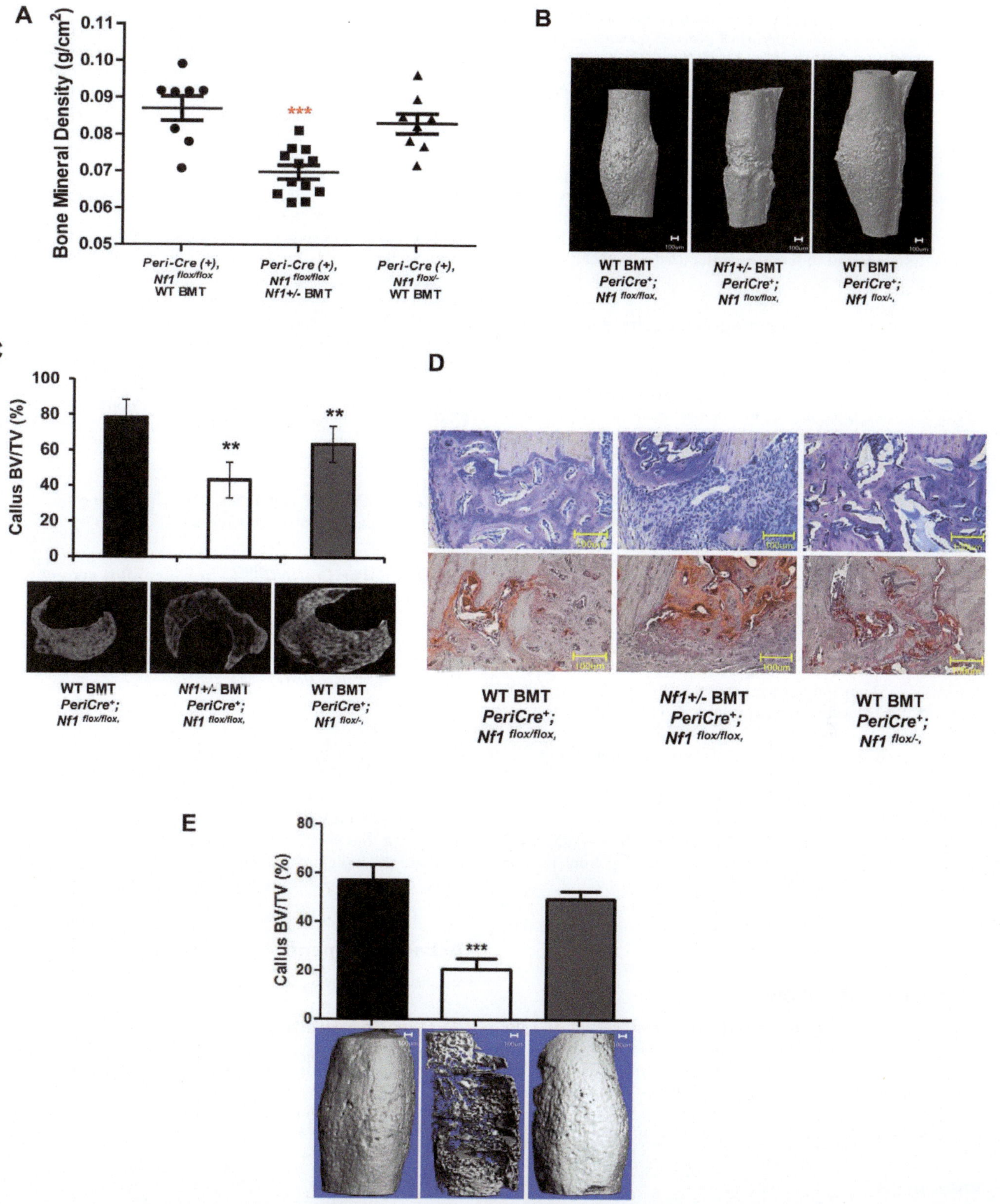

Figure 6. *Nf1+/−* bone marrow is necessary for skeletal deficits in *PeriCre; Nf1$^{flox/flox}$* and *Col2.3Cre; Nf1$^{flox/flox}$* mice. (**A**) Lethally irradiated *PeriCre; Nf1$^{flox/flox}$* and *PeriCre; Nf1$^{flox/-}$* mice were transplanted with *Nf1+/−* or WT bone marrow and monitored until 4 months following the transplantation. Tibia bone mineral density was measured 4 months after bone marrow transplantation (***$p<0.0001$). Mice then underwent tibial fracture four weeks before sacrifice. The genotypes are indicated. (**B**) 3-D reconstruction photographs from μCT scans of the fractured tibias. (**C**)

Representative μCT scan callus sections from fracture sites of *PeriCre; Nf1$^{flox/flox}$* and *PeriCre; Nf1$^{flox/-}$* mice transplanted with WT or *Nf1+/−* bone marrow (lower panel). The upper panel provides quantitative data of the callus BV/TV ratio (**p<0.01). (**D**) Representative photomicrographs of TRACP staining (upper panels 200×) and McNeal's staining (lower panels 200×) from *PeriCre; Nf1$^{flox/flox}$* and *PeriCre; Nf1$^{flox/-}$* tibiae reconstituted with WT or *Nf1+/−* bone marrow. (**E**) Upper panel shows callus BV/TV ratio from *Col2.3Cre*$^{+}$ mice transplanted with WT or *Nf1+/−* bone marrow (***P<0.0001) and lower panel are 3-D reconstruction photographs of μCT scans of the fractured tibias (*Col2.3Cre*$^{+}$ mice transplanted with WT or *Nf1+/−* bone marrow).

fractures. The mice were allowed to recover on a heated pad and then placed in recovery cages. Fracture repair was monitored by weekly radiography (pixRay-100, Bioptics, Phoenix, AZ) and cases where the internal fixation failed, (due to pin slippage, bending or breakage) the affected mouse was euthanized and excluded from subsequent analysis.

MSC and committed osteoprogenitor culture in murine specimens

MSCs were generated from each experimental group of mice as previously described [49]. Briefly, BM mononuclear cells (BMMNCs) were separated by low density gradient centrifugation from 6~8-week old mice. BMMNCs were then resuspended and cultured in mouse MesenCult basal medium containing MesenCult Supplement (Stem Cell Technologies Inc.) at a concentration of 2×10^6 cells/mL in a 10-cm tissue culture plate as previously described. When the cultures reached 80–90% confluency, cells were trypsinized and replated at a concentration of 5×10^5 cells/75 cm^2. MSCs at passage 5 to 10 were used for the following experiments. To culture committed osteoprogenitors, calvaria or femur distal metaphyses were resected and chopped finely with a scalpel. Bone chips were exposed to 0.25% trypsin for 1 hour and then passed through a 70-μm cell strainer (Falcon, Franklin Lakes, NJ, USA) to remove debris and matrix remnants. Cells were cultured in α-MEM medium and supplemented with 10% fetal bovine serum (FBS) and 1% penicillin–streptomycin at 37°C, 5% CO_2.

Bone marrow transplantation of hematopoietic cells

10^6 syngeneic WT or *Nf1+/−* bone marrow cells from WT GFP or *Nf1+/−* GFP mice were transplanted into young adult *PeriCre;Nf1$^{flox/flox}$* recipient mice following 1100 rads of ionizing radiation with two split doses [12]. The C57BL/6-TgN(ACT-bEGFP) 1Osb transgenic mouse line was obtained from Jackson Laboratory, Bar Harbor, Maine [58].

Statistical analysis. One way ANOVA and post *t*-test was used for all the statistical analysis in this study. P values less than 0.05 are considered as statistically significant.

Supporting Information

Figure S1 *PeriCre* is specifically expressed in the skeletal tissues of adult *PeriCre* transgenic mice. (**A**) Four-week old *PeriCre* transgenic (b,d) or control (a, c) mice were dissected and fixed in 4% paraformaldehyde. The whole bodies were washed in β-gal buffer 3×15 minutes at 4°C and then overnight with shaking. After a final wash in β-gal buffer, the whole bodies were stained with β-gal substrate at 37°C for 3 hrs. Periostin-Cre expression is reflected by blue LacZ staining. Representative cross sections from LacZ staining with H&E counterstaining are shown. *PeriCre* expression is reflected by blue staining. (**B**) Osteoblast cell cultures were prepared by digestion of the calvaria and incubated in alpha-MEM medium supplemented with 10%FBS, ascorbic acid, β-galactophospate, and dexathamosone. MSCs were prepared from bone marrow mononuclear cells. The cells were fixed in 4% paraformaldehyde in PBS and washed in β-gal buffer 3×15 minutes at 4°C. Cells were stained in β-gal substrate at 37°C for 3 hours. Blue staining represents LacZ positive osteoblasts or MSCs. (**C**) Neurofibromin expression in WT, *Nf1+/−*, and *Nf1−/−* MSCs and calvarial osteoblasts evaluated by western blot.

Figure S2 PCR of tail DNA. Differential expression of *Nf1*, *PeriCre*, *Loxp*, and recombinant *Cre* was confirmed by PCR.

Figure S3 *PeriCre^{+};Nf1$^{flox/-}$* mice exhibit reduced body size and weight. (**A**) Photographs of representative 4 month old mice from each genotype. (**B**) Body length was measured from the snout to the proximal end of the tail in 4 month old mice of each genotype. The number of animals analyzed were WT, n = 24; *Nf1+/−*, n = 20; *PeriCre^{+};Nf1$^{flox/flox}$*, n = 27; *PeriCre^{+};Nf1$^{flox/-}$*, n = 48. (**C**) Quantitative data of body weight of 4-month old mice of each genotypes.

Figure S4 The donor cells are presented in recipient mice. (**A**) Flow cytometric analysis of peripheral blood shows more than 95% cells are GFP positive. Colonies were observed under light microscope and fluorescent microscope. 100% of colonies are GFP positive. (**B**) Individual colonies were picked up from methylcellulose cultures and were subjected to PCR analysis.

Acknowledgments

We thank Lisa Tully for administrative support.

Author Contributions

Conceived and designed the experiments: XW FCY. Performed the experiments: XW YH SDR XL XY LJ PS. Analyzed the data: SC KSM AGR. Contributed reagents/materials/analysis tools: KSM AGR. Wrote the paper: XW FCY. Analyzed the data and involved in discussion: KSM GN AGR WC SJC TAG.

References

1. Cecchini MG, Hofstetter W, Halasy J, Wetterwald A, Felix R (1997) Role of CSF-1 in bone and bone marrow development. Mol Reprod Dev 46: 75–83; discussion 83–74.
2. Eriksen EF (2010) Cellular mechanisms of bone remodeling. Rev Endocr Metab Disord 11: 219–227.
3. Zhang J, Niu C, Ye L, Huang H, He X, et al. (2003) Identification of the haematopoietic stem cell niche and control of the niche size. Nature 425: 836–841.
4. Scadden DT (2006) The stem-cell niche as an entity of action. Nature 441: 1075–1079.
5. Wallace MR, Marchuk DA, Andersen LB, Letcher R, Odeh HM, et al. (1990) Type 1 neurofibromatosis gene: identification of a large transcript disrupted in three NF1 patients. Science 249: 181–186.
6. Atit RP, Mitchell K, Nguyen L, Warshawsky D, Ratner N (2000) The neurofibromatosis type 1 (Nf1) tumor suppressor is a modifier of carcinogen-induced pigmentation and papilloma formation in C57BL/6 mice. J Invest Dermatol 114: 1093–1100.
7. Atit RP, Crowe MJ, Greenhalgh DG, Wenstrup RJ, Ratner N (1999) The Nf1 tumor suppressor regulates mouse skin wound healing, fibroblast proliferation, and collagen deposited by fibroblasts. J Invest Dermatol 112: 835–842.

8. Bajenaru ML, Hernandez MR, Perry A, Zhu Y, Parada LF, et al. (2003) Optic nerve glioma in mice requires astrocyte Nf1 gene inactivation and Nf1 brain heterozygosity. Cancer Res 63: 8573–8577.
9. Cichowski K, Jacks T (2001) NF1 tumor suppressor gene function: narrowing the GAP. Cell 104: 593–604.
10. Sawada S, Florell S, Purandare SM, Ota M, Stephens K, et al. (1996) Identification of NF1 mutations in both alleles of a dermal neurofibroma. Nat Genet 14: 110–112.
11. Rasmussen SA, Overman J, Thomson SA, Colman SD, Abernathy CR, et al. (2000) Chromosome 17 loss-of-heterozygosity studies in benign and malignant tumors in neurofibromatosis type 1. Genes Chromosomes Cancer 28: 425–431.
12. Yang FC, Ingram DA, Chen S, Zhu Y, Yuan J, et al. (2008) Nf1-dependent tumors require a microenvironment containing Nf1+/− and c-kit-dependent bone marrow. Cell 135: 437–448.
13. Simmons GW, Pong WW, Emnett RJ, White CR, Gianino SM, et al. (2011) Neurofibromatosis-1 heterozygosity increases microglia in a spatially and temporally restricted pattern relevant to mouse optic glioma formation and growth. J Neuropathol Exp Neurol 70: 51–62.
14. Daginakatte GC, Gutmann DH (2007) Neurofibromatosis-1 (Nf1) heterozygous brain microglia elaborate paracrine factors that promote Nf1-deficient astrocyte and glioma growth. Hum Mol Genet 16: 1098–1112.
15. Zhu Y, Ghosh P, Charnay P, Burns DK, Parada LF (2002) Neurofibromas in NF1: Schwann cell origin and role of tumor environment. Science 296: 920–922.
16. Ajuebor MN, Hogaboam CM, Kunkel SL, Proudfoot AE, Wallace JL (2001) The chemokine RANTES is a crucial mediator of the progression from acute to chronic colitis in the rat. J Immunol 166: 552–558.
17. Rutkowski JL, Wu K, Gutmann DH, Boyer PJ, Legius E (2000) Genetic and cellular defects contributing to benign tumor formation in neurofibromatosis type 1. Hum Mol Genet 9: 1059–1066.
18. Ingram DA, Yang FC, Travers JB, Wenning MJ, Hiatt K, et al. (2000) Genetic and biochemical evidence that haploinsufficiency of the Nf1 tumor suppressor gene modulates melanocyte and mast cell fates in vivo. J Exp Med 191: 181–188.
19. Yang FC, Ingram DA, Chen S, Hingtgen CM, Ratner N, et al. (2003) Neurofibromin-deficient Schwann cells secrete a potent migratory stimulus for Nf1+/− mast cells. J Clin Invest 112: 1851–1861.
20. Johannessen CM, Reczek EE, James MF, Brems H, Legius E, et al. (2005) The NF1 tumor suppressor critically regulates TSC2 and mTOR. Proc Natl Acad Sci U S A 102: 8573–8578.
21. Kuorilehto T, Kinnunen P, Nissinen M, Alanne M, Leskela HV, et al. (2006) Vasculopathy in two cases of NF1-related congenital pseudarthrosis. Pathol Res Pract 202: 687–690.
22. Kuorilehto T, Nissinen M, Koivunen J, Benson MD, Peltonen J (2004) NF1 tumor suppressor protein and mRNA in skeletal tissues of developing and adult normal mouse and NF1-deficient embryos. J Bone Miner Res 19: 983–989.
23. Kuorilehto T, Poyhonen M, Bloigu R, Heikkinen J, Vaananen K, et al. (2005) Decreased bone mineral density and content in neurofibromatosis type 1: lowest local values are located in the load-carrying parts of the body. Osteoporos Int 16: 928–936.
24. Lammert M, Kappler M, Mautner VF, Lammert K, Storkel S, et al. (2005) Decreased bone mineral density in patients with neurofibromatosis 1. Osteoporos Int 16: 1161–1166.
25. Jacques C, Dietemann JL (2005) [Imaging features of neurofibromatosis type 1]. J Neuroradiol 32: 180–197.
26. Illes T, Halmai V, de Jonge T, Dubousset J (2001) Decreased bone mineral density in neurofibromatosis-1 patients with spinal deformities. Osteoporos Int 12: 823–827.
27. Heuze Y, Piot B, Mercier J (2002) [Difficult surgical management of facial neurofibromatosis type I or von Recklinghausen disease in children]. Rev Stomatol Chir Maxillofac 103: 105–113.
28. Stevenson DA, Moyer-Mileur LJ, Murray M, Slater H, Sheng X, et al. (2007) Bone mineral density in children and adolescents with neurofibromatosis type 1. J Pediatr 150: 83–88.
29. Stevenson DA, Zhou H, Ashrafi S, Messiaen LM, Carey JC, et al. (2006) Double inactivation of NF1 in tibial pseudarthrosis. Am J Hum Genet 79: 143–148.
30. Cohen MM, Jr. (2006) The new bone biology: pathologic, molecular, and clinical correlates. Am J Med Genet A 140: 2646–2706.
31. Yang FC, Chen S, Robling AG, Yu X, Nebesio TD, et al. (2006) Hyperactivation of p21 and PI3K cooperate to alter murine and human neurofibromatosis type 1-haploinsufficient osteoclast functions. J Clin Invest 116: 2880–2891.
32. Kolanczyk M, Kossler N, Kuhnisch J, Lavitas L, Stricker S, et al. (2007) Multiple roles for neurofibromin in skeletal development and growth. Hum Mol Genet 16: 874–886.
33. Elefteriou F, Benson MD, Sowa H, Starbuck M, Liu X, et al. (2006) ATF4 mediation of NF1 functions in osteoblast reveals a nutritional basis for congenital skeletal dysplasiae. Cell Metab 4: 441–451.
34. Wang W, Nyman J, Moss H, Gutierrez G, Mundy G, et al. (2010) Local low dose lovastatin delivery improves the bone healing defect caused by Nf1 loss-of-function in osteoblasts. J Bone Miner Res.
35. Kruzynska-Frejtag A, Wang J, Maeda M, Rogers R, Krug E, et al. (2004) Periostin is expressed within the developing teeth at the sites of epithelial-mesenchymal interaction. Dev Dyn 229: 857–868.
36. Yan W, Shao R (2006) Transduction of a mesenchyme-specific gene periostin into 293T cells induces cell invasive activity through epithelial-mesenchymal transformation. J Biol Chem 281: 19700–19708.
37. Lindsley A, Snider P, Zhou H, Rogers R, Wang J, et al. (2007) Identification and characterization of a novel Schwann and outflow tract endocardial cushion lineage-restricted periostin enhancer. Dev Biol 307: 340–355.
38. Takeda N, Manabe I, Uchino Y, Eguchi K, Matsumoto S, et al. (2010) Cardiac fibroblasts are essential for the adaptive response of the murine heart to pressure overload. J Clin Invest 120: 254–265.
39. Rios H, Koushik SV, Wang H, Wang J, Zhou HM, et al. (2005) periostin null mice exhibit dwarfism, incisor enamel defects, and an early-onset periodontal disease-like phenotype. Mol Cell Biol 25: 11131–11144.
40. Zhang W, Rhodes SD, Zhao L, He Y, Zhang Y, et al. (2011) Primary osteopathy of vertebrae in a neurofibromatosis type 1 murine model. Bone.
41. Warden SJ, Robling AG, Sanders MS, Bliziotes MM, Turner CH (2005) Inhibition of the serotonin (5-hydroxytryptamine) transporter reduces bone accrual during growth. Endocrinology 146: 685–693.
42. Stevenson DA, Birch PH, Friedman JM, Viskochil DH, Balestrazzi P, et al. (1999) Descriptive analysis of tibial pseudarthrosis in patients with neurofibromatosis 1. Am J Med Genet 84: 413–419.
43. Dacquin R, Starbuck M, Schinke T, Karsenty G (2002) Mouse alpha1(I)-collagen promoter is the best known promoter to drive efficient Cre recombinase expression in osteoblast. Dev Dyn 224: 245–251.
44. Marques P, Poutansant, Carbou (1951) Osseous manifestations of neurofibromatosis (Recklinghausen's disease). J Radiol Electrol Arch Electr Medicale 32: 608–609.
45. Sbihi A, Balafrej A, Iraqui-Hamdouch N, Hamdouch M, Baroudi A (1980) [Osseous manifestations of Recklinghausen's disease. The role of vertebral scalloping]. Maroc Med 2: 393–398.
46. Crawford AH, Jr., Bagamery N (1986) Osseous manifestations of neurofibromatosis in childhood. J Pediatr Orthop 6: 72–88.
47. Crawford AH (1989) Pitfalls of spinal deformities associated with neurofibromatosis in children. Clin Orthop Relat Res. pp 29–42.
48. Yu X, Chen S, Potter OL, Murthy SM, Li J, et al. (2005) Neurofibromin and its inactivation of Ras are prerequisites for osteoblast functioning. Bone.
49. Wu X, Estwick SA, Chen S, Yu M, Ming W, et al. (2006) Neurofibromin plays a critical role in modulating osteoblast differentiation of mesenchymal stem/progenitor cells. Hum Mol Genet 15: 2837–2845.
50. Jacks T, Shih TS, Schmitt EM, Bronson RT, Bernards A, et al. (1994) Tumour predisposition in mice heterozygous for a targeted mutation in Nf1. Nat Genet 7: 353–361.
51. Joseph NM, Mosher JT, Buchstaller J, Snider P, McKeever PE, et al. (2008) The loss of Nf1 transiently promotes self-renewal but not tumorigenesis by neural crest stem cells. Cancer Cell 13: 129–140.
52. Liu F, Woitge HW, Braut A, Kronenberg MS, Lichtler AC, et al. (2004) Expression and activity of osteoblast-targeted Cre recombinase transgenes in murine skeletal tissues. Int J Dev Biol 48: 645–653.
53. Munugalavadla V, Vemula S, Sims EC, Krishnan S, Chen S, et al. (2008) The p85alpha subunit of class IA phosphatidylinositol 3-kinase regulates the expression of multiple genes involved in osteoclast maturation and migration. Mol Cell Biol 28: 7182–7198.
54. O'Brien CA, Plotkin LI, Galli C, Goellner JJ, Gortazar AR, et al. (2008) Control of bone mass and remodeling by PTH receptor signaling in osteocytes. PLoS ONE 3: e2942.
55. Bonnarens F, Einhorn TA (1984) Production of a standard closed fracture in laboratory animal bone. J Orthop Res 2: 97–101.
56. Komatsu DE, Mary MN, Schroeder RJ, Robling AG, Turner CH, et al. Modulation of Wnt signaling influences fracture repair. J Orthop Res 28: 928–936.
57. Warden SJ, Komatsu DE, Rydberg J, Bond JL, Hassett SM (2009) Recombinant human parathyroid hormone (PTH 1–34) and low-intensity pulsed ultrasound have contrasting additive effects during fracture healing. Bone 44: 485–494.
58. Okabe M, Ikawa M, Kominami K, Nakanishi T, Nishimune Y (1997) 'Green mice' as a source of ubiquitous green cells. FEBS Lett 407: 313–319.

Anti-Osteoclastogenic Activity of Praeruptorin A via Inhibition of p38/Akt-c-Fos-NFATc1 Signaling and PLCγ-Independent Ca^{2+} Oscillation

Jeong-Tae Yeon[1]◔, Kwang-Jin Kim[1]◔, Sik-Won Choi[2], Seong-Hee Moon[2,3], Young Sik Park[4,5], Byung Jun Ryu[2], Jaemin Oh[6], Min Seuk Kim[7], Munkhsoyol Erkhembaatar[7], Young-Jin Son[1]*, Seong Hwan Kim[2,5]*

1 Research Institute of Basic Science, Sunchon National University, Suncheon, Republic of Korea, **2** Laboratory of Translational Therapeutics, Pharmacology Research Center, Division of Drug Discovery Research, Korea Research Institute of Chemical Technology, Daejeon, Republic of Korea, **3** Department of Biology, Chungnam National University, Daejeon, Republic of Korea, **4** Herbal Medicine Research Division, National Institute of Food & Drug Safety Evaluation, Cheongwon, Republic of Korea, **5** Graduate School of New Drug Discovery and Development, Chungnam National University, Daejeon, Republic of Korea, **6** Department of Anatomy & Institute for Skeletal Diseases, School of Medicine, Wongkwang University, Iksan, Republic of Korea, **7** Department of Oral Physiology, School of Dentistry, Wongkwang University, Iksan, Republic of Korea

Abstract

Background: A decrease of bone mass is a major risk factor for fracture. Several natural products have traditionally been used as herbal medicines to prevent and/or treat bone disorders including osteoporosis. Praeruptorin A is isolated from the dry root extract of *Peucedanum praeruptorum* Dunn and has several biological activities, but its anti-osteoporotic activity has not been studied yet.

Materials and Methods: The effect of praeruptorin A on the differentiation of bone marrow–derived macrophages into osteoclasts was examined by phenotype assay and confirmed by real-time PCR and immunoblotting. The involvement of NFATc1 in the anti-osteoclastogenic action of praeruptorin A was evaluated by its lentiviral ectopic expression. Intracellular Ca^{2+} levels were also measured.

Results: Praeruptorin A inhibited the RANKL-stimulated osteoclast differentiation accompanied by inhibition of p38 and Akt signaling, which could be the reason for praeruptorin A-downregulated expression levels of c-Fos and NFATc1, transcription factors that regulate osteoclast-specific genes, as well as osteoclast fusion-related molecules. The anti-osteoclastogenic effect of praeruptorin A was rescued by overexpression of NFATc1. Praeruptorin A strongly prevented the RANKL-induced Ca^{2+} oscillation without any changes in the phosphorylation of PLCγ.

Conclusion: Praeruptorin A could exhibit its anti-osteoclastogenic activity by inhibiting p38/Akt-c-Fos-NFATc1 signaling and PLCγ-independent Ca^{2+} oscillation.

Editor: Yin Tintut, University of California, Los Angeles, United States of America

Funding: This work was supported by the Korea Research Institute of Chemical Technology project's grant (SI-1304) and the Inter-ER Cooperation Projects (R0002019) of Korea Institute for Advancement of Technology, which were funded by the Korea Ministry of Knowledge Economy. MSK was supported by the Basic Science Research Program through the National Research Foundation of Korea (NRF-2012R1A1A1038381), funded by the Ministry of Education, Science and Technology (MEST). The funders had no role in study design, data collection and analysis, decision to publish, or preparation of the manuscript.

Competing Interests: The authors have declared that no competing interests exist.

* E-mail: sony@sunchon.ac.kr (YJS); hwan@krict.re.kr (SHK)

◔ These authors contributed equally to this work.

Introduction

Bone fracture is a public health problem because it occurs easily in patients with bone-related disorders including osteoporosis. As the elderly population is rapidly increasing, the medical costs of hospitalization caused by fractures have been become a serious social issue [1,2].

Bone homeostasis depends on the balance between osteoblastic bone formation and osteoclastic bone resorption, but an imbalance caused by an increased number of osteoclasts or overactivation can lead to impaired bone structure and low bone mass, which are common characteristics in patients with bone disorders [3,4]. Therefore, a method to pharmaceutically inhibit osteoclast differentiation is one of the therapeutic strategies for preventing and/or treating bone disorders and related fractures [5].

Clinically, osteoclast-targeting bisphosphonates have been widely used to treat patients with osteoporosis and/or prevent osteoporotic fracture. The orally available bisphosphonates principally inhibit the activation of osteoclasts by binding to hydroxyapatite [6], but recently bisphosphonate-related side effects including acute phase response, hypocalcaemia, secondary hyperparathyroidism, upper gastrointestinal tract problems, musculoskeletal pain, rental toxicity and osteonecrosis of the jaw have been reported [7]. Therefore, there have been several basic and clinical efforts to find anti-osteoporotic phytochemicals in order to minimize adverse side effects [8–10].

Praeruptorin A (Fig. 1A) is isolated from the dry root extract of *Peucedanum praeruptorum* Dunn, which has been used as an herbal medicine with several pharmacological activities [11–14]. Recently, praeruptorin A has been shown to suppress the lipopolysaccharide (LPS)-induced inflammatory response in RAW264.7 cells [15]. Since LPS is a potent stimulator of both inflammation and bone resorption [16,17] and several phytochemicals exhibit dual anti-inflammatory and anti-resorptive activities [18,19], in this study, the anti-osteoclastogenic activity of praeruptorin A was investigated. The functional involvement of praeruptorin A in osteoclast differentiation is not yet clearly understood.

Materials and Methods

Reagents

Praeruptorin A was purchased from Stanford Chemicals (CA). Mouse soluble receptor activator of nuclear factor-κB ligand (RANKL) and macrophage-colony stimulating factor (M-CSF) were purchased from R&D Systems (MN). Penicillin, streptomycin, cell culture medium, and fetal bovine serum (FBS) were purchased from Invitrogen Life Technologies (NY). The CCK-8 assay kit was from Dojindo Molecular Technologies (ML). Antibodies against c-Fos, NFATc1 and actin were from Santa Cruz Biotechnology (CA). Antibodies against p-p38, p38, p-JNK, JNK, p-ERK, ERK, Akt, p-Akt (Ser473), PLCγ and p-PLCγ were obtained from Cell Signaling Technology (MA).

Osteoclast Differentiation

This study was carried out in strict accordance with the recommendations in the Standard Protocol for Animal Study of Korea Research Institute of Chemical Technology (KRICT; Permit No. 2012-7D-02-01). The protocol (ID No. 7D-M1) was approved by the Institutional Animal Care and Use Committee of KRICT (IACUC-KRICT). All efforts were made to minimize suffering. In detail, after cervical dislocation, bone marrow cells were obtained from 5-wk-old male ICR mice (Damool Science, Daejeon, Korea) by flushing femurs and tibias with α-MEM supplemented with antibiotics (100 units/ml penicillin and 100 μg/ml streptomycin). Bone marrow cells were cultured for 1 day on a culture dish in α-MEM supplemented with 10% FBS and M-CSF (10 ng/ml). Non-adherent bone marrow cells were plated on a Petri dish and cultured for 3 days in the presence of M-CSF (30 ng/ml). After non-adherent cells were washed out, adherent cells were used as bone marrow-derived macrophages (BMMs). For osteoclastogenesis, BMMs (1×10^4 cells/well in a 96-well plate or 3×10^5 cells/well in a 6-well plate) were cultured in the presence of M-CSF (30 ng/ml) and RANKL (10 ng/ml) for 4 days.

Tartrate-resistant Acid Phosphatase (TRAP) Staining and Activity Assay

Cells were fixed with 3.7% formaldehyde for 5 min, permeabilized with 0.1% Triton X-100 for 5 min, and stained with the Leukocyte Acid Phosphatase Kit 387-A (Sigma-Aldrich, MO). TRAP-positive multinuclear cells with three or more nuclei were counted as osteoclasts. To measure TRAP activity, cells were treated with TRAP buffer (100 mM sodium citrate, pH 5.0, 50 mM sodium tartrate) including 3 mM *p*-nitrophenyl phosphate (Sigma-Aldrich) at 37°C for 5min. Reaction mixtures were transferred into a new plate containing an equal volume of 0.1 N NaOH, and optical density values were determined at 405 nm in a Wallac EnVision microplate reader (PerkinElmer, Finland).

Cytotoxicity Assay

BMMs were plated at a density of 1×10^4 cells/well on a 96-well plate in triplicate. After treatment with M-CSF (30 ng/ml) and praeruptorin A, cells were cultured for 3 days. Then, cell

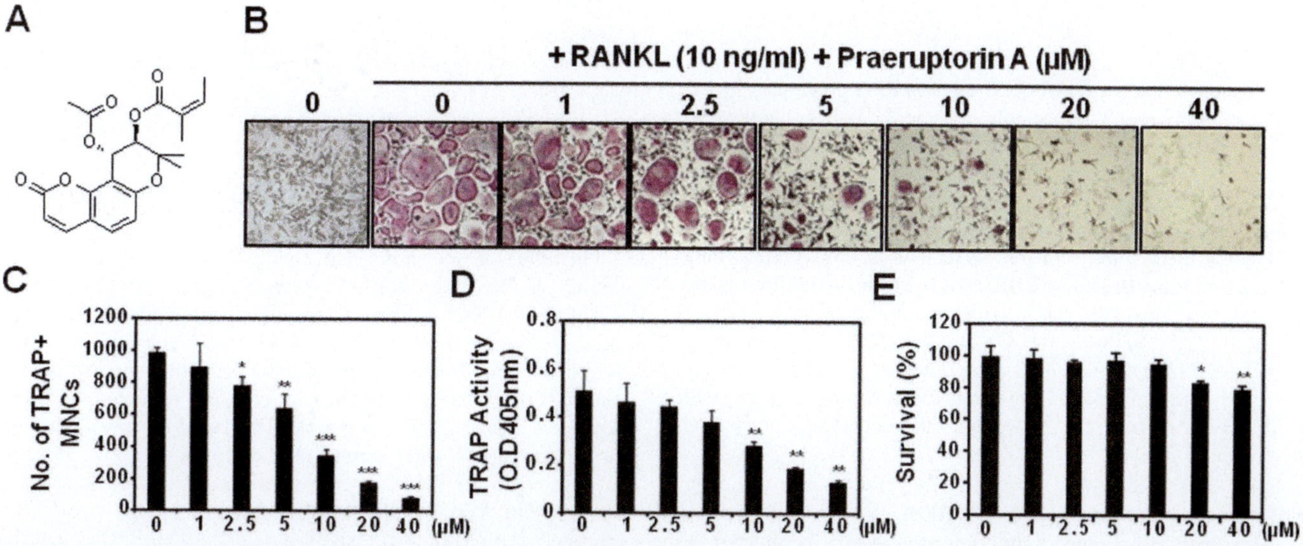

Figure 1. Effect of praeruptorin A on RANKL-induced osteoclast differentiation. (A) Chemical structure of praeruptorin A. (B) BMMs were pretreated with vehicle (0.1% DMSO) or praeruptorin A for 2 h and then incubated with RANKL (10 ng/ml) and M-CSF (30 ng/ml) for 4 days. Multinucleated cells were fixed, permeabilized, and stained with TRAP solution. Mature TRAP-positive multinucleated osteoclasts (MNCs) were photographed under a light microscope. TRAP-positive MNCs (nuclear number >3) were counted (C), and TRAP activity of osteoclasts was measured (D). (E) The effect of praeruptorin A on the viability of BMMs was evaluated by CCK-8 assay. *, $P<0.05$; **, $P<0.01$; ***$P<0.001$.

viability was measured with the CCK-8 kit according to the manufacturer's protocol.

Western Blot Analysis

Western blot analysis was performed as described previously [9,10]. Briefly, cells were washed, lysed, and centrifuged at 10,000× *g* for 15 min. After protein quantification of the supernatants by the BCA protein assay (Pierce, IL), proteins were denatured, separated on SDS-PAGE gels, and transferred onto PVDF membranes (Millipore, CA). After incubation with antibody, the membranes were developed using SuperSignal West Femto Maximum Sensitivity Substrate (Pierce) and visualized with the LAS-3000 luminescent image analyzer (Fuji Photo Film Co., Ltd., Japan). ImageJ software-based quantification of the detected bands was performed, and the relative, normalized ratio between the density of phosphorylated form and that of the protein itself or actin was presented in each figure.

NFATc1 Luciferase Activity Assay

Luciferase reporter plasmid, NFATc1-luc vector was purchased from Clontech (CA) and pRL-Renilla control vector was purchased from Promega (WI). The full-length human RANK cDNA was amplified from human leukocyte cDNA from Clontech (CA) and cloned into the HindIII-EcoRI site of pcDNA3.1 (Invitrogen). Recombinant human RANKL (hRNAKL) was purchased from R&D Systems (CA). For measurement of luciferase activity, human embryonic kidney HEK293T cells were plated at a density of 5×10^4 cells/well on a 48-well plate in triplicate for 1 day. Plasmids containing NFAT-luc (100 ng/well), pcDNA3.1-RANK (100 ng/well), and pRL-Renilla (20 ng/well) were transfected into HEK293T cells with Lipofectamine 2000 (Invitrogen, CA) according to the manufacturer's protocol. After 6 h, transfected HEK293T cells were treated with hRANKL (50 ng/mL) and praeruptorin A for 2 days. The luciferase activity was detected in cell extracts with the Dual-Luciferase Reporter Assay System (Promega, WI) and Wallac EnVision microplate reader (PerkinElmer). Luciferase activity assessed in triplicates was normalized to the average renilla luciferase activity.

Real-time PCR

Real-time PCR was performed as described previously [9,10]. Primers were chosen with the online Primer3 design program [20]. The primer sets used in this study are shown in Table 1. Briefly, total RNA was isolated with TRIzol reagent, and the first-strand cDNA was synthesized with the Omniscript RT kit (Qiagen) according to the manufacturer's protocol. SYBR green-based QPCR was performed with the Stratagene Mx3000P Real-Time PCR system and Brilliant SYBR Green Master Mix (Stratagene, CA). All reactions were run in triplicate, and data were analyzed by the $2^{-\Delta\Delta C}{}_T$ method [21]. Glyceraldehyde-3-phosphate dehydrogenase (GAPDH) was used as an internal standard gene. The statistical significance was determined by Student's *t*-test with GAPDH-normalized $2^{-\Delta\Delta C}{}_T$ values; differences were considered significant at $p<0.05$.

Retrovirus Preparation and Infection

Retrovirus preparation and infection were conducted as described previously [22]. Briefly, to obtain retroviral particles, pMX-IRES-green fluorescent protein (GFP; the control) or pMX-CA-NFATc1-GFP containing constitutively active (CA)-NFATc1 was transfected into Plat-E cells (Cell Biolabs, Inc., CA) using Lipofectamine 2000 reagent according to the manufacturer's protocol. After viral particles were collected from the culture

Table 1. Primer sequences used in this study.

Target Gene	Forward Primer (5′–3′)	Reverse Primer (5′–3′)
TRAP	GATGACTTTGCCAGTCAGCA	ACATAGCCCACACCGTTCTC
NFATc1	GGGTCAGTGTGACCGAAGAT	GGAAGTCAGAAGTGGGTGGA
OSCAR	AGGGAAACCTCATCCGTTTG	GAGCCGGAAATAAGGCACAG
Cathepsin K	GGCCAACTCAAGAAGAAAAC	GTGCTTGCTTCCCTTCTGG
DC-STAMP	CCAAGGAGTCGTCCATGATT	GGCTGCTTTGATCGTTTCTC
c-Src	CCAGGCTGAGGAGTGGTACT	CAGCTTGCGGATCTTGTAGT
GAPDH	AACTTTGGCATTGTGGAAGG	ACACATTGGGGGTAGGAACA

medium for 48 h, BMMs were incubated with those in the presence of M-CSF (30 ng/ml) and polybrene (10 μg/mL) for 8 h. For the osteoclast formation assay, BMMs were treated with RANKL (10 ng/ml), M-CSF (30 ng/ml) and praeruptorin A (10 μM) for 4 days.

Intracellular Ca^{2+} Measurement

Isolated BMMs were seeded at a density of 1×10^5 cells on the cover glass and cultured in the presence of RANKL (10 ng/ml) and M-CSF (30 ng/ml) for 24 h. Cells were incubated with vehicle (DMSO) or praeruptorin A (10 μM) for 2 h, treated with Fura-2, AM (5 μM), and then placed in the perfusion chamber to allow continuous perfusion of bath solution (140 mM NaCl, 5 mM KCl, 1 mM $MgCl_2$, 1 mM $CaCl_2$, 10 mM HEPES, and 10 mM glucose, pH 7.4, 310 mOsm) until each experiment was complete. Fluorescent dyes inside the cells were excited at wavelengths of 340 nm and 380 nm sequentially and the emitted fluorescence was passed through 510 nm cut-off filter. Each image was collected with a CCD camera and analyzed with MetaFluor software. All results were digitized to the mean of the ratio (340 nm/380 nm).

Statistical Analysis

All quantitative values are presented as mean ± SD. Statistical differences were analyzed using Student's *t*-test. A value of $p<0.05$ was considered significant.

Results

Praeruptorin A Inhibits RANKL-induced Osteoclast Differentiation

The effect of praeruptorin A on RANKL-induced osteoclastogenesis was evaluated in BMMs. Pre-treatment with praeruptorin A before RANKL treatment strongly prevented the RANKL-induced formation of TRAP-positive multinucleated cells in a dose-dependent manner (Fig. 1B and C). Consistent with these results, TRAP activity was also significantly inhibited by praeruptorin A above 10 μM (Fig. 1D). To clarify the possibility that the anti-osteoclastogenic activity of praeruptorin A could be due to its cytotoxicity in BMMs, we investigated the cytotoxic effect of praeruptorin A in BMMs. As shown in Fig. 1E, praeruptorin A exhibited significant cytotoxicity above 20 μM, suggesting that anti-osteoclastogenic activity of praeruptorin A without any cytotoxicity could be expected under 10 μM. Hoechst-stained nuclei supported no difference in cell cytotoxicity or spreading by praeruptorin A at 10 μM (Fig. S1). Therefore, the cells were treated with 10 μM of praeruptorin A in subsequent experiments to evaluate its anti-osteoclastogenic mechanism. At 10 μM, praeruptorin A also strongly inhibited osteoclast formation by inhibiting cell fusion; when it was added before fusion of preosteoclasts (or treated in the differentiation day 3; Fig. S2), the formation of multinucleated osteoclasts was significantly inhibited.

Praeruptorin A Inhibits RANKL-induced Activation of p38 and Akt

Anti-osteoclastogenic activity of praeruptorin A was confirmed by staining actin ring of mature osteoclasts (Fig. S3). This result was consistent with Fig. 1B. To elucidate the anti-osteoclastogenic mechanism of praeruptorin A, we investigated its effect on the activation of signaling molecules including JNK, p38, ERK, and Akt, which are known to play a role in the early stage of RANKL-induced osteoclast differentiation. After RANKL treatment, all signaling molecules were activated in 5–15 min, but pre-treatment with praeruptorin A 30 min before RANKL treatment attenuated the RANKL-induced phosphorylation of p38 and Akt within 15 min after RANKL treatment (Fig. 2A). The RANKL-induced activation of ERK and JNK were not changed by praeruptorin A.

Praeruptorin A Inhibits RANKL-induced Expression of c-Fos and NFATc1

Additionally, the inhibitory effect of praeruptorin A on the expression of transcription factors such as c-Fos and NFATc1 was evaluated by Western blot analysis. As shown in Fig. 2B, RANKL induced the expression of c-Fos and NFATc1 in the early and late stages of osteoclastogenesis, respectively. However, those inductions were inhibited by praeruptorin A. In particular, on day 3, the RANKL-induced expression of NFATc1 was strongly blocked by praeruptorin A.

Additionally, the inhibitory effect of praeruptorin A on the activation of NFATc1 was revealed by the NFATc1 luciferase activity assay (Fig. 2C); RANKL significantly induced the transcriptional activity of NFATc1 in HEK293T cells transfected with RANK plasmid and NFATc1 firefly-luciferase reporter plasmid, but the addition of 10 μM praeruptorin A significantly inhibited the RANKL-induced transcriptional activity of NFATc1.

Praeruptorin A Inhibits RANKL-induced mRNA Expression of Osteoclast-Specific Genes

The anti-osteoclastogenic activity of praeruptorin A was confirmed by evaluating the mRNA expression levels of osteoclast-specific genes. Consistent with the previous data, praeruptorin A significantly attenuated the RANKL-induced mRNA expressions of TRAP and NFATc1 (Fig. 3). Since NFATc1 can regulate the mRNA levels of osteoclast-related molecules including osteoclast-associated receptor (OSCAR), dendrite cell-specific transmembrane protein (DC-STAMP), cathepsin K and c-Src, we further investigated whether praeruptorin A could affect the mRNA expression of these genes during osteoclastogenesis. As expected, the mRNA expressions of these molecules were highly induced by RANKL, but praeruptorin A

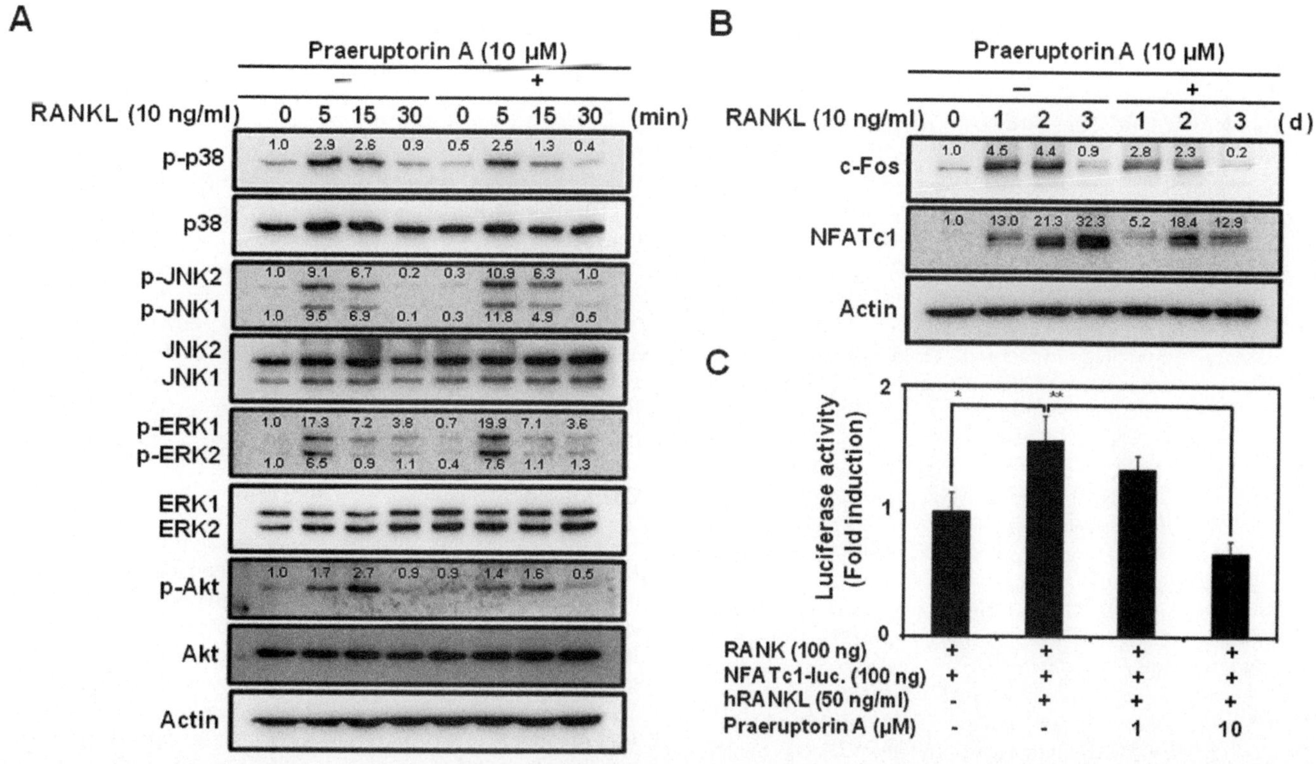

Figure 2. Effect of praeruptorin A on RANKL-induced activation or expression of osteoclast-specific signaling molecules and transcription factors. The effects of praeruptorin A on RANKL-induced phosphorylation of MAP kinases and Akt (A) and expression of transcription factors, c-Fos and NFATc1 (B), were evaluated by Western blot analysis. BMMs were pre-treated with praeruptorin A (10 μM) 2 h before treatment with RANKL (10 ng/ml) and M-CSF (30 ng/ml). Actin was used as an internal control. Densitometric analysis was performed using ImageJ software and the relative, normalized ratios of p-p38/p38, p-JNKs/JNKs, p-ERKs/ERK, p-Akt/Akt, c-Fos/actin and NFATc1/actin were presented. (C) The effect of praeruptorin A on the transcriptional activity of NFATc1 was evaluated by luciferase activity assay as described in 'Materials and Methods'. *, $P<0.05$; **, $P<0.01$.

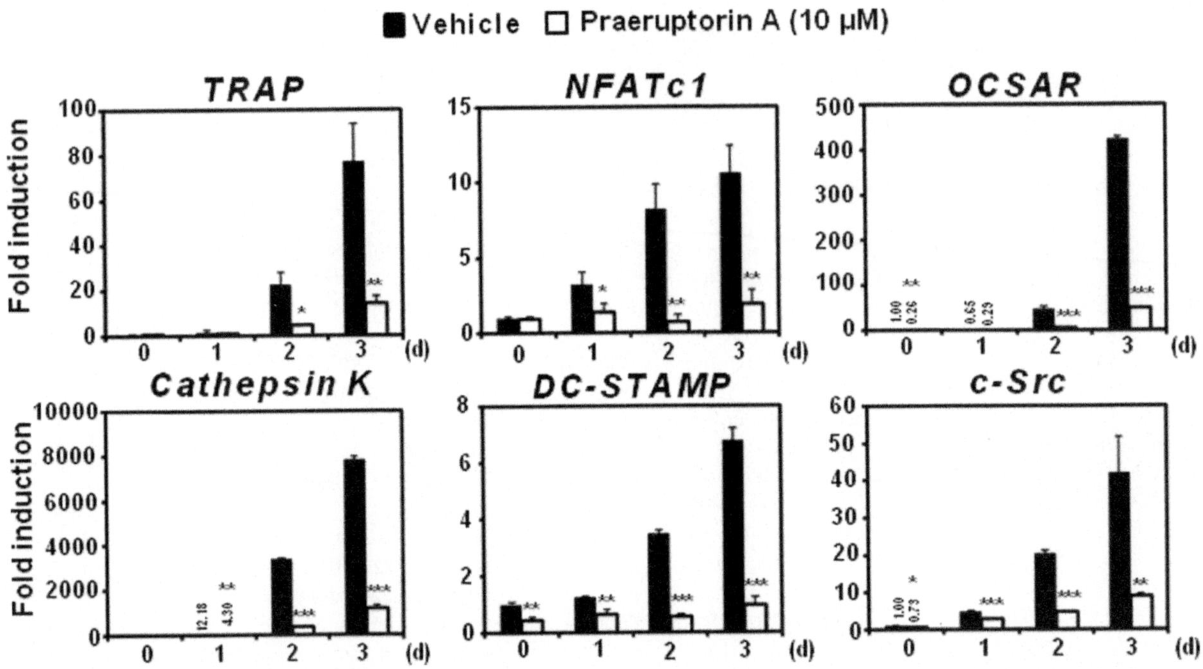

Figure 3. Effect of praeruptorin A on RANKL-induced mRNA expressions of osteoclastic-specific genes. BMMs were treated with vehicle (DMSO) or praeruptorin A (10 μM) for 2 h and then RANKL (10 ng/ml) was added into cells. The mRNA expression levels of osteoclastic-specific genes were analyzed by real-time PCR. *, $P<0.05$; **, $P<0.01$; ***$P<0.001$.

dramatically suppressed those inductions in a dose-dependent manner.

Ectopic NFATc1 Rescues Anti-osteoclastogenic Action of Praeruptorin A

The anti-osteoclastogenic action of praeruptorin A could result from its potential to block p38 and/or Akt signaling pathways that subsequently affect the expression and/or activity of c-Fos and the most distal transcription factor, NFATc1. To clarify this hypothesis, we investigated whether ectopic expression of the constitutively active form of NFATc1 (CA-NFATc1) could rescue the praeruptorin A-inhibited formation of TRAP-positive multinucleated osteoclasts. Based on GFP signaling, both the control GFP and CA-NFATc1-GFP plasmid were infected well, and the overexpression of NFATc1 was confirmed by Western blot analysis (Fig. 4D). Consistent with Fig. 1B, the formation of TRAP-positive multinucleated osteoclasts from BMM expressing the control GFP was strongly inhibited by praeruptorin A (upper images in Fig. 4A). However, even in the presence of praeruptorin A, TRAP-positive multinucleated osteoclasts were derived from BMMs over-expressing NFATc1 (bottom images in Fig. 4A). The ameliorating effect of NFATc1 on the praeruptorin A-mediated inhibition of osteoclast differentiation was also confirmed by counting the number of multinucleated osteoclasts, measuring the TRAP activity (Fig. 4B), and evaluating the mRNA expression levels of TRAP, OSCAR, cathepsin K and DC-STAMP (Fig. 4C). Additionally, Western blot analysis revealed that praeruptorin A strongly attenuated the Akt activation by the overexpression of activated NFATc1 (Fig. 4D). The overexpression of activated NFATc1 did not induce the phosphorylation of p38.

Praeruptorin A Inhibits Ca^{2+} Oscillation without Any Change in PLCγ Phosphorylation

Since several studies have reported the Ca^{2+} channel blocking activity of praeruptorin A [23,24], we further evaluated the effect of praeruptorin A on the RANKL-induced Ca^{2+} oscillation. As shown in Fig. 5A, when BMMs were treated with M-CSF plus RANKL for 24 h, Ca^{2+} oscillation was triggered, but not with M-CSF alone. However, additional treatment with praeruptorin A for 2 h before measuring Ca^{2+} oscillation completely inhibited the RANKL-induced Ca^{2+} oscillation.

We further examined the possibility that praeruptorin A could inhibit the RANKL-induced Ca^{2+} oscillation by blocking the RANKL-induced phosphorylation of PLCγ. In BMMs, the RANKL-induced phosphorylation of PLCγ was not changed by praeruptorin A.

Discussion

Osteoclasts are functionally essential for sustaining bone health. However, the overactivation of osteoclasts and/or their increased number can lead to diseases characterized to bone loss, which is a risk factor for fracture. In this study, praeruptorin A attenuated the RANKL-induced osteoclastogenesis in a dose-dependent manner without any cytotoxicity upto 10 μM. Anti-osteoclastogenic activity of praeruptorin A was independent on age, strain and sex of mouse (Fig. S4), and importantly, praeruptorin A significantly inhibited the fusion of preosteoclasts (Fig. S2) and the formation of resorptive pits by mature multinucleated osteoclasts (Fig. S5).

RANKL is the most essential cytokine for osteoclast differentiation (or osteoclastogenesis) [25]. The binding of RANKL to RANK, its receptor, triggers the activation of signaling molecules such as MAP kinases, Akt, and phospholipase Cγ (PLCγ) that subsequently induce the activation of transcription factors such as

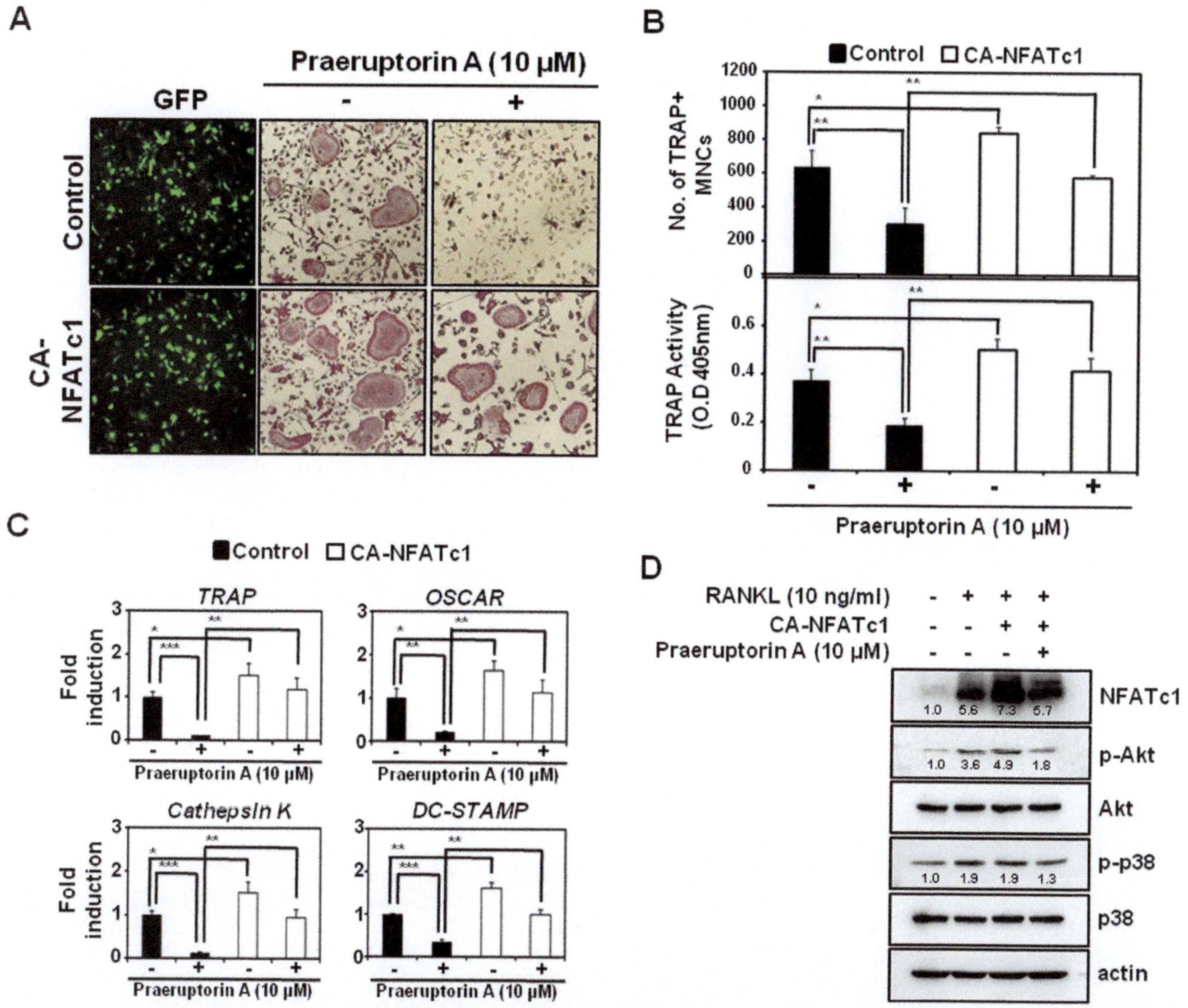

Figure 4. Effect of NFATc1 on anti-osteoclastogenic action of praeruptorin A. (A) BMMs were infected with retroviruses harboring the control GFP or Ca-NFATc1-GFP vectors. Transduced BMMs were cultured with RANKL (10 ng/ml) and M-CSF (30 ng/ml) in the presence of praeruptorin A (10 μM) or vehicle (DMSO). After incubation for 2 days, GFP expression was visualized under a fluorescence microscope. After 2 additional days, mature TRAP-positive multinucleated osteoclasts were visualized by TRAP staining. (B) TRAP-positive cells (nuclear number >3) were counted as osteoclasts, and TRAP activity was measured at 405 nm. On the differentiation day 2, the mRNA and protein expression levels of osteoclastogenesis-related molecules were analyzed by real-time PCR (C) and Western blot analysis, respectively (D). Densitometric analysis was performed using ImageJ software and the relative, normalized ratios of NFATc1/actin, p-Akt/Akt or p-p38/p38 were presented. *, $P<0.05$; **, $P<0.01$; ***$P<0.001$.

c-Fos and nuclear factor of activated T cells (NFATc1) to regulate the expression of genes required for osteoclast differentiation [26–28]. c-Fos is an essential factor for the induction of NFATc1, which is a master transcription factor that regulates the process of osteoclast differentiation by controlling osteoclast-specific genes [29–31].

Here, praeruptorin A attenuated the RANKL-induced phosphorylation of p38 without affecting JNK and ERK. A pharmacological inhibition experiment using the p38 inhibitor SB203580 revealed direct involvement of p38 in the RANKL-induced osteoclast differentiation [22,32,33]. Furthermore, a study using both p38 inhibitor SB203580 and over-expression of dominant negative MKK3 and MKK6, which are known as upstream kinases of p38, revealed that the p38 signaling pathway could mediate the induction of c-Fos and NFATc1 during RANKL-stimulated osteoclast differentiation [34].

Moreover, praeruptorin A also attenuated the RANKL-induced phosphorylation of Akt. Akt has been known to play a critical role in the survival of osteoclasts rather than in osteoclast differentiation through the phosphoinositide 3-kinase (PI3K) kinase signaling pathway [35,36]. However, a recent study showed the importance of the Akt-NFATc1 signaling axis in osteoclast differentiation [37]; inhibition of Akt phosphorylation by LY294002 resulted in the inhibition of osteoclast differentiation via modulation of RANKL-induced activation of NFATc1.

Thus, the anti-osteoclastogenic action of praeruptorin A could be due to its potential to inhibit both p38 and Akt signaling pathways that consequently downregulate the expression and/or

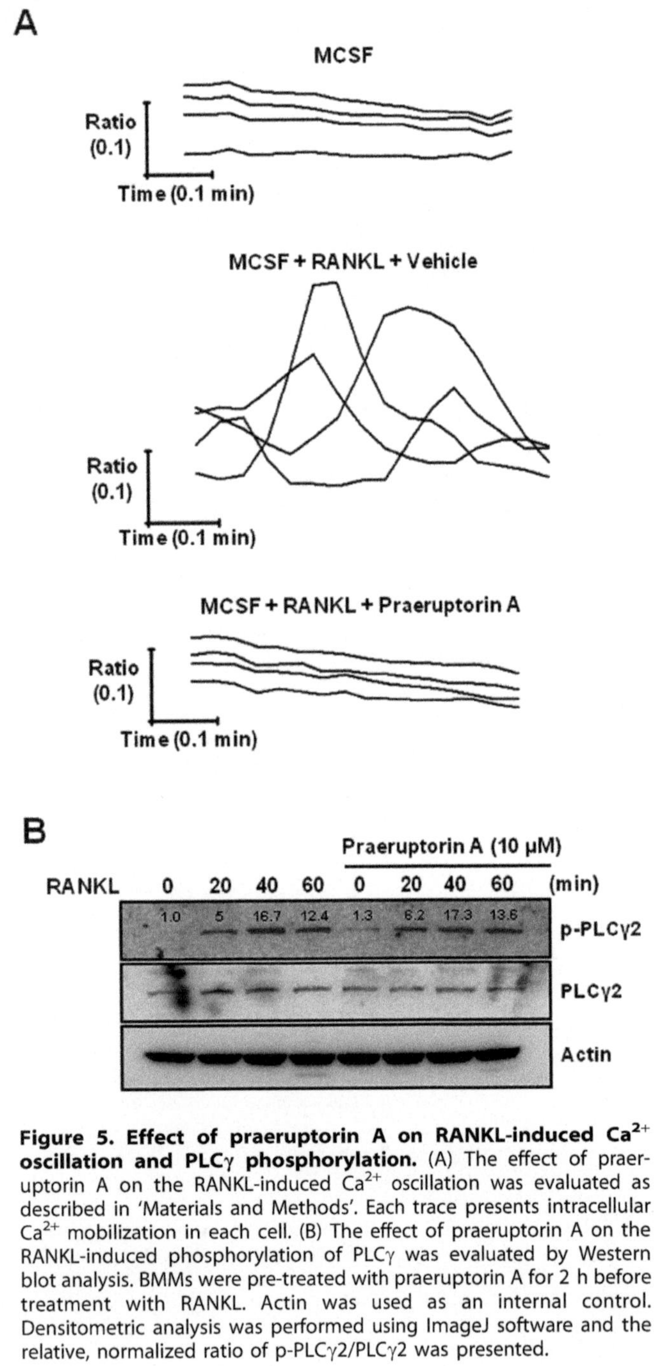

Figure 5. Effect of praeruptorin A on RANKL-induced Ca^{2+} oscillation and PLCγ phosphorylation. (A) The effect of praeruptorin A on the RANKL-induced Ca^{2+} oscillation was evaluated as described in 'Materials and Methods'. Each trace presents intracellular Ca^{2+} mobilization in each cell. (B) The effect of praeruptorin A on the RANKL-induced phosphorylation of PLCγ was evaluated by Western blot analysis. BMMs were pre-treated with praeruptorin A for 2 h before treatment with RANKL. Actin was used as an internal control. Densitometric analysis was performed using ImageJ software and the relative, normalized ratio of p-PLCγ2/PLCγ2 was presented.

activity of c-Fos and NFATc1. In particular, NFATc1, which is mainly regulated by c-Fos during osteoclastogenesis, plays a role as the most distal transcription factor required for regulating the expression of osteoclast-specific genes including TRAP, OSCAR, DC-STAMP, cathepsin K and c-Src [27,28,38]. TRAP is recognized as a marker of osteoclast differentiation and exhibits bone resorptive activity in the lysosomes [39]. OSCAR is a receptor that controls the PLCγ- Ca^{2+} signaling pathway, which is crucial for the activation of NFATc1 [40]. DC-STAMP and cathepsin K are well-known molecules for fusion and bone resorptive activity, respectively [38,41]. c-Src tyrosine kinase is also required for the maintenance of the osteoclast actin cytoskeleton and the control of bone resorption [42]. In our results, praeruptorin A significantly inhibited the RANKL-induced expression of c-Fos, NFATc1 and those osteoclast-specific genes. Additionally, praeruptorin A inhibited the RANKL-induced activation of NFATc1.

These results suggested that the downregulation of NFATc1 could be the outcome of the anti-osteoclastogenic action of praeruptorin A by inhibiting p38 and Akt signaling pathways. The hypothesis was proved by the ectopic expression of the constitutively active form of NFATc1; it significantly rescued the anti-osteoclastogenic action of praeruptorin A. The rescue of defected osteoclastogenesis by overexpression of NFATc1 has been reported in several studies [9,43]; for example, NFATc1-deficient embryonic stem cells failed to differentiate into osteoclasts after RANKL treatment, but the ectopic expression of NFATc1 rescued the abrogated osteoclast differentiation [30,44]. Additionally, praeruptorin A strongly attenuated the Akt activation by the overexpression of activated NFATc1, but that did not induce the phosphorylation of p38. These results suggested that the auto-amplification of NFATc1 during osteoclast differentiation could affect the activation of Akt, but not p38, and praeruptorin A has the potential to attenuate the NFATc1-mediated activation of Akt.

Furthermore, the overexpression of c-Fos did not significantly rescue the effect of praeruptorin A on osteoclast differentiation (Fig. S6), but the Western blot analysis revealed the involvement of NF-κB signaling in anti-osteoclastogenic action of praeruptorin A (Fig. S7). For degradation, IκBα was phosphorylated 5 min after RANKL treatment, and then free NF-κB p65 was translocated into nucleus in 15 to 30 min, but this activation of NF-κB by RANKL was shown to be attenuated by the pretreatment of praeruptorin A. The role of NF-κB in osteoclast differentiation has been described in several review articles [4,5].

In osteoclast differentiation, RANKL also triggers the activation of PLCγ, which subsequently leads to Ca^{2+} mobilization [45]. As well as activating MAP kinases and Akt, PLCγ-medicated Ca^{2+} mobilization affects the activation of NFATc1 required for regulating osteoclast-specific genes [27]. Importantly, several studies have reported the Ca^{2+} channel blocking activity of praeruptorin A [23,24]. These data clarify the hypothesis that praeruptorin A-mediated inhibition of Ca^{2+} oscillation via PLCγ could also downregulate the activity of NFATc1 during osteoclast differentiation. Interestingly, the RANKL-triggered Ca^{2+} oscillation was inhibited by praeruptorin A, but the RANKL-induced phosphorylation of PLCγ was not changed by praeruptorin A. These data suggest that the anti-osteoclastogenic activity of praeruptorin A involves inhibition of PLCγ-independent Ca^{2+} oscillation.

This is the first report of the anti-osteoclastogenic activity of praeruptorin A and its mode of action; praeruptorin A could inhibit the RANKL-induced osteoclast differentiation by inhibiting p38 and Akt signaling pathways and PLCγ-independent Ca^{2+} oscillation that consequently affect the expression and/or activity of the osteoclast-specific transcription factors, c-Fos and NFATc1. Also, NF-κB signaling was shown to be partly involved in the anti-osteoclastogenic action of praeruptorin A. In a further study, the binding molecules (or target proteins) of praeruptorin A might be identified, and the mechanism how praeruptorin A inhibits the fusion of preosteoclasts and the pit formation of mature osteoclasts might be elucidated.

Supporting Information

Figure S1 Effect of praeruptorin A on cell spreading during RANKL-induced osteoclast differentiation. BMMs (1×10^4 cells/well) were seeded in a 96-well plate, treated with the vehicle (0.1% DMSO) or praeruptorin A (10 μM) for 2 h in the presence of M-CSF (30 ng/ml), and incubated with RANKL (10 ng/ml) for 1 and 3 days. Then, cells were fixed, permeabilized, washed, and incubated with 10 μg/ml Hoechst 33342.

Figure S2 Effect of praeruptorin A on RANKL-induced osteoclast differentiation for the indicated periods. BMMs were cultured with praeruptorin A (10 μM) for various times periods (indicated the black arrow) in the presence of M-CSF and RANKL. After TRAP staining, TRAP-positive multinuclear cells (MNCs; nuclear number >3) were counted *, $P<0.05$; **, $P<0.01$; ***$P<0.001$.

Figure S3 Effect of praeruptorin A on the formation of actin rings during osteoclast differentiation. BMMs (1×10^4 cells/well) were seeded in a 96-well plate, treated with the vehicle (0.1% DMSO) or praeruptorin A (10 μM) for 2 h in the presence of M-CSF (30 ng/ml), and incubated with RANKL (10 ng/ml) for 4 days. Then, cells were fixed, permeabilized, washed, and stained with Hoechst 33342 and phalloidin-FITC for nucleus and actin rings, respectively.

Figure S4 (A) Effect of age, strain or sex on anti-osteoclastogenic action of praeruptorin A. BMMs were isolated from mice (male and female ICR strain, 5-week old; male and female C57BL6/N strain, 5-week old and 8-month old) and cultured with praeruptorin A in the presence of M-CSF and RANKL for 4 days. Osteoclast differentiation was visualized by TRAP staining. (B) Effect of age, strain or sex on anti-osteoclastogenic action of praeruptorin A. BMMs were isolated from mice (male and female ICR strain, 5-week old; male and female C57BL6/N strain, 5-week old and 8-month old) and cultured with praeruptorin A in the presence of M-CSF and RANKL for 4 days. After TRAP staining, TRAP-positive multinuclear cells (MNCs; nuclear number >3) were counted. TRAP activity and cell viability were also evaluated. *, $P<0.05$; **, $P<0.01$; ***$P<0.001$.

Figure S5 Anti-resorptive activity of praeruptorin A. (A) After co-culturing BMMs with osteoblasts for 7 days, multinucleated osteoclasts were replated on BioCoat Osteologic MultiTest slides and after 2 h incubation, cells were further incubated with praeruptorin A and RANKL for 6 h. Then, cells were stained for TRAP (upper images). (B) TRAP-positive multinucleated cells were counted. (C) After removing cells, the resorption pits (indicated by asterisks in bottom images) were observed under a light microscope. The relative resorbing areas were evaluated using the ImageJ program. ***$P<0.001$.

Figure S6 Effect of c-Fos on anti-osteoclastogenic action of praeruptorin A. BMMs were infected with retroviruses harboring the control GFP or c-Fos-GFP vectors. Transduced BMMs were cultured with RANKL (10 ng/ml) and M-CSF (30 ng/ml) in the presence of praeruptorin A (10 μM) or the vehicle (0.1% DMSO). (A) After incubation for 2 days, GFP expression was visualized under a fluorescence microscope (left images). After 2 additional days, mature TRAP-positive multinucleated osteoclasts were visualized by TRAP staining (middle and right images). TRAP-positive cells (nuclear number >3) were counted as osteoclasts (B), and TRAP activity was measured at 405 nm (C). *, $P<0.05$; **, $P<0.01$; ***$P<0.001$.

Figure S7 Effect of praeruptorin A on RANKL-induced activation of NF-κB signaling pathway. BMMs were treated with praeruptorin A (10 μM) for 30 min, stimulated with RANKL (10 ng/ml) for the indicated time. The expression levels of molecules in cytoplasmic or nuclear protein fractions were evaluated by Western blot analysis. Actin and lamin B1 were used for the loading control of cytosolic and nuclear proteins, respectively. Densitometric analysis was performed using ImageJ software and the relative, normalized ratios of IκBα/actin, p-IκBα/actin, cytosolic p65/actin or nuclear p65/lamin B1 were presented.

File S1 Materials and Methods.

Author Contributions

Conceived and designed the experiments: SHK YJS. Performed the experiments: JTY KJK SWC SHM YSP BJR JMO MSK ME. Analyzed the data: SHK YJS JTY KJK. Contributed reagents/materials/analysis tools: SHK YJS. Wrote the paper: SHK YJS.

References

1. Cooper C, Campion G, Melton LJ 3rd (1992) Hip fractures in the elderly: a world-wide projection. Osteoporos Int 2: 285–289.
2. Lippuner K, von Overbeck J, Perrelet R, Bosshard H, Jaeger P (1997) Incidence and direct medical costs of hospitalizations due to osteoporotic fractures in Switzerland. Osteoporos Int 7: 414–425.
3. Karsenty G, Wagner EF (2002) Reaching a genetic and molecular understanding of skeletal development. Dev Cell 2: 389–406.
4. Boyle WJ, Simonet WS, Lacey DL (2003) Osteoclast differentiation and activation. Nature 423: 337–342.
5. Del Fattore A, Teti A, Rucci N (2008) Osteoclast receptors and signaling. Arch Biochem Biophys 473: 147–160.
6. Fleisch H (2003) Bisphosphonates in osteoporosis. Eur Spine J 12 Suppl 2: S142–146.
7. Papapetrou PD (2009) Bisphosphonate-associated adverse events. Hormones (Athens) 8: 96–110.
8. Morabito N, Crisafulli A, Vergara C, Gaudio A, Lasco A, et al. (2002) Effects of genistein and hormone-replacement therapy on bone loss in early postmenopausal women: a randomized double-blind placebo-controlled study. J Bone Miner Res 17: 1904–1912.
9. Choi SW, Son YJ, Yun JM, Kim SH (2012) Fisetin Inhibits Osteoclast Differentiation via Downregulation of p38 and c-Fos-NFATc1 Signaling Pathways. Evid Based Complement Alternat Med 2012: 810563.
10. Choi SW, Moon SH, Yang HJ, Kwon DY, Son YJ, et al. (2013) Antiresorptive activity of bacillus-fermented antler extracts: inhibition of osteoclast differentiation. Evid Based Complement Alternat Med 2013: 748687.
11. Shen X, Chen G, Zhu G, Fong WF (2006) (+/−)-3'-O, 4'-O-dicynnamoyl-cis-khellactone, a derivative of (+/−)-praeruptorin A, reverses P-glycoprotein mediated multidrug resistance in cancer cells. Bioorg Med Chem 14: 7138–7145.
12. Wu JY, Fong WF, Zhang JX, Leung CH, Kwong HL, et al. (2003) Reversal of multidrug resistance in cancer cells by pyranocoumarins isolated from Radix Peucedani. Eur J Pharmacol 473: 9–17.
13. Ji Y, Rao MR (1996) [Effects of Peucedanum praeruptorum extractum on blood pressure, left ventricular hypertrophy and hemodynamic changes in left ventricular hypertrophied hypertensive rats]. Zhongguo Zhong Xi Yi Jie He Za Zhi 16: 676–678.
14. Zhang C, Li W, Xiao YQ (2005) [Comparative studies on pharmacological effects of the main chemical constituents of Peucedanum praeruptorum from He'nan and Jiangxi]. Zhongguo Zhong Yao Za Zhi 30: 1356–1358.
15. Yu PJ, Ci W, Wang GF, Zhang JY, Wu SY, et al. (2011) Praeruptorin A inhibits lipopolysaccharide-induced inflammatory response in murine macrophages through inhibition of NF-kappaB pathway activation. Phytother Res 25: 550–556.
16. Koide M, Okahashi N, Tanaka R, Kazuno K, Shibasaki K, et al. (1999) Inhibition of experimental bone resorption and osteoclast formation and survival by 2-aminoethanesulphonic acid. Arch Oral Biol 44: 711–719.

17. Inada M, Matsumoto C, Uematsu S, Akira S, Miyaura C (2006) Membrane-bound prostaglandin E synthase-1-mediated prostaglandin E2 production by osteoblast plays a critical role in lipopolysaccharide-induced bone loss associated with inflammation. J Immunol 177: 1879–1885.
18. Kim MH, Ryu SY, Choi JS, Min YK, Kim SH (2009) Saurolactam inhibits osteoclast differentiation and stimulates apoptosis of mature osteoclasts. J Cell Physiol 221: 618–628.
19. Lee SU, Choi YH, Kim YS, Min YK, Rhee M, et al. (2010) Anti-resorptive saurolactam exhibits in vitro anti-inflammatory activity via ERK-NF-kappaB signaling pathway. Int Immunopharmacol 10: 298–303.
20. Rozen S, Skaletsky H (2000) Primer3 on the WWW for general users and for biologist programmers. Methods Mol Biol 132: 365–386.
21. Livak KJ, Schmittgen TD (2001) Analysis of relative gene expression data using real-time quantitative PCR and the 2(-Delta Delta C(T)) Method. Methods 25: 402–408.
22. Yeon JT, Choi SW, Park KI, Choi MK, Kim JJ, et al. (2012) Glutaredoxin2 isoform b (Glrx2b) promotes RANKL-induced osteoclastogenesis through activation of the p38-MAPK signaling pathway. BMB Rep 45: 171–176.
23. Li JM, Chang TH, Sun XD, Hao LY, Wang YP, et al. (1994) Effect of dl-praeruptorin A on calcium current in ventricular cells of guinea pig. Zhongguo Yao Li Xue Bao 15: 525–527.
24. Song YL, Jing WH, Zhao HY, Yan R, Li PT, et al. (2012) Stereoselective metabolism of (+/−)-praeruptorin A, a calcium channel blocker from Peucedani Radix, in pooled liver microsomes of rats and humans. Xenobiotica 42: 231–237.
25. Takayanagi H (2005) Inflammatory bone destruction and osteoimmunology. J Periodontal Res 40: 287–293.
26. Feng X (2005) RANKing intracellular signaling in osteoclasts. IUBMB Life 57: 389–395.
27. Takayanagi H (2007) Osteoimmunology: shared mechanisms and crosstalk between the immune and bone systems. Nat Rev Immunol 7: 292–304.
28. Takayanagi H (2007) The role of NFAT in osteoclast formation. Ann N Y Acad Sci 1116: 227–237.
29. Grigoriadis AE, Wang ZQ, Cecchini MG, Hofstetter W, Felix R, et al. (1994) c-Fos: a key regulator of osteoclast-macrophage lineage determination and bone remodeling. Science 266: 443–448.
30. Takayanagi H, Kim S, Koga T, Nishina H, Isshiki M, et al. (2002) Induction and activation of the transcription factor NFATc1 (NFAT2) integrate RANKL signaling in terminal differentiation of osteoclasts. Dev Cell 3: 889–901.
31. Miyamoto T (2011) Regulators of osteoclast differentiation and cell-cell fusion. Keio J Med 60: 101–105.
32. Li X, Udagawa N, Itoh K, Suda K, Murase Y, et al. (2002) p38 MAPK-mediated signals are required for inducing osteoclast differentiation but not for osteoclast function. Endocrinology 143: 3105–3113.
33. Matsumoto M, Sudo T, Saito T, Osada H, Tsujimoto M (2000) Involvement of p38 mitogen-activated protein kinase signaling pathway in osteoclastogenesis mediated by receptor activator of NF-kappa B ligand (RANKL). J Biol Chem 275: 31155–31161.
34. Huang H, Chang EJ, Ryu J, Lee ZH, Lee Y, et al. (2006) Induction of c-Fos and NFATc1 during RANKL-stimulated osteoclast differentiation is mediated by the p38 signaling pathway. Biochem Biophys Res Commun 351: 99–105.
35. Gingery A, Bradley E, Shaw A, Oursler MJ (2003) Phosphatidylinositol 3-kinase coordinately activates the MEK/ERK and AKT/NFkappaB pathways to maintain osteoclast survival. J Cell Biochem 89: 165–179.
36. Wong BR, Besser D, Kim N, Arron JR, Vologodskaia M, et al. (1999) TRANCE, a TNF family member, activates Akt/PKB through a signaling complex involving TRAF6 and c-Src. Mol Cell 4: 1041–1049.
37. Moon JB, Kim JH, Kim K, Youn BU, Ko A, et al. (2012) Akt induces osteoclast differentiation through regulating the GSK3beta/NFATc1 signaling cascade. J Immunol 188: 163–169.
38. Kim K, Lee SH, Ha Kim J, Choi Y, Kim N (2008) NFATc1 induces osteoclast fusion via up-regulation of Atp6v0d2 and the dendritic cell-specific transmembrane protein (DC-STAMP). Mol Endocrinol 22: 176–185.
39. Angel NZ, Walsh N, Forwood MR, Ostrowski MC, Cassady AI, et al. (2000) Transgenic mice overexpressing tartrate-resistant acid phosphatase exhibit an increased rate of bone turnover. J Bone Miner Res 15: 103–110.
40. Nemeth K, Schoppet M, Al-Fakhri N, Helas S, Jessberger R, et al. (2011) The role of osteoclast-associated receptor in osteoimmunology. J Immunol 186: 13–18.
41. Delaisse JM, Andersen TL, Engsig MT, Henriksen K, Troen T, et al. (2003) Matrix metalloproteinases (MMP) and cathepsin K contribute differently to osteoclastic activities. Microsc Res Tech 61: 504–513.
42. Miyazaki T, Tanaka S, Sanjay A, Baron R (2006) The role of c-Src kinase in the regulation of osteoclast function. Mod Rheumatol 16: 68–74.
43. Lee SH, Kim T, Jeong D, Kim N, Choi Y (2008) The tec family tyrosine kinase Btk Regulates RANKL-induced osteoclast maturation. J Biol Chem 283: 11526–11534.
44. Asagiri M, Sato K, Usami T, Ochi S, Nishina H, et al. (2005) Autoamplification of NFATc1 expression determines its essential role in bone homeostasis. J Exp Med 202: 1261–1269.
45. Negishi-Koga T, Takayanagi H (2009) Ca2+-NFATc1 signaling is an essential axis of osteoclast differentiation. Immunol Rev 231: 241–256.

8

Dried Plum's Unique Capacity to Reverse Bone Loss and Alter Bone Metabolism in Postmenopausal Osteoporosis Model

Elizabeth Rendina[1], Kelsey D. Hembree[1], McKale R. Davis[1], Denver Marlow[2], Stephen L. Clarke[1], Bernard P. Halloran[3], Edralin A. Lucas[1], Brenda J. Smith[1]*

1 Department of Nutritional Sciences, Oklahoma State University, Stillwater, Oklahoma, United States of America, 2 Comparative Medicine Group, Kansas State University, Manhattan, Kansas, United States of America, 3 Veterans Affairs Medical Center, University of California San Francisco, San Francisco, California, United States of America

Abstract

Interest in dried plum has increased over the past decade due to its promise in restoring bone and preventing bone loss in animal models of osteoporosis. This study compared the effects of dried plum on bone to other dried fruits and further explored the potential mechanisms of action through which dried plum may exert its osteoprotective effects. Adult osteopenic ovariectomized (OVX) C57BL/6 mice were fed either a control diet or a diet supplemented with 25% (w/w) dried plum, apple, apricot, grape or mango for 8 weeks. Whole body and spine bone mineral density improved in mice consuming the dried plum, apricot and grape diets compared to the OVX control mice, but dried plum was the only fruit to have an anabolic effect on trabecular bone in the vertebra and prevent bone loss in the tibia. Restoration of biomechanical properties occurred in conjunction with the changes in trabecular bone in the spine. Compared to other dried fruits in this study, dried plum was unique in its ability to down-regulate osteoclast differentiation coincident with up-regulating osteoblast and glutathione (GPx) activity. These alterations in bone metabolism and antioxidant status compared to other dried fruits provide insight into dried plum's unique effects on bone.

Editor: Yi-Hsiang Hsu, Harvard Medical School, United States Of America

Funding: This project was funded in part by National Institutes of Health/National Center for Complementary and Alternative Medicine (NIH/NCCAM) (1R21AT006580) and the Oklahoma State University Business and Technology Development Program. The contents of this manuscript are solely the responsibility of the authors and do not necessarily represent the official views of the NCCAM or the National Institutes of Health. The funders had no role in study design, data collection and analysis, decision to publish, or preparation of the manuscript.

* E-mail: bjsmith@okstate.edu

Introduction

Bone remodeling is a dynamic process involving the orchestration of bone resorption, formation and mineralization. When the balance between these anabolic and catabolic events is altered or disrupted, skeletal quality can be compromised, resulting in an increase in fracture risk. An estimated 1.5 million osteoporotic-related fractures occur in the U.S. each year and more than 43 million Americans have been diagnosed with osteoporosis or osteopenia [1]. Furthermore, as the population demographics shift toward an older society, the prevalence of osteoporosis is projected to increase 20% by 2020 [1,2].

To date, the treatment options approved by the Food and Drug Administration exert their effects either by decreasing bone resorption or increasing formation of bone tissue. Anti-resorptive agents, such as bisphosphonates and denosumab decrease bone loss by inhibiting the differentiation and catabolic activity of osteoclasts in part by promoting osteoclast apoptosis [3]. Alternatively, intermittent parathyroid hormone (PTH) therapy (1–34 amino acid sequence) is considered anabolic in nature as it acts to increase bone formation and mineralization by up-regulating osteoblast differentiation and activity [4]. While anti-resorptive and anabolic treatment options have had a significant impact on osteoporosis management, they can be cost prohibitive and may be accompanied with undesirable side-effects such as osteonecrosis of the jaw, gastrointestinal distress, dizziness, and leg cramping [5,6]. Due to the projected increase in the prevalence of osteoporosis and the need for better treatment options, the search continues for alternative strategies to maintain and/ or restore skeletal health.

Post-menopausal bone loss remains the most common cause of osteoporosis [2]. During the first 5–10 years after menopause, a physiological state exists in which bone turnover (*i.e.*, both resorption and formation rate) is accelerated with the catabolic activity of osteoclasts favored over the anabolic activity of osteoblasts. The classic model used to study post-menopausal bone loss has been the ovariectomized (OVX) rat and mouse. This model has provided much insight into the effects of ovarian hormones, such as estrogen, progesterone, and follicle stimulating hormone (FSH), and their direct influence on bone metabolism [7–9]. Aside from these more direct effects on bone cells, estrogen's more recently recognized regulatory role in cellular inflammatory and oxidative processes has resulted in an increased interest in targeting these pathways for therapeutic purposes [10–12]. The detrimental effects of postmenopausal osteoporosis, along with the limited treatment options available to protect or reverse osteoporotic bone loss, has led investigators to explore the possibility of other potential treatment options.

Fruits and vegetables have been noted for a variety of health benefits including decrease in some cancer risks [13–18], improved cardiovascular health [19–23], and weight management [20,24,25]. Natural compounds such as those found in many fruits and vegetables exert anti-inflammatory and anti-oxidant activity that have the potential to attenuate bone loss. The up-regulation of antioxidant systems (*i.e.*, glutathione peroxidase or GPx) has been shown to suppress bone resorption associated with estrogen deficiency [26–29]. Dried plums (*Prunus domestica L.*), which have a high polyphenolic content and oxygen radical absorbance capacity (ORAC) score, have been shown to protect against and reverse bone loss in gonadal hormone deficient rat and mouse models of osteoporosis [30–34]. These studies with dried plum have consistently demonstrated that dried plum improves bone mineral density (BMD), trabecular bone microarchitecture, and biomechanical properties [30–34]. While dried plum has a number of components that may be exerting these osteoprotective effects, both *in vitro* [35,36] and *in vivo (unpublished data)* work by our laboratory suggests that the polyphenols are in large part responsible for these observations. Although the mechanism has yet to be fully described, dried plum's ability to restore bone mass appears to be associated with an increase or maintenance of bone formation in conjunction with suppression of bone resorption. These promising findings have led to the question of whether or not other dried fruits with known anti-oxidative properties can reverse bone loss to the extent of dried plum [31,33].

This study was designed to compare the efficacy of several dried fruits (*i.e.*, dried plum, apple, apricot, grape, and mango) in the restoration of bone in an osteopenic OVX mouse model and to provide further insight into these dried fruits' mechanism of action. The selection of dried fruits that were used in this study was based on the fruit undergoing similar processing to dried plum, being a rich source of antioxidants and/or having potential osteoprotective properties [37–39].

Materials and Methods

Animal Care and Diets

Female 12 week-old C57BL/6 mice (Charles River, Wilmington, MA) were housed in an environmentally controlled laboratory animal research facility. Following a 7-day acclimation period, mice were anesthetized using a ketamine/xylazine cocktail (80 mg ketamine and 8 mg xylazine/kg body weight) for either a sham-operation (Sham) or bilateral ovariectomy (OVX), and maintained on the control diet immediately following surgery for 2 weeks to induce bone loss. A subset of Sham and OVX animals (n = 6/group) served as baseline control groups, and were sacrificed after 2 weeks to confirm bone loss by whole body and spine BMD. Once bone loss had been established, mice were assigned to one of seven treatment groups (n = 8 mice/group): Sham control diet (AIN-93M), OVX control diet, or OVX mice consuming control diet supplemented with 25% (w/w) dried plum, dried apple, dried apricot, dried grape or dried mango for 8 weeks. Dried plum, apple, and apricot were provided by Mayan Sun Inc. (Yakima, Washington), while the dried grape and mango were prepared following a similar drying protocol in our laboratory. All diets were isocaloric and adjusted for macronutrient, calcium, phosphorus, and fiber content. Food intake and body weights were monitored and recorded weekly.

At the end of the study, animals were anesthetized using ketamine/xylazine, whole body dual-energy x-ray absorptiometry (DXA; LunarPIXI, GE Medical Systems, Madison, WI) scans were performed to determine whole body composition and bone density, and animals were exsanguinated via the carotid artery. A femur was cleaned of soft adhering tissue and the bone marrow was flushed with ice cold phosphate buffered saline (PBS) using a 25 mm gauge needle. Both the flushed femur and bone marrow were processed for RNA extraction. One tibia and the spine were also excised and cleaned of soft tissue. Bone densitometry of the spine was performed and both the tibia and 4th lumbar vertebra were analyzed for structural alterations by micro-computerized tomography (μCT). This study was carried out in strict accordance with the recommendations in the Guide for the Care and Use of Laboratory Animals of the National Institutes of Health. The protocol was approved by the Institutional Animal Care and Use Committee of Oklahoma State University (ACUP#HE096).

Bone Densitometry Assessment

In addition to whole body bone mineral area (BMA), content (BMC), and density (BMD), excised spines were also scanned on a plastic platform and a region of interest (ROI) was identified to include the 4th and 5th lumbar vertebra (i.e., L4 and L5). All DXA scans were analyzed using PIXImus Series Software version 1.4x.

Histology of the Proximal Tibia

Excised tibias were fixed in 10% neutral buffered formalin (NBF) for 48 hours and then transferred to 70% ethanol. Tibias were then decalcified in Cal-Rite (Thermo Scientific, Richard Allan Scientific) and processed by dehydration through sequential ethanol steps, cleared with toluene, and paraffin embedded. Tibias were cut in the sagittal plane (5 μm) using a microtome (Leica RM2165, Wetzlar, Germany), and sections stained with hematoxylin and eosin.

Microcomputed Tomography Analyses

Bone microarchitecture of the tibia and 4th lumbar vertebra was assessed by micro-computed tomography (μCT40, SCANCO Medical, Switzerland). The proximal tibial metaphysis and mid-diaphysis were used to analyze trabecular and cortical bone, respectively. Scans of the tibial metaphysis were performed at a resolution of 2048×2048 pixels. Semi-automated contours, starting 60 μm distal to the proximal growth plate, included a 750 μm volume of interest (VOI) of only secondary spongiosa for analysis of trabecular bone. Trabecular parameters evaluated included bone volume expressed per unit of total volume (BV/TV), trabecular number (Tb.N.), trabecular thickness (Tb.Th.), trabecular separation (Tb.Sp.) connectivity density (ConnDens) and structural model index (SMI). Analysis of cortical bone was performed by analyzing a 120 μm section at the mid-point of the tibia. Assessment of cortical bone parameters included cortical porosity, thickness, area, and medullary area of the tibial mid-diaphysis. The acquired images were analyzed at a threshold of 300, and a sigma of 0.7 and support of 1.0 were used for both trabecular and cortical bone of the tibia.

Analyses of the spine were performed by acquiring images at a resolution of 1024×1024 pixels, 80 μm from the dorsal and caudal growth plates. Similar to the tibial analysis, semi-automated contours were placed to assess secondary spongiosa within the VOI. The images were analyzed at a threshold of 340, and a sigma and support of 1.2 and 2.0, respectively.

Biomechanical Testing of Vertebra and Tibia with Finite Element Analysis

Finite element (FE) analysis software (SCANCO Medical) was used to evaluate alterations in biomechanical properties of the trabecular bone. Voxels from the VOI were converted into 8-node brick elements from micromechanical FE [40]. The elements in this FE model had linear, elastic and isotropic material properties. Simulated compression testing was applied on trabecular regions of the vertebral body and tibial metaphysis at a constant force. Total force, stiffness, and size-independent stiffness were determined.

Analysis of Plasma Antioxidant Capacity

Due to the potential influence dried fruits have on oxidative status, along with the impact this may have on osteoblast and osteoclast activity, plasma glutathione peroxidase (GPx) activity was determined using a commercially available kit from Cayman Chemical (Cat#703102, Ann Arbor, MI) [26,29,41,42]. All samples were diluted 1:2 and the assay was carried out according to the manufacture's protocol. The intra- and inter-assay coefficients for the GPx assay were 5.7% and 7.2%.

RNA Extraction and Quantitative Real-Time PCR

Alterations in the expression of genes associated with bone metabolism and apoptosis were assessed in bone by quantitative real-time PCR (qRT-PCR). Total RNA was extracted from pulverized-flushed femurs (Spex 6770 Freezer Mill, Metuchen, NJ) and bone marrow using Trizol Reagent and following the manufacturers protocol (Life Technology, Rockville, MD, USA). The hard tissue and bone marrow specimens were assessed separately because they represent an osteoblast rich cite and a cite in which osteoclasts reside [43]. RNA from the bone marrow was further purified with a second Trizol extraction. The A_{260}/A_{280} ratio was obtained using a Nanodrop Spectrophotometer (Rockland, DE) to determine quantity of RNA and gel electrophoresis was carried out to verify the quality of all RNA samples. qRT-PCR was then performed using 2 µg of total RNA pre-treated with DNase I and subjected to reverse-transcription (Superscript II, Invitrogen, Carlsbad, CA). cDNA (50 ng) was used for each qRT-PCR reaction and all reactions were assayed in duplicate using SYBR green chemistry (SABiosciences, Valencia, CA) on the Applied Biosystems 7900HT Fast Real-Time PCR System (Foster City, CA). All qRT-PCR results were evaluated by the comparative cycle number at threshold (C_T) method (User Manual #2, Applied Biosystems), using cyclophilin b (*Cyclo*) as the invariant control (**Table 1**).

Statistical Analysis

Statistical analyses were accomplished using SAS Version 9.2 (SAS Institute, NC). Comparisons were made between dietary treatment groups using one-way ANOVA, followed by *post hoc* analysis with Fischer's least square means separation test when F values were significant. Student's paired t-test was used for comparisons made between the sham-operated (Sham) and OVX groups at baseline. The percent change in trabecular bone was calculated by determining the difference between the OVX group mean BV/TV at baseline and BV/TV of individual animals within a given treatment at the final time point, and then dividing that value by the baseline value. All data are presented as mean ± standard error (SE) and α was set at 0.05.

Results

Body Weight, Body Composition, and Uterine Weights

At the end of the 2 week baseline period, there were no differences in initial body weight or body composition between the Sham and OVX animals (*data not shown*), but as anticipated after the 8 week treatment period the OVX group on control diet weighed significantly more than the Sham group (**Table 2**). The OVX control animals also had greater body fat mass and percent fat, while no alterations were observed in lean mass (**Table 2**). The dried plum, apple, and mango groups had lower body weight compared to the OVX control group and the mean body weight and body composition (*i.e.*, fat mass and percent fat) of the dried plum and apple groups were similar to the Sham. Although the dried apricot and grape diets did not prevent OVX-induced weight gain, animal consuming these diets had a lower fat mass and percent fat compared to OVX animals on control diet (**Table 2**). It is important to note that these body weight and body composition changes occurred despite no difference in food intake between any of the OVX groups.

The reduction in uterine weights in all OVX groups confirmed ovarian hormone deficiency was achieved with surgery and the absence of any estrogenic effects (*i.e.*, increase in uterine weight) associated with any of the dietary regimens (*data not shown*).

Bone Mineral Area, Content and Density

Two weeks post-surgery, DXA analysis confirmed a decrease ($p < 0.05$) in whole body (Sham = 49.8 ± 0.5 mg/ cm^2; OVX = 48.0 ± 0.6 mg/ cm^2) and spine (Sham = 47.3 ± 0.8 mg/ cm^2; OVX = 43.9 ± 0.8 mg/ cm^2) BMD in the OVX compared to the Sham baseline groups. After 8 weeks of treatment, the groups consuming the dried plum, apricot and grape supplemented diets had a higher whole body and spine BMD compared to the OVX cohort (**Table 2**). These improvements in whole body and spine BMD with dried plum were a result of increased BMC compared to the OVX animals on control diet. In contrast, the animals receiving the apricot supplemented diet exhibited an increase in whole body BMC, but to a lesser extent than that observed in the dried plum group. The increase in whole body and spine BMD in the group receiving the grape supplemented diet was not due to any statistically significant alterations in BMC compared to the OVX control animals.

Trabecular and Cortical Bone Microarchitecture

A representative micrograph from each treatment group is shown to depict gross-morphological alterations occurring in the proximal tibia after 8 weeks of dietary treatment (**Figure 1A**). To further examine the changes in the trabecular and cortical bone compartments of the tibia and lumbar vertebra, µCT scans of the proximal tibial metaphysis and the fourth lumbar vertebra were analyzed. At baseline, trabecular bone BV/TV tended to decrease in the proximal tibial metaphysis (Sham = 11.0 ± 0.5%, OVX = 8.8 ± 0.1%; $p = 0.0627$) and vertebral body (Sham = 12.7 ± 0.7%, OVX = 10.9 ± 0.6%; $p = 0.0521$), which is similar to previous reports in our laboratory with OVX-induced bone loss [30]. No alterations were observed in cortical bone at baseline (*data not shown*).

By the end of the 8 week dietary treatment period, the OVX animals on control diet had experienced an approximately 40% loss of trabecular bone (*i.e.*, BV/TV) at both the vertebral and tibial sites (**Figure 1B**). While the dried plum and apricot groups had a higher vertebral BV/TV (**Figure 1B**) and Tb.N. (**Table 3**) than the OVX control group ($p<0.05$), the only animals that had a similar BV/TV to the Sham were the mice on the dried plum diet. Based on comparisons to the OVX animals at baseline, dried plum had an anabolic effect on trabecular bone at the vertebral site (**Figure 2**) but only prevented bone loss at the proximal tibia. Vertebral Tb.Th. also increased in the dried plum group, an effect that was not observed with the other dietary treatments (**Table 3**). At the tibial site, dried plum was the only dietary treatment in which BV/TV (**Figure 1B**) and Tb.N. (**Table 3**) were

Table 1. List of Validated Primer Sequences used for qRT-PCR.

NCBI Gene Accession Reference	Symbol	Name	Sequence
NM_007431	*Alp*	Alkaline phosphatase	QF 5′- GGT ATG GGC GTC TCC ACA GT -3′
			QR 5′- GCC CGT GTT GTG GTG TAG CT -3′
NM_007523.2	*Bak1*	Bcl-2 homologous antagonist/killer-1	QF 5′- ACG AAC TCT TCA CCA CCA AGA TCG CCT -3′
			QR 5′- TCA AAC CAC GCT GGT AGA CGT ACA -3′
NM_001032298	*Ocn*	Osteocalcin	QF 5′- TGA GCT TAA CCC TGC TTG TGA CGA -3′
			QR 5′- AGG GCA CAG GTC CTA AAT AGT -3′
NM_009810	*Casp3*	Caspase-3	QF 5′- CAT AAG AGC ACT GGA ATG TCA TCT C -3′
			QR 5′- CCC ATG AAT GTC TCT CTG AGG TT -3′
NM_009811	*Casp9*	Caspase-9	QF 5′- CTG GGA CGC TCT GCT GAG T -3′
			QR 5′- CCA GAT CCT GCC TGC TGA AT -3′
NM_007742	*Col1a1*	Collagen Type 1	QF 5′- CGT CTG GTT TGG AGA GAG CAT -3′
			QR 5′- GGT CAG CTG GAT AGC GAC ATC -3′
NM_011149	*Cyclo*	Cyclophilin B	QF 5′- TGG AGA GCA CCA AGA CAG ACA -3′
			QR 5′- TGC CGG AGT CGA CAA TGA T -3′
NM_016791	*Nfatc1*	Nuclear factor of activated T-cells, cytoplasmic 1	QF 5′- GCG AAG CCC AAG TCT CTT TCC -3′
			QR 5′- GTA TGG ACC AGA ATG TGA -3′
NM_008764	*Opg*	Osteoprotegerin	QF 5′- TCC TGG CAC CTA CCT AAA ACA GCA -3′
			QR 5′- ACA CTG GGC TGC AAT ACA CA -3′
NM_011613	*Rankl*	Receptor activator for nuclear factor κ B ligand	QF 5′- CTG ATG AAA GGA GGG AGC AC -3′
			QR 5′- GAA GGG TTG GAC ACC TGA ATG -3′

comparable to the Sham animals. While no dietary treatment was able to reverse the OVX increase in tibial Tb.Sp., dried plum was similar to both the OVX control and Sham control groups (**Table 3**).

Consistent with the other μCT data reported in the vertebra, non-morphometric parameters revealed an OVX-dependent compromise in trabecular bone connectivity density, SMI, and density that both the dried plum and apricot diets were able to restore after 8 weeks (**Table 2**). In the tibia, only an OVX effect

Table 2. Body Weight and Composition, and Bone Densitometry of the Whole Body and Spine after 8 Weeks on Dietary Treatments.

	Sham	OVX-Control	OVX-Plum	OVX-Apple	OVX-Apricot	OVX-Grape	OVX-Mango
Final Body Weight (*g*)	24.9 ± 0.6^{d}	31.2 ± 0.7^{a}	26.1 ± 0.9^{cd}	26.1 ± 1.0^{cd}	29.1 ± 1.2^{ab}	29.1 ± 1.0^{ab}	28.2 ± 1.1^{bc}
Body Composition							
Lean Mass (g)	17.3 ± 0.4	18.7 ± 0.2	18.1 ± 0.5	18.0 ± 0.6	18.6 ± 0.5	18.3 ± 0.5	18.3 ± 0.5
Fat Mass (g)	6.2 ± 0.3^{c}	11.7 ± 0.6^{a}	6.1 ± 0.6^{c}	6.3 ± 0.4^{c}	9.1 ± 0.7^{b}	9.7 ± 0.6^{b}	8.7 ± 0.8^{b}
Percent Fat (%)	26.3 ± 0.6^{c}	38.3 ± 1.0^{a}	25.0 ± 1.3^{c}	25.6 ± 0.9^{c}	32.4 ± 1.4^{b}	34.5 ± 1.1^{b}	31.7 ± 1.6^{b}
Bone Densitometry							
Whole Body							
BMD (mg/cm²)	53.8 ± 0.5^{a}	47.3 ± 0.4^{e}	49.2 ± 0.5^{bc}	47.8 ± 0.4^{de}	49.8 ± 0.4^{b}	48.9 ± 0.5^{bcd}	48.3 ± 0.4^{cde}
BMC (mg)	564.1 ± 15.2^{a}	414.9 ± 14.1^{f}	513.2 ± 9.0^{b}	481.9 ± 10.0^{c}	480.2 ± 9.7^{cd}	445.2 ± 9.5^{ef}	450.4 ± 5.9^{de}
BMA (cm²)	10.5 ± 0.2^{a}	8.8 ± 0.3^{e}	10.4 ± 0.2^{a}	10.1 ± 0.2^{ab}	9.6 ± 0.2^{bc}	9.1 ± 0.2^{de}	9.3 ± 0.1^{cd}
Spine							
BMD (mg/cm²)	56.7 ± 1.6^{a}	44.1 ± 1.0^{c}	48.4 ± 0.8^{b}	46.0 ± 0.9^{bc}	47.35 ± 0.6^{b}	48.0 ± 1.3^{b}	45.6 ± 1.0^{bc}
BMC (mg)	17.0 ± 0.6^{a}	13.0 ± 0.6^{cd}	14.5 ± 0.2^{b}	12.3 ± 0.4^{d}	13.6 ± 0.3^{bc}	13.3 ± 0.3^{cd}	13.0 ± 0.4^{cd}
BMA (cm²)	0.30 ± 0.01^{a}	0.30 ± 0.01^{a}	0.30 ± 0.01^{a}	0.27 ± 0.01^{c}	0.29 ± 0.01^{ab}	0.28 ± 0.01^{bc}	0.29 ± 0.01^{abc}

Final body weight, body composition, and dual energy x-ray absorptiometry (DXA) scans of the whole body and spine after 8 weeks of sham-operated (Sham) and ovariectomized (OVX) mice fed control diet or OVX receiving control diet supplemented with either 25% (w/w) dried plum, apple, apricot, grape, or mango. Values are means ± SE, $n = 8$ mice in each group. Within a given row, groups that share the same superscript letter are not significantly different ($p<0.05$) from each other.

A.

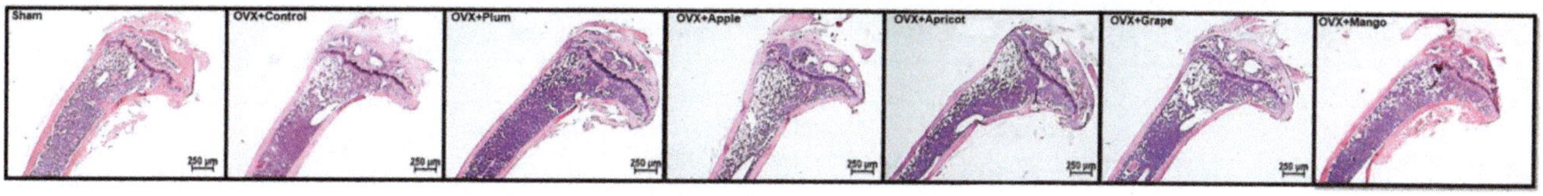

B.

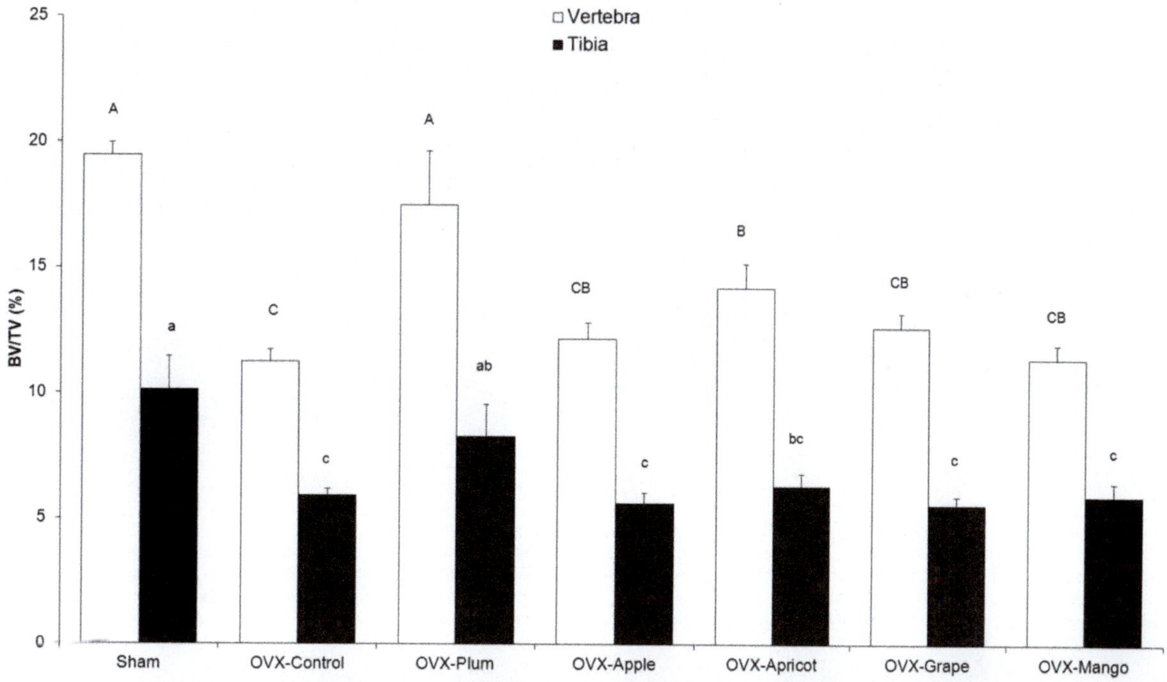

Figure 1. Histological Images of the Tibia and μCT Analyses of Trabecular Bone Volume in the Vertebra and Tibia. Representative images of the proximal tibia are shown with H&E stain following the 8 week treatment period (A). Comparisons of trabecular bone morphometric parameters in sham-operated (Sham) and osteopenic ovariectomized (OVX) mice fed control diet, or control diet supplemented with either 25% (w/w) dried plum, apple, apricot, grape, or mango. Trabecular bone microarchitectural of (B) bone volume/total volume (BV/TV) in the vertebral body (□) and proximal tibia (■). Bars represent the mean ± SE, $n = 6$ mice in each group. Bars that share the same superscript letter are not significantly different from each other ($p<0.05$).

was observed in connectivity density and apparent mean/ density; however, dried plum had an intermediate effect on SMI.

Analysis of cortical bone parameters of the tibial mid diaphysis revealed a reduced cortical thickness ($p<0.05$) in all OVX animals, regardless of the dietary regimen (**Table 3**). No difference was observed in cortical area between any of the OVX groups. No effect of OVX or dietary treatments was observed on medullary area after 8 weeks.

Biomechanical Properties of Trabecular Bone

Finite element (FE) analysis revealed decreased total force, stiffness, and size independent stiffness in the trabecular bone of the vertebral body of the OVX control animals compared to Sham (**Table 4**). However, all vertebral biomechanical parameters of the OVX groups receiving dried plum and apricot diets were completely reversed to the level of the Sham animals (**Table 4**). Dried grape was able to improve total force values compared to OVX control diet, however, not to the level of Sham (**Table 4**). Although a trend in total force ($p=0.0571$) and stiffness ($p=0.0554$) was observed in the tibia between groups, the only significant treatment effect was an increase in size independent stiffness in the dried plum group compared to all other groups (**Table 4**).

Plasma GPx Activity

Evaluation of systemic antioxidant activity revealed that the Sham and OVX control groups had similar plasma GPx activity, but the dried plum, grape, and mango groups significantly increased GPx activity compared to the OVX control (**Figure 3**). The apple and apricot diets appeared to have minimal to no impact on plasma antioxidant status compared to animals the groups receiving the control diet (**Figure 3**).

Osteoblast and Osteoclast Differentiation, Activity and Apoptosis

The relative abundance of mRNA encoding proteins associated with osteoclast differentiation and activity were assessed using total RNA prepared from bone marrow aspirates. The abundance of the mRNA encoding the osteoclastogenesis regulator, nuclear factor of activator T-cells cytoplasmic 1 (*Nfatc1*), was up-regulated in OVX control animals as would be expected compared to the Sham. The dried plum and apple diets suppressed the OVX-

Table 3. Bone Microarchitectural Parameters of the Lumbar Vertebra and Tibia.

	Sham	OVX-Control	OVX-Plum	OVX-Apple	OVX-Apricot	OVX-Grape	OVX-Mango
Vertebral Body							
Tb.N. (1/mm)	3.95 ± 0.06^{a}	2.96 ± 0.11^{c}	3.99 ± 0.26^{a}	3.08 ± 0.14^{bc}	3.50 ± 0.18^{b}	3.14 ± 0.11^{bc}	2.99 ± 0.10^{c}
Tb.Th. (mm)	0.049 ± 0.001^{a}	0.038 ± 0.001^{c}	0.043 ± 0.002^{b}	0.039 ± 0.001^{c}	0.040 ± 0.001^{bc}	0.040 ± 0.001^{bc}	0.038 ± 0.001^{c}
Tb.Sp.(mm)	0.20 ± 0.01^{d}	0.30 ± 0.01^{a}	0.21 ± 0.02^{cd}	0.29 ± 0.02^{a}	0.25 ± 0.02^{bc}	0.28 ± 0.01^{ab}	0.30 ± 0.01^{a}
ConnDens (1/mm^{3})	119.5 ± 6.7^{a}	85.1 ± 6.9^{b}	137.2 ±10.6^{a}	81.0 ± 6.3^{b}	119.4 ± 8.9^{a}	91.8 ± 6.8^{b}	88.8 ± 5.5^{b}
SMI	1.2 ± 0.1^{c}	1.8 ± 0.1^{a}	1.3 ± 0.2^{c}	1.7 ± 0.1^{ab}	1.5 ± 0.1^{bc}	1.6 ± 0.1^{ab}	1.8 ± 0.1^{a}
Tb.Density (mg/cm^{3})	299.4 ± 5.0^{a}	208.35 ± 11.2^{c}	282.9 ± 20.8^{a}	227.4 ± 7.0^{bc}	247.4 ± 9.6^{b}	234.1 ± 6.2^{bc}	223.1 ± 13.2^{bc}
Proximal Tibial Metaphysis							
Tb.N. (1/mm)	2.91 ± 0.29^{a}	1.86 ± 0.11^{b}	2.20 ± 0.23^{a}	1.75 ± 0.13^{b}	1.92 ± 0.16^{b}	1.72 ± 0.08^{b}	1.74 ± 0.15^{b}
Tb.Th. (mm)	0.034 ± 0.001^{a}	0.032 ± 0.001^{b}	0.033 ± 0.001^{ab}	0.032 ± 0.001^{ab}	0.033 ± 0.001^{ab}	0.032 ± 0.001^{ab}	0.034 ± 0.001^{ab}
Tb.Sp.(mm)	0.32 ± 0.03^{c}	0.51 ± 0.03^{ab}	0.44 ± 0.05^{bc}	0.55 ± 0.05^{a}	0.50 ± 0.05^{ab}	0.55 ± 0.24^{a}	0.56 ± 0.05^{a}
ConnDens (1/mm^{3})	69.2 ± 7.9^{a}	32.2 ± 5.1^{bc}	43.8 ± 13.2^{b}	25.7 ± 4.2^{bc}	30.8 ± 7.5^{bc}	15.9 ± 1.2^{c}	30.3 ± 4.8^{bc}
SMI	1.8 ± 0.2^{b}	2.4 ± 0.1^{a}	2.1 ± 0.1^{ab}	2.3 ± 0.1^{a}	2.2 ± 0.1^{a}	2.34 ± 0.1^{a}	2.27 ± 0.03^{a}
Tb.Density (mg/cm^{3})	137.3 ± 16.1^{a}	80.9 ± 9.6^{bc}	104.0 ± 17.8^{b}	66.8 ± 5.5^{c}	76.7 ± 7.2^{bc}	67.8 ± 4.3^{c}	72.0 ± 7.0^{c}
Tibia Diaphysis							
Cort.Th. (mm)	0.22 ± 0.04^{a}	0.20 ± 0.03^{bc}	0.21 ± 0.01^{ac}	0.20 ± 0.01^{b}	0.20 ± 0.01^{b}	0.20 ± 0.01^{b}	0.21 ± 0.01^{b}
Cort. Area (mm^{2})	0.62 ± 0.01^{a}	0.59 ± 0.01^{ab}	0.60 ± 0.02^{ac}	0.55 ± 0.01^{b}	0.58 ± 0.01^{ab}	0.54 ± 0.02^{b}	0.55 ± 0.01^{bc}
Cort.Med. Area (mm^{2})	0.86 ± 0.05	0.86 ± 0.04	0.89 ± 0.11	0.83 ± 0.01	0.84 ± 0.02	0.80 ± 0.03	0.75 ± 0.04
Porosity (%)	2.78 ± 0.1	2.99 ± 0.1	2.96 ± 0.1	3.14± 0.1	2.87 ± 0.05	2.84 ± 0.1	3.02 ± 0.1

Trabecular bone microarchitectural parameters include: bone volume/total volume trabecular number (Tb.N.), trabecular thickness (Tb.Th.), trabecular separation (Tb.Sp.), connectivity density (ConnsDens), structural model index (SMI), and trabecular density (Tb.Density) of the spine and proximal tibia. Cortical bone includes cortical thickness (Cort.Th.), cortical area (Cort. Area), medullary area (Cort.Med. Area) and cortical porosity of the of the tibial mid-diaphysis from sham-operated (Sham) and ovariectomized (OVX) mice fed control diet or OVX receiving control diet supplemented with either 25% (w/w) dried plum, apple, apricot, grape, or mango for 8 weeks. Values are means ± SE, n = 8 mice in each group. Within a given row, groups that share the same superscript letter are not significantly different ($p<0.05$) from each other.

induced increase in *Nfatc1* and restored the relative level of expression to that of the Sham group (**Figure 4A**). No alterations were observed in mRNA abundance of receptor activator for NF-κB ligand (*Rankl*) or osteoprotegerin (*Opg*) (*data not shown*).

To determine alterations in osteoblast activity, RNA from flushed femurs was used to assess gene expression. Type I collagen (*Colla1*) gene expression was increased by OVX and remained elevated in the dried plum, apple and mango groups (**Figure 4C**).

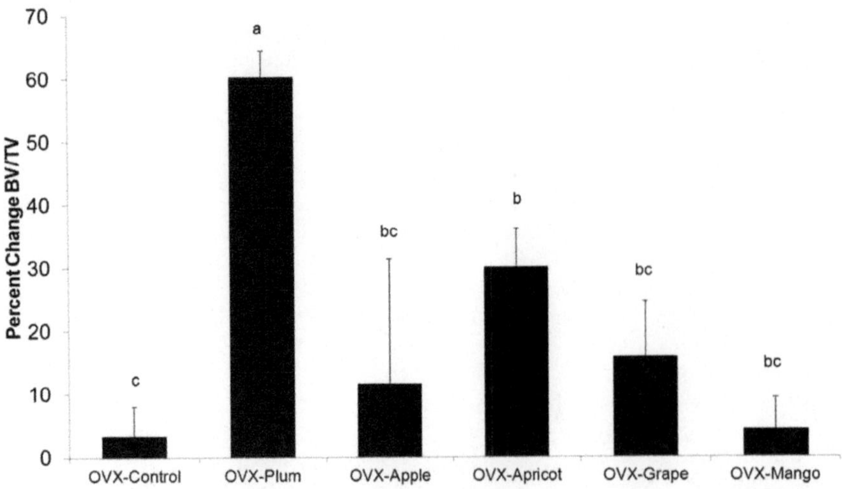

Figure 2. Percent Change in Vertebral Trabecular Bone Normalized to OVX-Control at Baseline. Percent change in vertebral BV/TV in ovariectomized (OVX) mice fed control diet, or control diet supplemented with either 25% (w/w) dried plum, apple, apricot, grape, or mango relative to baseline OVX controls. The percent change was calculated by determining the difference between the OVX group mean BV/TV at baseline and BV/TV of individual animals at the final time point, and then expressing that value relative to baseline. Bars represent the mean ± SE, n = 6 mice in each group. Bars that share the same superscript letter are not significantly different from each other ($p<0.05$).

Table 4. Biomechanical Properties of Trabecular Bone in the Lumbar Vertebra and Proximal Tibia.

	Sham	OVX-Control	OVX-Plum	OVX-Apple	OVX-Apricot	OVX-Grape	OVX-Mango
Vertebra							
Total Force (N)	1.6 ± 0.2[a]	0.6 ± 0.1[b]	1.7 ± 0.4[a]	0.9 ± 0.1[bc]	1.2 ± 0.2[ac]	1.1 ± 0.1[bc]	0.6 ± 0.1[b]
Stiffness (1×10^3N/m)	273.1 ± 32.0[ac]	113.6 ± 14.7[b]	308.2 ± 68.4[a]	166.5± 16.3[bd]	212.6 ± 26.0[cd]	187.2 ± 20.9[bc]	112.2 ± 11.5[b]
Size Independent Stiffness (N/m)	4.86 ± 0.52[a]	1.9 ± 0.2[c]	4.9 ± 1.1[a]	2.7 ± 0.2[bc]	3.4 ± 0.5[ab]	3.0 ± 0.3[bc]	1.8 ± 0.2[bc]
Tibia							
Total Force (N)	0.60 ± 0.24	0.46 ± 0.12	1.25 ± 0.41	0.39 ± 0.08	0.37 ± 0.17	0.36 ± 0.13	0.32 ± 0.16
Stiffness (1×10^3N/m)	271.6 ± 107.2	209.9 ± 51.8	562.0 ± 184.1	175.1 ± 36.6	168.8 ± 75.0	161.0 ± 59.8	142.9 ± 71.8
Size Independent Stiffness (N/m)	0.94 ± 0.36[b]	0.64 ± 0.15[b]	2.14 ± 0.71[a]	0.63 ± 0.14[b]	0.62 ± 0.29[b]	0.63 ± 0.22[b]	0.55 ± 0.29[b]

Finite element (FE) analysis of trabecular bone in the lumbar vertebra and proximal tibial metaphysis of sham-operated (Sham) and ovariectomized (OVX) mice fed control diet or OVX receiving control diet supplemented with either 25% (w/w) dried plum, apple, apricot, grape, or mango for 8 weeks. Values are means ± SE, $n = 6$ mice in each group. Within a given row, groups that share the same superscript letter are not significantly different ($p<0.05$) from each other.

No statistically significant alterations were detected in alkaline phosphatase (*Alp*) or osteocalcin (*Ocn*) due to OVX or dietary treatments at the end of the study, which was indicative of no transcriptional regulation of osteoblast activity or mineralization (**Figure 4B and 4D**).

Another plausible mechanism by which the dietary treatments altered bone formation and resorption in the OVX model was by regulating osteoblast and osteoclast apoptosis. In the osteoclast and osteoclast precursor rich bone marrow, Bcl-2 homologous antagonist/ killer 1 (*Bak1*), which promotes apoptosis by forming channels in outer mitochondrial membrane, mRNA abundance was up-regulated by all of the dried fruits except mango, compared to the levels of OVX control animals (**Figure 5A**). In hard tissue (*i.e.*, flushed femur), the essential proteases involved in the apoptotic process, caspase-9 (*Casp9*) and its downstream target caspase-3 (*Casp3*), gene expression was down-regulated in response to OVX, but no dietary treatment altered this response (**Figure 5C and 5D**).

Discussion

The bone densitometry data confirm that dried plum, and to a lesser extent apricot and grape, have the ability to protect bone in osteopenic OVX C57BL/6 mice. Evaluation of the bone microarchitectural parameters revealed that dried plum prevented the loss of trabecular bone in the proximal tibia and was the only fruit to exert an anabolic effect on the trabecular bone of the vertebra. These alterations in the vertebral trabecular bone of animals receiving dried plum coincided with improved biomechanical properties, including bone strength and stiffness. These improvements in the biomechanical and structural properties suggest that dried plum supplementation results in enhanced bone quality.

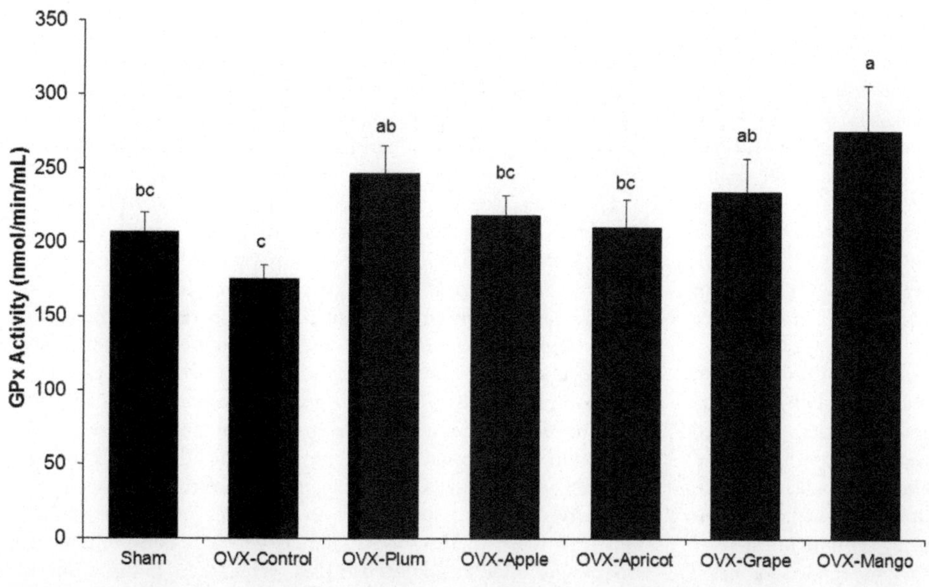

Figure 3. Alterations in Plasma Glutathione Peroxidase Activity (GPx) with Dried Fruit Treatments. Comparisons of plasma GPx in sham-operated (Sham) and ovariectomized (OVX) mice fed control diet, or control diet supplemented with either 25% (w/w) dried plum, apple, apricot, grape, or mango for 8 weeks. Bars represent the mean ± SE, $n = 8$ mice in each group. Bars that share the same superscript letter are not significantly different from each other ($p<0.05$).

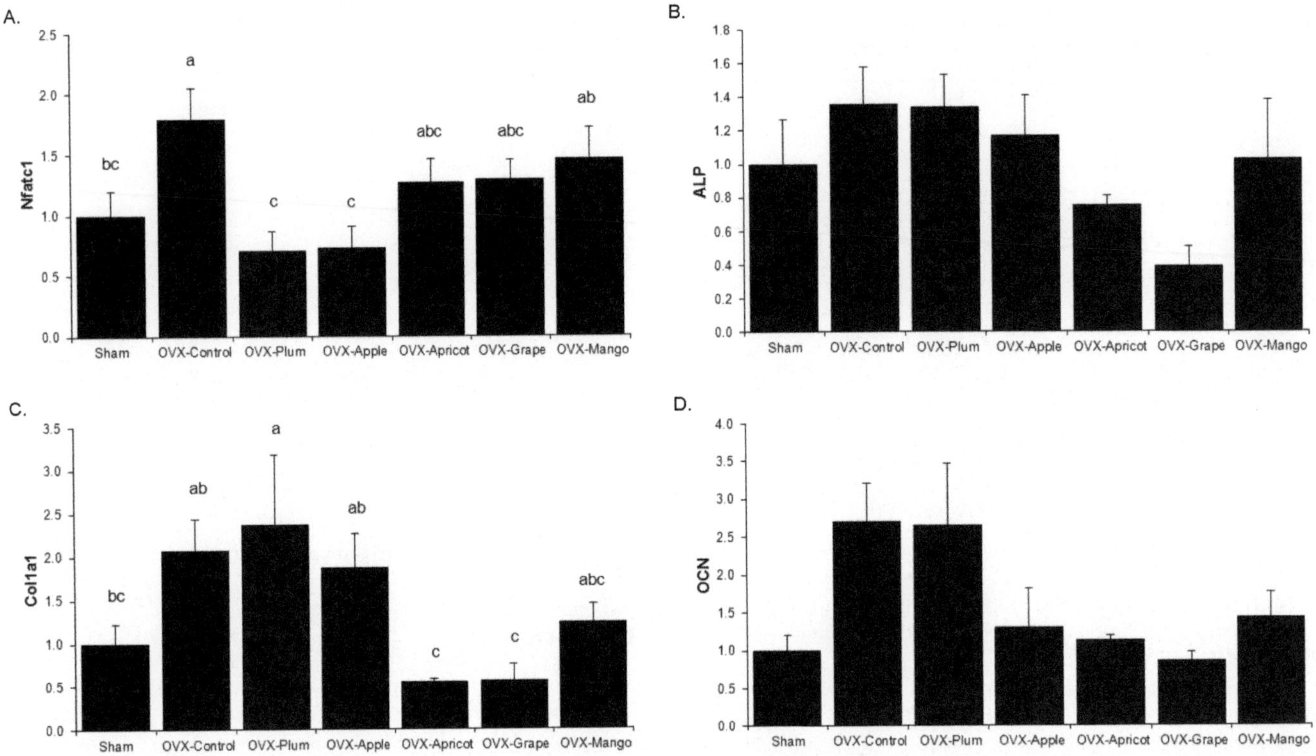

Figure 4. qRT-PCR Analyses of Genes Involved in Osteoclastogenesis and Osteoblast Activity. Bone marrow (A) was analyzed for relative mRNA abundance of the osteoclastgensis gene nuclear factor of activated T-cells (*Nfatc1*), while the flushed femur (B-D) was used to assess genes involved in osteoblast activity and function: alkaline phosphatase (*Alp*), type 1 collagen (*Col1a1*), and osteocalcin (*Ocn*) in sham-operated (Sham) and ovariectomized (OVX) mice fed control diet, or control diet supplemented with either 25% (w/w) dried plum, apple, apricot, grape, or mango. Bars represent the mean ± SE, $n = 6$ mice in each group. Bars that share the same superscript letter are not significantly different from each other ($p<0.05$).

Due to the role of oxidative stress in bone loss resulting from estrogen deficiency and reports by others that natural compounds in foods can increase plasma GPx in conjunction with improved bone indices, GPx activity was assessed [27–29]. The groups supplemented with dried plum, grape and mango groups experienced an increase plasma GPx activity compared to the OVX-control group; however, the lack of a skeletal response in the mango group suggests the favorable effects of dried plum on bone are not solely dependent on GPx antioxidant activity. Our results do not rule out that other antioxidant systems (*e.g.*, catalase activity and superoxide dismutase) altered in response to dried fruit consumption are responsible for the positive effects observed on bone, but these systems warrant further investigation before conclusions regarding the role of antioxidant systems in this context can be made [26,44].

Due to the apparent novelty of dried plum to not only prevent catabolic activity but also have anabolic effects on bone at some skeletal sites, the relative mRNA abundance of key genes involved in the regulation osteoblast and osteoclast differentiation and activity were assessed. Dried plum decreased osteoclastogenesis through the attenuation of *Nfatc1* gene expression, while simultaneously up-regulating osteoblast activity by enhancing *Col1a1* mRNA. This data is consistent with previous reports of dried plum's dual anti-resorptive and anabolic actions which represents an uncoupling of bone turnover in favor of accrual of new bone tissue [30,35]. Although *Rankl* expression was not altered in this study, NFATc1 is the key transcription factor that regulates osteoclastogenesis and is a downstream target of RANK-RANKL signaling. Taken together, these data suggest that dried plum did not regulate *Rankl* at a transcriptional level in this study. Interestingly, dried apple also decreased *Nfatc1* and *Col1a1* transcription, but these alterations in mRNA were not accompanied with beneficial effects on BMD or trabecular bone volume at this time point. These findings raise the issue that dried plum has additional effects, perhaps in part tied to its influence on antioxidant systems that ultimately lead to its unique ability to restore bone

The concept that dried plum and other fruits could be altering osteoblast and osteoclast via apoptosis was also explored in this study. Our data show that OVX decreased *Bak1* gene expression in the bone marrow compared to Sham, suggesting estrogen withdrawal not only promotes osteoclastogenesis by up-regulating *Nfatc1* but also attempts to suppress mitochondria-mediated apoptosis. Dried plum, apple, apricot, and grape prevented the OVX-induced decrease in *Bak1* gene expression, which indicates that the dried plum and apple groups not only suppressed the formation of osteoclasts but may prohibit the OVX-induced decrease in apoptosis. Conversely, in the hard tissue there were no effects of dietary treatments on the relative abundance of *Casp3* and -*9* mRNA in the OVX animals which is consistent with a decrease in osteoblast apoptosis [28]. While these findings provide some evidence of apoptotic regulation by dried plum in the current study, the discrepancies between the early apoptosis marker *Bak1* versus the later apoptosis markers, *Casp9* and *Casp3,* suggest a possible difference in transcriptional regulation of apoptosis in bone marrow and mineralized bone.

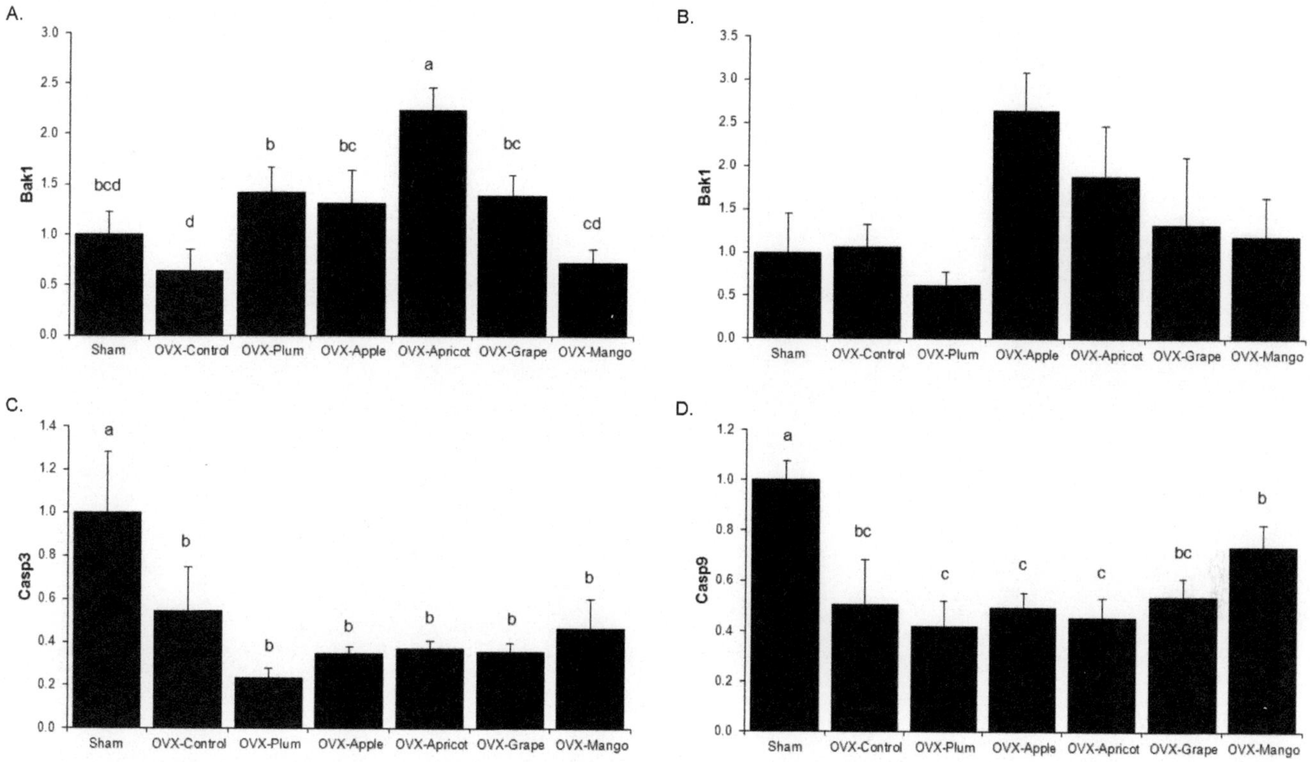

Figure 5. Relative mRNA Abundance of Apoptotic Genes. The relative mRNA abundance of apoptotic genes was assessed in the bone marrow (A) and flushed femur (B–D). Genes of interest including, B-cell lymphoma homologous antagonist/killer (*Bak1*), caspase -3 (*Casp3*) and 9 (*Casp9*) from sham-operated (Sham) and ovariectomized (OVX) mice fed control diet, or control diet supplemented with either 25% (w/w) dried plum, apple, apricot, grape, or mango. Bars represent the mean ± SE, $n = 6$ mice in each group. Bars that share the same superscript letter are not significantly different from each other ($p<0.05$).

Dried plum's ability to both prevent bone loss and restore bone has been postulated to be due to the high polyphenol content or perhaps the unique polyphenolic compound profile acting as antioxidant and/or anti-inflammatory agent [34]. A recent report from our laboratory showed that an extract of the total polyphenols from dried plum reduced osteoclastogenesis and up-regulated osteoblast differentiation and activity, both under normal and inflammatory conditions [35,36]. Thus it stands to reason that fruits with similar polyphenolic profiles might be able to exert comparable actions on the skeleton. Dried plum ('Improved French') is rich in hydroxycinnamic acids including, neochlorogenic, cryptochlorogenic, and chlorogenic acid [45,46]. Of the fruits tested in the present study, a large portion of apricot's polyphenolic compounds are made up of neochlorogenic and chlorogenic acid, similar to dried plum [45,47]. Although apricot and, to a lesser extent, apple have similar polyphenolic compounds, dried plum is unique in its combination and overall content of the polyphenols [45,48]. Additionally, dried plums are a good source of other nutrients with known effects on bone, including oligofructose, magnesium, vitamin K, boron and potassium [49,50]. This study suggests that dried plum may represent a unique combination of nutrients and polyphenolic compounds that is responsible for the observed anabolic activity of the skeleton. However, further investigation of the bioactive components is needed and it is premature to draw any specific conclusions at this time.

In summary, this is the first study to demonstrate the extent to which dried plum restores bone in osteopenic OVX animals compared to apple, apricot, grape and mango supplementation. The potency of dried plum was unique in the sense that it not only prevented bone loss, but also induced an anabolic response in the vertebra. These structural changes coincided with local up-regulation of indicators of osteoblast activity and the down-regulation of osteoclastogenesis. These alternations in mediators of bone metabolism occurred in conjunction with enhanced systemic GPx activity. While this study provides new insight into the alterations in bone metabolism as it relates to dried plum, it is clear that further delineation of these mechanisms is warranted. A limitation of this study is that most of the data presented here provide evidence for transcriptional regulation of osteogenesis and it remains to be observed whether dried plum affects osteoblastogenesis and osteoclastogenesis on a translational level as well. Furthermore, the bioactive component(s) in dried plum remain to be identified and ongoing studies are designed to determine whether it is a single component or the unique combination of nutrients and phytochemicals in dried plum that is responsible for the osteoprotective effects. The continued investigation of how dried plum is able to mediate these effects on bone is important in optimizing this potential dietary strategy for osteoporosis prevention and may provide insight for the development of novel interventions for postmenopausal bone loss.

Author Contributions

Conceived and designed the experiments: ER BPH EAL SLC BJS. Performed the experiments: ER KDH DM MRD SLC EAL BJS. Analyzed the data: ER KDH BJS. Contributed reagents/materials/analysis tools: ER BJS SLC EAL. Wrote the paper: ER KDH MRD DM SLC BPH EAL BJS.

References

1. NOF (2002) America's Bone Health: The State of Osteoporosis and Low Bone Mass in Our Nation.
2. The Surgeon General (2004) Bone Health and Osteoporosis: A Report of the Surgeon General.
3. Reszka AA, Halasy-Nagy JM, Masarachia PJ, Rodan GA (1999) Bisphosphonates act directly on the osteoclast to induce caspase cleavage of mst1 kinase during apoptosis. A link between inhibition of the mevalonate pathway and regulation of an apoptosis-promoting kinase. J Biol Chem 274: 34967-34973.
4. Deal C (2004) The use of intermittent human parathyroid hormone as a treatment for osteoporosis. Curr Rheumatol Rep 6: 49-58.
5. Cosman F (2008) Parathyroid hormone treatment for osteoporosis. Curr Opin Endocrinol Diabetes Obes 15: 495-501.
6. Purcell PM, Boyd IW (2005) Bisphosphonates and osteonecrosis of the jaw. Med J Aust 182: 417-418.
7. Gallagher AC, Chambers TJ, Tobias JH (1996) Androgens contribute to the stimulation of cancellous bone formation by ovarian hormones in female rats. Am J Physiol 270: E407-E412.
8. Wronski TJ, Lowry PL, Walsh CC, Ignaszewski LA (1985) Skeletal alterations in ovariectomized rats. Calcif Tissue Int 37: 324-328.
9. Barbagallo M, Carbognani A, Palummeri E, Chiavarini M, Pedrazzoni M, et al. (1989) The comparative effect of ovarian hormone administration on bone mineral status in oophorectomized rats. Bone 10: 113-116.
10. Farage MA, Neill S, MacLean AB (2009) Physiological changes associated with the menstrual cycle: a review. Obstet Gynecol Surv 64: 58-72.
11. Clowes JA, Riggs BL, Khosla S (2005) The role of the immune system in the pathophysiology of osteoporosis. Immunol Rev 208: 207-227.
12. Cenci S, Weitzmann MN, Roggia C, Namba N, Novack D, et al. (2000) Estrogen deficiency induces bone loss by enhancing T-cell production of TNF-alpha. J Clin Invest 106: 1229-1237.
13. Chou CC, Yang JS, Lu HF, Ip SW, Lo C, et al. (2010) Quercetin-mediated cell cycle arrest and apoptosis involving activation of a caspase cascade through the mitochondrial pathway in human breast cancer MCF-7 cells. Arch Pharm Res 33: 1181-1191.
14. Heinonen OP, Albanes D, Virtamo J, Taylor PR, Huttunen JK, et al. (1998) Prostate cancer and supplementation with alpha-tocopherol and beta-carotene: incidence and mortality in a controlled trial. J Natl Cancer Inst 90: 440-446.
15. Hwang ES, Bowen PE (2005) Effects of lycopene and tomato paste extracts on DNA and lipid oxidation in LNCaP human prostate cancer cells. Biofactors 23: 97-105.
16. Kuriyama S, Shimazu T, Ohmori K, Kikuchi N, Nakaya N, et al. (2006) Green tea consumption and mortality due to cardiovascular disease, cancer, and all causes in Japan: the Ohsaki study. JAMA 296: 1255-1265.
17. Lippman SM, Klein EA, Goodman PJ, Lucia MS, Thompson IM, et al. (2009) Effect of selenium and vitamin E on risk of prostate cancer and other cancers: the Selenium and Vitamin E Cancer Prevention Trial (SELECT). JAMA 301: 39-51.
18. Stoner GD, Kresty LA, Carlton PS, Siglin JC, Morse MA (1999) Isothiocyanates and freeze-dried strawberries as inhibitors of esophageal cancer. Toxicol Sci 52: 95-100.
19. Adrian M, Chanut E, Laurant P, Gaume V, Berthelot A (2008) A long-term moderate magnesium-deficient diet aggravates cardiovascular risks associated with aging and increases mortality in rats. J Hypertens 26: 44-52.
20. Basu A, Lucas EA (2007) Mechanisms and effects of green tea on cardiovascular health. Nutr Rev 65: 361-375.
21. Clerici C, Setchell KD, Battezzati PM, Pirro M, Giuliano V, et al. (2007) Pasta naturally enriched with isoflavone aglycons from soy germ reduces serum lipids and improves markers of cardiovascular risk. J Nutr 137: 2270-2278.
22. Peters U, Poole C, Arab L (2001) Does tea affect cardiovascular disease? A meta-analysis. Am J Epidemiol 154: 495-503.
23. Rotondo S, Di Castelnuovo A, de Gaetano G (2001) The relationship between wine consumption and cardiovascular risk: from epidemiological evidence to biological plausibility. Ital Heart J 2: 1-8.
24. Devareddy L, Hooshmand S, Collins JK, Lucas EA, Chai SC, et al. (2008) Blueberry prevents bone loss in ovariectomized rat model of postmenopausal osteoporosis. J Nutr Biochem 19: 694-699.
25. Droke EA, Hager KA, Lerner MR, Lightfoot SA, Stoecker BJ, et al. (2007) Soy isoflavones avert chronic inflammation-induced bone loss and vascular disease. J Inflamm (Lond) 4: 17.
26. Lean JM, Jagger CJ, Kirstein B, Fuller K, Chambers TJ (2005) Hydrogen peroxide is essential for estrogen-deficiency bone loss and osteoclast formation. Endocrinology 146: 728-735. en.2004-1021 [pii];10.1210/en.2004-1021 [doi].
27. Badescu L, Badulescu O, Badescu M, Ciocoiu M (2012) Mechanism by Sambucus nigra Extract Improves Bone Mineral Density in Experimental Diabetes. Evid Based Complement Alternat Med 2012: 848269.10.1155/2012/848269 [doi].
28. Kim WK, Ke K, Sul OJ, Kim HJ, Kim SH, et al. (2011) Curcumin protects against ovariectomy-induced bone loss and decreases osteoclastogenesis. J Cell Biochem 112: 3159-3166. 10.1002/jcb.23242 [doi].
29. Abujazia MA, Muhammad N, Shuid AN, Soelaiman IN (2012) The effects of virgin coconut oil on bone oxidative status in ovariectomised rat. Evid Based Complement Alternat Med 2012: 525079. 10.1155/2012/525079 [doi].
30. Rendina E, Lim YF, Marlow D, Wang Y, Clarke SL, et al. (2012) Dietary supplementation with dried plum prevents ovariectomy-induced bone loss while modulating the immune response in C57BL/6J mice. J Nutr Biochem 23: 60-68. S0955-2863(10)00265-2 [pii];10.1016/j.jnutbio.2010.10.010 [doi].
31. Deyhim F, Stoecker BJ, Brusewitz GH, Devareddy L, Arjmandi BH (2005) Dried plum reverses bone loss in an osteopenic rat model of osteoporosis. Menopause 12: 755-762.
32. Franklin M, Bu SY, Lerner MR, Lancaster EA, Bellmer D, et al. (2006) Dried plum prevents bone loss in a male osteoporosis model via IGF-I and the RANK pathway. Bone 39: 1331-1342.
33. Bu SY, Lucas EA, Franklin M, Marlow D, Brackett DJ, et al. (2007) Comparison of dried plum supplementation and intermittent PTH in restoring bone in osteopenic orchidectomized rats. Osteoporos Int 18: 931-942.
34. Arjmandi BH, Lucas EA, Juma S, Soliman A, Stoecker BJ, et al. (2001) Dried Plum prevents ovarectomy-induced bone loss in rats. JANA 4: 50-56.
35. Bu SY, Lerner M, Stoecker BJ, Boldrin E, Brackett DJ, et al. (2008) Dried Plum Polyphenols Inhibit Osteoclastogenesis by Downregulating NFATc1 and Inflammatory Mediators. Calcif Tissue Int .
36. Bu SY, Hunt TS, Smith BJ (2008) Dried plum polyphenols attenuate the detrimental effects of TNF-alpha on osteoblast function coincident with up-regulation of Runx2, Osterix and IGF-I. J Nutr Biochem.
37. Kono R, Okuno Y, Inada K, Tokuda A, Hashizume H, et al. (2011) A Prunus mume extract stimulated the proliferation and differentiation of osteoblastic MC3T3-E1 cells. Biosci Biotechnol Biochem 75: 1907-1911. JST.JSTAGE/bbb/110264 [pii].
38. Hsu YL, Liang HL, Hung CH, Kuo PL (2009) Syringetin, a flavonoid derivative in grape and wine, induces human osteoblast differentiation through bone morphogenetic protein-2/extracellular signal-regulated kinase 1/2 pathway. Mol Nutr Food Res 53: 1452-1461. 10.1002/mnfr.200800483 [doi].
39. Hooshmand S, Chai SC, Saadat RL, Payton ME, Brummel-Smith K, et al. (2011) Comparative effects of dried plum and dried apple on bone in postmenopausal women. Br J Nutr 106: 923-930. S000711451100119X [pii];10.1017/S000711451100119X [doi].
40. Keyak JH, Meagher JM, Skinner HB, Mote CD Jr (1990) Automated three-dimensional finite element modelling of bone: a new method. J Biomed Eng 12: 389-397.
41. Muthusami S, Ramachandran I, Muthusamy B, Vasudevan G, Prabhu V, et al. (2005) Ovariectomy induces oxidative stress and impairs bone antioxidant system in adult rats. Clin Chim Acta 360: 81-86.
42. Manolagas SC (2010) From estrogen-centric to aging and oxidative stress: a revised perspective of the pathogenesis of osteoporosis. Endocr Rev 31: 266-300.
43. Lee BS, Holliday LS, Ojikutu B, Krits I, Gluck SL (1996) Osteoclasts express the B2 isoform of vacuolar H(+)-ATPase intracellularly and on their plasma membranes. Am J Physiol 270: C382-C388.
44. Rahman I, Biswas SK, Kirkham PA (2006) Regulation of inflammation and redox signaling by dietary polyphenols. Biochem Pharmacol 72: 1439-1452.
45. Neveu V, Perez-Jimenez J, Vos F, Crespy V, du CL, et al. (2010) Phenol-Explorer: an online comprehensive database on polyphenol contents in foods. Database (Oxford) 2010: bap024. 10.1093/database/bap024 [doi].
46. Piga A, Del CA, Corda G (2003) From plums to prunes: influence of drying parameters on polyphenols and antioxidant activity. J Agric Food Chem 51: 3675-3681.
47. Schmitzer V, Slatnar A, Mikulic-Petkovsek M, Veberic R, Krska B, et al. (2011) Comparative study of primary and secondary metabolites in apricot (Prunus armeniaca L.) cultivars. J Sci Food Agric 91: 860-866. 10.1002/jsfa.4257 [doi].
48. Vrhovsek U, Rigo A, Tonon D, Mattivi F (2004) Quantitation of polyphenols in different apple varieties. J Agric Food Chem 52: 6532-6538. 10.1021/jf049317z [doi].
49. Fang N, Yu S, Prior RL (2002) LC/MS/MS characterization of phenolic constituents in dried plums. J Agric Food Chem 50: 3579-3585. jf0201327 [pii].
50. Dikeman CL, Bauer LL, Fahey GC Jr (2004) Carbohydrate composition of selected plum/prune preparations. J Agric Food Chem 52: 853-859. 10.1021/jf034858u [doi].

9

Hip Fractures and Bone Mineral Density in the Elderly—Importance of Serum 25-Hydroxyvitamin D

Laufey Steingrimsdottir[1]*, Thorhallur I. Halldorsson[1], Kristin Siggeirsdottir[2], Mary Frances Cotch[4], Berglind O. Einarsdottir[2], Gudny Eiriksdottir[2], Sigurdur Sigurdsson[2], Lenore J. Launer[3], Tamara B. Harris[3], Vilmundur Gudnason[2,5], Gunnar Sigurdsson[2,5]

1 Unit for Nutrition Research, University of Iceland and Landspitali University Hospital, Reykjavik, Iceland, **2** Icelandic Heart Association Research Institute, Kopavogur, Iceland, **3** Intramural Research Program, Laboratory of Epidemiology, Demography and Biometry, National Institute of Aging, Bethesda, Maryland, United States of America, **4** Division of Epidemiology and Clinical Applications, National Eye Institute, Bethesda, Maryland, United States of America, **5** University of Iceland, Reykjavik, Iceland

Abstract

Background: The significance of serum 25-hydroxyvitamin D [25(OH)D] concentrations for hip fracture risk of the elderly is still uncertain. Difficulties reaching both frail and healthy elderly people in randomized controlled trials or large cohort studies may in part explain discordant findings. We determined hazard ratios for hip fractures of elderly men and women related to serum 25(OH)D, including both the frail and the healthy segment of the elderly population.

Methods: The AGES-Reykjavik Study is a prospective study of 5764 men and women, age 66–96 years, based on a representative sample of the population of Reykjavik, Iceland. Participation was 71.8%. Hazard ratios of incident hip fractures and baseline bone mineral density were determined according to serum concentrations of 25(OH)D at baseline.

Results: Mean follow-up was 5.4 years. Compared with referent values (50–75 nmol/L), hazard ratios for hip fractures were 2.24 (95% CI 1.63, 3.09) for serum 25(OH)D <30 nmol/L, adjusting for age, sex, body mass index, height, smoking, alcohol intake and season, and 2.08 (95% CI 1.51, 2.87), adjusting additionally for physical activity. No difference in risk was associated with 30–50 nmol/L or ≥75 nmol/L in either model compared with referent. Analyzing the sexes separately, hazard ratios were 2.61 (95% CI 1.47, 4.64) in men and 1.93 (95% CI 1.31, 2.84) in women. Values <30 nmol/L were associated with significantly lower bone mineral density of femoral neck compared with referent, z-scores -0.14 (95% CI −0.27, −0.00) in men and −0.11 (95% CI −0.22, −0.01) in women.

Conclusions: Our results lend support to the overarching importance of maintaining serum 25(OH)D above 30 nmol/L for bone health of elderly people while potential benefits of having much higher levels could not be detected.

Editor: Bin He, Baylor College of Medicine, United States of America

Funding: This study was funded by the National Institutes of Health, USA contract N01- AG-12100, and the National Institute on Aging Intramural Research Program, the National Eye Institute USA (Z01-EY000401), National Institutes of Health, Hjartavernd (The Icelandic Heart Association), and Althingi (Icelandic Parliament). The funders had no role in study design, data collection and analysis, decision to publish, or preparation of the manuscript.

Competing Interests: The authors have declared that no competing interests exist.

* E-mail: laufey@hi.is

Introduction

The importance of vitamin D for skeletal health has long been recognized, and serum 25-hydroxyvitamin D [25(OH)D] is the generally accepted indicator of vitamin D status. Still, optimal serum concentration for bone health is a subject of active debate and intensive research [1]. The Institute of Medicine recently recommended serum levels of 40–50 nmol/L for most adults, based on multiple skeletal outcomes [2], while other experts have suggested levels as high as 75 to 100 nmol/L [3,4].

Several functional indicators are used for vitamin D adequacy as it relates to bone health of the elderly, including bone mineral density and prevention of bone loss [5,6], as well as surrogate measures such as maximal calcium absorption and suppression of parathyroid hormone levels [4,7]. However, fracture prevention, and the levels of 25(OH)D associated with decreased fracture risk may be a more relevant and clinically useful functional marker, as it relates directly to health and quality of life of the elderly. Still, associations between circulating 25(OH)D concentrations and incident fractures in old age remain uncertain [5,6,8]. While several prospective cohort studies have reported higher risk for fractures at lower 25(OH)D concentrations [3,9–14], others show no such association [15–17]. Further, the reported thresholds of significance for fracture risk are quite varied, ranging from 30–40 nmol/L (11) to a high of 90–100 nmol/L [3].

Hip fracture risk of the elderly is a function of multiple factors, including bone mineral density, muscle strength and balance, all of which have been related to vitamin D status and function [9,18]. In nine out of ten instances, hip fracture is sustained through a fall [19], and risk of falling has been related to vitamin D status [20].

Adding to this uncertainty, Randomized controlled trials (RCTs), often considered to provide the highest quality evidence, have not shown a consistent benefit from vitamin D supplements for hip bone mineral density (BMD) or fracture prevention, except possibly in the institutionalized elderly [21] or when given in combination with calcium [22]. Conversely, a recent meta-analysis of RCTs, estimating actual intake of vitamin D rather than prescribed dose, concluded that intakes ≥800 IU/day may be somewhat favorable in the prevention of hip fractures and other non-vertebral fractures in adults 65 years or older [23].

Given the social and economic burden of hip fractures in the elderly, prevention and risk reduction are of prime importance. Sufficient doses of vitamin D for skeletal health in old age need particular elucidation. However, high-risk groups, such as the frail elderly, may be difficult to reach in large cohort studies or RCTs of community-living adults, which in turn may have contributed to the discordant findings of previous studies.

Here we report on the risk of incident hip fractures in the elderly related to circulating 25(OH)D concentrations and bone mineral density in participants in the large prospective AGES-Reykjavik Study, selected at random from the general population.

Methods

Participants

The Ages Gene/Environment Susceptibility (AGES) -Reykjavik Study [24] is a follow-up of the population based Reykjavik Cohort Study, initiated in 1967.

A total of 27,281 men and women, all Caucasians, born in 1907–1935 and residing in Reykjavik and nearby communities were selected at random from the national registry. From these, 19,381 attended the study during the period 1967 to 1991 [25]. From the 11,549 cohort members still alive when AGES-Reykjavik Study examinations began in September 2002, 8,030 individuals were randomly chosen and invited to the study. From these, 5,764 participants, age 66–96 years (mean age 76 years), had enrolled in the AGES-Reykjavik Study by January 2006 (71.8% of invited), with continuous recruitment throughout the period. Participants were offered free taxi rides to the clinic at every visit and personal assistance from the drivers in order to better reach those with limited mobility.

Ethics statement

Written informed consent was obtained from all participants, and the study was approved by the Icelandic National Bioethics Committee (VSN: 00-063) and the National Institute on Aging Intramural Institutional Review Board (MedStar IRB for the Intramural Research Program, Baltimore, MD).

Clinical data collection

Extensive data were collected in the AGES-Reykjavik Study during a series of clinical examinations, according to standardized study protocols by staff of the Icelandic Health Association. Data were gathered on smoking, alcohol intake and consumption frequency of selected foods, including milk and dairy products, using a validated food frequency questionnaire [26]. Physical activity was assessed by self-reported level of physical activity during the last 12 months, where participants were asked how frequently in times per month, week or day they engaged in moderate or vigorous activity, giving examples of this level of activity for clarification. Participants got personal assistance in answering questions. Quantitative computed tomography (QCT) -scanning was performed for BMD measurements.

Of the 5,764 participants of AGES-Reykjavik, 303 did not meet the inclusion criteria, e.g., lacking serum 25(OH)D measurements, leaving 5461 individuals included in the study, all with available fracture data. Of these, 679 individuals did not undergo QCT scanning, leaving 4782 individuals for the analysis of BMD and vitamin D status.

Measurement of serum 25(OH)D

Blood was collected during the first clinic visit to AGES-study, from September 2002 to January 2006, and fasting serum samples were kept frozen at −80°C on-site in the IHA laboratory. Quantitative determination of total 25(OH) D (D_2 and D_3) was conducted by means of a direct, competitive chemiluminescence immunoassay (CLIA), using the LIAISON 25 OH Vitamin D Total assay (DiaSorin, Inc., Stillwater, Minnesota). The inter assay coefficient of variation was <6.5%, using a previously frozen serum pool as the control sample and <12.7% when the calculated data were from measurements using Liaison quality controls.

Bone mineral density measurements

During the first clinic visit, QCT measurements, providing true volumetric density, were taken on the left hip, using a 4-detector CT system (Sensation, Siemens Medical Systems, Erlangen, Germany). Using a standardized protocol, scans were obtained encompassing the proximal femur from a level 1 cm above the acetabulum to a level 5 mm inferior to the lesser trochanter with 1 mm slice thickness. To calibrate CT Hounsfield units to equivalent bone mineral concentration, all subjects were scanned with a calibration phantom (Image Analysis, Columbia, KY, USA). Further procedures and quality assessments have been described in detail elsewhere [24,27].

The variables used in the present study are volumetric integral BMD (mg/cm^3), reflecting both trabecular and cortical bone mass, of the femoral neck and trochanteric region separately. Reasons for exclusion from the QCT were inability to lie supine, body weight over 150 kg or having undergone hip replacement surgery.

Fractures

Hip fracture data were recorded, verified and confirmed from medical and radiological records as previously described [28]. Incident fractures were recorded from participants' enrollment into the study until 31st of December 2009, with a mean follow-up time of 5.4 years (SD 1.5). Hip fractures were defined according to International Classification of Diseases version 10, diagnostic codes S72.0, S72.1, S72.2 (WHO 1994). The AGES-Reykjavik Study fracture registration has been shown to have a capture rate of about 97% for hip fracture [28].

Statistical analyses

The mean and standard deviation (SD) were used to describe continuous variables and percentages were used for dichotomous variables. Serum 25(OH)D was categorized, *a priori*, into four groups of <30, ≥30–50, ≥50–75 and ≥75 nmol/L. The group ≥50–75 nmol/L (sufficient level) was used as referent, to establish whether beneficial effects could be detected at higher levels (≥75 nmol/L) and to compare with lower levels, (30–50 nmol/L) and (<30 nmol/L), concentrations that have been considered inadequate and depleted, according to the Institute of Medicine [2]. The absolute BMD values (in mg/cm^3) of the femoral neck and trochanteric area were transformed into a gender-specific z-score, based on the internal distribution in our study population. The z-score for femoral neck was used as the primary outcome measure when examining the association between 25(OH)D and BMD, which was performed as a secondary analysis.

Cox Proportional Hazard Model was used when examining the association between 25(OH)D and bone fractures; and linear regression when examining the association with bone mineral density. As a measure of association we used χ^2-test (Type III) for dichotomous outcomes and t-test for continuous outcomes under the null hypothesis that all 25(OH)D groups were equal (p for effect). For testing linear trend, ordinal values (0,1,2,3) for serum 25(OH)D were entered in the regression model. All of the analyses were carried out using SAS statistical software (version 9.2, SAS Institute, Cary, NC).

In our analyses we selected *a priori* and included the following set of covariates: age (continuous, no missing), sex (binary, no missing) height (continuous, 0.1% missing), current smoking (binary, 2.5% missing), body mass index (BMI) (<18.5, 18.5–24.9, 25–29.9, 30–34.9, 35–39.9 and 40+, 0.1% missing), current alcohol intake (0, 1–25, 26–50 and 50+ g/day, 3% missing), season (winter: Dec, Jan, Feb, spring: Mar, Apr, May, summer: June, July, Aug, autumn: Sept Oct Nov, no missing), current physical activity (never, rarely, occasionally, moderate, high, 4.0% missing). As self reported milk and dairy product intake and serum 25(OH)D at baseline were essentially uncorrelated (Spearman $r = 0.06$), milk and dairy product intake was not included as covariate. The proportion of subjects missing data on one or more covariate was 4.4%. Due to the relatively low number of missing values for most covariates, missing values were replaced with median (continuous) and most frequent (dichotomous) values. Two models were used for covariate adjustment: Model A adjusting for age, sex, smoking, BMI, height, alcohol intake and season of blood sample collection; and Model B, additionally adjusting for physical activity.

To check the robustness of our findings with respect to imputation for missing covariates and length of follow-up we 1) ran all analyses using complete case analyses (all subjects with missing covariates excluded); and 2) examined the association between baseline 25(OH)D with hip fractures, excluding all fractures occurring within 6 months from baseline.

Results

A total of 261 hip fractures were encountered during a mean follow-up time of 5.4 years (SD 1.5). Characteristics of the study participants by sex and serum 25(OH)D are shown in **Table 1**. Fourteen per cent of men and 19% of women had serum 25(OH)D concentrations below 30 nmol/L, and 21% and 14% had concentrations ≥75 nmol/L, men and women respectively. There were significant negative trends associated with 25(OH)D category for the following variables in both men and women: BMI, % physically inactive, % drinking no alcohol and % smoking, while positive trends were found for BMD. There was no significant association between level of serum 25(OH)D and mean age for men or women.

For males the mean (SD) integral BMD was 254 (51)mg/cm^3 for femoral neck and 250 (50)mg/cm^3 for trochanter. The corresponding values for females were 244 (50)mg/cm^3 and 226 (48)mg/cm^3. The mean (SD) serum 25(OH)D was 57 (25)nmol/L and 51 (24)nmol/L for males and females, respectively.

Table 2 shows hip fracture hazard ratios according to serum 25(OH)D categories for all participants and for men and women separately. Compared with referent values of 50–75 nmol/L, the risk for hip fractures more than doubled in all subjects with levels below 30 nmol/L, values remaining relatively stable through adjustment models. Adjusting for age, height and BMI, current smoking, season of blood sampling and alcohol intake, the hazard ratio was 2.24 (95% CI 1.63, 3.09) and with further adjustment for physical activity it was 2.08 (95% CI 1.51, 2.87). No increase in risk was associated with serum concentrations 30–50 nmol/L compared with referent values and neither was there any difference in risk associated with values ≥75 nmol/L in either adjustment model. When the sexes were analyzed separately, hazard ratio for men was 2.61 (95% CI 1.47, 4.64), compared with 1.93 (95% CI 1.31, 2.84) for women in the fully adjusted model. Again risk ratios did not change significantly between the different adjustment models in either sex. Values between 30–50 nmol/L and values ≥75 nmol/L were not associated with changes in risk compared with referent values in either sex.

Based on the prevalence of hip fractures in the 50–75 nmol/ group for all subjects (4.0%) we estimated the excess number of fractures, i.e. expected minus observed fractures, in the <30 nmol/L group. Expected fractures were 38, or 0.04*938 (number of subjects with <30 nmol/L), while 77 fractures were observed. This suggests that 15% (or 39 excess fractures out of 261 in total) may be attributable to poor (<30 nmol/L) serum 25(OH) D status.

Associations between 25(OH)D concentrations and BMD at baseline in femoral neck are shown in **Table 3**, with BMD reported as z-scores. Using the values 50–75 nmol/L as referent, values below 30 nmol/L were consistently associated with slightly lower BMD z-score. In Model A, adjusting for age, height, BMI, smoking, alcohol intake and season, the adjusted difference in z-score was −0.18 (95% CI −0.31, −0.04) in men and −0.13 (95% CI −0.23, −0.03) in women. In model B, additionally adjusting for physical activity, the corresponding values were −0.14 (95% CI −0.27, −0.00) and −0.11 (95% CI −0.22, −0.01), men and women, respectively. No significant difference in risk was associated with other categories of 25(OH)D concentrations, except for a small increase at concentrations ≥75 nmol/L. Taking both sexes together, there was an increase of 0.10 (95% CI 0.02, 0.18) in Model A, with values remaining stable through further adjustment. When sexes were analyzed separately, only BMD z-scores for males remained significantly higher in the ≥75 nmol/L group than in the referent. Comparable values were found for BMD in trochanter associated with 25(OH)D concentrations in both sexes (data not shown). A total of 679 participants in the study did not undergo QCT scanning. Associations between hip fractures and 25(OH)D concentrations in the 4782 individuals with available scanning data were found to be similar to those observed in the larger group of 5461 participants.

Figure 1 shows the percentage of incident hip fractures according to baseline values of 25(OH)D in all participants, during a mean follow-up time of 5.4 years, mean time to event 3.4 years (SD1.8). A total of 10.6% of those with values below 15 nmol/L experienced a fracture, while corresponding proportions were 7.6% and 4.4% for those with values from 15–30 nmol/L and 30–50 nmol/L, respectively. There was non-significant change in the percentage at higher 25(OH)D values. However, mean time to fracture was not significantly different between the 25(OH)D groups, 3.1 years (SD 1.8) in the lowest category, compared with 3.9 years (SD 3.9), 3.3 years (SD 1.3) and 3.5years (SD 1.6) in the higher categories.

Finally we found little evidence to suggest that imputing values for missing covariates may have contributed to residual confounding. As an example, when comparing the referent with <30 nmol/L for both sexes using model B (Table 2) the hazard ratio for hip fracture was 2.08 (1.51, 2.87) and was essentially unchanged 2.08 (1.49, 2.91) when subjects with missing covariate information were excluded. Correspondingly when all individuals with hip fracture events occurring within 6 months ($n = 14$) were excluded (using

Table 1. Characteristics of male and female participants at baseline according to categories of serum 25-hydroxyvitamin D (N = 5461), mean and SD.

	Serum 25-hydroxyvitamin D (nmol/L)				
	<30	**30-<50**	**50-<75**	**≥75**	**P value[1]**
Males (n = 2346)					
n (%)	337 (14%)	638 (28%)	886 (38%)	485 (21%)	
Femoral neck BMD, mg/cm^3	245 (59)	253 (51)	254 (50)	259 (53)	0.0005
Trochanter BMD, mg/cm^3	242 (51)	248 (51)	252 (47)	255 (51)	0.0002
Age in years	76.7 (5.8)	76.8 (5.5)	76.7 (5.4)	76.8 (5.4)	0.65
Height, cm	175.1 (6.2)	175.1 (6.2)	175.5 (6.2)	175.8 (6.2)	0.03
BMI, kg/m^2	27.2 (4.3)	27.3 (3.9)	26.7 (3.7)	26.3 (3.5)	<0.0001
% Physically inactive	61	46	37	34	<0.0001
% Not drinking alcohol	34	30	24	27	0.002
% Current smokers	23	12	8	9	<0.0001
Females (n = 3125)					
n (%)	601 (19%)	992 (32%)	1103 (35%)	429 (14%)	
BMD for femoral neck (mg/cm^3)	240 (50)	245 (52)	245 (49)	248 (48)	0.03
BMD for trochanter (mg/cm^3)	221 (49)	227 (50)	227 (46)	229 (45)	0.02
Age in years	76.8 (5.6)	76.7 (5.8)	76.3 (5.7)	76.7 (5.6)	0.20
Height, cm	160.3 (5.7)	160.7 (5.6)	161.1 (5.9)	160.8 (6.1)	0.006
BMI, kg/m^2	28.1 (5.5)	27.8 (4.9)	26.6 (4.4)	26.2 (4.3)	<0.0001
% Physically inactive	66	50	45	42	<0.0001
% Not drinking alcohol	54	41	35	37	<0.0001
% Current smokers	18	12	11	10	0.0001

[1]T-test for trend for continuous covariates with serum 25-hydroxyvitamin D entered as ordinal values.
Chi-square test for dichotomous covariates.

imputed covariate values), the hazard ratio was 2.10 (1.51, 2.93). There was no trend with respect to time to fracture across categories of 25(OH)D. As an example the mean time to event was 3.1 years (SD 1.8) in the lowest (<30 nmol/L) compared with 3.3 years (SD 1.3) in the referent category (50 -<75 nmol/L).

Discussion

In this prospective cohort study of 5461 elderly people experiencing a sizable number of hip fractures (n = 261), the estimated risk of hip fracture was twice as high in individuals with serum 25(OH)D concentrations below 30 nmol/L, using 50–75 nmol/L as a referent and adjusting for a series of relevant cofactors. The risk increase associated with low 25(OH)D levels was somewhat higher for men than women, but remained stable and highly significant in both sexes through various adjustments. No statistically significant difference in risk was associated with other categories of 25(OH)D concentrations, for levels either between 30 and 50 nmol/L or above 75 nmol/L, compared with the referent values.

The relevance of vitamin D status for hip fracture risk has been considered uncertain in large systematic reviews of vitamin D and bone health [5,6]. Indeed, several cohort studies have found no associations between hip fracture risk and vitamin D [15–17], while some studies have reported risk protection by quite high serum 25(OH)D concentrations, up to 100 nmol/L [3,10]. Still others show tendencies for increased risk at low levels below 30–40 nmol/L, with no further protection at higher concentrations [9,11,13]. According to a large multi-center study from Norway [14] there is a moderate increase in risk for hip fractures among those in the lowest quartile for baseline 25(OH)D (≤42.1 nmol/L) compared with the highest ≥67.9 nmol/L), with a hazard ratio of 1.34. Also, RCTs are not unequivocal in their conclusions, regarding either the efficacy or ideal dose of vitamin D supplements for fracture prevention [21,22,29]. Elucidating the significance of vitamin D for hip fracture risk of the elderly is of great public health significance, considering the public health costs, high mortality and human suffering related to hip fractures [30]. As vitamin D of varying doses is widely used in clinical practice to lower the risk of osteoporotic fractures, it is of prime importance to determine whether relatively high 25(OH)D concentrations are needed for risk protection, concentrations which generally require larger doses of vitamin D supplementation than the 800 IU currently recommended for the elderly by the Institute of Medicine [2] and recently endorsed in a review of randomized controlled trials [31]. Even though these higher doses are not considered toxic, adverse effects, such as increased risk of kidney stones, have been indicated in studies like the Women's Health Initiative [32]. The study of Sanders et al. [33] further alerts to possible adverse outcomes associated with large doses, as they reported increased risk for falls and fractures in a group of elderly people receiving 500,000 IU of vitamin D annually for 3 to 5 years.

Table 2. Hazard ratios for hip fractures according to serum 25-hydroxyvitamin D categories among all subjects (N = 5461), and stratified by sex.

		Unadjusted	Model A[2]	Model B[3]
		HR (95% CI)	HR (95% CI)	HR (95% CI)
All Subjects	cases/n (%)			
<30 nmol/L	77/938 (8.2%)	2.14 (1.57, 2.94)	2.24 (1.63, 3.09)	2.08 (1.51, 2.87)
30–50 nmol/L	71/1620 (4.4%)	1.10 (0.80, 1.52)	1.13 (0.82, 1.56)	1.11 (0.80, 1.53)
50–75 nmol/L	80/1989 (4.0%)	1.00	1.00	1.00
≥75 nmol/L	33/914 (3.6%)	0.91 (0.61, 1.37)	0.90 (0.60, 1.35)	0.94 (0.62, 1.41)
P for effect[1]		<0.0001	<0.0001	<0.0001
Males	cases/n (%)			
<30 nmol/L	25/337 (7.4%)	2.61 (1.49, 4.58)	2.81 (1.59, 4.96)	2.61 (1.47, 4.64)
30–50 nmol/L	24/604 (3.8%)	1.35 (0.77, 2.36)	1.52 (0.86, 2,67)	1.49 (0.84, 2.63)
50–75 nmol/L	25/886 (2.8%)	1.00	1.00	1.00
≥75 nmol/L	14/485 (2.9%)	0.99 (0.51, 1.90)	0.97 (0.50, 1.88)	1.02 (0.53, 1.97)
P for effect[1]		0.003	0.001	0.006
Females	cases/n (%)			
<30 nmol/L	52/601 (8.7%)	1.89 (1.29, 2.76)	2.06 (1.40, 3.02)	1.93 (1.31, 2.84)
30–50 nmol/L	47/992 (4.7%)	0.97 (0.66, 1.44)	1.01 (0.68, 1.50)	0.99 (0.67, 1.47)
50–75 nmol/L	55/1103 (5.0%)	1.00	1.00	1.00
≥75 nmol/L	19/429 (4.4%)	0.94 (0.56, 1.58)	0.86 (0.51, 1.46)	0.89 (0.53, 1.51)
P for effect[1]		0.001	0.0002	0.001

Abbreviations: HR Hazard Ratio, CI confidence interval.
[1]Chi-square test (type 3).
[2]Adjusted for age at recruitment, sex (when all subjects are included), height, body mass index, current smoking, season of blood sampling and alcohol intake.
[3]Additionally adjusted for current physical activity

Differences in previous study outcomes have been explained in part by the different populations under study as well as possible differences in confounder adjustments [5]. Specifically, the frail and sickly may not be included or reached in all community-based studies of the elderly, but lower vitamin D status is consistently reported among the frail compared with those more physically active and in better health [3,9]. Thus, the segment of the elderly population having the lowest 25(OH)D levels may not be included in many cohort studies and the significance of very low values thus overlooked or minimized [9,11]. In our study, which was based on a random sample from the general population, the participation rate was high, or 71.8%, and the distribution of 25(OH)D concentration was quite wide, with comparable proportions of the population having values below 30 nmol/L and above 75 nmol/L. A significant proportion of all hip fractures in our study (15%), may thus be attributed to poor or deficient (<30 nmol/L) serum 25(OH)D. Interestingly, this is a comparable proportion to that reported from combined calcium and vitamin D supplementation for reducing fracture risk [34]. Possibly the relatively high calcium intake in our population, due to widespread use of milk and dairy products, may contribute to this effect [7].

The fracture incidence observed in our study, where both sexes were taken together for improved statistical power, also strongly indicates that there is a nonlinear relationship between circulating 25(OH)D and fracture risk, with only small gains being associated with serum levels above 50 nmol/L. The highest incidence was observed in the group with 25(OH)D values below 15 nmols, with steeply decreasing proportion with increased circulating vitamin D up to 50 nmol/L, but little differences above those concentrations.

While appropriate adjustments were made for season in our analysis, seasonal variation in 25(OH)D values was less pronounced in the present study than previously reported for younger populations in Reykjavik, geographically located at 64° N [7]. The difference in mean values obtained in summer and winter was only 4 nmol/L in this elderly population. The relative lack of seasonal variation indicates that vitamin D intake may play a more important role for vitamin D status in this population compared with younger people. Indeed, cod liver oil, either as liquid or capsules, is a common supplement in Iceland, with 61% of this population reporting taking the supplement daily and 13% several times per week, according to AGES questionnaire. However, intake of milk or dairy products at baseline was not associated with vitamin D status in our study. Notably, milk or dairy products were not fortified with vitamin D during the study period.

We measured volumetric QCT-BMD rather than areal BMD, but similar associations have been shown between fractures and BMD using these two measures [35,36]. Similar to many previous studies [3,12] we found a slight but significant positive trend between BMD in femoral neck and serum concentrations of 25(OH)D in both sexes. Again, only levels below 30 nmol/L were consistently significantly different from the referent, which is in concordance with our results regarding increases in hip fracture risk below 30 nmol/L. However, according to earlier studies the observed difference of 0.10-0.16 BMD z-scores might be expected to be associated with only modest increases in fracture risk [37,38]. The two-fold increase in risk associated with low 25(OH)D in our study supports the contention that the relationship between vitamin D and fracture risk may indeed be non-linear [1]. It has been suggested that vitamin D may reduce fracture rates through

Table 3. Differences in z-score (number of SD from age corrected mean) of femoral neck bone mineral density according to serum 25-hydroxyvitamin D categories at baseline (N = 4782).

	Unadjusted	Model A[2]	Model B[3]
	Δ(95% CI)	Δ (95% CI)	Δ (95% CI)
Femoral neck BMD(z-score)			
All (N = 4782)			
<30 nmol/L	−0.13 (−0.21, −0.04)	−0.15 (−0.23, −0.07)	−0.13 (−0.21, −0.05)
30–50 nmol/L	−0.02 (−0.09, 0.05)	−0.04 (−0.11, 0.03)	−0.03 (−0.10, 0.03)
50–75 nmol/L	Referent	Referent	Referent
≥75 nmol/L	0.08 (−0.01, 0.16)	0.10 (0.02, 0.18)	0.09 (0.01, 0.17)
P for effect[1]	0.0006	<0.0001	0.0001
Males (n = 2104)			
<30 nmol/L	−0.18 (−0.31, −0.04)	−0.18 (−0.31, −0.04)	−0.14 (−0.27, −0.00)
30–50 nmol/L	−0.02 (−0.13, 0.08)	−0.04 (−0.15, 0.07)	−0.03 (−0.13, 0.08)
50–75 nmol/L	Referent	Referent	Referent
≥75 nmol/L	0.10 (−0.02, 0.21)	0.12 (0.01, 0.24)	0.11 (−0.01, 0.22)
P for effect[1]	0.004	0.0009	0.01
Females (n = 2678)			
<30 nmol/L	−0.10 (−0.21, 0.01)	−0.13 (−0.23, −0.03)	−0.11 (−0.22, −0.01)
30–50 nmol/L	−0.01 (−0.11, 0.08)	−0.04 (−0.12, 0.05)	−0.03 (−0.12, 0.05)
50–75 nmol/L	Referent	Referent	Referent
≥75 nmol/L	0.06 (−0.06, 0.18)	0.07 (−0.04, 0.19)	0.07 (−0.04, 0.18)
P for effect[1]	0.14	0.01	0.03

Abbreviations: CI confidence interval.
[1]F-test (type 3).
[2]Adjusted for age at recruitment, sex (when all subjects are included), height, body mass index, current smoking, season of blood sampling and alcohol intake.
[3]Additionally adjusted for current physical activity.

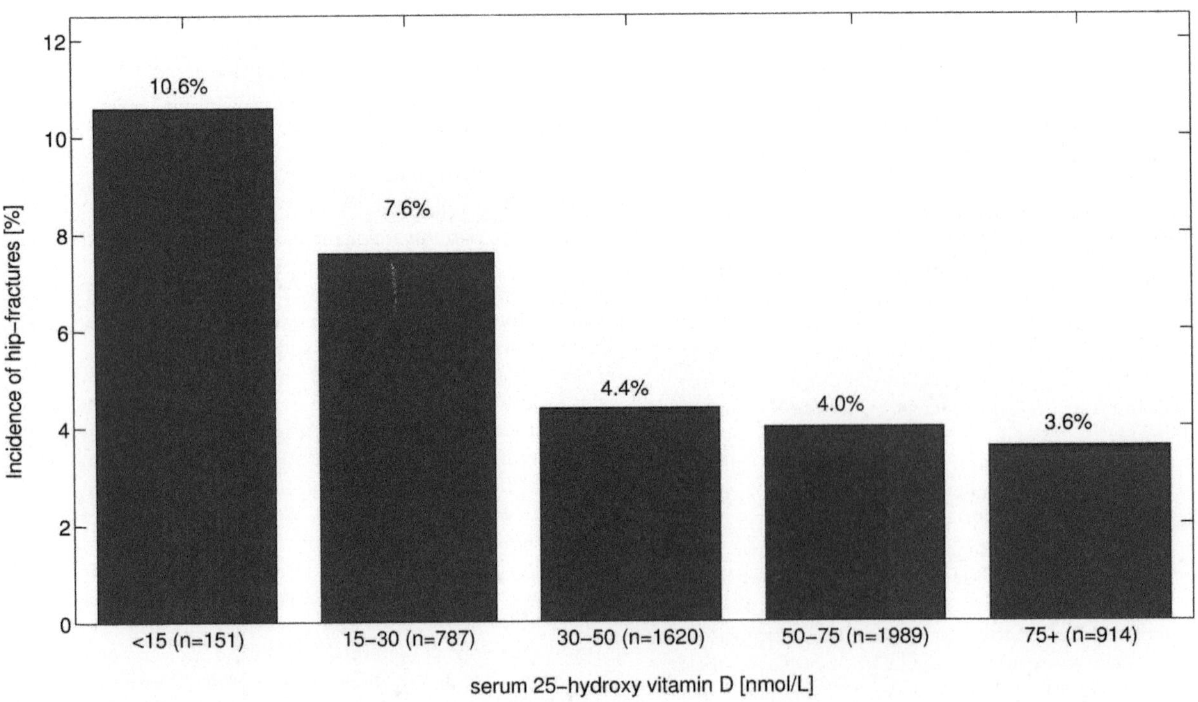

Figure 1. Hip fracture incidence (%) during a follow-up of 5.4 years (SD1.5) among AGES participants (N = 5461) according to serum baseline categories of 25(OH)D. Unadjusted values.

additional mechanisms, independent of bone density [39]. Specifically, vitamin D supplements may effectively decrease the risk of falling, especially in the institutionally elderly, possibly through actions involving balance and muscle strength [20,40].

It is well known that elderly men have higher mean BMD and lower risk for hip fractures than women [14,27], as confirmed in our study. However, the risk increase associated with low 25(OH)D concentrations was comparable in men and women suggesting that vitamin D status is no less important for lowering fracture risk among elderly men than women.

Concerns have been raised over assays for 25(OH)D giving varying results, casting doubt on the comparability of specific values for vitamin D status [41]. Our study employed a common assay method for 25(OH)D, widely used in clinical settings. Thus we believe that our results are clinically relevant, even though the levels measured by the CLIA method may be systematically lower than those measured by HPLC. Furthermore, systematic errors in absolute serum levels should only affect interpretations of our findings in terms of absolute cut-off values but should not affect the magnitude and strength of the observed association.

The length of follow-up may also be a concern, as single baseline vitamin D values may not represent status many years later [42]. Indeed, the study by Looker [13] showed that vitamin D concentrations predicted major osteoporotic fracture risk only for 10 years of follow up. Importantly, our mean follow-up time was 5.4 years, with mean time to event 3.4 years. Frail individuals may also be selectively advised to take vitamin D supplements, diminishing observed risk. However, results from our 25(OH)D analysis were not available until at the end of follow up, and thus our subjects could not be informed of their status earlier.

The main strength of our study is the large number of elderly people, displaying a wide variation in serum 25(OH)D values, and sustaining a total of 261 hip fractures. Thus, robust associations could be obtained between vitamin D status and fracture risk. The main limitation to our study, however, is the single baseline measurement of 25(OH)D. Also, as this is an observational study, some residual confounding cannot be excluded. However, as hazard ratios for hip fracture were quite similar in unadjusted and fully adjusted data in both sexes, residual confounding is not likely to substantially affect our main results.

To conclude: Our results lend support to the overarching importance of maintaining serum 25(OH)D above 30 nmol/L for bone health of elderly people while potential benefits of having much higher levels could not be detected.

Acknowledgments

We thank all the participants of the AGES-Reykjavik Study and the clinic staff at the Icelandic Heart Association for their invaluable contribution.

Author Contributions

Conceived and designed the experiments: LS TIH VG GS. Performed the experiments: BOE GE KS SS MFC. Analyzed the data: LS TIH GS. Contributed reagents/materials/analysis tools: KS MFC LJL TBH VG. Wrote the paper: LS TIH GS.

References

1. Dawson-Hughes B (2013) What is the optimal dietary intake of vitamin D for reducing fracture risk? Calcif Tissue Int 92: 184–190.
2. Ross AC, Manson JE, Abrams SA, Aloia JF, Brannon PM, et al. (2011) The 2011 report on dietary reference intakes for calcium and vitamin D from the Institute of Medicine: what the clinicians need to know. J Clin Endocrinol Metab 96: 53–58.
3. Bischoff-Ferrari HA, Giuvannucci E, Willett WC, Dietrich T, Dawson-Hughes B (2006) Estimation of optimal serum concentrations of 25-hydroxyvitamin D for multiple health outcomes. Am J Clin Nutr 84: 18–28.
4. Holick MF (2007) Vitamin D deficiency. N Engl J Med 357: 266–281.
5. Cranney A, Horsley T, O'Donnell S, Weiler H, Puil L, et al. (2007) Effectiveness and safety of vitamin D in relation to bone health. Evid Rep Technol Assess 158:1–235.
6. Chung M, Balk EM, Brendel M, Ip S, Lau J, et al. (2009) Vitamin D and calcium: a systematic review of health outcomes. Evid Rep Technol Assess 183:1–420.
7. Steingrimsdottir L, Gunnarsson O, Indridason OS, Franzson L, Sigurdsson G (2005) Relationship between serum parathyroid hormone levels, vitamin D sufficiency, and calcium intake. JAMA 294: 2336–2341.
8. Avenell A, Gillespie WJ, Gillespie LD, O'Connell D (2009) Vitamin D and vitamin D analogues for preventing fractures associated with involutional and post-menopausal osteoporosis. Cochrane Database Syst Rev 2: CD000227. doi:10.1002/14651858.CD000227.pub3.
9. Gerdhem P, Ringsberg KAM, Obrant KJ, Akesson K (2005) Association between 25-hydroxy vitamin D levels, physical activity, strength and fractures in the prospective population-based OPRA study of elderly women. Osteoporos Int 16: 1425–1431.
10. Looker AC, Mussolino ME (2008) Serum 25-hydroxyvitamin D and hip fracture risk in older US white adults. J Bone Miner Res 23: 143–150.
11. Melhus H, Snellman G, Gedeborg R, Byberg L, Berglund L, et al. (2010) Plasma 25-hydroxyvitamin D levels and fracture risk in a community-based cohort of elderly men in Sweden. J Clin Endocrinol Metab 95: 2637–2645.
12. Robinson-Cohen C, Katz R, Hoofnagle AN, Cauley JA, Furberg CD, et al. (2011) Mineral metabolism markers and the long-term risk of hip fracture: The cardiovascular health study. J Clin Endocrinol Metab 96: 2189–2193.
13. Looker AC (2013) Serum 25-hydroxyvitamin D and risk of major osteoporotic fractures in older U.S adults. J Bone Miner Res 28: 997–1006.
14. Holvik K, Ahmed LA, Forsmo S, Forsmo S, Gjesdal CG, et al. (2013) Low serum levels of 25-hydoxyvitamin D predict hip fracture in the elderly. A NOREPOS study. J Clin Endocrinol Metab 98: 3341-3350. doi:10.1210/jc.2013-1468.
15. Roddam AW, Neale R, Appelby P, Allen NE, Tipper S, et al. (2007) Association between plasma 25-hydroxyvitamin D levels and fracture risk – the EPIC-Oxford study. Am J Epidemiol 166: 1327–1336.
16. Cauley JA, Parimi N, Ensrud KE, Bauer DC, Cawthon PM, et al. (2010) Serum 25-hydroxyvitamin D and the risk of hip and nonspine fractures in older men. J Bone Miner Res 25: 545–553.
17. Barbour KE, Houston DK, Cummings SR, Boudreau R, Prasad T, et al. (2012) Calciotropic hormones and the risk of hip and nonspine fractures in older adults: The Health ABC Study. J Bone Miner Res 27: 1177–1185.
18. Muir SW, Montero-Odasso M (2011) Effect of vitamin D supplementation on muscle strength, gait and balance in older adults: A systematic review and meta-analysis. J Am Geriatr Soc 59: 2291–2300.
19. Schwartz AV, Villa ML, Prill M, Kelsey JA, Galinus JA, et al. (1999) Falls in older Mexican-American women. J Am Geriatr Soc 47: 1371–1378.
20. Kalyani RR, Stein B, Valiyil R, Manno R, Maynard JW, et al. (2010) Vitamin D treatment for the prevention of falls in older adults: systematic review and meta-analysis. J Am Geriatr Soc 58: 1299–1310.
21. Lai JK, Lucas RM, Clements MS, Roddam AW, Banks E (2010) Hip fracture risk in relation to vitamin D supplementation and serum 25-hydroxyvitamin D levels: A systematic review and meta-analysis of randomised controlled trials and observational studies. BMC Public Health 10: 331. doi 10.1186/1471-2458-10-331.
22. The DIPART (vitamin D Individual Patient Analysis of Randomized Trials) Group (2010) Patient level pooled analysis of 68 500 patients from seven major vitamin D fracture trials in US and Europe. BMJ 340:b5463. doi:10.1136/bmj.b5463.
23. Bischoff-Ferrari HA, Willett WC, Orav EJ, Lips P, Meunier PJ, et al. (2012) A pooled analysis of vitamin D dose requirements for fracture prevention. N Engl J Med 367: 40–49.
24. Harris TB, Launer LJ, Eiriksdottir G, Kjartansson O, Jonsson PV, et al. (2007) Age, Gene/Environment Susceptibility-Reykjavik Study: multidisciplinary applied phenomics. Am J Epidemiol 165: 1076–1087.
25. Bjornsson G, Bjornsson OJ, Davidsson D, Kristjansson BT, Olafsson O, et al. (1982) Report abc XXIV. Health Survey in the Reykjavik Area. – Women. Stages I-III, 1968–1969, 1971–1972 and 1976–1978. Participants, Invitation, Response etc. The Icelandic Heart Association, Reykjavik.
26. Eysteinsdottir T, Thorsdottir I, Gunnarsdottir I, Steingrimsdottir L (2012) Assessing validity of a short food-frequency questionnaire on present dietary intake of elderly Icelanders. Nutr J 11:12. doi:10.1186/1475-2891-11-12
27. Sigurdsson G, Aspelund T, Chang M, Jonsdottir B, Sigurdsson S, et al. (2006) Increasing sex difference in bone strength in old age: The Age, Gene/Environment Susceptibility-Reykjavik study (AGES-REYKJAVIK). Bone 39: 644–651.
28. Siggeirsdottir K, Aspelund T, Sigurdsson G, Mogensen B, Chang M, et al. (2007) Inaccuracy in self-report of fractures may underestimate association with health outcomes when compared with medical record based fracture registry. Eur J Epidemiol 22: 631–639.

29. Grimnes G, Joakimsen R, Figenschau Y, Torjesen PA, Almås B, et al. (2012) The effect of high-dose vitamin D on bone mineral density and bone turnover markers in postmenopausal women with low bone mass-a randomized controlled 1-year trial. Osteoporos Int 23: 201–211.
30. Johnell O (2006) Review: Vitamin D plus calcium, but not vitamin D alone, prevents osteoporotic fractures in older people. Evid Based Med 11: 13. doi:10.1136/ebm.11.1.13
31. Bouillon R, Van Schoor NM, Gielen E, Boonen S, Mathieu C, et al. (2013) Optimal vitamin D status: a critical analysis on the basis of evidence-based medicine. J Clin Endocrinol Metab 98:E1283-304. doi: 10.1210/jc.2013-1195.
32. Jackson RD, LaCroix AZ, Gass M, Wallace RB, Robbins J, et al. (2006) Women's Health Initiative Investigators. Calcium plus vitamin D supplementation and the risk of fractures. N Engl J Med 354: 669–683.
33. Sanders KM, Stuart AL, Williamson EJ, Simpson JA, Kotowicz MA, et al. (2010) Annual high-dose oral vitamin D and falls and fractures in older women: a randomized controlled trial. JAMA. 303: 1815–1822.
34. Boonen S, Lips P, Bouillon R, Bischoff-Ferrari HA, Vanderschueren D, et al. (2007) Need for additional calcium to reduce the risk of hip fracture with vitamin d supplementation: evidence from a comparative metaanalysis of randomized controlled trials. J Clin Endocrinol Metab 92: 1415–1423.
35. Rianon NJ, Lang TF, Siggeirsdottir K, Sigurdsson G, Eiriksdottir G, et al. (2014) Fracture risk assessment in older adults using a combination of selected quantitative computed tomography bone measures. A sub-analysis of the Age, Gene/Environment Susceptibility-Reykjavik Study. J Clin Densitom 17: 25–31.
36. Black DM, Bouxsein ML, Marshall LM, Cummings SR, Lang TF, et al. (2008) Osteoporotic Fractures in Men (MrOS) Research Group. Proximal femoral structure and the prediction of hip fracture in men: a large prospective study using QCT. J Bone Miner Res 23: 1326–1333.
37. Cummings SR, Black DM, Nevitt MC, Browner W, Cauley J, et al. (1993) Bone density at various sites for prediction of hip fractures. The Study of Osteoporotic Fractures Research Group. Lancet 341: 72–75.
38. Marshall D, Johnell O, Wedel H (1996) Meta-analysis of how well measures of bone mineral density predict occurrence of osteoporotic fractures. BMJ 312: 1254–1259.
39. Rabenda V, Bruyère O, Reginster JY (2011) Relationship between bone mineral density changes and risk of fractures among patients receiving calcium with or without vitamin D supplementation: a meta-regression. Osteoporos Int 22: 893–901.
40. Cameron ID, Gillespie LD, Robertson MC, Murray GR, Hill KD, et al. (2012) Interventions for preventing falls in older people in care facilities and hospitals. Cochrane Database Syst Rev doi: 10.1002/14651858.CD005465.pub3.
41. Snellman G, Melhus H, Gedeborg R, Byberg L, Berglund L, et al. (2010) Determining vitamin D status: a comparison between commercially available assays. PLoS One doi: 10.1371/journal.pone.0011555.
42. Jorde R, Sneve M, Hutchinson M, Emaus N, Figenschau Y, et al. (2010) Tracking of serum 25-hydroxyvitamin D levels during 14 years in a population-based study and during 12 months in an intervention study. Am J Epidemiol 171: 903–908.

Polymorphisms in the Inflammatory Genes *CIITA*, *CLEC16A* and *IFNG* Influence BMD, Bone Loss and Fracture in Elderly Women

Maria Swanberg[1,2], Fiona E. McGuigan[1], Kaisa K. Ivaska[3], Paul Gerdhem[4,5], Kristina Åkesson[1,6]*

1 Clinical and Molecular Osteoporosis Research Unit, Department of Clinical Sciences, Lund University, Sweden, **2** Neurodegeneration and Inflammation Genetics Unit, Department of Experimental Medical Science, Lund University, Sweden, **3** Department of Cell Biology and Anatomy, Institute of Biomedicine, University of Turku, Turku, Finland, **4** Department of Clinical Science, Intervention and Technology, Karolinska Institute, Stockholm, Sweden, **5** Department of Orthopaedics, Karolinska University Hospital, Stockholm, Sweden, **6** Department of Orthopaedics, Skåne University Hospital, Malmö, Sweden

Abstract

Osteoclast activity and the fine balance between bone formation and resorption is affected by inflammatory factors such as cytokines and T lymphocyte activity, mediated by major histocompatibility complex (MHC) molecules, in turn regulated by the MHC class II transactivator (MHC2TA). We investigated the effect of functional polymorphisms in the MHC2TA gene (*CIITA*), and two additional genes; C-type lectin domain 16A (*CLEC16A)*, in linkage disequilibrium with *CIITA* and Interferon-γ (*IFNG*), an inducer of *CIITA;* on bone density, bone resorption markers, bone loss and fracture risk in 75 year-old women followed for up to 10 years (OPRA n = 1003) and in young adult women (PEAK-25 n = 999). *CIITA* was associated with BMD at age 75 (lumbar spine p = 0.011; femoral neck (FN) p = 0.049) and age 80 (total body p = 0.015; total hip p = 0.042; FN p = 0.028). Carriers of the *CIITA* rs3087456(G) allele had 1.8–3.4% higher BMD and displayed increased rate of bone loss between age 75 and 80 (FN p = 0.013; total hip p = 0.030; total body $p = 3.8E^{-5}$). Despite increasing bone loss, the rs3087456(G) allele was protective against incident fracture overall (p = 0.002), osteoporotic fracture and hip fracture. Carriers of *CLEC16A* and *IFNG* variant alleles had lower BMD ($p < 0.05$) and ultrasound parameters and a lower risk of incident fracture (*CLEC16A*, p = 0.011). In 25-year old women, none of the genes were associated with BMD. In conclusion, variation in inflammatory genes *CIITA*, *CLEC-16A* and *INFG* appear to contribute to bone phenotypes in elderly women and suggest a role for low-grade inflammation and MHC class II expression for osteoporosis pathogenesis.

Editor: Stacey Cherny, University of Hong Kong, Hong Kong

Funding: This work was supported by grants from the Swedish Research Council www.vr.se (K2009-53X-14691-07-3, K2010-77PK-21362-01-2), FAS www.fas.se (Grant 2007–2125), Greta and Johan Kock Foundation www.kockskastiftelsen.se, A. Påhlsson Foundation, A. Osterlund Foundation, Knut and Alice Wallenberg Foundation www.wallenberg.com/kaw, the H Järnhardt foundation, King Gustav V and Queen Victoria Foundation, Åke Wiberg Foundation, Thelma Zoegas Foundation, Malmö University Hospital Research Foundation, Research and Development Council of Region Skåne, Sweden, the Swedish Medical Society www.slf.se. The funders had no role in study design, data collection and analysis, decision to publish, or preparation of the manuscript.

Competing Interests: The authors have declared that no competing interests exist.

* E-mail: Kristina.Akesson@med.lu.se

Introduction

Osteoporosis is a common disease in our ageing society and affects one in three women during the course of their lifetime. The disease is characterized by quantitative and qualitative changes to bone tissue and results in increased risk of fractures [1]. The etiology of osteoporosis is complex and contains both genetic and environmental risk factors, as well as interactions between them. As much as 80% of the population variance in bone mineral density (BMD) is genetically determined and results from many common alleles conferring small risk increments [2]. Genes may be phenotype specific or pleiotropic within the context of osteoporosis or shared with other complex diseases [2,3].

The role of the immune system is well established in conditions that are primarily inflammatory such as rheumatoid arthritis (RA), systemic lupus erythematosus (SLE) and multiple sclerosis (MS), however, systemic inflammatory processes are involved in other complex diseases such as obesity, diabetes and cardiovascular disease, and possibly also osteoporosis [4–6]. These diseases are generally more prevalent with increasing age and shared common risk factors have been identified [5,6]. While patients with some chronic inflammatory disorders are more likely to develop osteopenia, osteoimmunological interplay also constitutes part of normal physiological processes in bone.

The interplay between the immune system and bone metabolism includes molecular and cellular interactions between haematopoietic cells, lymphocytes, osteoblasts and osteoclasts, which are derived from the monocyte-macrophage lineage [2,3]. These interactions involve major histocompatibility complex (MHC) molecules and cytokines that have dual roles in bone homeostasis [3,7,8]. Antigen presentation on MHC molecules and the resulting activating patterns are crucial to the degree and type of immune response. Macrophage lineage cells are thus capable of both eliciting and modulating the inflammatory response by presenting MHCII molecules and activating T lymphocytes. The MHCII transactivator (MHC2TA) assembles transcription factors at promoter sites and is the master regulator of MHCII expression [9]. Expression of MHC2TA is crucial for proper antigen presentation [10] and is in turn induced by the cytokine interferon-γ (IFNγ).

Allelic variation in MHCII molecules contributes to several diseases including MS [11], RA [12,13] and osteoarthritis [14,15] while Genome-wide association studies (GWAS) of bone density and fracture have identified the human leukocyte antigen (HLA) region on chromosome 6p21, which encodes many immune-related genes including MHCII [16,17]. In the HLA region, the common rs3130340(T) allele was found to be associated with reduced BMD at the spine and increased risk of low trauma fractures [17]. Combining GWAS and gene expression data, Farber performed weighted gene co-expression network analysis (WGCNA) and identified a co-expression module highly enriched for genes involved in immune processes [18]. In addition, association studies have identified the pro-inflammatory interleukin 6 (IL6) gene as a determinant for low BMD [19–22], while in a previous study of the pro-inflammatory cytokine macrophage migration inhibitory factor (*MIF*) gene we reported association of *MIF* polymorphisms with bone loss and increased levels of bone resorption markers in elderly women [23].

A more pro-inflammatory profile characterized by increased levels of IFNγ and changes in cytokine regulation is evident in perimenopausal women and may induce bone loss. For example, activated T lymphocytes produce tumor necrosis factor-α (TNFα), an instrumental cytokine contributing to increased osteoclast activity and subsequent loss of bone density [24]. Studies in mice report a key role for MHC2TA in ovariectomy-induced bone loss, where the increased production of IFNγ increased MHC2TA expression, leading to lymphocyte activation and production of TNFα [25]. Based on the link between bone and inflammation, we hypothesize that polymorphisms of genes in the IFNγ-MHC2TA-MHCII pathway have implications for susceptibility to postmenopausal and senile osteoporosis. To date, this has not been explored as a determinant of bone loss and fracture with advancing age or at the time of maximal bone mass. In this study, we therefore analyzed polymorphisms in three genes encoding proteins regulating adaptive immune responses; MHC2TA (*CIITA*; 16p13), C-type lectin domain 16A (*CLEC16A*; 16p13) and IFNγ (*IFNG*; 12q14).

The rational for selecting these genes for analysis is based on considerable evidence. For example, null mutations in *CIITA* cause severe immunodeficiency [10] while common functional polymorphisms in the gene affect MHCII expression levels and susceptibility to inflammatory and complex diseases [26–33]. *CLEC16A* is located adjacent to and in linkage disequilibrium (LD) with *CIITA*, motivating analysis of this gene in conjunction with *CIITA*. Furthermore, CLECs play important roles in adaptive immunity by shaping the cytokine profile [34] and associations between *CLEC16A*, both in conjunction and independent of *CIITA* have been reported in several inflammatory conditions [31,35–38]. IFNγ induces MHCII expression through *CIITA* and polymorphisms in *IFNG* are associated with differential gene expression and disease susceptibility [39]. In postmenopausal women, the production of pro-inflammatory cytokines such as IFNγ is increased [40] and studies in ovariectomized mice have shown increased production of IFNγ, enhanced activation of T lymphocytes through MHC2TA and increased bone loss [25].

To address the genetic impact of polymorphisms in genes with possible effects on osteoimmunological interactions involving MHCII, T-lymphocytes and osteoclast activation, we studied both young and elderly women; 1003 75-year old women followed for up to 10 years and 999 25-year old women in order to capture age-related differences on BMD, bone loss and incident fracture risk.

Methods

Study Subjects

The Malmö Osteoporotic Prospective Risk Assessment (OPRA) cohort is a longitudinal population-based cohort of Caucasian women aged 75 years who were randomly selected from the Malmö city files between 1995 and 1999. No exclusion criteria were applied. A total of 1604 women were invited, 1044 (65%) attended at baseline and 715 women completed the 5 year follow-up visit.

In this study, BMD was measured at baseline and 5 years, with additional measurements available in 371 women at 10 years for hip and total body. Bone resorption markers were measured in serum at baseline and at the 1-, 3-, and 5-year follow-up visits. Information on medication, smoking and illness was collected by a questionnaire. Of the 1044 women at baseline, 145 (14%) were smokers, 208 (20%) were former smokers, 69 had diabetes, 48 were using hormone replacement therapy (HRT) or bisphosphonates at baseline (119 were using one or both of these medications at baseline or sometime during the 5 year follow-up period). Full details of this cohort have been reported previously [41].

The PEAK-25 cohort is a population-based cohort of Caucasian women aged 25 years living in Malmö. Initially, 2394 women randomly selected from the city files between 1999 and 2004 were invited, 1059 (44%) attended the full investigation. The exclusion criteria used were pregnancy or recent childbirth (n = 102, 7.6% of non-participants). Of those who participated, 56% were non-smokers 26% were current smokers and 18% were previous smokers. Full details of this cohort have been reported previously [42].

All participants gave written informed consent and the Lund University Ethics Committee approved the study. This study was performed according to the principles of the Helsinki declaration.

The data reported in this analysis is based on women for whom genotype and phenotype data was available, corresponding to 1003 women from the OPRA cohort at baseline and 999 women from the PEAK-25 cohort. Clinical characteristics of the women attending the baseline visit are shown in Table 1.

Marker Selection

Polymorphisms in *CIITA*, *CLEC16A* and *INFG* were selected based on previously reported associations with inflammatory disorders, other diseases or differential gene expression [29–31,33,35–37,39,43,44]. The SNPs have not previously been identified in GWAS of osteoporosis related traits. Marker details and criteria for selection are shown in Table 2.

Genotyping

Total genomic DNA was isolated from blood using the QIAamp 96 DNA blood kit (Qiagen, Valencia, CA, USA) according to the manufacturer's instructions.

Genotyping of *CLEC16A* (rs6498169) and *INFG* polymorphisms rs2069705 and rs2069727 was performed using Taqman SNP genotyping Assay (Applied Biosystems, Foster City, CA, USA). PCR was conducted in a Dual 384-well GeneAmp PCR system 9700 (Applied Biosystems), with an endpoint plate read on ABI 7900HT (Appied Biosystems) using the SDS 2.2.2 software. Polymorphisms for *CIITA* (rs3087456 and rs4774), *CLEC16A* (rs2903692 and rs725613) and *INFG* (rs2069718) were genotyped by Sequenom's iPlex Gold system (Sequenom, San Diego, CA). The overall success rate for both methods was >98 for all polymorphisms. Approximately 3% of the samples from each cohort were genotyped in duplicate with 100 percent concordance.

Table 1. Baseline clinical characteristics of the OPRA and PEAK-25 cohorts.

	OPRA (n = 1003)			PEAK-25 (n = 999)		
Variable	**Mean**	**±SD**	**(Range)**	**Mean**	**±SD**	**(Range)**
Age (years)	75.2	0.1	(75.0–75.9)	25.5	0.2	(25.0–25.9)
Weight (kg)	67.8	11.5	(41–110)	64.6	11.1	(40–135)
Height[a] (cm)	164.1	5.5	(145–180)	167.6	6.1	(150–187)
BMD (g/cm²)[b]						
Total body	1.007	0.097	(0.718–1.422)	1.174	0.073	(0.969–1.478)
Femoral neck	0.748	0.130	(0.153–1.230)	1.055	0.124	(0.746–1.604)
Total hip	0.849	0.149	(0.498–1.416)			
Lumbar spine	0.993	0.195	(0.518–1.855)	1.217	0.129	(0.824–1.868)
Ultrasound[c]						
BUA	102	10	(56–136)	118	11	(59–149)
SoS	1523	27	(1425–1643)	1575	32	(1498–1706)
Stiffness	72	13	(31–112)	99	15	(42–150)

[a]Height at age 20 (OPRA), Height at baseline visit, age 25 (PEAK25).
[b]BMD n = 904–946 (OPRA), n = 996–999 (PEAK-25).
[c]QUS n = 853 (OPRA), n = 853 (PEAK-25).

All polymorphisms conformed to Hardy-Weinberg equilibrium. Allele and genotype frequencies are reported in Supplementary Table S1.

Bone Density

The areal BMD was measured with dual-energy x-ray absorptiometry (DXA) by Lunar DPX-L for OPRA and Lunar Prodigy for PEAK-25 (Lunar Corporation WI, USA and GE Health Lunar Densitometry, WI, USA) at all sites (total body (TB), femoral neck (FN), total hip (TH) and lumbar spine L2–L4 (LS)). Analyses of OPRA scans were made with software versions 1.33 and 1.35 at baseline, 4.7b at five years and 4.7e at 10 years. The total hip scans were all analyzed with version 4.7b. There was no drift in phantom measurement results during the study period. Analyses of PEAK-25 scans were made with software versions 2.05, 2.15, 3.60, 5.70 and 7.70. DXA calibrations were performed daily using a manufacturer supplied phantom and the precision error (coefficient of variation) was total body; 0.94, LS; 1.45 and FN; 4.01 [45].

The rate of bone loss (RBL) between age 75 and 80 represents the annual change in BMD between the scan at baseline (BMD_{BL}) and the 5-year follow-up (BMD_{5Y}). It was calculated as $[(BMD_{5Y}\text{-}BMD_{BL})/BMD_{BL}/\text{years between scans}*100]$. The LS BMD at age 80 and LS RBL are not reported since previously we showed that LS BMD increased likely due to the presence of osteophytes, degenerative changes and compressive fractures common in women of this age [46]. Weight and BMD at age 75, 80 and 85 along with RBL is presented in Supplementary Table S3.

Quantitative Ultrasound

Quantitative ultrasound measurement speed of sound (SoS), broadband ultrasound attenuation (BUA) and stiffness index (SI, derived from of BUA and SoS) were assessed in both cohorts using a Lunar Achilles® system (Lunar Corporation, Madison, WI, USA). The right calcaneus was measured unless precluded by a previous history of injury or fracture. Precision was 1.5 for BUA and SOS [47] and calibrations were performed daily.

Fracture

Fractures in the OPRA cohort were self-reported for adult fractures (age 20–75) at the time of inclusion in the study and were verified from radiological files as previously reported [48]. In addition, incident fractures during the follow-up period (until November 2006) were recorded and verified by reviewing the related medical records [49]. The majority of fractures sustained (>99%) were attributable to low energy trauma. Fractures were classified as being osteoporotic if affecting the hip, distal radius, spine or proximal humerus.

Table 2. Markers used in the study and allele frequency in the OPRA cohort.

SNP ID	Location Chr (bp)	Common allele (frequency)	Minor allele (frequency)	Selection criteria
CIITA				
rs3087456	16 (10970902)	A (0.765)	G (0.235)	Association with inflammatory disease and differential gene expression. [29,30,33]
rs4774	16 (11000848)	G (0.689)	C (0.311)	
CLEC16A				
rs725613	16 (11169683)	T (0.660)	G (0.340)	Associated with type 1 diabetes and multiple sclerosis. [31,35,73–75]
rs2903692	16 (11238783)	G (0.678)	A (0.322)	
rs6498169	16 (11249329)	A (0.604)	G (0.396)	Associated with multiple sclerosis and rheumatoid arthritis [31,36,76]
IFNG				
rs2069727	12 (68548223)	T (0.532)	C (0.468)	Located 3′ near gene
rs2069718	12 (68550162)	C (0.582)	T (0.418)	Association with SLE. Located in intron 3 [39]
rs2069705	12 (68555011)	T (0.626)	C (0.374)	Association with SLE. Located 5′ upstream of gene [39]

Biochemistry

The serum bone markers C-terminal cross-linking telopeptide of type I collagen (S-CTX) and serum tartrate-resistant acid phosphatase 5b (S-TRACP5b) were analyzed in the OPRA cohort. S-TRACP5b was determined with BoneTRAP® assay (SBA Sciences/Immunodiagnostic Systems IDS Inc., Bolton, UK) and S-CTX was determined with Elecsys β-CrossLaps immunoassay (Roche Diagnostics, Indianapolis, IN). Details of the assays have been reported previously [46].

Longitudinal measures of bone resorption markers at baseline, 1-, 3-, and 5-years (age 80) were used. Among the 1003 women included in this study, data for all time points was available from 614 subjects for S-TRACP5b and from 606 subjects for S-CTX. Subgroups were created according to whether women had constantly low or constantly or high levels of S-CTX or S-TRACP5b over 5 years, as described previously. Those in the lowest or highest tertiles at three or more time points were considered to have constantly low or high levels, respectively, over the 5-year period. All others were classified into the intermediate group [50]. Among the 1003 women included in this study, 93 were constantly high and 108 constantly low for S-TRACP5b and 121 constantly high and 117 constantly low for S-CTX. Women using potent estrogen or bisphosphonates were excluded from the analyses (S-TRACP5b n = 76, S-CTX n = 77) since these medications have been shown to decrease S-CTX levels [51,52].

Routine biochemistry measured C-reactive protein (CRP, mg/L) in plasma, erythrocyte sedimentation rate (ESR, mm/h) in blood and leukocytes (BLC 10^9/L) in blood at 10-year follow-up.

Statistics

Deviation from Hardy-Weinberg equilibrium was calculated by the chi-square test. Linkage disequilibrium (LD) was evaluated within each gene and between *CIITA* and *CLEC-16A* using the Haploview program (http://www.broad.mit.edu/mpg/haploview/) and taking into consideration both D and r^2. Haplotypes were constructed for *CLEC16A* and *IFNG* using PHASE version 2.02 [53], and estimated haplotypes with a frequency >0.10 and a >0.8 probability of correct assignment were used for analysis.

ANOVA was used to determine associations between genotypes, bone density and rate of bone loss.

Bone resorption marker values were log-transformed prior to analysis due to non-normal distribution. The t-test was used for comparing mean S-CTX and S-TRACP5b values, and the Pearson Chi-Square test was used for analyzing consistently high and low levels of markers and association of polymorphisms with fracture incidence.

Linear regression was used to identify confounding factors for BMD, RBL and ultrasound and where indicated, multinomial logistic regression was used to adjust for total body BMD and weight at baseline in fracture analyses. Age was not included for adjustment since all the women within each cohort were of the same age.

The following covariates were used in the analyses of the OPRA cohort. BMD at baseline: weight (baseline), diabetes, current use of bisphosphonates (BPs) or potent estrogen (E) and smoking exposure (cigarettes per day*years smoking); BMD at 5-year follow-up: weight (5-year follow-up) and smoking exposure; BMD at 10-year follow-up: weight (10-year follow-up); RBL: use of E and/or BPs at baseline or during follow-up; QUS: weight (baseline), current use of BPs or E and smoking exposure. Exclusion of estrogen or bisphosphonate users from the analysis (n = 82) did not appreciably alter the results overall.

When indicated, weight change between baseline and 5-year follow-up visit was also used as covariate for RBL. Covariates used in the PEAK-25 cohort were height, weight and smoking for BMD; weight and smoking for ultrasound phenotypes.

Interaction between polymorphisms may contribute to opposite or synergistic effects on the phenotype of interest. To this end we performed pairwise interactions between SNPs to explore the effect on differences in BMD and QUS. Using general linear model-ANOVA (GLM-ANOVA), the model included an interaction term, covariates and assumed a co-dominant genetic model. In the results, p-values are reported for the interaction overall while in the tables mean BMD values defined by SNP_1-SNP_2 carriers compared to SNP_1-SNP_2 non-carriers are presented.

A priori power analyses indicated that the sample size of our studies allowed a >80% power to detect a difference in BMD of 0.1 standard deviations among genotype groups, while maintaining a type I error at 5%. This is based on the assumption of a SD of 0.13 g/cm^2 in BMD, which allows detection of a 0.065 g/cm^2 difference between genotype groups assuming a minor allele frequency of 0.21 or greater. Similarly, the OPRA study had >80% power to detect relative risks for fracture of at least 1.2.

All statistical analyses were performed using SPSS for Windows 18.0 (SPSS Inc., Chicago, IL) and associations with a p-value of <0.05 were considered nominally significant. The phenotypes and several of the markers studied are not independent (i.e. are correlated or in LD), therefore applying a Bonferroni correction would be over-stringent. We therefore report the uncorrected p-values and acknowledge the fact that multiple tests were performed.

Results

CIITA

The 2 SNPs in *CIITA* were not in strong LD with each other (D'<0.36, r^2<0.02) or with the 3 SNPs in the adjacent *CLEC16A* gene (D'<0.45, r^2<0.04). Haplotype estimates predicted 3 common (>10%) haplotypes (Supplementary Table S2). Haplotype analysis for *CIITA* did not add appreciably to the overall information obtained from genotype analyses (data not shown).

Bone Density and Bone Loss

In the OPRA cohort of elderly women, there was a moderate association between *CIITA* and BMD. Carriers of the rare rs3087456(G) allele displayed higher FN BMD at age 75 (baseline) and interaction between variant alleles rs3087456(G) and rs4774(C) was observed, resulting in higher LS BMD. At age 80 (5-year follow-up), FN BMD and TB BMD were also higher in rs3087456(G) carriers and an interaction between rs3087456(G) and rs4774(C) was associated with higher BMD at all sites (Table 3). At 10-year follow-up (n = 376), interaction between rs3087456(G) and rs4774(C) variant alleles was observed, with higher BMD at the FN (p = 0.019) TH (p = 0.027) and TB (p = 0.004) compared to common homozygotes (rs3087456(G): FN +0.4%, TH +1.7%, TB +1.8%; rs4774(C): FN +1.9%, TH +2.5%, TB +1.5%), data not shown.

The QUS results were in line with those for BMD with rs3087456(G) carriers having higher mean values for stiffness (72.9/70.6; p = 0.030) and BUA (102.6/101.1; p = 0.045).

Homozygotes for the rare *CIITA* allele rs3087456(G) had higher annual rates of bone loss (RBL) at the FN (p = 0.013), TH (p = 0.030) and TB (p = 0.00016). TB RBL was also higher for rs4774(C) homozygotes (p = 3.8E-5). This association was independent of weight change for FN and TB, but not for TH

Table 3. Associations between BMD and *CIITA, CLEC16A* and *IFNG* in the OPRA cohort.

Gene	SNP (rare allele)/haplotype	Site	Age	BMD mean[1] (g/cm^2)	P-value*
CIITA	rs3087456(G)	FN	75	0.740/0.761	0.049
	rs3087456(G)*rs4774(C)	LS	75	0.967/0.992	0.011[2]
	rs3087456(G)	FN	80	0.702/0.726	0.041
	rs3087456(G)*rs4774(C)	FN	80	0.692/0.717	0.020[3]
	rs3087456(G)*rs4774(C)	TH	80	0.784/0.803	0.042
	rs3087456(G)	TB	80	0.989/1.009	0.015
	rs3087456(G)*rs4774(C)	TB	80	0.981/1.005	0.027
CLEC16A	Haplotype 1[4]	LS	75	1.002/0.983	0.037
	Haplotype 1[4]	FN	80	0.716/0.706	0.035
	Haplotype 1[4]	TH	80	0.802/0.794	0.039
	rs6498169	TB	80	0.997/1.002/0.985	0.037
IFNG	Haplotype 4[5]	TH	75	0.854/0.846	0.035
	rs2069727*rs2069705	LS	75	0.973/1.007/0.989 0.993/1.002/0.962	0.027

*Only associations where p<0.05 are reported.
[1]BMD values are reported as follows: For single SNP analysis (non-carrriers/carriers or common homozygotes/heterozygotes/variant homozygotes); For haplotypes (non-carriers/carriers); For interactions in allelic models (non-carriers of both variant alleles/carriers of both variant alleles); For interactions in genotypic models, values are given for each marker as common homozygotes/heterozygotes/variant homozygotes since no individuals were carriers of both variant alleles.
[2]For rs3087456 * rs4774 genotypic model, p = 0.011.
[3]For rs3087456 * rs4774 genotypic model, p = 0.028.
[4]CLEC16A haplotype 1: rs725613(T)/rs2903692(G)/rs6498169(A).
[5]IFNG haplotype 4: rs2069727(T)/rs2069718(T)/rs2069705(C).

(Table 4). In addition, there was interaction between SNPs rs3087456*rs4774 for TB RBL (p = 8.7E-5, adjusted 0.002).

CIITA was not associated with body weight at baseline, but to weight change between age 75 and 80 (rs3087456, p = 0.016, genotypic model). Women with the rs3087456(G/G) genotype had a mean weight loss of 2.8 kg compared to 1.4 kg for women with the rs3087456(A/A) genotype.

Bone resorption markers were not associated with *CIITA* genotype, neither was blood biochemistry (CRP, ESR) or blood leukocyte count.

Fracture

Among the OPRA participants, 51% (n = 507) had suffered at least one fracture between age 20 and 75, with no significant difference between the *CIITA* genotype groups. Incident fracture after age 75 was confirmed for 350 women (35%), resulting predominantly (99%) from low energy trauma. One or more osteoporotic fractures (at the hip, vertebra, distal radius or proximal humerus) occurred in 282 individuals (28%), of whom 110 (11%) had hip fracture.

The rs3087456(G) allele was protective against incident fracture overall, osteoporotic fractures and hip fracture (Table 5). The protective effect was significant even after correction for BMD and body weight at age 75 (Table 5).

Table 4. *CIITA* association with rate of bone loss between age 75 and 80.

Site	Marker	Mean BMD (g/cm^2)[1]	P-value[2]	Adjusted P-value[3]
Femoral neck	rs3087456	−1.398/−1.498/−2.096	0.013	0.036
Total Hip	rs3087456	−1.123/−1.333/−1.599	0.030	NS
Total Body	rs3087456	−0.299/−0.250/−0.356	0.00016	0.0011
Total Body	rs4774	−0.286/−0.266/−0.348	0.000038	0.00069

[1]CC/CV/VV (c = common, v = variant allele).
[2]Genotypic model.
[3]Adjusted for weight change between age 75 and 80.

CLEC16A

LD between the *CLEC16A* SNPs was stronger between rs725613 and rs2903692 (D' = 0.95, $r^2 = 0.84$) than with rs6498169 (D'≥0.90, $r^2 \geq 0.27$). Three common (>10%) haplotypes were predicted (Supplementary Table S2).

Bone Density and Bone Loss

Carriers of *CLEC16A* haplotype 1 (rs725613(T)/rs2903692(G)/rs6498169(A)) had lower LS BMD at baseline (−2%) and lower BMD at the 5 year follow-up at the FN (−1.3%) and TH (−1.5%) (Table 3). Women with genotype rs6498169(G/G) displayed lower TB BMD at 5-year follow-up (0.98 vs 1.00, p = 0.037) compared to the rs6498169(A/A) or (A/G) genotypes. For bone loss between age 75 and 80, women with the rs2903692(A/A) genotype displayed reduced TB RBL (−1.30 vs −1.51, p = 0.033).

The rs2903692 marker was also associated with QUS parameters, as carriers of the rare (A) allele had lower stiffness values (71.2 vs 72.0; p = 0.040) while BUA was lowest in the (G/A) heterozygotes (GG: 101.9, GA: 101.5, AA: 101.9; p = 0.045).

Carriers of *CLEC16A* haplotype 1 had higher blood leucocyte counts at 10 years compared to non-carriers (BLC 7.0 vs 6.3×10^9/L, p = 0.002), while bone markers were not significantly associated.

Table 5. Association of *CIITA and CLEC16* polymorphisms with incident fractures between age 75 and 80 in the OPRA cohort.

Polymorphism	Genotype	Women without fracture (%)	Women with fracture (%)	p-value (adjusted)[1]	Odds Ratio (95% confidence interval)
Any fracture					
*CIITA_* rs3087456	AA	349 (61)	223 (39)	0.002	
	AG/GG	294 (71)	122 (29)	(0.005)	0.657 (0.491–0.879)
CLEC16A_rs725613	TT	264 (61)	171 (39)	0.011	
	TG/GG	380 (69)	175 (32)	(0.013)	0.699 (0.526–0.928)
Hip fracture					
CIITA_ rs3087456	AA	498 (87)	74 (13)	0.025	
	AG/GG	381 (92)	35(8)	(0.038)	0.626 (0.402–0.975)
CLEC16A_rs725613	TT	392 (90)	43 (10)	NS	
	TG/GG	489 (88)	66 (12)	(NS)	
Osteoporotic fracture[2]					
CIITA_ rs3087456	AA	395 (69)	177 (31)	0.021	
	AG/GG	315 (76)	101 (24)	(0.047)	0.732 (0.538–0.996)
CLEC16A_rs725613	TT	297 (68)	138 (32)	0.027	
	TG/GG	415 (75)	140 (25)	(0.022)	0.705 (0.522–0.951)

[1]P-values calculated by χ^2; adjusted for variables weight and TB BMD at 75y (Any fracture, Osteoporotic fracture) or weight and FN BMD at 75y (Hip fracture).
[2]Osteoporotic fracture sites include hip, vertebrae, distal radius, proximal humerus.

Fracture

Carriage of the rare *CLEC16A* rs725613(G) allele or *CLEC16A* haplotype 7 (rs725613(G)/rs2903692(A)/rs6498169(A)) was similarly protective against incident fracture overall, including after correction for TB BMD and body weight. The rs725613(G) allele was also protective of osteoporotic fractures, but not hip fracture specifically (Table 5).

IFNG

The three markers in *IFNG* were in LD (D′ = 0.99, r^2>0.45) and 3 common haplotypes were predicted (Supplementary Table S2).

Bone Density and Bone Loss

None of the individual genotypes were associated with BMD at baseline or follow-up; however carriers of haplotype 4 (rs2069727(T)/rs2069718(T)/rs2069705(C)) had 1% lower baseline BMD at the hip. Interaction between rs2069727*rs2069705 was also observed at the lumbar spine (Table 3).

For the QUS phenotypes, there were small but significant differences in mean values. The variant alleles for all 3 *IFNG* SNPs, but not their derived haplotypes, were associated with increased BUA, the most significant being rs2069727(C) (p = 0.00003). Carriers of rs2069705(G) and *IFNG* haplotype 4 had lower SoS values (p = 0.003). The rs2069727(C) and rs2069718(C/T) genotypes were associated with slightly higher stiffness values with both a single-marker and interactive model (p = 0.033-0.05). There was no association between polymorphisms in the *IFNG* gene and bone loss, fracture, bone markers or blood biochemistry.

Young Adult Women – the PEAK-25 Cohort

In young adult women representing peak bone mass, there was no association between *CIITA, CLEC16A or IFNG* SNPs and BMD. Small differences (<0.4%) between the genotype groups were observed between *CIITA* rs4774 and the QUS phenotype SoS (p = 0.031).

Discussion

This study suggests that inflammatory genes play a role in regulating bone mass and bone loss and influence the risk of incident fractures in elderly women. Specifically, we report association between polymorphisms in the inflammatory genes *CIITA*, *CLEC16A* and *IFNG* with BMD, ultrasound parameters, annual rate of bone loss and incident fractures in 75-year old women followed for 10 years. These results support inflammation and, specifically, MHCII expression as key components in postmenopausal or senile osteoporosis.

The reported association of *CIITA* and *IFNG* polymorphisms to BMD in elderly women is contrasted by the absence of association in young adult women, which suggests differential effects of these genes across the life span. It also supports our hypothesis that low-grade systemic inflammatory processes are elements of normal ageing in women, possibly due to the link between estrogen and cytokine levels. Estrogen receptors are expressed on both lymphocytes and mononuclear cells [54], making them responsive to changes in estrogen levels. Estrogen deficiency leads to increased immune activation mediated by antigen presenting cells (APCs) and cytokines (IFNγ, IL-7 and transforming growth factor-β), resulting in increased TNFα production from activated T lymphocytes [24]. By increasing both the production and sensitivity to RANKL, TNFα has potent effects on osteoclasts [24]. Polymorphisms affecting immune activation processes could therefore have an impact during periods with generally higher pro-inflammatory profile, such as old age and illness. We interpret the discrepant results between the elderly and young adult women as a reflection of differences in duration of exposure to low-grade systemic inflammation. The potentially deleterious effects of inflammation should be more pronounced if the systemic inflammatory processes have continued for years. This could also explain why, despite numerous GWAS of osteoporosis related phenotypes [16–18,55–71], these SNPs have not previously been identified; GWAS are not able to identify gene-environment interactions while the top 15 SNPs associated with BMD account for <3% of the variance of BMD [16].

Our observed results in elderly women - an association between functional polymorphisms in *CIITA*, BMD and fracture- is supported by previous reports evaluating the impact of the MHC2TA protein on molecular interactions and pathways. MHC2TA regulation of osteoclasts has been described in murine cells where it negatively regulated NFATc1 (nuclear factor of activated T-cells, cytoplasmic 1) and OSCAR by sequestering CBP/p300 from their promoter regions [72]. Decreased expression of *CIITA* would in this context lead to increased formation of osteoclasts. However, alternative mechanisms are also suggested since transgenic mice overexpressing *CIITA* display a hyper-osteoclastogenic phenotype and increased activation of signaling downstream of RANK (*E. Benasciutti and S. Cenci, personal communication)*.

Based on our observations in this study and from earlier results from us and co-workers on expression levels [33], we postulate that the studied *CIITA* polymorphisms have osteoclast-stimulating effects that override the direct, inhibitory effect of IFNγ on osteoclasts [25]. Mechanistically this may be explained by estrogen deficiency after menopause, leading to increased production of IFNγ [24,25] and an induction of *CIITA* expression in cells of the monocyte/macrophage lineage. The resulting MHC2TA protein acts as a transcriptional transactivator at MHCII promoters, and induces expression of MHCII molecules on antigen presenting cells [9]. The T cell pool then increases due to inhibited T cell apoptosis by the increased amount of IFNγ and more T cells become activated by binding MHCII molecules. The activated T cells produce TNF, which could stimulate osteoclast activity through induction of RANKL, and increase osteoclast number through stimulating cytokines. The increase in osteoclast activity could then lead to decreased BMD and increased risk of fracture. The observed protective effect from the *CIITA* rs3087456(G) allele is associated with lower expression of *CIITA* and MHCII [33], which could slow down the process of T cell- and osteoclast stimulation and result in higher BMD and reduced fracture risk.

In the present study, the inverse effect of *CIITA* variant alleles on rate of bone loss compared to BMD and fracture is however somewhat contradictory. Individuals carrying *CIITA* variant alleles (mainly *CIITA* rs3087456(G)) lost more bone mineral density between age 75 and 80, but had higher BMD at age 75, 80 and 85 and, importantly, were protected from incident fracture during this time. *CIITA* variant alleles thus had a net positive effect on bone density and bone strength in elderly women at all time-points, despite also being associated with a higher rate of bone loss. Gene effects on bone turnover were not reflected by the bone resorption markers S-CTX and S-TRACP5b, however, the low numbers with consistently high or low turnover may have masked such effects. Furthermore, markers indicate turnover (and the potential effect of inflammatory processes on it) only at the time of sample collection and may not be able to capture the long-term effects of inflammation.

In addition to *CIITA*, *CLEC16A* and to a lesser extent *INFG* were associated with bone mass phenotypes. However, the contribution to fracture risk is less clear; *CLEC16A* was associated with a significantly reduced fracture risk, although less than *CIITA*, while *INFG* was not. A potential explanation would be that the *CLEC16A* marker most strongly associated with fracture (rs725613), is located closest to, and is in weak LD with *CIITA*.

The strengths of the study include the comprehensive and extended evaluation of the women in the OPRA-cohort, including detailed fracture information and bone turnover markers. We also have the possibility to make direct comparisons of ageing effects through the large cohort of young adult women in the PEAK-25 cohort. In this study, the reported association with bone phenotypes and overall fracture risk in the elderly women support the relevance of inflammatory genes affecting MCHCII expression in the pathogenesis of osteoporosis.

The study has some limitations, notably the large number of tests performed. Taking this into consideration and applying a conservative Bonferroni correction, the results can be considered to fall short of p<0.05. Performing adjustment at least for the 8 markers tested, association with BMD is non-significant, whereas association of CIITA with total body RBL, fracture and hip fracture is still significant. Importantly however the direction of effect of the SNPs within each gene is consistent indicating biological plausibility for the observations and importantly, both cohorts are of sufficient size to be confident of detecting true genotype related differences in the phenotypes analysed.

Replication studies are needed in order to fully evaluate the effect of the studied SNPs on osteoporosis-related phenotypes. Thus, replication in a similarly aged cohort to OPRA is necessary to corroborate the findings. Secondly, routine biochemistry including leukocyte count, CRP and ESR as clinical indicators of inflammation was only available on all OPRA participants at age 85. The finding that *CLEC16A* haplotypes were associated with higher counts of blood leukocytes with a similar trend for single markers, suggests that it would have been interesting to have complete longitudinal data. Thirdly, longitudinal data for the young adult women would be potentially interesting (including follow-up extending into the perimenopausal years) in order to facilitate evaluation of the natural course of inflammatory influence with normal ageing and transition to an estrogen deplete state. In a study comparing levels of IFNγ in young, perimenopausal and elderly women, the levels of IFNγ increased at menopause compared to young women, but fell to even lower levels in the elderly [40]. These results strongly argue for testing the studied *CIITA* and *IFNG* polymorphisms in cohorts of perimenopausal women for comparison.

We conclude that expression-related polymorphisms in the inflammatory genes *CIITA* and *CLEC16A* are associated with BMD and fracture in elderly women. These findings illustrate the importance of inflammation and MHCII expression in particular in the pathogenesis of reduced bone strength in the elderly.

Supporting Information

Table S1 Allele and genotype frequencies for *CIITA*, *CLEC16A* and *IFNG* in the OPRA and PEAK25 cohorts.

Table S2 *CIITA*, *CLEC16A* and *IFNG* haplotype frequencies in the OPRA and PEAK25 cohorts.

Table S3 Weight and BMD at age 75, 80 and 85 years (y) in the OPRA cohort (n = 1003) and rate of bone loss (RBL) between 75 and 80 y.

Acknowledgments

Thanks are extended to Lisa Jansson for genotyping support, to the research nurses at the Clinical and Molecular Osteoporosis Research Unit, Malmö and to all the women who kindly participated in the study.

Author Contributions

Conceived and designed the experiments: MS KÅ. Performed the experiments: MS. Analyzed the data: MS. Wrote the paper: MS FEM KVI PG KÅ. Conduct of study: MS. Data collection: PG KÅ. Data interpretation: MS FEM KÅ.

References

1. Cummings SR, Melton LJ (2002) Epidemiology and outcomes of osteoporotic fractures. Lancet 359: 1761–1767.
2. Ferrari S (2008) Human genetics of osteoporosis. Best Pract Res Clin Endocrinol Metab 22: 723–735.
3. Takayanagi H (2007) Osteoimmunology: shared mechanisms and crosstalk between the immune and bone systems. Nat Rev Immunol 7: 292–304.
4. Hofbauer LC, Brueck CC, Shanahan CM, Schoppet M, Dobnig H (2007) Vascular calcification and osteoporosis–from clinical observation towards molecular understanding. Osteoporos Int 18: 251–259.
5. Holmberg AH, Johnell O, Nilsson PM, Nilsson J, Berglund G, et al. (2006) Risk factors for fragility fracture in middle age. A prospective population-based study of 33,000 men and women. Osteoporos Int 17: 1065–1077.
6. Sennerby U, Farahmand B, Ahlbom A, Ljunghall S, Michaelsson K (2007) Cardiovascular diseases and future risk of hip fracture in women. Osteoporos Int 18: 1355–1362.
7. Dewhirst FE, Stashenko PP, Mole JE, Tsurumachi T (1985) Purification and partial sequence of human osteoclast-activating factor: identity with interleukin 1 beta. J Immunol 135: 2562–2568.
8. Takayanagi H, Ogasawara K, Hida S, Chiba T, Murata S, et al. (2000) T-cell-mediated regulation of osteoclastogenesis by signalling cross-talk between RANKL and IFN-gamma. Nature 408: 600–605.
9. Nagarajan UM, Bushey A, Boss JM (2002) Modulation of gene expression by the MHC class II transactivator. J Immunol 169: 5078–5088.
10. Steimle V, Otten LA, Zufferey M, Mach B (1993) Complementation cloning of an MHC class II transactivator mutated in hereditary MHC class II deficiency (or bare lymphocyte syndrome). Cell 75: 135–146.
11. Allen M, Sandberg-Wollheim M, Sjogren K, Erlich HA, Petterson U, et al. (1994) Association of susceptibility to multiple sclerosis in Sweden with HLA class II DRB1 and DQB1 alleles. Hum Immunol 39: 41–48.
12. Stastny P (1976) Mixed lymphocyte cultures in rheumatoid arthritis. J Clin Invest 57: 1148–1157.
13. Zanelli E, Breedveld FC, de Vries RR (2000) HLA class II association with rheumatoid arthritis: facts and interpretations. Hum Immunol 61: 1254–1261.
14. Pattrick M, Manhire A, Ward AM, Doherty M (1989) HLA-A, B antigens and alpha 1-antitrypsin phenotypes in nodal generalised osteoarthritis and erosive osteoarthritis. Ann Rheum Dis 48: 470–475.
15. Nakajima M, Takahashi A, Kou I, Rodriguez-Fontenla C, Gomez-Reino JJ, et al. (2010) New sequence variants in HLA class II/III region associated with susceptibility to knee osteoarthritis identified by genome-wide association study. PLoS One 5: e9723.
16. Rivadeneira F, Styrkarsdottir U, Estrada K, Halldorsson BV, Hsu YH, et al. (2009) Twenty bone-mineral-density loci identified by large-scale meta-analysis of genome-wide association studies. Nat Genet 41: 1199–1206.
17. Styrkarsdottir U, Halldorsson BV, Gretarsdottir S, Gudbjartsson DF, Walters GB, et al. (2008) Multiple genetic loci for bone mineral density and fractures. N Engl J Med 358: 2355–2365.
18. Farber CR (2010) Identification of a gene module associated with BMD through the integration of network analysis and genome-wide association data. J Bone Miner Res 25: 2359–2367.
19. Chung HW, Seo JS, Hur SE, Kim HL, Kim JY, et al. (2003) Association of interleukin-6 promoter variant with bone mineral density in pre-menopausal women. J Hum Genet 48: 243–248.
20. Ferrari SL, Ahn-Luong L, Garnero P, Humphries SE, Greenspan SL (2003) Two promoter polymorphisms regulating interleukin-6 gene expression are associated with circulating levels of C-reactive protein and markers of bone resorption in postmenopausal women. J Clin Endocrinol Metab 88: 255–259.
21. Ferrari SL, Garnero P, Emond S, Montgomery H, Humphries SE, et al. (2001) A functional polymorphic variant in the interleukin-6 gene promoter associated with low bone resorption in postmenopausal women. Arthritis Rheum 44: 196–201.
22. Murray RE, McGuigan F, Grant SF, Reid DM, Ralston SH (1997) Polymorphisms of the interleukin-6 gene are associated with bone mineral density. Bone 21: 89–92.
23. Swanberg M, McGuigan F, Ivaska KK, Gerdhem P, Lerner UH, et al. (2010) Polymorphisms in the macrophage migration inhibitory factor gene and bone loss in postmenopausal women. Bone 47: 424–429.
24. Weitzmann MN, Pacifici R (2006) Estrogen regulation of immune cell bone interactions. Ann N Y Acad Sci 1068: 256–274.
25. Cenci S, Toraldo G, Weitzmann MN, Roggia C, Gao Y, et al. (2003) Estrogen deficiency induces bone loss by increasing T cell proliferation and lifespan through IFN-gamma-induced class II transactivator. Proc Natl Acad Sci U S A 100: 10405–10410.
26. Bronson PG, Caillier S, Ramsay PP, McCauley JL, Zuvich RL, et al. (2010) CIITA variation in the presence of HLA-DRB1*1501 increases risk for multiple sclerosis. Hum Mol Genet 19: 2331–2340.
27. Bronson PG, Goldstein BA, Ramsay PP, Beckman KB, Noble JA, et al. (2011) The rs4774 CIITA missense variant is associated with risk of systemic lupus erythematosus. Genes Immun.
28. Grunewald J, Idali F, Kockum I, Seddighzadeh M, Nisell M, et al. (2010) Major histocompatibility complex class II transactivator gene polymorphism: associations with Lofgren's syndrome. Tissue Antigens 76: 96–101.
29. Lindholm E, Melander O, Almgren P, Berglund G, Agardh CD, et al. (2006) Polymorphism in the MHC2TA gene is associated with features of the metabolic syndrome and cardiovascular mortality. PLoS One 1: e64.
30. Martinez A, Alvarez-Lafuente R, Mas A, Bartolome M, Garcia-Montojo M, et al. (2007) Environment-gene interaction in multiple sclerosis: human herpesvirus 6 and MHC2TA. Hum Immunol 68: 685–689.
31. Martinez A, Perdigones N, Cenit MC, Espino L, Varade J, et al. (2010) Chromosomal region 16p13: further evidence of increased predisposition to immune diseases. Ann Rheum Dis 69: 309–311.
32. Skinningsrud B, Husebye ES, Pearce SH, McDonald DO, Brandal K, et al. (2008) Polymorphisms in CLEC16A and CIITA at 16p13 are associated with primary adrenal insufficiency. J Clin Endocrinol Metab 93: 3310–3317.
33. Swanberg M, Lidman O, Padyukov L, Eriksson P, Akesson E, et al. (2005) MHC2TA is associated with differential MHC molecule expression and susceptibility to rheumatoid arthritis, multiple sclerosis and myocardial infarction. Nat Genet 37: 486–494.
34. Geijtenbeek TB, Gringhuis SI (2009) Signalling through C-type lectin receptors: shaping immune responses. Nat Rev Immunol 9: 465–479.
35. Hakonarson H, Grant SF, Bradfield JP, Marchand L, Kim CE, et al. (2007) A genome-wide association study identifies KIAA0350 as a type 1 diabetes gene. Nature 448: 591–594.
36. Hafler DA, Compston A, Sawcer S, Lander ES, Daly MJ, et al. (2007) Risk alleles for multiple sclerosis identified by a genomewide study. N Engl J Med 357: 851–862.
37. Marquez A, Varade J, Robledo G, Martinez A, Mendoza JL, et al. (2009) Specific association of a CLEC16A/KIAA0350 polymorphism with NOD2/CARD15(–) Crohn's disease patients. Eur J Hum Genet 17: 1304–1308.
38. Zuvich RL, Bush WS, McCauley JL, Beecham AH, De Jager PL, et al. (2011) Interrogating the complex role of chromosome 16p13.13 in multiple sclerosis susceptibility: independent genetic signals in the CIITA-CLEC16A-SOCS1 gene complex. Hum Mol Genet.
39. Kim K, Cho SK, Sestak A, Namjou B, Kang C, et al. (2010) Interferon-gamma gene polymorphisms associated with susceptibility to systemic lupus erythematosus. Ann Rheum Dis 69: 1247–1250.
40. Deguchi K, Kamada M, Irahara M, Maegawa M, Yamamoto S, et al. (2001) Postmenopausal changes in production of type 1 and type 2 cytokines and the effects of hormone replacement therapy. Menopause 8: 266–273.
41. Gerdhem P, Brandstrom H, Stiger F, Obrant K, Melhus H, et al. (2004) Association of the collagen type 1 (COL1A 1) Sp1 binding site polymorphism to femoral neck bone mineral density and wrist fracture in 1044 elderly Swedish women. Calcif Tissue Int 74: 264–269.
42. McGuigan FE, Larzenius E, Callreus M, Gerdhem P, Luthman H, et al. (2007) Variation in the BMP2 gene: bone mineral density and ultrasound in young adult and elderly women. Calcif Tissue Int 81: 254–262.
43. Pravica V, Perrey C, Stevens A, Lee JH, Hutchinson IV (2000) A single nucleotide polymorphism in the first intron of the human IFN-gamma gene: absolute correlation with a polymorphic CA microsatellite marker of high IFN-gamma production. Hum Immunol 61: 863–866.
44. Morrison BA, Ucisik-Akkaya E, Flores H, Alaez C, Gorodezky C, et al. (2010) Multiple sclerosis risk markers in HLA-DRA, HLA-C, and IFNG genes are associated with sex-specific childhood leukemia risk. Autoimmunity 43: 690–697.
45. Lenora J, Akesson K, Gerdhem P (2010) Effect of precision on longitudinal follow-up of bone mineral density measurements in elderly women and men. J Clin Densitom 13: 407–412.
46. Lenora J, Ivaska KK, Obrant KJ, Gerdhem P (2007) Prediction of bone loss using biochemical markers of bone turnover. Osteoporos Int 18: 1297–1305.
47. Karlsson MK, Obrant KJ, Nilsson BE, Johnell O (1998) Bone mineral density assessed by quantitative ultrasound and dual energy X-ray absorptiometry. Normative data in Malmo, Sweden. Acta Orthop Scand 69: 189–193.
48. Gerdhem P, Akesson K (2007) Rates of fracture in participants and non-participants in the Osteoporosis Prospective Risk Assessment study. J Bone Joint Surg Br 89: 1627–1631.

49. Ivaska KK, Gerdhem P, Vaananen HK, Akesson K, Obrant KJ (2010) Bone turnover markers and prediction of fracture: a prospective follow-up study of 1040 elderly women for a mean of 9 years. J Bone Miner Res 25: 393–403.
50. Ivaska KK, Lenora J, Gerdhem P, Akesson K, Vaananen HK, et al. (2008) Serial assessment of serum bone metabolism markers identifies women with the highest rate of bone loss and osteoporosis risk. J Clin Endocrinol Metab 93: 2622–2632.
51. Okabe R, Nakatsuka K, Inaba M, Miki T, Naka H, et al. (2001) Clinical evaluation of the Elecsys beta-CrossLaps serum assay, a new assay for degradation products of type I collagen C-tlopeptides. Clin Chem 47: 1410–1414.
52. Seibel MJ (2006) Biochemical Markers of Bone Turnover Part II: Clinical Applications in the Management of Osteoporosis. Clin Biochem Rev 27: 123–138.
53. Stephens M, Smith NJ, Donnelly P (2001) A new statistical method for haplotype reconstruction from population data. Am J Hum Genet 68: 978–989.
54. Weusten JJ, Blankenstein MA, Gmelig-Meyling FH, Schuurman HJ, Kater L, et al. (1986) Presence of oestrogen receptors in human blood mononuclear cells and thymocytes. Acta Endocrinol (Copenh) 112: 409–414.
55. Cho YS, Go MJ, Kim YJ, Heo JY, Oh JH, et al. (2009) A large-scale genome-wide association study of Asian populations uncovers genetic factors influencing eight quantitative traits. Nat Genet 41: 527–534.
56. Duncan EL, Danoy P, Kemp JP, Leo PJ, McCloskey E, et al. (2011) Genome-wide association study using extreme truncate selection identifies novel genes affecting bone mineral density and fracture risk. PLoS Genet 7: e1001372.
57. Guo Y, Tan LJ, Lei SF, Yang TL, Chen XD, et al. (2010) Genome-wide association study identifies ALDH7A1 as a novel susceptibility gene for osteoporosis. PLoS Genet 6: e1000806.
58. Guo Y, Zhang LS, Yang TL, Tian Q, Xiong DH, et al. (2010) IL21R and PTH may underlie variation of femoral neck bone mineral density as revealed by a genome-wide association study. J Bone Miner Res 25: 1042–1048.
59. Hsu YH, Zillikens MC, Wilson SG, Farber CR, Demissie S, et al. (2010) An integration of genome-wide association study and gene expression profiling to prioritize the discovery of novel susceptibility Loci for osteoporosis-related traits. PLoS Genet 6: e1000977.
60. Karasik D, Hsu YH, Zhou Y, Cupples LA, Kiel DP, et al. (2010) Genome-wide pleiotropy of osteoporosis-related phenotypes: the Framingham Study. J Bone Miner Res 25: 1555–1563.
61. Koller DL, Ichikawa S, Lai D, Padgett LR, Doheny KF, et al. (2010) Genome-wide association study of bone mineral density in premenopausal European-American women and replication in African-American women. J Clin Endocrinol Metab 95: 1802–1809.
62. Kung AW, Xiao SM, Cherny S, Li GH, Gao Y, et al. (2010) Association of JAG1 with bone mineral density and osteoporotic fractures: a genome-wide association study and follow-up replication studies. Am J Hum Genet 86: 229–239.
63. Paternoster L, Lorentzon M, Vandenput L, Karlsson MK, Ljunggren O, et al. (2010) Genome-wide association meta-analysis of cortical bone mineral density unravels allelic heterogeneity at the RANKL locus and potential pleiotropic effects on bone. PLoS Genet 6: e1001217.
64. Styrkarsdottir U, Halldorsson BV, Gretarsdottir S, Gudbjartsson DF, Walters GB, et al. (2009) New sequence variants associated with bone mineral density. Nat Genet 41: 15–17.
65. Timpson NJ, Tobias JH, Richards JB, Soranzo N, Duncan EL, et al. (2009) Common variants in the region around Osterix are associated with bone mineral density and growth in childhood. Hum Mol Genet 18: 1510–1517.
66. Xiong DH, Liu XG, Guo YF, Tan LJ, Wang L, et al. (2009) Genome-wide association and follow-up replication studies identified ADAMTS18 and TGFBR3 as bone mass candidate genes in different ethnic groups. Am J Hum Genet 84: 388–398.
67. Kiel DP, Demissie S, Dupuis J, Lunetta KL, Murabito JM, et al. (2007) Genome-wide association with bone mass and geometry in the Framingham Heart Study. BMC Med Genet 8 Suppl 1: S14.
68. Kou I, Takahashi A, Urano T, Fukui N, Ito H, et al. (2011) Common variants in a novel gene, FONG on chromosome 2q33.1 confer risk of osteoporosis in Japanese. PLoS One 6: e19641.
69. Liu YZ, Pei YF, Liu JF, Yang F, Guo Y, et al. (2009) Powerful bivariate genome-wide association analyses suggest the SOX6 gene influencing both obesity and osteoporosis phenotypes in males. PLoS One 4: e6827.
70. Richards JB, Rivadeneira F, Inouye M, Pastinen TM, Soranzo N, et al. (2008) Bone mineral density, osteoporosis, and osteoporotic fractures: a genome-wide association study. Lancet 371: 1505–1512.
71. Zhao LJ, Liu XG, Liu YZ, Liu YJ, Papasian CJ, et al. (2010) Genome-wide association study for femoral neck bone geometry. J Bone Miner Res 25: 320–329.
72. Kim JH, Kim K, Youn BU, Jin HM, Kim N (2010) MHC class II transactivator negatively regulates RANKL-mediated osteoclast differentiation by downregulating NFATc1 and OSCAR. Cell Signal 22: 1341–1349.
73. Awata T, Kawasaki E, Tanaka S, Ikegami H, Maruyama T, et al. (2009) Association of type 1 diabetes with two Loci on 12q13 and 16p13 and the influence coexisting thyroid autoimmunity in Japanese. J Clin Endocrinol Metab 94: 231–235.
74. Wu X, Zhu X, Wang X, Ma J, Zhu S, et al. (2009) Intron polymorphism in the KIAA0350 gene is reproducibly associated with susceptibility to type 1 diabetes (T1D) in the Han Chinese population. Clin Endocrinol (Oxf) 71: 46–49.
75. Zoledziewska M, Costa G, Pitzalis M, Cocco E, Melis C, et al. (2009) Variation within the CLEC16A gene shows consistent disease association with both multiple sclerosis and type 1 diabetes in Sardinia. Genes Immun 10: 15–17.
76. Rubio JP, Stankovich J, Field J, Tubridy N, Marriott M, et al. (2008) Replication of KIAA0350, IL2RA, RPL5 and CD58 as multiple sclerosis susceptibility genes in Australians. Genes Immun 9: 624–630.

11

Skeletal Site-Related Variation in Human Trabecular Bone Transcriptome and Signaling

Satya S. Varanasi[1]⁹, Ole K. Olstad[2]⁹, Daniel C. Swan[3], Paul Sanderson[4], Vigdis T. Gautvik[2,6], Sjur Reppe[2,6], Roger M. Francis[5], Kaare M. Gautvik[2,6,7], Harish K. Datta[1]*

1 Musculoskeletal Research Group, Institute of Cellular Medicine, Medical School, Newcastle University, Newcastle Upon Tyne, United Kingdom, 2 Department of Clinical Biochemistry, Oslo University Hospital, Ullevål, Norway, 3 Bioinformatics Support Unit, Institute for Cell and Molecular Biosciences, Medical School, Newcastle University, Newcastle Upon Tyne, United Kingdom, 4 Department of Orthopaedic Surgery, Newcastle General Hospital, Newcastle Upon Tyne, United Kingdom, 5 Institute for Ageing and Health, Newcastle University, Newcastle Upon Tyne, United Kingdom, 6 Institute of Basic Medical Sciences, University of Oslo, Oslo, Norway, 7 Department of Clinical Chemistry, Lovisenberg Deacon Hospital, Oslo, Norway

Abstract

Background: The skeletal site-specific influence of multiple genes on bone morphology is recognised, but the question as to how these influences may be exerted at the molecular and cellular level has not been explored.

Methodology: To address this question, we have compared global gene expression profiles of human trabecular bone from two different skeletal sites that experience vastly different degrees of mechanical loading, namely biopsies from iliac crest and lumbar spinal lamina.

Principal Findings: In the lumbar spine, compared to the iliac crest, the majority of the differentially expressed genes showed significantly increased levels of expression; 3406 transcripts were up- whilst 838 were down-regulated. Interestingly, all gene transcripts that have been recently demonstrated to be markers of osteocyte, as well as osteoblast and osteoclast-related genes, were markedly up-regulated in the spine. The transcriptome data is consistent with osteocyte numbers being almost identical at the two anatomical sites, but suggesting a relatively low osteocyte functional activity in the iliac crest. Similarly, osteoblast and osteoclast expression data suggested similar numbers of the cells, but presented with higher activity in the spine than iliac crest. This analysis has also led to the identification of expression of a number of transcripts, previously known and novel, which to our knowledge have never earlier been associated with bone growth and remodelling.

Conclusions and Significance: This study provides molecular evidence explaining anatomical and micro-architectural site-related changes in bone cell function, which is predominantly attributable to alteration in cell transcriptional activity. A number of novel signaling molecules in critical pathways, which have been hitherto not known to be expressed in bone cells of mature vertebrates, were identified.

Editor: Jörg Hoheisel, Deutsches Krebsforschungszentrum, Germany

Funding: The support of the EU project OSTEOGENE (No. FP6-502491) was under FP6 programme and partially funded by Newcastle University and Newcastle University Hospital Trust is thankfully acknowledged. The funders had no role in study design, data collection and analysis, decision to publish, or preparation of the manuscript.

Competing Interests: The authors have declared that no competing interests exist.

* E-mail: h.k.datta@ncl.ac.uk

⁹ These authors contributed equally to this work.

Introduction

Mechanical loading, and the associated mechanical stress, shows immense skeletal site-related variation [1,2]. A stark example of such profound differences in the extent of the mechanical loading is that of the lumbar spine (LS), where normally far greater loading is experienced than at such skeletal sites as skull or iliac crest (ILC) [3]. There are therefore marked differences in bone density, micoarchitecture and bone composition at different skeletal sites, which reflect evolutionary adaptation of the skeleton [4–6]. A focus of recent interest is how environmental and genetic factors influence bone mineral density (BMD). The genotypic influence on skeleton have largely been focused on the phenotype relating to bone density, and only a handful studies have investigated bone geometry or bone quality indirectly by looking at the risk of fracture [7]. Genetic factors influence bone mass and between 50–90% of variation in BMD is inherited [7]. These BMD determinants are known to be polygenic, and objective evidence for this is provided by candidate gene SNPs (single nucleotide polymorphisms), quantitative trait locus and family linkage studies [7–20]. Previous studies have identified multiple candidate genes and chromosomal regions which influence bone mass and are linked to osteoporosis-related phenotypes [10–20]. These studies have also provided evidence for the presence of gender- and skeletal site-specific regulation and variation of BMD [10–20]. However, the nature of polygenic influences and the resulting complexity of molecular interaction mediating these effects in the development, attainment and subsequent maintenance of bone mineral density (BMD) are unclear.

Bone is a heterogeneous tissue and its histological classification, based on macroscopic texture of cross sections, classifies the tissue into compact (or cortical) and cancellous (or trabecular) subtypes. The trabeculae, within cancellous bone, while may appear to be disorganized are in fact arranged to provide maximum strength and are aligned in the direction to support maximum mechanical stress. Trabecular bone has a porous network of irregular cavities, and being less dense than compact bone, constitutes only a small fraction of total bone mass, but provide approximately 90% of the total bone surface area representing about 80% of the exchangeable calcium pool. It is this much larger surface area that makes trabecular bone metabolically more active than compact bone. The question as to how mechanical loading, and the associated mechanical stress, affects particular histological type of bone at different sites in the skeleton is of interest. To date many studies have been performed examining the mechanical stress related changes in the bone strength, microarchitecture and even cellular changes [1–6]. The effect of differences in the mechanical loading on the underlying complex molecular architecture of bone, which is critical for bone function, has never been investigated. Therefore, to address this question we have performed a global gene transcriptome investigation on human male cancellous bone from two anatomical sites, exposed to marked differences in mechanical and functional demands.

Results

Raw data Analysis

In view of high degree of molecular homogeneity in the overall transcript expression between these sites (>95%), the data from the three lumbar vertebrae, namely L2, L3 and L4, were grouped for analysis (Table S1). If filtration on absents (or presents) is used to remove transcripts that have absent call in all the arrays then 40,450 transcripts were found, and the number of transcripts expressed in all of the bone biopsies is approximately 14,300. The Venn analysis revealed 9177 gene transcripts to be uniquely expressed in the LS as opposed to 713 gene transcripts in the ILC. A statistical comparison of global gene expression in lamina of lumbar vertebrae (L2, L3 and L4) and ILC revealed differential expression of 4244 gene transcripts with significant differences (fold change ≥2.0, p-value ≤0.05). It was seen that compared with ILC, in LS region 3406 transcripts were up-regulated and 838 were down regulated. However, the number of differentially expressed transcripts between the skeletal sites was found to be 1733 for an adjusted p-value <0.05 and fold change >2; 1025 probesets are up-regulated in LS versus ILC, 708 probesets are

Table 1. Top up-regulated genes showing up-regulation >50 fold in lamina of lumbar vertebrae (LS) in comparison with iliac crest (ILC).

Probe Set ID	Gene Title	Gene Symbol	p-value LS vs. ILC	FC Absolute LS vs. ILC	S.D
206373_at	zic1 family member (odd-paired homolog, Drosophia)	Zic1	8.95E-08	202.03	1.78
217404_s_at	collagen, type II, alpha 1 (primary osteoarthritis, spondyloepiphyseal dysplasia, congenital)	COL2A1	1.6E-5	167.51	2.95
205713_s_at	cartilage oligomeric matrix protein	COMP	1.08E-11	166.98	1.15
209904_at	troponin C type 1 (slow)	TNNC1	0.003	157.67	4.79
206227_at	cartilage intermediate layer protein, nucleotide pyrophosphohydrolase	CILP	6.84E-11	154.45	1.25
214087_s_at	myosin binding protein C, slow type	MYBPC1	1.87E-04	134.89	3.41
204737_s_at	myosin, heavy chain 6, cardiac muscle, alpha (cardiomyopathy, hypertrophic 1) myosin, heavy chain 7, cardiac muscle, beta	MYH6///MYH7	0.002	112.49	4.18
204810_s_at	creatine kinase, muscle	CKM	0.002	96.48	4.07
209888_s_at	myosin, light chain 1, alkali; skeletal, fast	MYL1	8.70E-04	84.64	3.58
209742_s_at	myosin, light chain 2, regulatory, cardiac, slow	MYL2	0.002	82.85	3.88
213201_s_at	troponin T type 1 (skeletal, slow)	TNNT1	0.002	79.48	3.99
209621_s_at	PDZ and LIM domain 3	PDLIM3	3.82E-05	77.27	2.68
213782_s_at	myozenin 2	MYOZ2	0.002	74.63	3.89
212654_at	tropomyosin 2 (beta)	TPM2	3.23E-04	69.76	3.14
213492_at	collagen, type II, alpha 1 (primary osteoarthritis, spondyloepiphyseal dysplasia, congenital)	COL2A1	4.40E-05	68.00	2.49
222043_at	Clusterin	CLU	1.32E-09	62.26	1.31
203872_at	actin, alpha 1, skeletal muscle	ACTA1	0.00307	60.50	3.85
219728_at	Myotilin	MYOT	8.21E-04	58.01	3.31
205054_at	Nebulin	NEB	0.001	57.24	3.31
204179_at	Myoglobin	MB	0.001	56.32	3.51
228224_at	proline/arginine-rich end leucine-rich repeat protein	PRELP	2.74E-09	55.65	1.19
219106_s_at	kelch repeat and BTB (POZ) domain containing 10	KBTBD10	0.002	50.02	3.41

FC, fold change; SD, standard deviation.

downregulated in LS compared to ILC. Examination of Gene Ontology (GO) terms show a statistically significant over representation for a number of GO terms ($p<0.005$) including biological and cell adhesion, extracellular matrix formation and skeletal development (Table S2).

Bone cells related transcriptomes

The detailed analysis of the data reveals some profound and consistent changes in the transcriptomes that are characteristically associated with skeletal tissues, which were up-regulated in the LS when compared with ILC (Table 1 & 2). Bone related genes, such as SOST, MEPE and matrix Gla protein were among the most up-regulated, but also novel and genes with uncharacterised gene function, such as Zic1, cDNA clone ZA88B06 and DKFZP434C153 protein showed high differential expression. The comparison of transcripts characteristically associated with osteoblasts, osteoclast and osteocytes, revealed profound difference between the ILC and LS (Table 3). Interestingly, whilst transcripts of enzymes, matrix proteins and humoral factors, reflecting activities of osteoblasts, osteoclasts and osteocytes showed up-regulation in the LS, the cell structure components of these cells, namely PTHR2, CTR and PDPN, respectively, showed similar expression in both sites. The array data was validated by qRT-PCR of RNA from five ILC and equal number of randomly selected LS biopsies. The verification was carried out by determining expression of select group of differential expressed transcripts. The transcripts were selected to reflect respective expression activities of each of the three bone cell types, for osteoclast CATK, for osteoblast Col1α and for osteocytes SOST, DMP1 and MEPE (Table 3 & 4). The increased expression in the LS compared with ILC suggested increased transcriptional activity of the three bone cells rather than any changes in their numbers. OSCAR and PTHR2 expression seen in the array data were substantiated by qRT-PCR, which reflects lack of site-related significant differences in actual number of osteoclast and osteoblast respectively. Thus, the major molecular differences between the two distinct bone sites were strictly associated with osteocyte and osteoblast related transcripts encoding matrix (secretory) proteins and key master regulatory genes encoding transcription factors, e.g. RUNX2.

Pathways analysis and novel gene identification

The differential analysis revealed that the top three pathways, i.e., with the highest number of differentially expressed transcripts, were TNF receptor signaling pathway, BMP signaling and Proteogylcan syndecan-mediated signaling (Tables S3 to S6; Figures 1, 2, & 3). The details of the gene transcripts for the signaling mediated by TNF receptor, BMP and Proteogylcan syndecan-mediated pathway (Figures 1, 2 & 3) is given in Tables S4, S5 and S6, respectively. The majority of the post-receptor transcripts of these pathways were found to show up-regulation in the LS when compared with ILC. The analysis also reveals a number of hitherto unidentified and unknown transcripts which are involved in the signaling.

Probesets with a 5-fold or more change in expression were analysed with Ingenuity Pathway Analysis (IPA), a list of 268 eligible entities for IPA analysis. The most significant biological function classification was in skeletal and muscular development and function with the most significant subclass being skeletal development (corrected p-value of 2.22×10^{-9}) (Table S7). Network analysis of the data set suggested one interaction network with skeletal and muscular system development and function including the genes Akt, COL1A1, CTGF, EGFR, EGR1, ERK, IGFBP3, ITGA4, Jnk, MYH11, NF-kB, (complex), PDGFBB, PI3K, Pka, POSTN, PTPRK, SOX9, SPARC, TGFB2, TIMP3 (Figure 4).

Table 2. Selected skeletal genes showing significant up-regulation on expression in the lamina of lumbar vertebrae (LS) compared with iliac crest (ILC).

Probe Set ID	Gene Title	Gene Symbol	*p*-value LS *vs. ILC*	FC Absolute LS *vs. ILC*	S.D.
223869_at	Sclerosteosis	SOST	1.90E-08	40.79	1.35
208175_s_at	dentin matrix acidic phosphoprotein	DMP1	1.35E-05	13.59	1.37
221150_at	matrix, extracellular phosphoglycoprotein with ASARM motif (bone)	MEPE	2.60E-05	9.22	1.30
231766_s_at	collagen, type XII, alpha 1	COL12A1*	2.51E-04	12.77	1.82
231879_at	collagen, type XII, alpha 1	COL12A1*	0.00182	4.141	1.23
225664_at	collagen, type XII, alpha 1	COL12A1*	2.39E-07	13.26	1.05
209101_at	connective tissue growth factor	CTGF	2.41E-07	11.77	1.05
238481_at	matrix Gla protein	MGP*	8.48E-07	20.55	1.24
202291_s_at	matrix Gla protein	MGP*	7.42E-09	12.45	0.85
232267_at	G protein-coupled receptor 133	GPR133	2.30E-10	14.34	0.72
219522_at	four jointed box 1 (Drosophila)	FJX1	8.63E-06	7.75	1.02
1561754_at	Full length insert cDNA clone ZA88B06	ZA88B06	1.41E-04	4.05	0.93
241902_at	mohawk homeobox	MKX*	2.55E-04	7.82	1.46
239468_at	mohawk homeobox	MKX*	5.28E-06	6.55	0.88
213591_at	aldehyde dehydrogenase 7 family, member A1	ALDH7A1	5.40E-05	8.08	1.24
208950_s_at	aldehyde dehydrogenase 7 family, member A1	ALDH7A1	5.76E-04	2.22	0.60

FC, fold change; SD, standard deviation.
*Multiple probe sets.

Table 3. Comparison of differences in the absolute expression of osteoblast, osteoclast and osteocyte-related gene transcripts in lamina of lumbar vertebrae (LS) and iliac crest (ILC).

Cell type	Probe Set ID	Gene Symbol	Gene Title	FC (LS vs. ILC)
Osteocytes	208175_s_at	DMP1	dentin matrix acidic phosphoprotein	13.59
	221150_at	MEPE	matrix, extracellular phosphoglycoprotein with ASARM motif (bone)	9.22
	221166_at	FGF23	fibroblast growth factor 23	3.52
	223869_at	SOST	sclerosteosis	40.79
	204879_at	PDPN*	podoplanin	6.43
	208233_at	PDPN*	podoplanin	2.82
	221898_at	PDPN*	podoplanin	5.90
	226658_at	PDPN*	podoplanin	2.75
Osteoblasts	202310_s_at	COL1A1*	collagen, type I, alpha 1	6.13
	202311_s_at	COL1A1*	collagen, type I, alpha 1	3.99
	1556499_s_at	COL1A1*	collagen, type I, alpha 1	2.19
	206956_at	BGLAP	bone gamma-carboxyglutamate (gla) protein (osteocalcin)	3.78
	209875_s_at	SPP1	secreted phosphoprotein 1 (osteopontin, bone sialoprotein I, early T-lymphocyte activation 1)	2.97
	212667_at	SPARC*	secreted protein, acidic, cysteine-rich (osteonectin)	5.86
	200665_s_at	SPARC*	secreted protein, acidic, cysteine-rich (osteonectin)	4.01
	209875_s_at	SPP1	secreted phosphoprotein 1 (osteopontin, bone sialoprotein I, early T-lymphocyte activation 1)	2.97
	207370_at	IBSP*	integrin-binding sialoprotein (bone sialoprotein, bone sialoprotein II)	3.97
	236028_at	IBSP*	Integrin-binding sialoprotein (bone sialoprotein, bone sialoprotein II)	7.35
	236859_at	RUNX2*	runt-related transcription factor 2	3.80
	221283_at	RUNX2*	runt-related transcription factor 2	2.74
	236858_s_at	RUNX2*	runt-related transcription factor 2	2.21
	205289_at	BMP2*	bone morphogenetic protein 2	2.71
	205290_s_at	BMP2*	bone morphogenetic protein 2	2.60
	239769_at	CDH11*	Cadherin 11, type 2, OB-cadherin (osteoblast)	3.00
	207173_x_at	CDH11*	cadherin 11, type 2, OB-cadherin (osteoblast)	2.85
	205911_at	PTHR1	parathyroid hormone receptor 1	4.29
	206772_at	PTHR2	parathyroid hormone receptor 2	−1.59
Osteoclasts	202450_s_at	CTSK	cathepsin K	4.04
	1554503_a_at	OSCAR	osteoclast associated, immunoglobulin-like receptor	−1.28
	207886_s_at	CALCR*	calcitonin receptor	1.59
	207887_s_at	CALCR*	calcitonin receptor	1.04
	204638_at	ACP5	acid phosphatase 5, tartrate resistant	2.03

FC, fold change.
*Multiple probe sets.

Discussion

The global transcriptosome first ever analysis of human lamellar LS and ILC revealed that whilst most of the transcripts showed a similar level of expression, a limited number of functionally associated subsets showed marked anatomical site-related differences. Interestingly, between L2, L3 and L4 vertebrae from different subjects there was a higher overall molecular homogeneity when compared with ILC from the same person. Therefore for further comparison the three vertebrae were treated as one group. Similarly, high degree of overall molecular homogeneity in gene expression was seen between symmetrical sites in ILC [20] underscoring the importance of function as a major determinant of bone cell gene expression .and adaptability. The number of gene transcripts and the extent of their up-regulation was much higher in the lamina of spinal vertebra when compared with ILC. The analysis of up-regulated genes showed that these were related to changes in key cellular and molecular components and strongly associated with essential biological functions in bone. The gene transcripts, reflecting respective transcriptional activities of osteocytes, osteoblasts and osteoclasts from vertebrae when compared with ILC, were found to be consistently up-regulated in the vertebrae and magnitude of the increased expression was quite similar. In contrast, the gene transcripts that reflect osteocytes, osteoblasts and osteoclasts number showed insignificant or less marked skeletal site-related variation. This conclusion was based on an analysis of the data evaluating osteocyte-, osteoblast- and osteoclast-specific structural transcripts, namely podoplanin in osteocytes, parathyroid hormone receptor in osteoblasts and osteocytes and calcitonin receptor and osteoclast-associated

Table 4. The validation of the array data was carried out by qRT-PCR of select number of transcripts for equal number of iliac crest (ILC) and lumbar spine (LS) samples (n = 5).

Gene	Affymetrix Absolute Fold Change (ILC vs. LS)	qRT-PCR RQ (ILC vs. LS)
COL1A1	−7.2	−22.8
SOST	−53	−90.7
DMP1	−42	−33.0
MEPE	−23.5	−40.7
CTSK	−8.2	−15.8
ZIC1	−86.7	−666
PTHR2	1.5	1.7
OSCAR	1.7	1.4

receptor in osteoclasts. We postulate that these transcripts provide estimate of the cell numbers with the reasonable assumption that each cell type in vertebra and ILC express on average similar number of the marker molecules. Since these transcripts were found to show only minor differences in vertebra and ILC when compared with other activity related transcripts (Table 3 & 4), we interpret that the observed increase in the respective activities of the three bone cell types were predominantly due to increase in the relative cell activity rather than reflecting a change in absolute cell number. Interestingly, the most profound up-regulation in the spinal vertebrae was observed for transcripts reflecting osteocyte activity, namely in SOST, DMP1, and MEPE.

In light of the recent observations, the data analysis allows us to suggest possible mechanisms for the existing evidence of increased bone turnover, based on the described molecular differences in osteoblast- and osteoclast-related bone remodelling in lamellar bone of LS when compared with ILC. It is generally accepted that mechanical stress induced by weight-bearing exercise increases osteoblast activity, and that the absence of mechanical stimulation resulting from prolonged immobilization or microgravity causes severe bone loss [21,22]. In recent years a number of observations suggest, based on *in vitro* studies and animal transgenic models, that osteocytes act as mechano-sensory cells and that lacuno-canaliculi carry signaling molecules that are responsible for maintenance of bone structure and mass [23]. Osteocytes are interconnected by a network that involves their dendritic processes within lacunae to osteoblasts; that mirrors the CNS neuronal network, but comprehensive identity of all relevant signaling molecules in bone remains to be identified [24,25]. We believe that the present data show that osteocytes are more metabolically active than hitherto understood and play a central role in the determination and maintenance of bone structure [24–26]. The bone matrix secludes and isolates osteocytes which have an extensive interaction and also connect to other surrounding cells via an elaborate network of dendritic processes which may have the potential to modulate bone resorption [26].

We hypothesize that significantly higher transcriptional activity within specific functional osteocyte networks in the spinal vertebra, when compared with ILC, is reflective of the increased stress experienced at the LS [3]. The mechanical stress, both due fluid shear stress and tissue strain, in bone is now thought to be mainly detected by osteocytes (Figure 5) [24–29]. Osteocytes are involved in mechano-sensing as well as in mechano-transduction of the stress into biochemical signal [24–29]. The increased expression of osteocyte-related transcripts, such as SOST, DMP1, MEPE, in the spine relative to the ILC, provides for the first time evidence of mechanical stress-related *in vivo* increase in osteocyte transcriptional activity. The osteocyte activity, resulting from excess mechanical loading, increases the respective activities of osteoblasts and osteoclasts, as evident from increase in the expression of matrix proteins (COL1A, SPARC, and IBSP) and osteoclast-specific enzymes (CTSK and ACP5) (Table 3 & 4; Figure 5). These genes, i.e., characteristically associated with osteocyte, osteoblasts and osteoclasts, showing markedly increased expression, encode secretory proteins. Further evidence of skeletal site-related difference in the bone remodelling activity due to mechanical stress, that seem to be orchestrated by osteocyte, is provided by the PathwayArchitect™ analysis (Figures 2, 3 and 4; Tables S4, S5 and S6). The analysis shows that top pathways, in terms of differential expression in the lamina of LS as compared with the ILC, are those involved in the bone formation by osteoblasts (BMP signalling pathway, Proteoglycan Syndecan signalling) and bone-resorption by osteoclast (TNF receptor signalling, and other network groups, e.g. adherence/adhesion). The most likely explanation in the observed increase in transcriptional activity in the osteocyte, as well as osteoblasts and osteoclasts, in the spine is likely to be a higher degree of local mechanical stress [3]. The data presented provides support for the proposal that osteocytes modulate respective bone-formation and bone-resorptive activities of osteoblasts and osteoclasts, and thereby regulate and maintain of bone mass. These observations add to our understanding about the central role of osteocytes in the maintenance of bone mass in health and in the pathogenesis of osteoporosis.

The comparison of the relative expression of the transcripts led to identification of a number of novel and uncharacterised genes, whose function in bone cell biology is not yet known [30,31]. In addition, the pathways analysis revealed the known key signaling molecules (Figs. 1, 2 & 3 and corresponding Tables S4, S5 & S6), and led to the identification some novel pathways specific intracellular putative proteins. Further studies, such as cell protein expression, protein-protein interaction and knock-in and knock-out functional studies are required to establish the role of these novel proteins. In conclusion, taken together the data show that at the transcriptional level bone has a strong ability to adapt to functional demands, and osteocyte play a critical role in the process. The adaptive response involves "growth and developmental processes", probably made possible through their "high sensitivity to synaptic processes" and "matrix" engineering properties.

Methods

Subject selection

The participants numbered thirteen Caucasian men who were all from North East England, U.K., who were undergoing spinal decompression laminectomies or spinal fusions of the LS. This study was conducted according to the principles expressed in the Declaration of Helsinki. The study was approved by the Institutional Review Board of Northumberland Local Research Ethics Committee, Blyth, Northumberland NE24 2AG (REC Reference: 04/Q0902/29), and all subjects gave their informed written consent. Underlying secondary causes of osteoporosis were excluded by medical history, physical examination and laboratory investigations. Men with a history of treatment with antiresoptive agents, steroid, anticonvulsant and anticoagulant were excluded [32] (Text S1). The mean±SD (range) of age, weight and height respectively were 53.9±10.7 (35.0-69.0)yr, 86.6±8.6 (84.0-

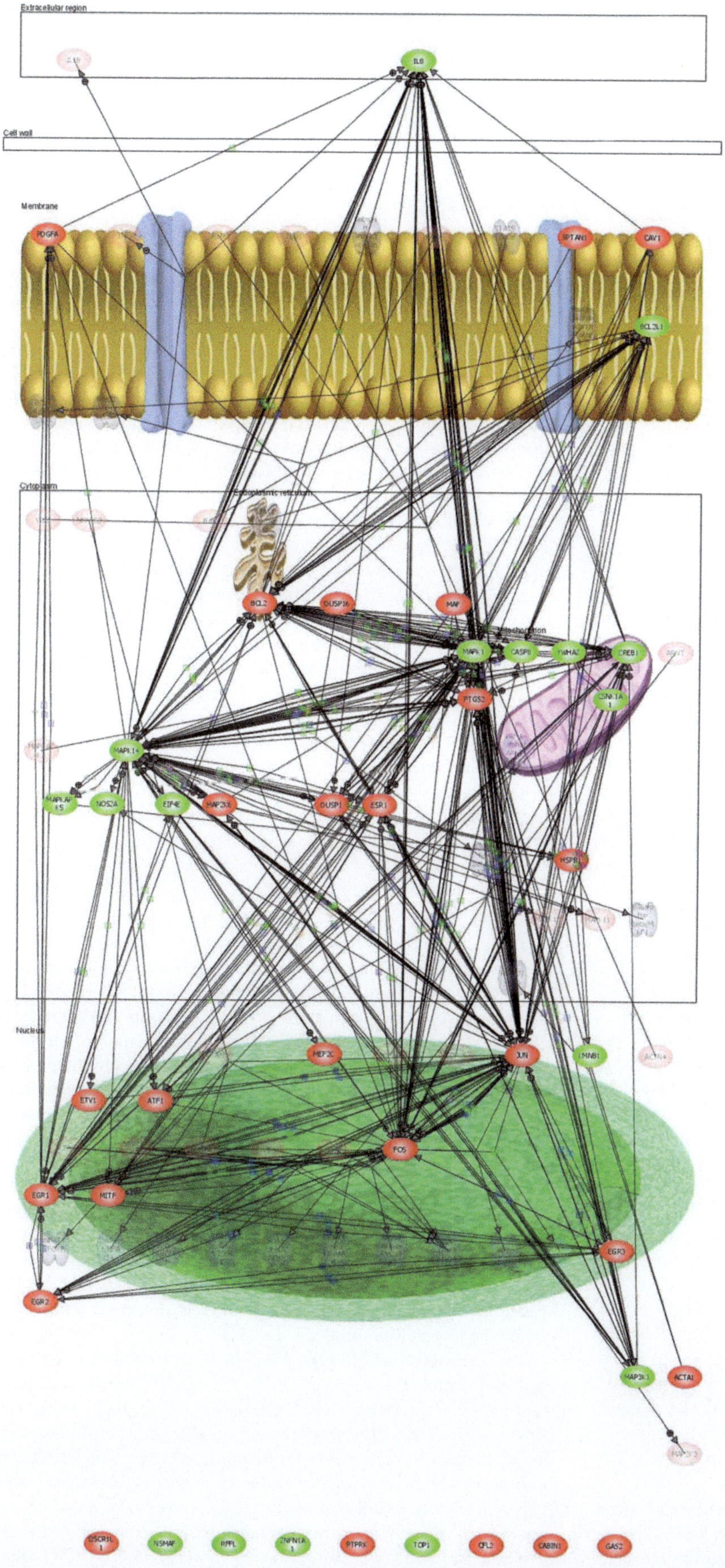
Extracellular region
IL6
Cell wall
Membrane
PDGFA
SPTAN1
CAV1
BCL2L1
Cytoplasm
Endoplasmic reticulum
BCL2
DUSP16
MAF
Mitochondrion
MAPK1
CASP8
YWHAZ
CREB1
PTGS2
CSNK1A1
MAPK14
MAPKAPK5
NOS2A
EIF4E
MAP2K6
DUSP1
ESR1
HSPB1
Nucleus
MEF2C
JUN
LMNB1
ETV1
ATF1
FOS
EGR1
MITF
EGR3
EGR2
MAP3K1
ACTA1
DSCR1L1
NSMAF
PFPL
TNFRSF1A
PTPRK
TOP1
CFL2
CABIN1
GAS2

Figure 1. TNF receptor signaling in trabecular bone. Direct interaction network models were constructed by Pathway Architect analysis of the differentially expressed transcript in the lumbar spine and iliac crest trabecular bone. Up-regulated transcripts are indicated red whilst the down-regulated are shown in green. Arrows link interacting genes and positive (+) and negative (−) associations are marked respectively. Green boxes denote regulation, blue boxes binding and orange circles indicating phosphorylation.

108.2)kg and 176.4±6.3 (167.0-184)cm, respectively. The mean±SD (range) for BMD, given as areal density, for LS, total hip, and femoral neck respectively were 1.067±0.332 (0.760-1.387), 1.047±0.153 (0.820-1.271) and 0.870±0.153 (0.620-1.202) gm/cm^2, respectively. None of the subjects had history of low trauma fractures (Table S8 and Text S1).

All bone biopsies were trabecular and taken from a specific site in the ILC site, 2 cm backwards from the anterior superior iliac spine. Further consistency was achieved by ensuring that only one senior surgeon supervised all biopsies with explicit instructions to avoid attached tissues, specifically muscle. Similarly spinal biopsies were all trabecular and all were from lamina processes of the lumbar vertebrae two, three and four. A total of 24 biopsies were obtained for analysis from 13 men, 19 from the lamina of the LS and 5 from the ILC.

Biochemical and BMD measurements

Serum testosterone, sex-hormone-binding globulins, follicular stimulating hormone and luteinizing hormone were measured by commercially available radioimmunoassays (SAS laboratory, Royal Victoria Infirmary, Newcastle upon Tyne). All bone density measurements were performed by DXA using a Hologic QDR 2000 Bone Densitometer (Hologic, Waltham, MA). In vivo precision for measurement with this system is 1.0% at the LS (L1-L4) and 1.5% for the femoral neck. BMD results were obtained as an areal density in g/cm^2, but were also given as T- and Z- scores. The T-score is the number of standard deviation units above or below the mean for normal young men, whilst the Z-score is the number of standard deviation units above or below the age-related normal men (calculated using the manufacturer's standard normal reference database). The results of laboratory investigations for all these subjects were within normal laboratory ranges.

Extraction of RNA

The trabecular bone from the laminar and ILC that were excess to the surgical requirement were collected as biopsies of size approximately 0.25 to 1 cm^3. The biopsies were immediately frozen and stored in liquid nitrogen for later extraction of RNA. The frozen bone biopsies were pulverized with a mortar in liquid nitrogen with their content of marrow intact. RNA was then extracted by homogenization in Trizol (Life Technologies, Invitrogen, cat no 15596) 1 ml/100 mg, then following the manufacturers procedure. RNA was further purified using the RNeasy kit (Qiagen) to remove organic components and finally re-suspended in RNAse free deionsed water and quantified using the Nanodrop spectrophotometer. The total RNA integrity was checked using Agilent 2100 BioAnalyzer (Agilent Technologies, Inc.) prior to cDNA synthesis. In addition, the quality of the RNA was controlled according to the Affymetrix test manual by measuring the ratio between 3′ and 5′ end for GAPDH mRNA (ratio always<2.0)

Microarray analysis

Double-stranded cDNA and biotin-labeled cRNA probes were made from 5 μg total RNA using the Superscript Choice system (Invitrogen) and the Enzo Bioarray respectively. Procedures were performed according to recommendations from Affymetrix [20,31]. This cRNA was hybridized to Affymetrix Human Genome U133 Plus 2.0 Array containing cDNA oligonucleotides representing more than 54,000 probe sets for 38,000 different genes followed by washing and staining on the GeneChips Fluidics Station 450 (Affymetrix) according to manufacturer's instructions. The chips were scanned on the Affymetrix GeneChip® 3000 scanner. The quality of the RNA and probe was controlled by an Affymetrix based test measuring the ratio between 5′ and 3′ mRNAs for β-actin and GAPDH and found to be highly satisfactory. The datasets originating from the specimens were first processed by the Affymetrix Mas5.0 software, and signal values representing the expression level of each transcript were generated. Each sample was normalized as recommended by Affymetrix by multiplying all signal values with a scaling factor that results in an average signal value of 500 for all genes that are classified as "present" calculated by the Affymetrix MAS 5.0 program. The scaling factor is set by examining all the probe sets on the array to compute a trimmed mean signal and derive a scale factor for the array so that: Target signal = Scale factor × Trimmed mean signalprobe array. Thus, the scale factor standardizes the trimmed mean signal of the array to the target signal. The patients were coded, and all analyses were carried out blindly. Both samples from each patient were analyzed in the same kit for cRNA probe synthesis and hybridized to chips from the same batch. One chip was used for each sample (cRNA synthesis) as the variability between chips and cRNA syntheses is significantly lower than the potential variability derived from different biological samples.

Data Analysis

The overview of differentially expressed genes in the LS relative to ILC in male controls was generated by the use of Affymetrix software, which made it possible to compare data from two arrays. The statistical analysis is based on 22 different cDNA oligonucleotides to measure quantitatively one mRNA transcript, and each cDNA probe is distributed as 22 different "micro-spots". Thus, 22 signals for each mRNA transcript (probeset) are generated and enables the Affymetrix software GCOS to compute p-values for differential expression when two transcripts on two different arrays are compared. The Wilcoxon's Signed Rank test uses the differences between Perfect Match and Mismatch probe signal intensities, as well as the differences between Perfect Match intensities and background to compute each p-value difference. From Wilcoxon's Signed Rank test, a total of three, one-sided p-values are computed for each probe set. The most conservative value is chosen to determine the "change call". That is the value closest to 0.5 signifying that no change is detected. These are combined to give one final p-value.

Data from HGU-1333 plus 2 Affymetrix GeneChip arrays was imported into GeneSpring GX 11 and summarised and normalised with MAS5 and GC-RMA. Flag data from the MAS5 analysis was used to derive a probeset list where at least 19 out of 25 samples had a present or marginal call. This left 20796 probesets, which was further reduced to 20764 probesets after Affymetrix control probesets were removed from the list. This list was used for all downstream statistical analysis. An unpaired t-test between LS and ILC samples was used to detect differential

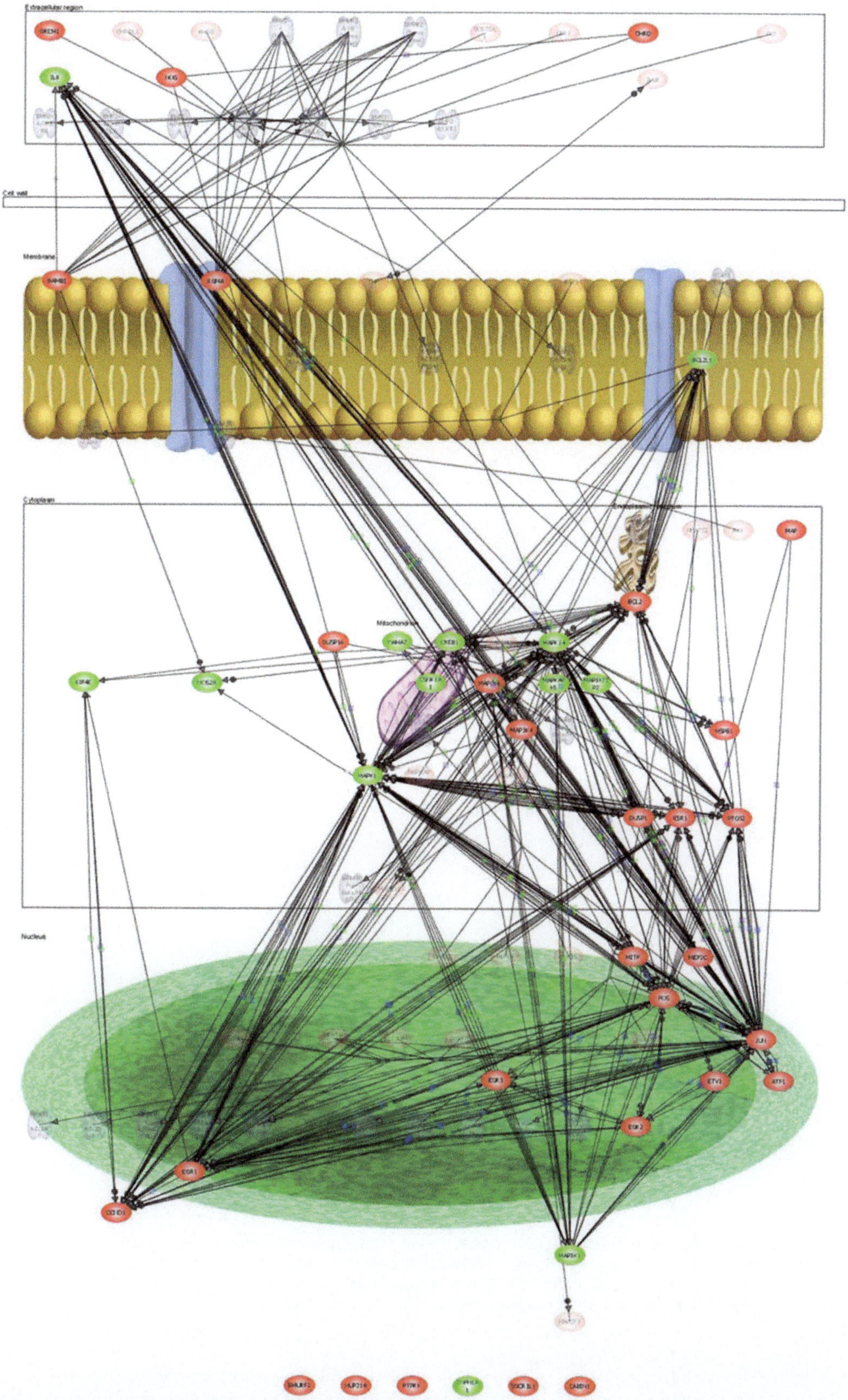

Figure 2. BMP signaling in trabecular bone. In this interaction network model, constructed by Pathway Architect analysis software of differential expressed genes between iliac crest and the lumbar spine, up-regulated transcripts are indicated red whilst the down-regulated are shown in green. Arrows link interacting genes and positive (+) and negative (−) associations are marked respectively. Green boxes denote regulation, blue boxes binding and orange circles indicating phosphorylation.

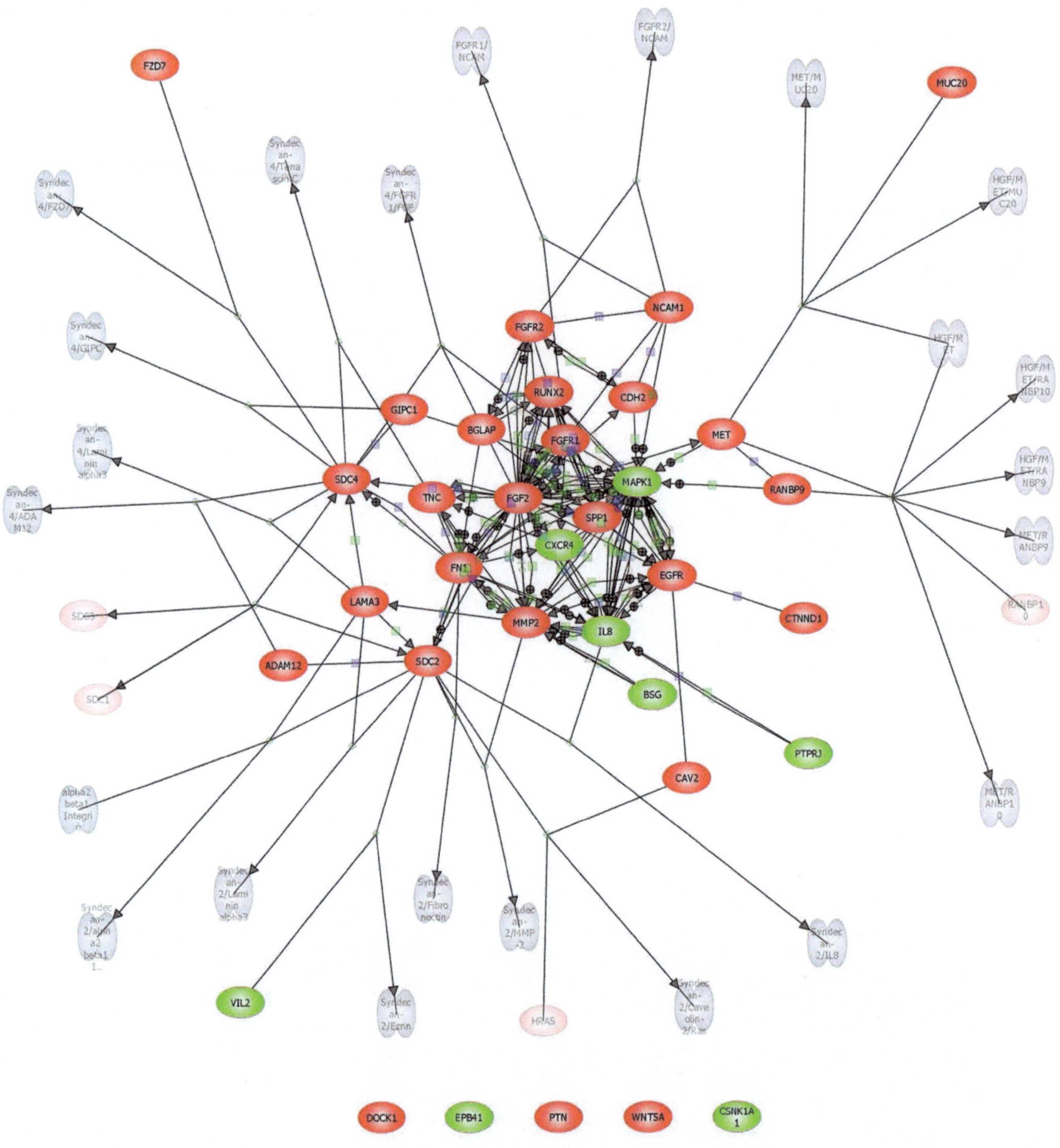

Figure 3. Proteogylcan Syndecan-mediated signaling in trabecular bone. Direct interaction network models constructed by Pathway Architect analysis of the differentially expressed transcript in the lumbar spine and iliac crest trabecular bone. Up-regulated transcripts are indicated red whilst the down-regulated are shown in green. Arrows link interacting genes and positive (+) and negative (−) associations are marked respectively. Green boxes denote regulation, blue boxes binding and orange circles indicating phosphorylation.

expression. Probesets reported as being differentially expressed if they satisfy a corrected p-value cutoff of <0.05 when performing multiple testing correction with Benjamini-Hochberg False Discovery Rate (FDR).

Pathway analysis was also carried out with Ingenuity Pathway Analysis 8.5 (Ingenuity Systems http://www.ingenuity.com) on probesets differentially expressed in lumbar and ILC biopsies. Canonical pathways analysis identified the pathways from the Ingenuity library of pathways that were most significant to the data set. The significance of the association between the data set and the canonical pathway was measured in 2 ways: 1) A ratio of the number of molecules from the data set that map to the pathway divided by the total number of molecules that map to the canonical pathway is displayed. 2) Fisher's exact test was used to

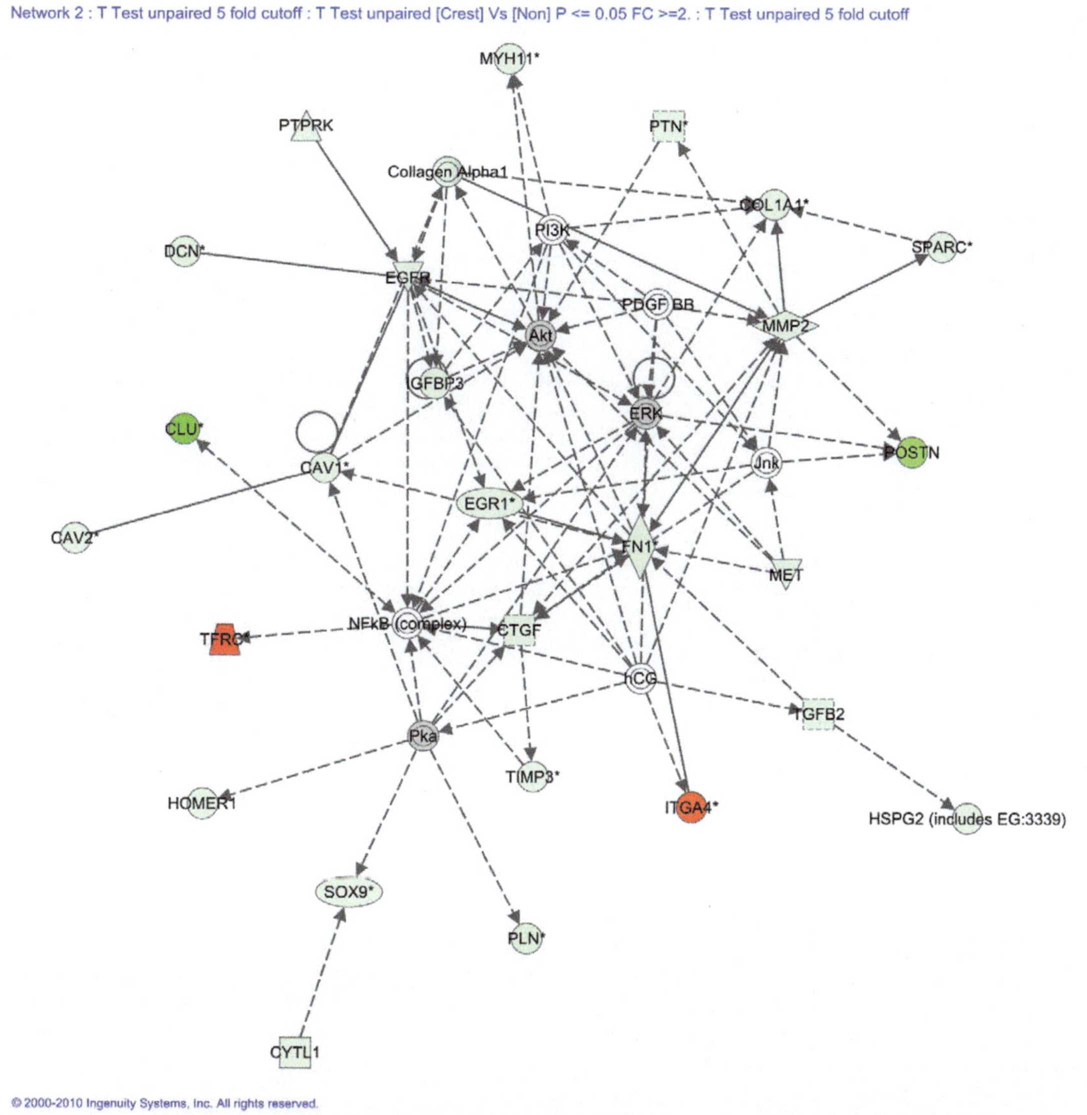

Figure 4. Network enriched for genes involved in skeletal system. Molecules are represented as nodes, and the biological relationship between two nodes is represented as an edge (line). The intensity of the node color indicates the degree of down- (red) or up- (green) regulation where lumbar spine is compared with iliac crest. Nodes are displayed using various shapes that represent the functional class of the gene product. Direct relationships are shown in solid arrows, indirect relationships in dashed arrows. Genes with no colour are added to the network by Ingenuity Pathway Analysis as part of the network generation algorithm.

calculate a p-value determining the probability that the association between the genes in the dataset and the canonical pathway is explained by chance alone.

Affymetrix identifiers and fold change information was loaded into IPA and each identifier was mapped to its corresponding object in Ingenuity's Knowledge Base. A 5-fold cutoff of fold change was set to identify molecules whose expression was significantly differentially regulated. These molecules, called Network Eligible molecules, were overlaid onto a global molecular network developed from information contained in Ingenuity's Knowledge Base. Networks of Network Eligible Molecules were then algorithmically generated based on their connectivity. The Functional Analysis of a network identified the biological functions and/or diseases that were most significant to the molecules in the network. The network molecules associated with biological functions and/or diseases in Ingenuity's Knowledge Base were considered for the analysis. Right-tailed Fisher's exact test was used to calculate a p-value determining the probability that each biological function and/or disease assigned to that network is due to chance alone. All edges of the pathways generated are supported by at least one reference from the literature, from a textbook, or from canonical information stored in the Ingenuity Pathways Knowledge Base. Human, mouse, and rat orthologs of a gene are stored as separate objects in the Ingenuity Pathways Knowledge Base, but are represented as a single node in the network.

ArrayAssist (Stratagene) was further used to created a raw data set and identify differential gene expression. The change in relative expression of the remaining set of transcripts was assessed using t-tests with Benjamin-Hochberg (false discovery rate, FDR) correction (2-fold minimum cut-off and $p<0.05$). These transcripts, i.e., showing $FC \geq 2$ in bone biopsies taken from ILC and

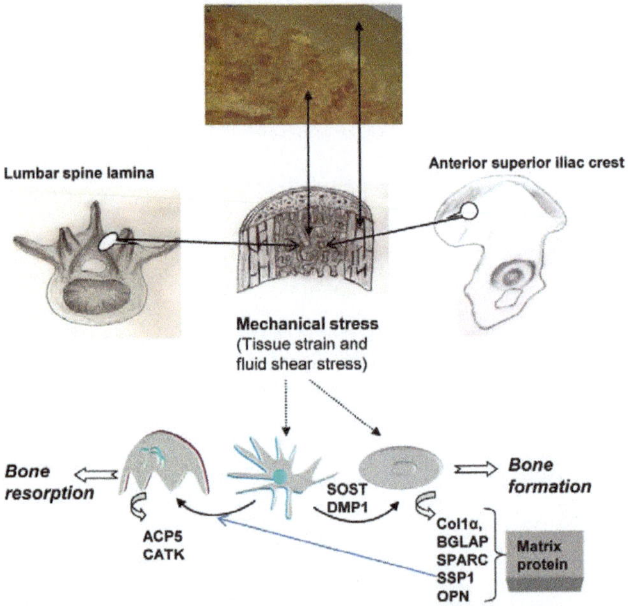

Figure 5. Role of osteocytes in mechanotransduction in trabecular bone. The increased mechanical stress is detected by mechanosensors, a function which is primarily performed by the osteocytes (~90% of the total cell number). The increased mechanical stress is mechano-transduced into intracellular biochemical signals by osteocytes and results in increased transcriptional activity of range of genes (SOST, MEPE and DMP1). Osteocytes also transmute mechanical stress into intercellular biochemical signals to modulate the respective activities of the osteoclasts and osteoblasts.

LS, were further analysed by PathwayArchitect^{TM} software (Stratagene). This analysis utilizes existing relevant literature for pathway analysis and visualization and permits identification of shared common direct regulators or downstream targets. PathwayArchitect^{TM} analysis software can identify gene-gene interaction, gene regulation and their key functions in the complex pathways.

The guidelines described in MIAME (Minimal Information About a Microarray Experiment) has been followed in writing this paper. The primary data has been submitted to the European Bioinformatics Institute (EMBL-EBI) ArrayExpress repository. The experiment name is "Skeletal Site-Related Variation in Human Bone Transcriptome" and Signalling ArrayExpress accession number is: E-MEXP-2219.

Quantitative RT-PCR

The Affymetrix gene expression data were validated for selected transcripts using the TaqMan gene expression assays and the Applied Biosystems Prism 7900 HT sequence detection system. Five 500 ng total RNA from each donor was reverse transcribed using Omniscript (Qiagen Ltd.), and cDNA representing 2.5 ng total RNA was used in each PCR reaction. The PCR reactions were run in duplicates. The relative changes of each transcript, using GAPDH (glyceraldehyde-3-phosphate dehydrogenase) as endogenous control, were calculated using the $2(\Delta\Delta C(T)$ method [33], and the gene expression results are given as RQ (relative quantitation).

Supporting Information

Table S1 Anatomical-site related comparison of overall molecular homogeneity between different skeletal sites.

Table S2 Examination of Gene Ontology (GO) terms shows an overrepresentation for a number of GO terms ($p<0.005$) including cell adhesion, extracellular matrix formation and skeletal development.

Table S3 Top 30 signalling pathways identified by comparing differential transcript expression in the lumbar spine versus iliac crest (4244 gene transcripts with FC $\geq$2, p-value $\leq$0.05).

Table S4 TNF receptor signalling pathway gene transcripts identification based on differential expression in lamina lumbar spine and iliac crest; the analysis was carried out using Pathway Architect Software and the pathway generated is shown in Fig. 2.

Table S5 BMP signalling pathway gene transcripts identification based on the differential expression in iliac crest and in the lamina of lumbar spine; the analysis was carried out using Pathway Architect Software and the pathway generated is shown in Fig. 3.

Table S6 Proteoglycan Syndecan signalling events identification based on analysis of differential expression in the lamina of lumbar spine and iliac crest; the analysis was carried out using Pathway Architect Software and the pathway generated is shown in Fig. 4.

Table S7 Probesets with a 5-fold or more change in expression were analysed with Ingenuity Pathway Analysis (IPA), a list of 268 eligible entities for IPA analysis. The most significant biological function classification was in skeletal and muscular development and function.

Table S8 Anthropometric indices age and bone density of individual subjects.

Text S1 Details of clinical evaluation, including medical history and laboratory investigations, used for the subject selection.

Acknowledgments

We are grateful to all the volunteers for participating in the study and to the theatre staff of Freeman Hospital and Newcastle General Hospital for their help in collecting the bone biopsy samples. We would like to thank Lynn Conroy of Musculoskeletal Unit, Freeman Hospital, for bone mineral assessment and Dr. Paul Genever and the Technology Facility at the University of York for access to the Analysis Software.

Author Contributions

Conceived and designed the experiments: KMG HKD. Performed the experiments: SSV OKO VTG. Analyzed the data: SSV OKO DCS HKD. Contributed reagents/materials/analysis tools: DCS SR RMF HKD. Wrote the paper: HKD. Performed subject clinical assessment: PS RMF KMG. Took biopsies: PS. Clinical assessment of the subjects: HKD.

References

1. Lanyon LE (1984) Functional strain as a determinant of bone remodeling. Calcif Tissue Int 36: S56–S61.
2. Rubin CT, Lanyon LE (1985) Regulation of bone mass by mechanical strain magnitude. Calcif Tissue Int 37: 411–417.
3. Mannion AF, Adams MA, Dolan P (2000) Sudden and unexpected loading generates high forces on the LS. Spine 25: 842–852.
4. Turner CH, Pavalko FM (1998) Mechanotransduction and functional response of the skeleton to physical stress: the mechanisms and mechanics of bone adaptation. J Orthop Sci 3: 346–355.
5. Huiskes R, Ruimerman R, van Lenthe GH, Janssen JD (2000) Effects of mechanical forces on maintenance and adaptation of form in trabecular bone. Nature 405: 704–706.
6. Aerssens J, Boonen S, Joly J, Dequeker J (1997) Variations in trabecular bone composition with anatomical site and age: potential implications for bone quality assessment. J Endocrinol 155: 411–421.
7. Peacock M, Turner CH, Econs MJ, Foroud T (2002) Genetics of osteoporosis. Endocr Rev 23: 303–326.
8. Koller DL, Econs MJ, Morin PA, Christian JC, Hui SL, et al. (2000) Genome screen for QTLs contributing to normal variation in bone mineral density and osteoporosis. J Clin Endocrinol Metab 85: 3116–3120.
9. Karasik D, Myers RH, Cupples LA Hannan MT, Gagnon DR, et al. (2002) Genome screen for quantitative trait loci contributing to normal variation in bone mineral density: the Framingham Study. J Bone Miner Res 17: 1718–1727.
10. Peacock M, Koller DL, Hui S, Johnston CC, Foroud T, et al. (2004) Peak bone mineral density at the hip is linked to chromosomes 14q and 15q. Osteoporos Int 15: 489–496.
11. Ralston SH, Galwey N, Mackay I, Albagha OM, Cardon L, et al. (2005) Loci for regulation of bone mineral density in men and women identified by genome wide linkage scan: the FAMOS study. Hum Mol Genet 2005;14: 943–951.
12. Richards JB, Rivadeneira F, Inouye M, Pastinen TM, Soranzo N, et al. (2008) Bone mineral density, osteoporosis, and osteoporotic fractures: a genome-wide association study. Lancet 371: 1505–1512.
13. Styrkarsdottir U, Halldorsson BV, Gretarsdottir S, Gudbjartsson DF, Walters GB, et al. (2008) Multiple genetic loci for bone mineral density and fractures. N Engl J Med 358: 2355–2365.
14. Xiong DH, Shen H, Zhao LJ, Xiao P, Yang TL, et al. (2006) Robust and comprehensive analysis of 20 osteoporosis candidate genes by very high-density single-nucleotide polymorphism screen among 405 white nuclear families identified significant association and gene–gene interaction. J Bone Miner Res 21: 1678–1695.
15. Orwoll ES, Belknap JK, Klein RF (2001) Gender specificity in the genetic determinants of peak bone mass. J Bone Miner Res 16: 1962–1971.
16. Naganathan V, Macgregor A, Snieder H, Nguyen T, Spector T, et al. (2003) Site and gender specificity of inheritance of bone mineral density. J Bone Miner Res 18: 1531–1538.
17. Peacock M, Koller DL, Lai D, Hui S, Foroud T, et al. (2005) Sex-specific quantitative trait loci contribute to normal variation in bone structure at the proximal femur in men. Bone 37: 467–473.
18. Ioannidis JP, Ng MY, Sham PC, Zintzaras E, Lewis CM, et al. (2207) Meta-analysis of genome-wide scans provides evidence for sex- and site-specific regulation of bone mass. J Bone Miner Res 22: 173–183.
19. Enjuanes A, García-Giralt N, Supervía A, Nogués X, Ruiz-Gaspà S, et al. (2006) A new SNP in a negative regulatory region of the CYP19A1 gene is associated with lumbar spine (BMD) in postmenopausal women. Bone 38: 738–743.
20. Reppe S, Stilgren L, Olstad OK, Brixen K, Nissen-Meyer LS, et al. (2006) Gene expression profiles give insight into the molecular pathology of bone in primary hyperparathyroidism. Bone 39: 189–198.
21. Lorentzon M, Eriksson AL, Nilsson S, Mellström D, Ohlsson C (2004) The COMT val158met polymorphism is associated with peak BMD in men. J Bone Miner Res 19: 2005–2011.
22. Semb H (1969) Experimental limb disuse and bone blood flow. Acta Orthop Scand 40: 552–562.
23. Zerath E (1998) Effects of microgravity on bone and calcium homeostasis. Adv Space Res 21: 1049–1058.
24. Bonewald L (2006) Osteocytes as Multifunctional Cells. Journal of Musculoskeletal and Neuronal Interactions 6: 331–333.
25. Datta HK, Ng FW, Walker J, Tuck SP, Varanasi SS (2008) The cell biology of bone metabolism. J Clin Path 61: 577–587.
26. Zhao S, Zhang YK, Harris S, Ahuja SS, Bonewald LF (2002) MLO-Y4 osteocyte-like cells support osteoclast formation and activation. J Bone Miner Res 17: 2068–2079.
27. Lanyon LE (1993) Osteocytes, strain detection, bone modelling and remodeling. Calcif Tissue Int 53: S102–S107.
28. Datta HK, Wu JJ, Tuck SP, Walker J (2008) Emerging evidence of osteocytes as mechanosensors and regulators of mineralisation. European Musculoskeletal Review 3: 48–52.
29. Bonewald LF, Johnson ML (2008) Osteocytes, mechanosensing and Wnt signaling. Bone 42: 606–615.
30. Datta HK, Varanasi SS, Olstad OK, Gautvik V, Sanderson P, et al. (2009) ASBMR 31st Annual Meeting Abstract SU0078.
31. Kalogeropoulos M, Varanasi SS, Olstad OK, Sanderson P, Gautvik V, et al. (2010) Zic1 Transcription Factor in Bone: Neural Developmental Protein Regulates Mechanotransduction in Osteocytes. FASEB J. In press.
32. Al-oanzi ZH, Tuck SP, Raj N, Harrop JS, Summers G, et al. (2006) Assessment of Vitamin D Status in Male Osteoporosis. Clin Chem 52: 248–54.
33. Livak KJ, Schmittgen TD (2001) Real-time quantitative PCR and the 2(Delta Delta C(T) method. Methods 25: 402–408.

Hip Structural Parameters over 96 Weeks in HIV-Infected Adults Switching Treatment to Tenofovir-Emtricitabine or Abacavir-Lamivudine

Hila Haskelberg[1]*, Nicholas Pocock[2], Janaki Amin[1], Peter Robert Ebeling[3], Sean Emery[1], Andrew Carr[2], on behalf of the STEAL Study Group

1 The Kirby Institute, University of New South Wales, Sydney, Australia, **2** St. Vincent's Hospital, Sydney, Australia, **3** North West Academic Centre, University of Melbourne, Melbourne, Australia

Abstract

Background: Therapy with tenofovir is associated with lower bone mineral density (BMD), higher markers of bone turnover and increased fracture risk in HIV-infected adults. Bone structural parameters generated by hip structural analysis may represent a separate measure of bone strength, but have not been assessed in HIV.

Methods: Dual-energy X-ray absorptiometry (DXA) scans from 254 HIV-infected adults randomised to simplify their existing dual nucleoside analogue reverse transcriptase inhibitor therapy to coformulated tenofovir-emtricitabine or abacavir-lamivudine were analysed using DXA-derived hip structural analysis software. Hip structural parameters included femoral strength index, section modulus, cross-sectional area, and cross-sectional moment of inertia. We used one-way ANOVA to test the relationship between nucleoside analogue type at baseline and structural parameters, multivariable analysis to assess baseline covariates associated with femoral strength index, and t-tests to compare mean change in structural parameters over 96 weeks between randomised groups.

Results: Participants taking tenofovir at baseline had lower section modulus (-107.3 mm^2, $p=0.001$), lower cross-sectional area (-15.01 mm^3, $p=0.001$), and lower cross-sectional moment of inertia ($-2{,}036.8$ mm^4, $p=0.007$) than those receiving other nucleoside analogues. After adjustment for baseline risk factors, the association remained significant for section modulus ($p=0.008$) and cross-sectional area ($p=0.002$). Baseline covariates significantly associated with higher femoral strength index were higher spine T-score ($p=0.001$), lower body fat mass ($p<0.001$), lower bone alkaline phosphatase ($p=0.025$), and higher osteoprotegerin ($p=0.024$). Hip structural parameters did not change significantly over 96 weeks and none was significantly affected by treatment simplification to tenofovir-emtricitabine or abacavir-lamivudine.

Conclusion: In this population, tenofovir use was associated with reduced composite indices of bone strength as measured by hip structural analysis, but none of the structural parameters improved significantly over 96 weeks with tenofovir cessation.

Trial Registration: ClinicalTrials.gov NCT00192634

Editor: Yi-Hsiang Hsu, Harvard Medical School, United States of America

Funding: This work was supported by The Kirby Institute (formerly the National Centre in HIV Epidemiology and Clinical Research) funded by the Australian Government Department of Health and Ageing. The Kirby Institute is affiliated with the Faculty of Medicine, University of New South Wales. The funders had no role in study design, data collection and analysis, decision to publish, or preparation of the manuscript.

Competing Interests: Hila Haskelberg and Janaki Amin declare no conflict of interest. Nicolas Pocock received consultancy fees from Merck, Sanofi Aventis and Servier; and has served on an advisory board for Merck. Peter Ebeling's institution has received research funding from Merck; consultancy fees from Gilead Sciences and GlaxoSmithKline/ViiV Healthcare; and has served on an advisory board for Merck. Sean Emery has received research grant support from Abbvie, Gilead Sciences, Merck Research Laboratories, Pfizer, and ViiV Healthcare. Andrew Carr has received research funding from ViiV Healthcare, and Merck; consultancy fees from Gilead Sciences, ViiV Healthcare, MSD and Roche; lecture and travel sponsorships from Gilead Sciences, MSD, and ViiV Healthcare; and has served on advisory boards for Gilead Sciences, MSD, and ViiV Healthcare.

* E-mail: hhaskelberg@kirby.unsw.edu.au

Introduction

Low bone mineral density (BMD) and higher rates of fractures have been reported in HIV-infected adults compared with general population controls [1,2], and have been particularly associated with tenofovir (TDF) therapy [3]. BMD as measured by dual-energy X-ray absorptiometry (DXA) is the gold standard for clinical assessment of bone fragility. The relationship between decreased BMD and increased risk of fractures is well established [4]. BMD, however, only accounts for about 50% of fracture risk [5] and does not describe other components of bone quality such as geometric configuration, which can be estimated by DXA-derived hip structural analysis (HSA) [6,7]. HSA software

Table 1. Hip structural parameters included in this analysis [8].

Measure	Derivation	Comments
Femoral strength index	Calculated as strength/stress, where, strength = 185–0.34 (age - 45) and stress is moment*y/CSMI+force/CSA	Indicates the bone's resistance to fracture from forces generated during a fall on the greater trochanter
Hip axis length (HAL, mm)	The distance along the femoral neck axis, extending from the bone edge at the base of the trochanter to the bone edge at the inner pelvic brim	Suggested to be a measure of the degree to which the femur extends beyond the pelvis, increasing risk for impact, though relationship to fractures is unclear
Buckling ratio	Ratio of the outer radius to the cortical thickness	Indicator of cortical stability under compressive loads
Section Modulus (Z, mm^3)	CSMI divided by half the width of the femoral neck	A measure of bending strength
Cross-sectional area (CSA; mm^2)	Represents the area of mineral packed together in the defined cross section of the femoral neck	Proportional to bone's ability to resist axial compressive force
Cross-sectional moment of inertia (CSMI; mm^4)	calculated using the mass distribution derived from the absorption curve	Bone's ability to resist bending forces

generates a femoral strength index, an integral measure that combines BMD, femur geometry, age, height and weight and aims to reflect the bone's ability to withstand forces generated during a fall [8].

A cross-sectional analysis of hip osteoporotic fractures and composite indices of femoral neck strength in healthy women found decreased measures of femoral neck strength in women with fractures [9]. In addition, structural parameters were found to predict hip fracture in postmenopausal women after adjusting for both clinical risk factors and BMD [10–13]. Yet the role of these measures as independent predictors of hip fracture remains controversial, particularly in men [14].

Studies of osteoporosis and fractures in HIV-infected adults have mainly focused on BMD; the effects of HIV and its treatment on other measures of bone quality are unclear. Walker Harris et al. [15] have recently found in a cross-sectional study that HIV/HCV-co-infected men had significantly lower measures of hip strength at the narrow neck and shaft when compared to healthy controls. Lower lean body mass accounted for most of the differences between groups after adjusting for race, age, smoking status, height, and weight [15]. In a longitudinal study of perinatally HIV-infected youth (n = 31; 9–18 y), neither bone geometry nor strength was significantly different compared with healthy controls [16].

In the STEAL study, patients randomized to simplify their existing dual nucleoside reverse transcriptase inhibitor (NRTI) therapy to coformulated tenofovir-emtricitabine (TDF-FTC) had greater BMD decreases and greater bone turnover marker increases over 96 weeks than those who were randomised to abacavir-lamivudine (ABC-3TC) [17]. STEAL provides an opportunity to examine bone structure cross-sectionally and longitudinally, and in particular any effect of TDF. We hypothesised that there would be a significant difference between TDF-FTC and ABC-3TC in measures of bone structure, as assessed by DXA-derived Hip Structural Analysis. The aim of this analysis was to estimate and compare changes in bone structural parameters by randomised arm from baseline to 96 weeks. A secondary objectives was were to determine the relationship between femoral strength index and baseline clinical and biochemical characteristics, and to explore the relationship between markers of bone turnover and changes in the above measures of bone structure

Methods

Study design

STEAL was an open-label, prospective, randomized, non-inferiority study that compared simplification of current NRTIs to fixed-dose combination TDF-FTC or ABC-3TC over 96 weeks in 357 adults with plasma HIV viral load <50 copies/mL [17]. The supporting CONSORT checklist and STEAL protocol are available as supporting information; see Checklist S1, and Protocol S1

Ethics Statement

The study was approved by each site's Human Research and Ethics Committee and registered at Clinicaltrials.gov (NCT00192634). The specific ethics committees that gave approval for the STEAL study are: St Vincent's Hospital Human Research Ethics Committee (HREC), South Eastern Sydney/Illawarra Area Health Service HREC, Harbour HREC of Northern Sydney Central Coast Health, North Coast Area Health Service HREC, Sydney West Area Health Service HREC, Sydney South West Area Health Service HREC, Alfred Hospital EC, Southern Health HREC, Melbourne Health HREC, The Prince Charles Hospital HREC, Cairns & Hinterland Health Service District EC, Gold Coast Health Service District HREC, Royal Brisbane and Women's Hospital HREC, Flinders Clinical Research EC, Royal Adelaide Hospital Research EC, Royal Perth Hospital EC. Each participant signed a written informed consent before enrolment.

DXA and hip structural analysis

DXA measurements of the right hip and lumbar spine BMD were performed for each participant at baseline, week 48, and week 96, using a standardized protocol. The following were recorded: hip and spine BMD, T-scores and Z-scores, total body fat tissue and lean tissue masses. DXA instruments varied between study sites and for this analysis, only data from GE-Lunar scanners were used.

Archived lunar image files of the right femur were analysed by a trained individual blinded to antiretroviral therapy, using the HSA software Lunar Prodigy enCORE 2011 version 13.60.033 (GE Healthcare). The HSA software provides a line of pixels traversing the bone axis which gives a projection of the surface area of bone in the cross section. The results reported in this analysis are from the femoral neck. The HSA software automatically assesses all cross sections in the femoral neck and identifies the plane that is

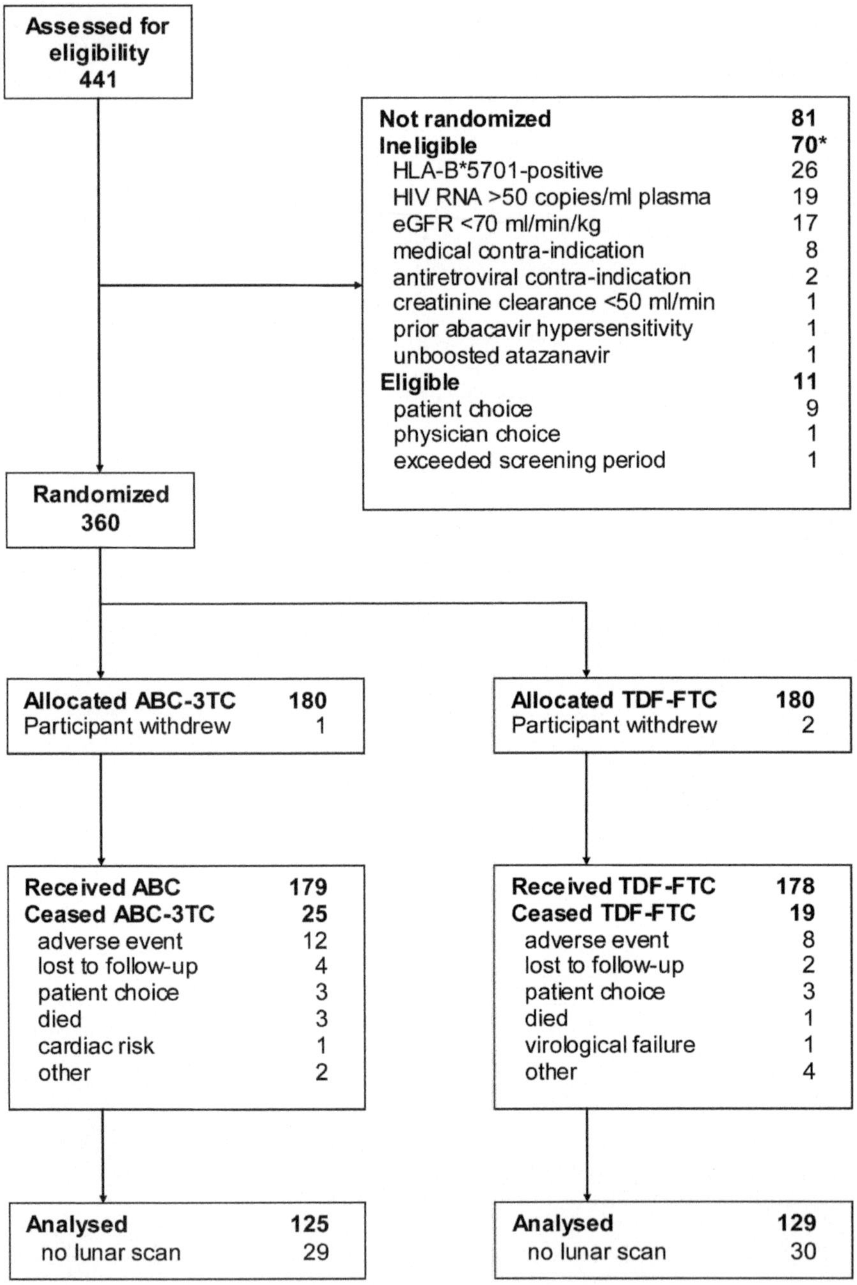

Figure 1. Patient disposition.

the weakest, by calculating the mass distribution derived from an X-ray absorption curve [8]. Specifically, the following structural parameters were obtained: hip axis length (HAL, mm), femoral strength index, buckling ratio, section modulus (Z, in mm^3), cross-sectional moment of inertia (CSMI, in mm^4), and cross sectional area (CSA, in mm^2) (Table 1).

Laboratory markers

Plasma and serum samples were collected at baseline and at weeks 12, 24, 48, 72 and 96 (following a 10-hour overnight fast, except at week 12) and stored at $-70°C$. Markers of bone resorption (C-terminal cross-linking telopeptide of type 1 collagen [βCTX]), bone formation (procollagen type 1 N-terminal propeptide [P1NP]; bone-specific alkaline phosphatise [BALP]) and regulators of bone turnover (osteoprotegerin [OPG] and receptor activator of nuclear factor kappa ligand [RANKL]) were evaluated. The following were assessed at baseline only: interleukin-6, oestradiol, free testosterone and 25-hydroxy vitamin D. Assays are described elsewhere [18]. BTMs were batch-tested after study completion in one laboratory.

Statistical analyses

All analyses were performed on the per-protocol data so as to evaluate the biological effects of exposure to randomised therapy. "Per-protocol" is defined as available data collected on partici-

Table 2. Baseline characteristics.

	NRTI at study entry			Randomization		
Baseline characteristics	**ABC (n = 53)**	**TDF (n = 74)**	**Other (n = 127)**	**ABC-3TC (n = 125)**	**TDF-FTC (n = 129)**	**Main Study (n = 357)**
Age (years)	48.7±8.4	42.8±8.5	44±8.4	45.8±8.9	44.3±8.4	45.1±8.6
Male (%)	98	99	98	99	98	98
Ethnicity – white (%)	92	88	79	84	85	86
HIV duration (years)	13.4±5.6	8.7±5.7	9.9±5.7	10.0±5.7	10.5±6.1	10.2±6.0
CD4+ count	613±257	609±257	612±248	629±259	595±245	612±282
ART exposure						
NRTI duration (years)	8.0±4.1	4.1±3.1	5.8±2.8	5.8±3.5	5.8±3.5	5.8±3.6
Current protease inhibitor (%)	26	28	19	24	22	23
Anthropometric factors						
Weight (kg)	76.8±11.5	72.9±12.2	77.7±12.8	76.0±12.9	76.2±12.2	76.8±12.6
Fat mass (kg)	16.2±6.8	14.9±7.2	16.5±7.7	15.7±7.3	16.2±7.5	16.8±7.9
Bone mineral density						
Right hip (g/cm^2)	1.06±0.14	1.00±0.11	1.04±0.13	1.04+0.13	1.02+0.13	
Lumbar Spine (g/cm^2)	1.26±0.14	1.16±0.15	1.21±0.16	1.2±0.16	1.2±0.15	
Bone turnover markers						
βCTx (ng/L)	256±152	314±157	226±134	252±154	265±145	
BALP (μg/L)	16.8±8.4	23.6±11.6	17.9±10.3	19.3±10.1	19.4±11.2	
P1NP (μg/L)	45.7±19.1	67.7±22.8	50.1±21.9	53.1±23.9	55.7±22.6	
OPG (pmol/L)	3.8±1.1	4.0±1.4	3.8±1.1	3.9±1.3	3.8±1.1	
RANKL (pmol/L)	0.2±0.3	0.2±0.2	0.3±0.5	0.2±0.3	0.2±0.4	
Hip structural parameters						
Femoral strength index	1.68±0.43	1.57±0.34	1.60±0.38	1.60±0.37	1.62±0.39	
Hip axis length (mm)	118.1±6.9	116.8±7.1	118.9±8.5	118.2±7.4	118.1±8.2	
Buckling ratio	3.9±1.6	4.4±1.5	4.2±1.8	4.2±1.7	4.2±1.7	
Section modulus (mm^3)	873±196	766±147	836±180	832±175	815±182	
Cross-sectional area (mm^2)	174±28	159±20	169±26	167±25	167±26	
Cross-sectional moment of inertia (mm^4)	16235±5032	14198±3387	15705±4222	15473±4127	15283±4368	

Note. Results are expressed as mean ± standard deviation or %.
Abbreviations: **ABC-3TC**, abacavir-lamivudine; **BALP**, bone-specific alkaline phosphatase; **βCTx**, C-terminal cross-linking telopeptide of type 1 collagen; **BMD**, bone mineral density; **NNRTI**, non-nucleoside reverse transcriptase inhibitor; **NRTI**, nucleoside reverse transcriptase inhibitor; **OPG**, osteoprotegerin; **P1NP**, procollagen type 1 N-terminal propeptide; **RANKL**, Receptor Activator of Nuclear Factor Kappa Ligand; **TDF-FTC**, tenofovir-emtricitabine.

pants while on randomised strategy as defined in the STEAL protocol.

The associations between baseline covariates (including demographic, HIV-related factors, antiretroviral therapy, body composition, bone remodelling regulators, sex hormones, and vitamin D), and absolute baseline femoral strength index were analysed using linear regression. Multivariable model was built using backward, stepwise methods. Covariates that achieved a p-value <0.1 in univariate analysis were assessed for inclusion in the model. In an exploratory analysis, one-way ANOVA was used to assess the relationship between type of NRTI at study entry (ABC, TDF, or other) and all structural measures at baseline. To test this relationship further, linear regression models were a-priori adjusted for covariates known to be related to bone status i.e. age, sex, ethnicity, smoking, height, total body fat mass, total body lean mass, and HIV infection duration to account for possible associations with hip structural analysis outcomes. Structural parameters at week 48 and week 96 were compared with baseline using paired t-tests. Randomized groups were compared for changes in structural measures by t-tests at 48 weeks and 96 weeks. Results are reported as regression coefficients i.e. differences between groups. Statistical significance was defined as a 2-sided α of 0.05. Statistical analyses were performed with STATA (StataCorp. 2011. Stata Statistical Software: Release 12. College Station, TX: StataCorp LP USA).

Results

Patient disposition is outlined in Figure 1. Of 357 participants enrolled in the parent study, 285 had GE-lunar Prodigy scans data available at baseline; 17 discontinued ABC-3TC and 14 discontinued TDF-FTC by week 96. Therefore, the analysed per-protocol population comprised the remaining 254 participants (71% of main study population). Baseline characteristics of the population analysed were similar to those of all study participants [19] and well balanced between arms (Table 2). At study entry, 29% of the participants (n = 74) were taking TDF-containing regimen, 21% (n = 53) were on ABC-containing regimen and 50%

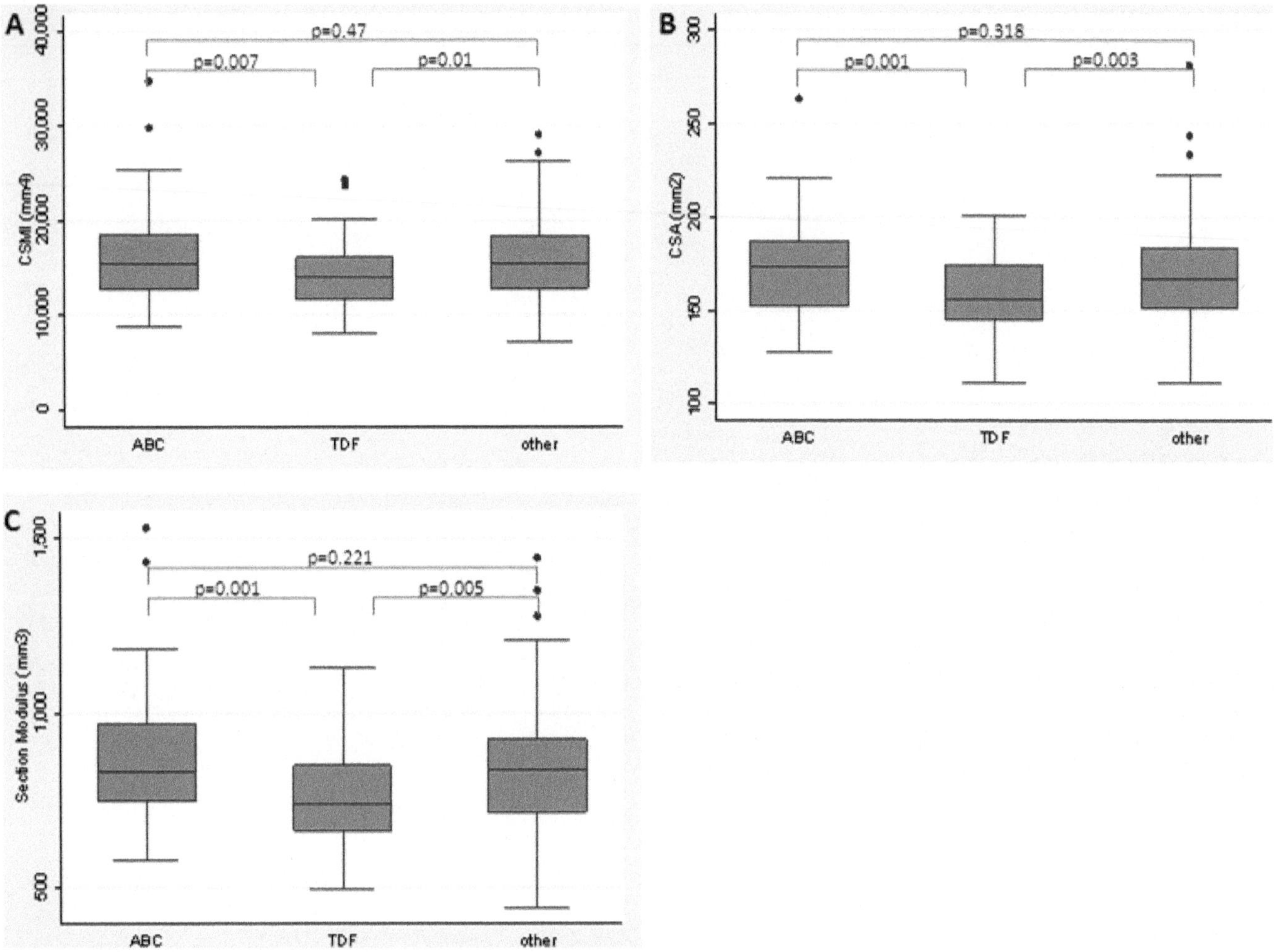

Figure 2. Hip structural parameters at baseline by type of NRTI at study entry (A) CSMI (bone's ability to resist bending), (B) CSA (bone's ability to resist axial compressive force) and (C) section modulus (bending strength). Abbreviations: CSA, cross-sectional area; CSMI, cross-sectional moment of inertia.

(n = 127) were taking other NRTIs (typically two of the following: 3TC, FTC, zidovudine, didanosine, stavudine).

Hip structural parameters at baseline

Baseline CSMI, CSA, and section modulus were all significantly different across the three sub-groups of NRTI types at baseline [CSMI: $F(2,208) = 26.98$, $p = 0.013$; CSA: $F(2,251) = 6.59$, $p = 0.002$; section modulus: $F(2,251) = 6.51$, $p = 0.002$].

Compared to the ABC group, participants that entered the study on TDF had lower baseline CSMI (coefficient: -2036.8 mm^4; 95% CI: -3520.8 to -552.7; $p = 0.007$), lower CSA (-15.01 mm^2; 95% CI: -23.8 to -6.2; $p = 0.001$), and lower section modulus (-107.3 mm^3; 95% CI: -169.1 to -45.4; $p = 0.001$) (Figure 2). After adjustment, the association remained significant for CSA (-13.7 mm^2; 95% CI: -21.3 to -6.2; $p = 0.002$) and section modulus (-83.1 mm^3; 95% CI: -135.5 to -30.6; $p = 0.008$), but not for CSMI (-1168.85 mm^4; 95% CI: -2366.9 to 29.2; $p = 0.159$).

Baseline covariates significantly associated with higher femoral strength index at baseline in multivariable analysis were higher spine T-score (p trend = 0.001), lower body fat mass (p trend < 0.001), lower bone alkaline phosphatase (BALP; $p = 0.025$), and higher osteoprotegerin (OPG; $P = 0.024$; Table 3).

Changes in hip structural parameters over 96 weeks

For all structural measures besides HAL, there was no significant difference between baseline and week 48 or between baseline and week 96 for the whole cohort. The absolute increase in HAL from baseline was statistically significant at week 48 though not at week 96 [(diff: 0.25; 95% confidence intervals [CI]: 0.09 to 0.41; $p = 0.002$); (diff: 0.16; 95% CI: -0.005 to 0.33; $p = 0.058$, respectively]. There was no difference between randomised arms in absolute change at week 48 or week 96 (Table 4).

Analysing the effect of randomisation by the NRTI sub-groups, patients that were on ABC at baseline and switched to TDF (n = 24) had significantly greater decreases of CSA (coeff: -6.7 mm^2; 95% CI: -12.3 to -1.0; $p = 0.021$) and CSMI (coeff: -675.1 mm^4; 95% CI: -1298.4 to -51.7; $p = 0.034$) at week 48 compared with those who continued on ABC (n = 26). There were no significant differences from baseline to week 96. No significant change was found for 74 patients on TDF at baseline who either stayed on TDF or switched to ABC.

Table 3. Covariates associated with femoral strength index at baseline

Covariate	Univariate analysis					Multivariate model (n = 228)			
	N	**Coef. femoral strength index**	**95% Conf. Interval**	**P>|z|**	**overall P value**	**Coef. femoral strength index**	**95% Conf. Interval**	**P>|z|**	**overall P value**
HIV RNA (copies/ml)	254	0	(−0.00 to 0.00)	0.09		0	(−0.00 to 0.00)	0.191	
No PI - NNRTI*	195	0				0			
PI	59	−0.12	(−0.23 to −0.01)	0.027		−0.09	(−0.20 to 0.01)	0.079	
Spine BMD wk0 - quartiles									
0.788–1.061*	54	0				0			
1.062–1.180	60	0.17	(0.03 to 0.31)	0.016		0.15	(0.01 to 0.28)	0.034	
1.181–1.292	71	0.22	(0.09 to 0.35)	0.001		0.27	(0.14 to 0.40)	<0.001	
1.293–1.798	69	0.2	(0.06 to 0.33)	0.004	0.005	0.18	(0.06 to 0.31)	0.005	**0.003**
Total body lean tissue mass wk0 - quartiles									
32464–51980 g*	67	0				0			
51981–56673 g	57	0	(−0.13 to 0.14)	0.977		0.03	(−0.10 to 0.16)	0.677	
56674–61811 g	62	−0.1	(−0.23 to 0.03)	0.129		−0.05	(−0.18 to 0.08)	0.436	
61812–79671 g	68	−0.09	(−0.21 to 0.04)	0.191	0.09	−0.04	(−0.17 to 0.10)	0.614	0.391
Total body fat tissue mass wk0 - quartiles									
1110–10590 g*	69	0				0			
10591–15428 g	59	−0.17	(−0.29 to −0.04)	0.008		−0.19	(−0.32 to −0.07)	0.002	
15429–20942 g	64	−0.25	(−0.37 to −0.13)	<0.001		−0.31	(−0.43 to −0.19)	<0.001	
20943–46433 g	62	−0.36	(−0.48 to −0.24)	<0.001	<0.001	−0.38	(−0.50 to −0.25)	<0.001	**<0.001**
Alkaline phosphatase (mmol/l)	253	0	(−0.00 to −0.00)	0.039		0	(−0.00 to 0.00)	0.886	
BALP Wk0	228	0	(−0.01 to 0.00)	0.066		−0.01	(−0.01 to −0.00)	**0.03**	
OPG Wk0	228	0.04	(0.00 to 0.09)	0.032		0.04	(0.00 to 0.08)	**0.038**	
RANK-L Wk0	228	0.15	(0.02 to 0.28)	0.021		0.13	(0.01 to 0.25)	**0.032**	

Table 4. Mean change in hip structural parameters over 96 weeks by randomisation

Hip structural parameters	Abacavir-lamivudine	Tenofovir-emtricitabine	Mean difference (95% confidence interval)	*P*
Femoral strength index	−0.02	−0.01	0.01 (−0.05 to 0.07)	0.704
Hip axis length (mm)	0.3	0.03	−0.27 (−0.6 to 0.6)	0.109
Buckling ratio	−0.06	−0.3	−0.2 (−0.7 to 0.1)	0.220
Section modulus (mm^3)	2.2	0.2	−2.0 (−16.8 to 12.7)	0.787
Cross-sectional area (mm^2)	1.3	−0.2	−1.5 (−3.8 to 0.6)	0.155
Cross-sectional moment of inertia (mm^4)	−42.4	−3.8	38.6 (−276 to 353)	0.810

Discussion

To our knowledge, this is the first longitudinal study to investigate DXA-derived structural properties of the femoral neck in HIV-infected adults. In this cohort of predominantly young HIV-infected men, participants that were taking TDF at study entry had decreased composite indices of bone strength, as estimated by hip structural analysis, compared to ABC and other NRTIs. Independent baseline factors associated with lower femoral hip strength index at baseline included lower bone formation markers and lower body fat mass. The majority of structural parameters did not improve over 96 weeks of follow-up and nor were they significantly affected by treatment simplification to TDF-FTC or ABC-3TC.

Most studies of HIV-infected adults have shown that they are at greater risk of fractures when compared with healthy population controls [1,2], yet the pathogenesis of HIV-associated bone disease is multifactorial and not fully understood. In the STEAL cohort, four participants experienced fractures, two in each treatment arm [17]. In a number of randomized controlled studies, the initiation or a switch to ART was associated with 6–12 months of bone loss, which then stabilizes [17,19]. In post-menopausal women, treatment with a bisphosphonate resulted in significant improvements in hip geometric parameters after one [20] and two years [21] of treatment. The finding in our cohort that most of the structural indices did not significantly change following ART switch, supports the finding by Tuck et al. that some bone geometrical measures are relatively stable over time in men [14]. Furthermore, our data also corroborate a recent population-based study (n = 1760), which found that a decline in BMD was counteracted by an increase in bone size, resulting in only a small decrease of up to 0.5% in composite indices of hip strength (as measured by DXA-derived hip structural analysis), resulting in a partial preservation of bone strength in men from peak value to age 90 years [22].

In our study, higher OPG was independently associated with higher femoral strength index. The RANKL/RANK/OPG signalling pathway has a critical role in bone remodelling; specifically, OPG inhibits bone resorption [23]. Our results are consistent with the Framingham Offspring Study in HIV-uninfected adults (n = 1165 men), which found that increased OPG was independently positively associated with indices of hip strength in men [24]. Higher OPG levels may reflect a compensatory reaction to accelerated bone resorption and deterioration of cortical bone [25]. This may also explain the observation that there were no significant changes over the 2 years of follow-up in majority of structural parameters in our cohort. We also found that lower body fat mass was an independent predictor of higher femoral strength index, which is consistent with the index's formula – negative correlation between the strength (resistance to fracture forces) relative to load (forces placed on the hip during a fall).

Unlike the previous cross-sectional study of hip geomerty in HIV/HCV co-infected adults [15], we found no association between any of the structural parameters and lower lean mass. However, it is difficult to directly compare the two studies. Firstly, chronic hepatitis C monoinfection has been independently associated with unbalanced bone turnover and reduced bone quality [26]. Secondly, the population studied by Walker-Harris was mostly African-American (86%) while 85% of our cohort was Caucasian and probably less than 10% had HCV co-infection. And finally, the participants in the HIV/HCV cohort were evaluated at three locations at the proximal femur using a Hologic scanner, which employs a different HSA method to assess strength at the femoral neck than the Lunar software used in our study.

Despite being younger with shorter duration of HIV and shorter exposure to ART, participants that were on TDF at study entry had significantly lower CSA (bone's ability to resist bending) and section modulus (bending strength) at baseline than those receiving other NRTIs. Switching from TDF lead to an increase in BMD [27], in our study, however, TDF cessation did not lead to a significant improvement in any structural parameter of the hip over 96 weeks. The Study of Osteoporotic Fractures (n = 7474) found that that a 1 SD decrease in CSA increased the risk of incident hip fracture by 1.80–1.93, depending on which covariates were included in the model [13]. There is a body of literature demonstrating a greater effect of TDF-based regimens on decreasing BMD [17,19,28] and increased fracture risk [3]. As the reduced composite indices of bone strength that were found with TDF, did not improve after treatment switch, it may imply that prevention of loss in bone strength is more important than switching treatment to improve these bone measures. It was recently found by Bedimo at el. [3] that cumulative exposure to TDF was an independent predictor of increased risk of osteoporotic fractures (yearly HR 1.12; 95% CI 1.03–1.21). The possible effects of long-term exposure to TDF on bone structure require further investigation in patients initiating antiretroviral therapy.

Our study has several limitations. There is an inherent limitation in using DXA, which produces two-dimensional images, to assess three-dimensional measures of hip geometry and the calculated strength indices [6]. Furthermore, relative changes in the cortical versus cancellous bone are not detected by DXA. However, the DXA-derived HSA method is currently more available and affordable than the three-dimensional techniques (such as finite element modelling), and allows the evaluation of femoral neck structure in additional to BMD. Our finding regarding the association to TDF was only found in the uncontrolled cross-sectional analysis at baseline. Another limitation is the generalizability of our findings: our cohort comprised mainly Caucasian men and we only analysed data from GE-Lunar scanners, therefore limiting our ability to extend our findings to different populations or to other methods that assess hip strength. Lastly, the short follow-up period and small sample size precluded the investigation of fracture risk. Nevertheless, our study includes a comprehensive set of bone-related data - bone turnover markers, BMD and hip structure, which allows us a greater understanding of the skeletal status of this cohort.

To conclude, HIV-infected adults who were on TDF at study entry, had reduced composite indices of bone strength (as assessed by hip structural analysis), compared with other NRTIs groups. Treatment simplification to TDF-FTC or ABC-3TC had no significant effect on hip structural parameters over 96 weeks of follow-up. This study suggests that hip structural parameters may not improve with TDF cessation in our cohort's age group and their assessment does not add any predictive value to BMD in clinical management of HIV-infected adults. Yet, differences in the length, width, and angle of the femoral neck may increase fracture risk with ageing; further longer prospective studies of bone structure in larger cohorts of individuals with HIV may shed more light on the pathogenesis of bone disease in HIV-infection.

Supporting Information

Checklist S1 The supporting CONSORT checklist.

Protocol S1 STEAL main study protocol.

Acknowledgments

The content is solely the responsibility of the authors and the views expressed in this publication do not necessarily represent the position of the Australian Government.

STEAL Study Group (as listed in [17])

STEAL study investigators – Anthony Allworth, Jonathan Anderson, David Baker, Mark Bloch, Mark Boyd, John Chuah, David Cooper, Stephen Davies, Linda Dayan, William Donohue, Nicholas Doong, Dominic Dwyer, John Dyer, Robert Finlayson, Michelle Giles, David Gordon, Mark Kelly, Nicholas Medland, Richard Moore, David Nolan, David Orth, Jeffrey Post, John Quin, Tim Read, Norman Roth, Darren Russell, David Shaw, David Smith, Don Smith, Alan Street, Ban Kiem Tee, Ian Woolley.

We extend our grateful thanks to all the participants and the study co-ordinators.

Author Contributions

Conceived and designed the experiments: HH, NP, AC. Performed the experiments: HH, NP. Analyzed the data: HH. Contributed reagents/materials/analysis tools: NP. Wrote the paper: HH. All authors reviewed all data and analyses, and reviewed the manuscript.

References

1. Hansen A-BE, Gerstoft J, Kronborg G, Larsen CS, Pedersen C, et al. (2012) Incidence of low and high-energy fractures in persons with and without HIV infection: a Danish population-based cohort study. AIDS 26: 285–293 210.1097/QAD.1090b1013e32834ed32838a32837.
2. Triant VA, Brown TT, Lee H, Grinspoon SK (2008) Fracture prevalence among human immunodeficiency virus (HIV)-infected versus non-HIV-infected patients in a large U.S. healthcare system. J Clin Endocrinol Metab 93: 3499–3504.
3. Bedimo R, Maalouf NM, Zhang S, Drechsler H, Tebas P (2012) Osteoporotic fracture risk associated with cumulative exposure to tenofovir and other antiretroviral agents. AIDS 26: 825.
4. Kanis JA (2002) Diagnosis of osteoporosis and assessment of fracture risk. Lancet 359: 1929–1936.
5. Marshall D, Johnell O, Wedel H (1996) Meta-analysis of how well measures of bone mineral density predict occurrence of osteoporotic fractures. BMJ 312: 1254–1259.
6. Beck T (2003) Measuring the structural strength of bones with dual-energy X-ray absorptiometry: principles, technical limitations, and future possibilities. Osteoporosis International 14: 81–88.
7. Lou Bonnick S (2007) Hsa: Beyond bmd with dxa. Bone 41: S9–S12.
8. Yoshikawa T, Turner C, Peacock M, Slemenda C, Weaver C, et al. (1994) Geometric structure of the femoral neck measured using dual-energy X-ray absorptiometry. Journal of Bone and Mineral Research 9: 1053–1064.
9. Li G-W, Chang S-X, Xu Z, Chen Y, Bao H, et al. (2013) Prediction of hip osteoporotic fractures from composite indices of femoral neck strength. Skeletal radiology 42: 195–201.
10. LaCroix A, Beck T, Cauley J, Lewis C, Bassford T, et al. (2010) Hip structural geometry and incidence of hip fracture in postmenopausal women: what does it add to conventional bone mineral density? Osteoporosis International 21: 919–929.
11. Faulkner KGK, Wacker WKW, Barden HSH, Simonelli CC, Burke PKP, et al. (2006) Femur strength index predicts hip fracture independent of bone density and hip axis length. Osteoporosis international 17: 593–599.
12. Bergot C, Bousson V, Meunier A, Laval-Jeantet M, Laredo J (2002) Hip fracture risk and proximal femur geometry from DXA scans. Osteoporosis International 13: 542–550.
13. Kaptoge S, Beck TJ, Reeve J, Stone KL, Hillier TA, et al. (2008) Prediction of incident hip fracture risk by femur geometry variables measured by hip structural analysis in the study of osteoporotic fractures. Journal of Bone and Mineral Research 23: 1892–1904.
14. Tuck S, Rawlings D, Scane A, Pande I, Summers G, et al. (2011) Femoral Neck Shaft Angle in Men with Fragility Fractures. Journal of Osteoporosis 2011.
15. Walker Harris V, Sutcliffe CG, Araujo AB, Chiu GR, Travison TG, et al. (2012) Hip bone geometry in HIV/HCV-co-infected men and healthy controls. Osteoporosis International 23: 1779–1787.
16. Macdonald H, Chu J, Nettlefold L, Maan E, Forbes J, et al. (2013) Bone geometry and strength are adapted to muscle force in children and adolescents perinatally infected with HIV. Journal of musculoskeletal & neuronal interactions 13: 53–65.
17. Martin A, Bloch M, Amin J, Baker D, Cooper DA, et al. (2009) Simplification of antiretroviral therapy with tenofovir-emtricitabine or abacavir-Lamivudine: a randomized, 96-week trial. Clinical Infectious Diseases 49: 1591.
18. Haskelberg H, Hoy JF, Amin J, Ebeling PR, Emery S, et al. (2012) Changes in Bone Turnover and Bone Loss in HIV-Infected Patients Changing Treatment to Tenofovir-Emtricitabine or Abacavir-Lamivudine. PLoS One 7: e38377.
19. McComsey GA, Kitch D, Daar ES, Tierney C, Jahed NC, et al. (2011) Bone Mineral Density and Fractures in Antiretroviral-Naive Persons Randomized to Receive Abacavir-Lamivudine or Tenofovir Disoproxil Fumarate-Emtricitabine Along With Efavirenz or Atazanavir-Ritonavir: AIDS Clinical Trials Group A5224s, a Substudy of ACTG A5202. Journal of Infectious Diseases 203: 1791.
20. Lewiecki EM, Keaveny TM, Kopperdahl DL, Genant HK, Engelke K, et al. (2009) Once-monthly oral ibandronate improves biomechanical determinants of bone strength in women with postmenopausal osteoporosis. Journal of Clinical Endocrinology & Metabolism 94: 171–180.
21. Bonnick S, Beck T, Cosman F, Hochberg M, Wang H, et al. (2009) DXA-based hip structural analysis of once-weekly bisphosphonate-treated postmenopausal women with low bone mass. Osteoporosis international 20: 911–921.
22. Alwis G, Karlsson C, Stenevi-Lundgren S, Rosengren BE, Karlsson MK (2012) Femoral Neck Bone Strength Estimated by Hip Structural Analysis (HSA) in Swedish Caucasians Aged 6–90 Years. Calcified Tissue International 90: 174.
23. Hofbauer LC, Schoppet M (2004) Clinical implications of the osteoprotegerin/RANKL/RANK system for bone and vascular diseases. JAMA: The Journal of the American Medical Association 292: 490–495.
24. Samelson EJ, Broe KE, Demissie S, Beck TJ, Karasik D, et al. (2008) Increased Plasma Osteoprotegerin Concentrations Are Associated with Indices of Bone Strength of the Hip. Journal of Clinical Endocrinology & Metabolism 93: 1789–1795.
25. Szulc P, Hawa G, Boutroy S, Vilayphiou N, Schoppet M, et al. (2011) Cortical Bone Status Is Associated with Serum Osteoprotegerin Concentration in Men: The STRAMBO Study. Journal of Clinical Endocrinology & Metabolism 96: 2216–2226.
26. Gaudio A, Pennisi P, Muratore F, Bertino G, Ardiri A, et al. (2012) Reduction of volumetric bone mineral density in postmenopausal women with hepatitis C virus-correlated chronic liver disease: A peripheral quantitative computed tomography (pQCT) study. European Journal of Internal Medicine 23: 656–660.
27. Bloch M, Tong W, Hoy J, Richardson R, Baker D, et al. (2012) Improved Low Bone Mineral Density and Bone Turnover Markers with Switch from Tenofovir to Raltegravir in Virologically Suppressed HIV-1+ Adults at 48 Weeks: The TROP Study. Conference of Retrovirus and Opportunistic Infection. Washington.
28. Stellbrink HJ, Orkin C, Arribas JR, Compston J, Gerstoft J, et al. (2010) Comparison of changes in bone density and turnover with abacavir-lamivudine versus tenofovir-emtricitabine in HIV-infected adults: 48-week results from the ASSERT study. Clinical Infectious Diseases 51: 963.

13

Repression of Osteoblast Maturation by ERRα Accounts for Bone Loss Induced by Estrogen Deficiency

Marlène Gallet[1], Soraya Saïdi[2], Eric Haÿ[2], Johann Photsavang[3], Caroline Marty[2], Juliette Sailland[1], Julie Carnesecchi[1], Violaine Tribollet[1], Bruno Barenton[1], Christelle Forcet[1], Marie-Christine Birling[4], Tania Sorg[4], Olivier Chassande[3], Martine Cohen-Solal[2], Jean-Marc Vanacker[1]*

1 Institut de Génomique Fonctionnelle de Lyon, Université de Lyon, Centre national de la recherche scientifique UMR5242, Ecole Normale Supérieure de Lyon, Lyon, France, **2** Institut National de la Santé et de la Recherche Médicale U606, Hôpital Lariboisière, Paris, France, **3** Institut National de la Santé et de la Recherche Médicale U1026, Bordeaux, France, **4** Institut Clinique de la Souris, Illkirch-Graffenstaden, France

Abstract

ERRα is an orphan member of the nuclear receptor family, the complete inactivation of which confers resistance to bone loss induced by ageing and estrogen withdrawal to female mice in correlation with increased bone formation *in vivo*. Furthermore ERRα negatively regulates the commitment of mesenchymal cells to the osteoblast lineage *ex* vivo as well as later steps of osteoblast maturation. We searched to determine whether the activities of ERRα on osteoblast maturation are responsible for one or both types of *in vivo* induced bone loss. To this end we have generated conditional knock out mice in which the receptor is normally present during early osteoblast differentiation but inactivated upon osteoblast maturation. Bone ageing in these animals was similar to that observed for control animals. In contrast conditional ERRαKO mice were completely resistant to bone loss induced by ovariectomy. We conclude that the late (maturation), but not early (commitment), negative effects of ERRα on the osteoblast lineage contribute to the reduced bone mineral density observed upon estrogen deficiency.

Editor: Franky L. Chan, The Chinese University of Hong Kong, Hong Kong

Funding: This work was supported by Agence Nationale de la Recherche (grant ANR-GENOPAT-012), Ligue contre le Cancer (comité Rhône) and Association pour la Recherche sur le Cancer. The funders had no role in study design, data collection and analysis, decision to publish, or preparation of the manuscript.

* E-mail: jean-marc.vanacker@ens-lyon.fr

Introduction

Bone remodeling is a dynamic process in which resorption exerted by osteoclasts is compensated for by formation exerted by osteoblasts. Although normally tightly regulated, this equilibrium can be disrupted under various circumstances [1,2]. For instance, during ageing mesenchymal cells (MCs, the osteoblast progenitors) become more prone to differentiate into adipocytes than into osteoblast, *in fine* leading to a relative excess osteoclast activity. In contrast estrogen deficiency in post-menopause women results in derepressed osteoclast differentiation and activity that is not compensated for by a similarly increased osteoblast activity. Ageing and menopause thus both lead to increased bone fragility (*i.e.* osteoporosis) and enhanced fracture risk. Given the global ageing of the world population, osteoporosis and its consequences now represent a major public health problem, in particular in females. Treatments against post-menopause osteoporosis have up to now generally aimed at reducing osteoclast activities, in particular via hormone replacement therapies [3–5]. Due to controversial side effects of the latter treatments, the possibility of enhancing osteoblast differentiation and/or activities (bone anabolism) could appear as a promising approach [6,7].

MCs differentiation into osteoblast has increasingly been characterized including at the level of the sequential expression of functional markers. Two transcription factors, Runx2 and Osx, are instrumental in the first steps of this cascade and precede and/or regulate the expression of later markers, which reflect osteoblast maturation. These include collagen 1a (Col1a), alkaline phosphatase (ALP), osteocalcin and osteopontin [8].

ERRα belongs to the nuclear receptor family, the members of which act as transcription factors [9]. Although no natural ligand has been identified to date for ERRα (which is thus referred to as "orphan receptor"), synthetic compounds have been isolated that modulate its activities and/or protein stability [10–13]. High expression of ERRα in various human cancer types is correlated to poor prognosis (reviewed in [14]). Furthermore the receptor has been shown to promote tumorigenicity and angiogenesis in human carcinoma cells xenografted onto Nude mice ([15–17], reviewed in [18]), suggesting that inhibition of ERRα could be beneficial in cancer treatment [19]. Several reports have demonstrated that ERRα is a key positive regulator of various metabolic functions, controlling lipid uptake, fatty acid oxidation, the tricarboxylic acid cycle, oxidative phosphorylation and mitochondrial biogenesis (reviewed in [20,21]). In addition, ERRα impacts on MCs differentiation, promoting commitment towards the adipocyte pathway [22] while inhibiting the osteoblast one [23,24]. Indeed, when set in differentiation *ex vivo*, MCs originating from ERRα knock-out (ERRαKO) mice display a higher and earlier expression of Runx2, Col1a, ALP and osteocalcin, associated with increased mineralization capacities. Mechanistically ERRα has been suggested to modulate Wnt signaling [25] whereas the closely related ERRγ receptor (which also represses osteoblast differentiation) impairs Runx2 transcriptional activities [26]. In addition to these early effects on MCs commitment, ERRα may impact on later steps of osteoblast differentiation. Indeed, the enhanced *ex* vivo differentiation of ERRαKO-originating MCs can be reverted by re-expression of the receptor after the onset of differentiation, suggesting that ERRα-deficient MCs still display a certain level of plasticity [24]. Furthermore, the expression of osteopontin, an inhibitor of mineralization and late marker of osteoblast differentiation, is down regulated in ERRα-deficient osteoblasts, in contrast to other earlier markers. *In vivo* studies have shown that the bone mineral density of female ERRαKO mice is not reduced upon ageing, in contrast to the situation in wild type animals [23,24]. Furthermore, these mice also resist to the bone loss resulting from estrogen withdrawal (obtained by ovariectomy). These phenomena are associated with an increased bone formation rate without any modification in bone resorption, indicating that osteoblasts, not osteoclasts, are the major cellular effectors mediating these resistances. In contrast, male ERRαKO mice were indistinguishable from wild type animals both in terms of bone ageing and sensitivity to androgen deficiency. Inactivating ERRα may thus be beneficial in females to protect bone against the deleterious impacts of ageing and estrogen deficiency by promoting bone anabolism (reviewed in [27]).

It is unknown whether only one or both the early and late (as defined above) effects of ERRα on osteoblast differentiation contribute to which *in vivo* resistance. To investigate this question, we have used the Cre-Lox technology to engineer mice in which ERRα is specifically inactivated during the late phase of osteoblast differentiation. We here report that female conditional ERRαKO mice resist to bone loss induced by ovariectomy but not to the one induced by natural ageing. ERRα thus contributes to estrogen deficiency-induced bone loss through its inhibitory activities on osteoblast maturation. Moreover, our results describe an animal model in which age-related and hormone-deficiency-related bone loss in females can be clearly uncoupled.

Results

To generate a conditional knock-out mouse model for ERRα, we used ERRα$^{fl/fl}$ mice in which ERRα exon 2 was flanked by loxP sites. These animals were crossed with Col1a-Cre mice [28]. The latter animals express the Cre recombinase under the control of a collagen 1a promoter fragment, which is selectively active in early osteoblasts, only after the onset of differentiation. The resulting mice (ERRα$\Delta^{OB}\Delta^{OB}$, Col1a$^{Cre/+}$) are thus predicted to be inactivated for ERRα only in maturing osteoblasts and not in mesenchymal stem cells or early committed osteoblast progenitors (Fig. 1A). Genotyping using specific primer sets detected the floxed allele in all tissues tested, whereas recombination only occurred in bone (long bone and skull) but not in "soft" (*i.e.* bone-free) tissues (Fig. 1B). This recombination appears only partial at the organ level likely due to the unavoidable presence of osteoclasts and non-bone contaminating cells (*e.g.* blood cells) as well as to the heterogeneity in the stages of maturation in which osteoblasts are in bone. ERRα$^{fl/fl}$ and ERRαΔ^{OB}/Δ^{OB},Col1a$^{Cre/+}$ mice are hereafter referred to as control and conditional knock-out (cKO) mice, respectively.

Due to the above-mentioned tissue heterogeneity, a decrease of ERRα expression could not be measured in bone *in vivo*. We thus turned to an *ex vivo* model in which pre-osteoblasts from mice calvaria (cranial vault) were set in culture and allowed to differentiate into osteoblasts. At the beginning of differentiation,

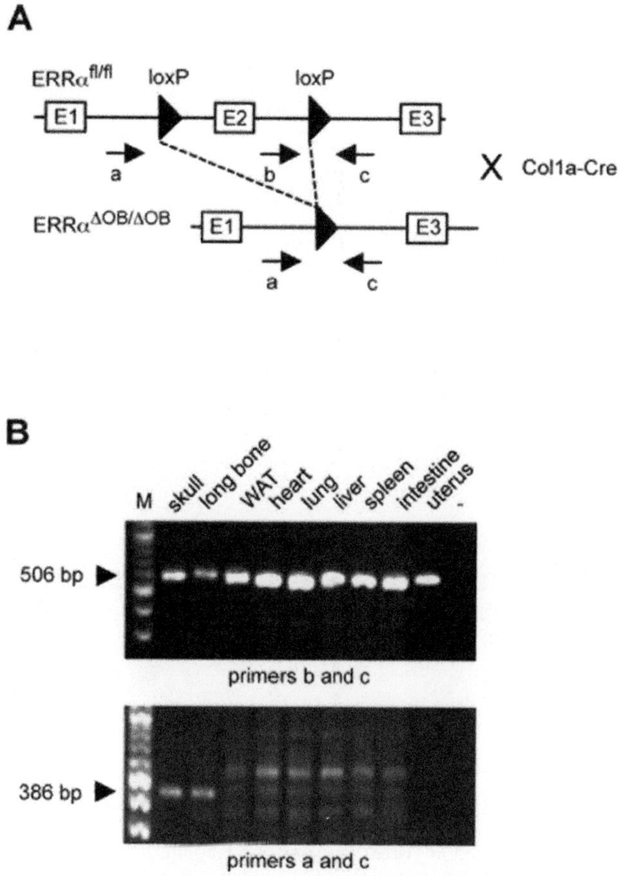

Figure 1. Validation of ERRα conditional knock-out approach. **A.** General strategy used. Exon 2 (E2; encoding the first zinc finger in the DNA binding domain) of the ERRα gene was flanked by loxP sites in ERRα$^{fl/fl}$ mice (here after referred to as control [c] mice). Crossing these mice with Col1a-Cre animals resulted in ERRα$\Delta^{OB}\Delta^{OB}$,Col1a$^{Cre/+}$ mice (hereafter referred to as conditional knock-out [cKO] animals), which display E2 deletion specifically in maturing osteoblasts. Location of PCR primers (see sequences in Material and Methods section) for the detection of the various alleles is depicted. Note that the gene structure is not drawn to scale. **B.** Genotyping of ERRα alleles. PCR using the indicated primers were performed using DNA extracted from the indicated organs. Upper panel, detection of the floxed allele (506 bp) in all organs tested; lower panel, detection of the recombinant allele (386 bp) in skull vault and long bone. M: size marker; −: blank PCR (no DNA).

ERRα protein was equally (albeit weakly) detected in cells from control and cKO mice (Fig. 2A). After five days of differentiation, ERRα expression was enhanced in control cells as expected [29] whereas it was dramatically lower in cKO-originating cells. ERRα loss appeared only partial, which can be due to the heterogeneity of the cell culture that also contains fibroblasts. We thus examined the expression of ERRα by immunofluorescence in cells expressing Col1a (*i.e.* differentiating osteoblasts) (Fig. 2B). In control cultures, ERRα was expressed in the nucleus of these cells, as expected. However, in cKO-originating cells, the receptor was undetectable in Col1a-expressing cells, demonstrating a complete deletion of ERRα in maturing osteoblasts.

We next analyzed the differentiation parameters of these cells. We found that, in the absence of ERRα (cKO-originating cells), alkaline phosphatase (ALP) activity was enhanced as compared to control cells, as evidenced by a greater number of labeled foci and

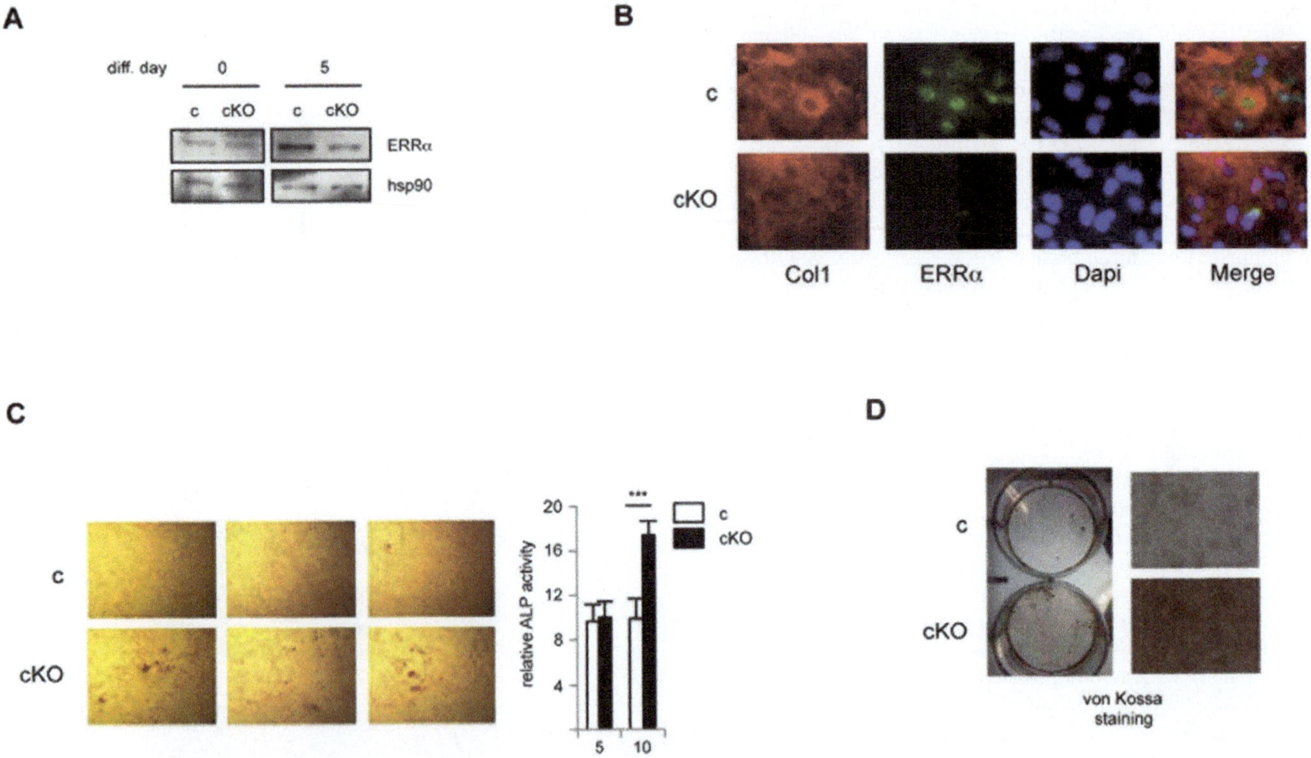

Figure 2. Conditional inactivation of ERRα enhances late osteoblast functions. Pre-osteoblasts from control (c) or conditional knock-out (cKO) mice were isolated from calvaria and allowed to differentiate *ex vivo*. **A.** Expression of ERRα detected in western blot after the indicated differentiation period. Hsp90 was used as a loading control. **B.** Lack of ERRα expression in Col1a-expressing cKO cells. After 6 days of differentiation, cells were fixed and stained with Dapi, anti-Col1a or anti-ERRα antibodies as indicated. **C.** Alkaline phosphatase activity was detected by whole cell cultures staining after 10 days of differentiation (left panel), or by *in vitro* enzymatic assay relative to protein content (right panel) after the indicated days of differentiation. The latter panel depicts a typical experiment (out of three) performed in triplicate. Data are expressed as average with error bars representing S.D. **D.** Mineralization activity was detected by von Kossa staining after 15 days of differentiation. Whole culture wells are presented on the left panels, field enlargements on the right ones.

global enzymatic activity (Fig. 2C). Mineralizing activity was also dramatically enhanced in cKO cultures as compared to control ones (Fig. 2D). In the absence of ERRα, the expression (measured by real time PCR) of middle to late differentiation markers such as Col1a, ALP and osteocalcin (Ocn) was transiently enhanced (after 5 days of differentiation) and thereafter normalized, suggesting a time-dependent effect of the receptor (Fig. 3A). In contrast, expression of osteopontin, an ERRα direct target gene [30], was reduced after 10 days of differentiation. Interestingly these variations of expression are identical to those observed when analyzing cells originating from complete (*i.e.* not conditional) ERRαKO mice [24]. Reintroduction of ERRα by lentiviral infection reversed the expression of the differentiation markers (Fig. 3B). However, the expression of Runx2, an early differentiation inducer (the expression of which precedes that of Col1a; [8]) was not modified in cKO-originating cells as compared to control ones nor upon reintroduction of ERRα. Since Runx2 activates the expression of Col1a, ALP and Ocn [8], this may altogether suggest that ERRα counteracts Runx2 activity. In this hypothesis, ERRα would act similarly to the closely related ERRγ [26]. To investigate this possibility, we performed cotransfection experiments in C3H10T1/2 (mesenchymal) cells (Fig. 3C). Runx2 activated expression driven by its cognate response element (OSE; [31]). However coexpression of ERRα or ERRγ completely blunted this effect. As a control, we verified that both ERRγ and ERRα were capable of activating transcription from their common response element (ERRE), even if ERRα requires the presence of the PGC-1α coactivator in these cells. Noteworthy, Runx2 did not impact on ERR activities under these conditions. Similar results were obtained in C2C12 cells, which are more committed than C3H10T1/2 (data not shown).

Altogether this shows that *i)* ERRα is specifically inactivated in cKO cells only after the onset of osteoblast differentiation *ex vivo*, *ii)* the absence of the receptor under these conditions promotes late osteoblast differentiation without impacting on early commitment and differentiation steps. This validates the present cKO model as a tool to study the *in vivo* effects of ERRα on osteoblast maturation (as opposed to early MSC commitment).

The absence of ERRα in complete KO mice protects female (but not male) animals against age-induced as well as against ovariectomy-induced bone loss [24]. We thus first investigated whether cKO mice were also protected from age-related bone loss. To this end bone structural parameters were determined by X-ray microtomography (microCt) comparing 14 wk and 24 wk old females (Fig. 4). We observed an equal reduction of bone volume (BV/TV, Fig. 4A), bone mineral density (BMD, Fig. 4B) and trabecular number (Tb N, Fig. 4C) in both genotypes upon ageing. Trabecular spacing (Tb Sp, Fig. 4D) was also equally enhanced, reflecting the decreased number of trabeculae, in spite of constant trabecular thickness (Tb Th, Fig. 4E), not expected to decrease upon ageing. Noteworthy all these parameters displayed identical values between control and cKO mice at a given age, indicating

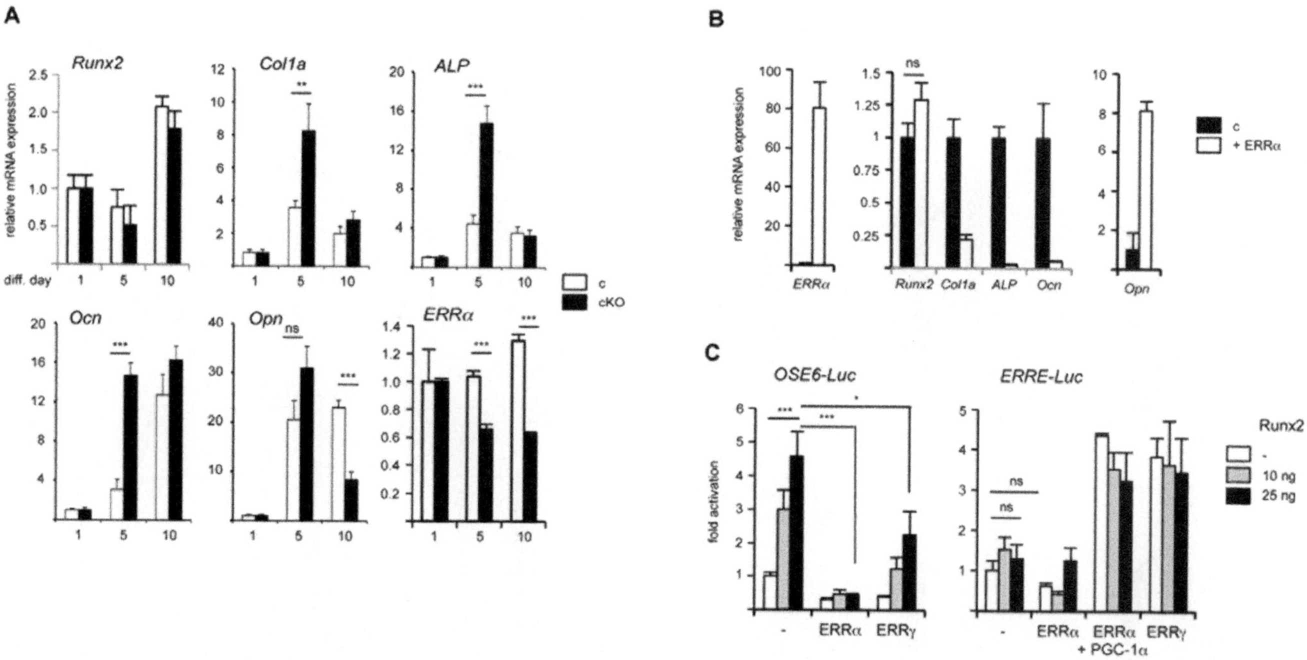

Figure 3. ERRα represses osteoblast differentiation markers. A. Evaluation of the expression of osteoblast differentiation markers by real time PCR at the indicated time after differentiation of mouse calvarial cells. ALP: alkaline phosphatase; Ocn: osteocalcin; Opn: osteopontin. A single representative experiment (out of three, performed in triplicate) is shown. Data are expressed relative to differentiation day 1 with error bars representing S.D. **B.** Reintroduction of ERRα in cKO cells normalizes the expression of differentiation parameters. Lentivirus encoding human ERRα was used to infect mouse calvarial cells induced in osteoblastic differentiation. RNAs were extracted after differentiation day 5. Data are expressed relative to control-infected cells (empty lentivirus: c) as mean +/− s.e.m. Differences for each gene are significant ($p<0.005$) except where indicated. Experiments were performed in triplicate with n = 4. **C.** ERRα represses Runx2 transcriptional activities. C3H10T1/2 cells were transfected with OSE6-Luc (Runx2-responsive) or ERRE-Luc (ERRα-responsive) plasmid together with the indicated amount of Runx2, and fixed amounts of ERRα or ERRγ, as indicated. CMV-renillaLuc was added as a transfection efficiency control and PGC-1α-encoding plasmid was added together with ERR for the right panel as indicated. Results are expressed as fold activation over transfection with activator and expressed as the average of a typical triplicate experiment (out of three) with error bars representing S.D. *: $p<0.05$; **: $p<0.01$; ***: $p<0.005$; ns: non significant.

that ERRα inactivation after the onset of osteoblast differentiation does not protect against age-induced bone loss.

We next studied the bone structural parameters two weeks after gonadectomy on control and cKO animals (Fig. 5). Female mice of both genotype responded identically to ovariectomy (ovx) in terms of reduced uterine thickness (Fig. 5A). In control female mice, we observed the expected decrease in bone volume (Fig. 5B), bone mineral density (Fig. 5C) and trabecular thickness (Fig. 5F) upon ovx. As also expected the number of trabeculae was unchanged (Fig. 5D) and a non-significant trend toward enhanced spacing between trabeculae was observed (Fig. 5E). Strikingly, none of these parameters were modified in ovariectomized cKO mice as compared to sham-operated animals. The divergent response to ovx of control and cKO mice can also be viewed on the reconstructed 3D structures of trabecular bones (see Movies S1, S2, S3, and S4). This situation is in full contrast with the one prevailing in male mice in which orchidectomy (orx) led to dramatically reduced bone volume (Fig. 5G) and mineral density (Fig. 5H) both in control and cKO mice. We concluded that inactivating ERRα during osteoblast maturation completely protects against bone loss induced by hormonal deficiency, selectively in females.

Discussion

Amongst other, ageing is associated with bone loss, leading to osteoporosis (understood as bone fragility syndrome) and increased fracture risk. Due to the global ageing of the human population worldwide, osteoporosis is now a major health problem, being the most common metabolic disorder of old age in humans [1,2]. During ageing bone formation by osteoblasts is impaired due a decreased number and activity of osteoblasts, and concomitantly bone resorption by osteoclasts is increased. Whereas both males and females are subjected to age-associated osteoporosis, the situation is further aggravated in females after menopause. The cessation of ovarian function, resulting in highly decreased circulating levels of estrogens, indeed leads to unimpaired osteoclast differentiation and activity which is not compensated for by an equivalent rise in osteoblast activity [32]. Although age-related- and estrogen-deficiency-related bone loss essentially originates in different cell compartments, it is expected that enhancing bone anabolism (*i.e.* promoting bone formation by osteoblasts) could be an efficient mean to counteract osteoporosis in general [6,7].

In this line, we and others have shown that genetic inactivation of the orphan nuclear receptor ERRα in mice leads to resistance to bone loss induced by ovariectomy (used as a model for estrogen-deficiency, thus mimicking menopause) or ageing [23,24]. Interestingly these phenotypes were not associated with a decrease in osteoclast activity suggesting that ERRα does not modulate bone resorption *in vivo* at least under the above-mentioned challenging conditions. In contrast, ERRαKO animals displayed a higher bone formation rate as compared to wild type ones, altogether strongly suggesting that ERRα contributes to bone loss exclusively through the effects it exerts in osteoblasts. It should however be mentioned that ERRα has been shown to be required for

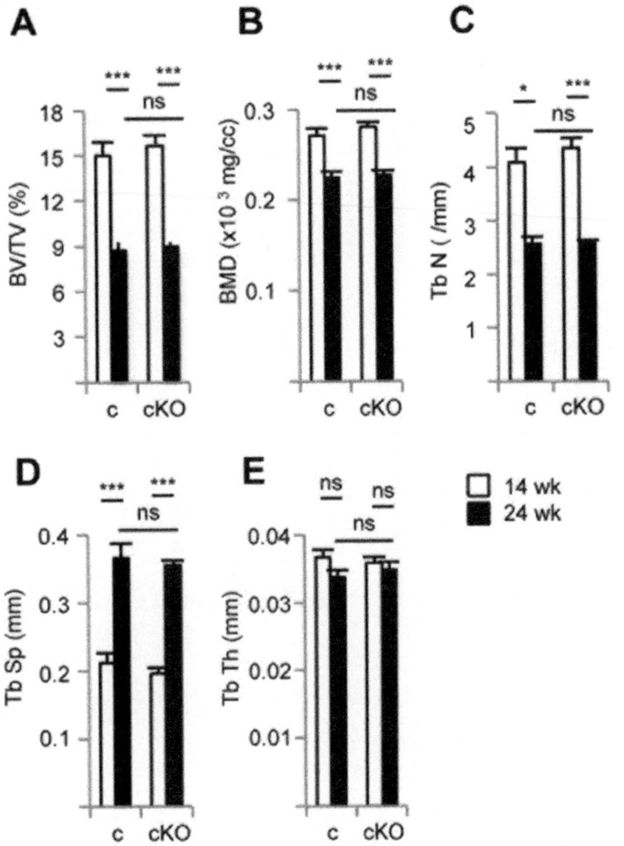

Figure 4. Conditional inactivation of ERRα *in vivo* does not impact bone ageing. Bone volume fraction (BV/TV; **A**), bone mineral density (BMD; **B**), trabecular number (Tb N; **C**), trabecular spacing (Tb Sp; **D**) and trabecular thickness (Tb Th; **E**) were determined by microCT-scan at 14 (white bars) and 24 wk (black bars) in the femur of female control (c) and conditional ERRα knock-out (cKO) mice (n = 6 to 11 per group). Error bars represent s.e.m. *: $p<0.05$; ***: $p<0.005$; ns: non significant.

osteoclast differentiation and/or activities in response to bone loss induced by rosiglitazone, a thiazolidinedione prescribed for the treatment of insulin resistance and diabetes [33].

The actual role of ERRα in osteoblast differentiation *in vitro* (inducer or inhibitor of differentiation?) is controversial and has been thoroughly discussed in our recently published review [27]. However, the absence of ERRα has been associated to an increased capacity of mesenchymal cells (MCs) to differentiate in osteoblasts *ex vivo* [23,24]. Conversely MCs were less prone to differentiate into adipocytes in the absence of the receptor [22] leading to reduced fat marrow in ERRαKO animals [23] suggesting that ERRα is an early switch factor influencing MCs differentiation towards the adipocyte pathway at the expense of the osteoblastic one. ERRα has been suspected of additional effects in later steps of osteoblast maturation which may be mediated by osteopontin (opn), a downstream positive target of the receptor [30]. Indeed opn has been shown to reduce bone mineralization and its absence in KO mice confers resistance to ovx-induced bone loss [34], as does inactivation of ERRα.

The conditional KO approach described in the present report allows us to discriminate between the early (MCs commitment) and late (osteoblast maturation) effects of ERRα. To inactivate a floxed ERRα allele, we indeed expressed the Cre recombinase

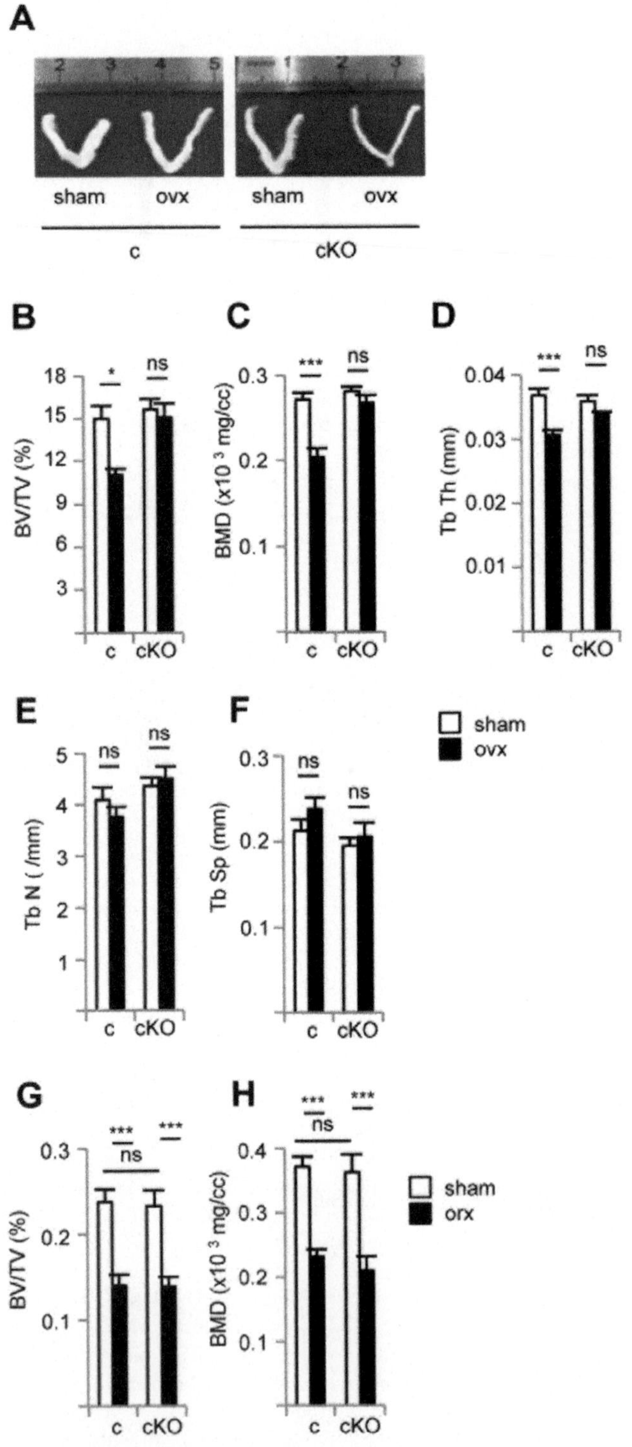

Figure 5. Conditional inactivation of ERRα *in vivo* protects against ovariectomy-induced bone loss. A. Photograph of uteri in sham-operated or ovariectomized (ovx) control (c) or cKO mice. **B–F.** Same parameters as in Fig. 3 were determined in females either sham-operated (white bars) or two weeks after ovariectomy (ovx; black bars). BV/TV (**G**) and BMD (**H**) were determined in male mice either sham-operated (white bars) or four weeks after orchidectomy (orx; black bars). All mice (n = 6 to 10 per group) were 14 wk old at the end of the experiment. Error bars represent s.e.m. *: $p<0.05$; ***: $p<0.005$; ns: non significant.

under the control of a Col1a promoter fragment, driving expression during mid stages of osteoblast differentiation, *i.e.* well after MCs commitment to the osteoblastic lineage [28]. As a consequence we observed a decrease in ERRα expression only during mid to late stages of osteoblast maturation *ex vivo*, whereas the receptor is normally present in pre-osteoblasts. Consistently the expression of Runx2, an early differentiation marker and inducer [8], was normally regulated during cKO pre-osteoblast differentiation in contrast to what observed in complete ERRαKO mice, where a marked increase of Runx2 expression had been observed [23,24]. However, the expression of mid- to late markers of osteoblast differentiation was deregulated in cKO-originating cells, in a manner similar to that observed in complete ERRαKO animals. In this respect our data suggest that ERRα may reduce osteoblast differentiation by antagonizing Runx2 transactivation capacities, in a manner similar to that demonstrated for the closely related ERRγ receptor [26].

Age-induced bone loss in cKO mice was similar to the one measured in control animals. This excludes that the activities of ERRα during osteoblast maturation may mediate age-dependent bone loss. It is tempting to rather speculate that the activities of ERRα as a repressor of MCs commitment to the osteoblastic lineage are involved in this phenomenon. However, we cannot formally exclude the impact of a yet uncharacterized primary activity of ERRα outside the bone compartment that would result in age-related bone loss. Investigating the bone response of ERRα cKO animals to gonadectomy revealed that males were normally sensitive whereas females were completely protected from bone loss. This situation is actually identical to the one observed in complete ERRαKO mice and confirms a gender-dependent effect of the receptor in bone. More importantly our results demonstrate that ERRα contributes to ovariectomy-induced bone loss via its activities on osteoblast maturation, and not through the regulation of MCs commitment. These results are summarized on Figure 6.

Together with data published by other laboratories, our results suggest that ERRα could be a promising target for the design of innovative therapies against bone loss, specifically in females. In this respect, we previously demonstrated that expression of the receptor in bone is not modified according to the estrogen status in mice [35]. Although ERRα is an orphan receptor, several synthetic compounds have been identified that modulate its activities and impact on its stability [10–14]. A pharmacological approach could thus be considered to specifically impact on the receptor. However complete inhibition of the receptor can be expected to lead to various undesired side effects on metabolism. For instance, given the role of ERRα as a switch factor in MCs commitment, its inhibition, while promoting osteoblast differentiation, would likely affect adipogenesis and thereby lipid storage and consumption. A more reliable approach would consist in impacting only the late osteoblast activities of the receptor, although this would solely be efficient against estrogen deficiency-induced bone loss. Such a compound, modulating a specific subset of the receptor's activities, is still to be identified.

Materials and Methods

Animals

Col1a-Cre mice have been described elsewhere [28]. $ERR\alpha^{fl/fl}$ (Esrra<tm1ICS> mouse line) animals have been generated in the Institut Clinique de la Souris (Illkirch-Graffenstaden). For genotyping, DNA extracted from organs using conventional methods was PCR amplified using Eurobio kit. PCR cycle used: 94°C, 30 sec; 62°C, 30 sec; 72°C, 1 min. PCR products were analysed on 1.2% agarose gels.

Primers Used for Genotyping

a: 5′-GCCCCCCTTGGCCCCCCTTAGCCCCCTCCC-3′

b: 5′-CCCTGCTTCTGTGCCCTTTGC-3′

c: 5′-CCACCACTGCCCAGCTTCAC-3′

For surgery, animals were anesthetized with sodium pentobarbital. Testes were ligatured and cut through an incision in the scrotum. Ovaries were removed through an incision in the flanks. Animals were sacrificed 2 wk after operation.

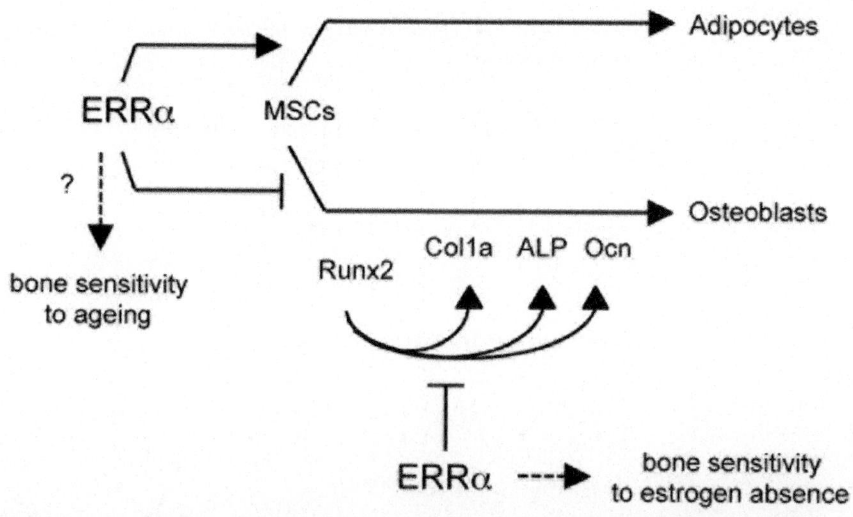

Figure 6. *In vivo* and *ex vivo* effects of ERRα on bone. ERRα impairs the later steps of osteoblastic differentiation. The results presented here show that these activities are involved in bone loss induced by estrogen deficiency and may involve the repression of Runx2- driven transcriptional activities. In contrast, these activities are not involved in bone sensitivity to ageing. Data published by other show that ERRα also promotes the early commitment of mesenchymal stem cells (MSCs) toward the adipocytic pathway while restricting the osteoblastic one. We hypothesize that these early activities are responsible, at least in part, for bone loss induced by ageing. See text for details and references.

All animal experiments were performed in the Plateau de Biologie Expérimentale de la Souris (PBES; ENS Lyon) under animal care procedures, conducted in accordance with the guidelines set by the European Community Council Directives (86/609/EEC) and approved by the ENS Lyon ethical committee. Animals were in C57black6 background and had access to food and water *ad libitum*. Mice were sacrificed by cervical dislocation at 10 a.m.

X-ray Microcomputed Tomography Analysis

3D microarchitecture of the femur was evaluated using a high-resolution (8 μm) microtomographic imaging system (eXplore Locus, GE, USA). A 3D region within the secondary spongiosa in the proximal metaphysis of the femur was reconstructed, beginning 500 μm proximal to the growth plate and extending to 1.5 mm. Cortical bone was reconstructed from a 1 mm thick region of interest centered on the diaphysis, 5 mm distal from the proximal growth plate. Morphometric parameters were computed using the Advanced Bone Analysis Microview Software (GE).

Calvarial Cell Cultures

Calvariae were isolated from 1–5 day old mice and digested for 1 hr in collagenase (Sigma). After centrifugation, cell pellet was set in culture in six-well plates in αMEM supplemented with 10% fetal calf serum (FCS), 1% penicillin/streptomycin. Cells were induced to differentiate into osteoblasts with 50 μg/ml L-ascorbic acid and 10 mM β-glycerophosphate. Culture medium was replaced every 2 to 3 days. For immunofluorescence, cells were fixed in 4% paraformaldehyde for 10 min, then permeabilized with 0.5% Triton, 0.3% BSA in PBS for 5 min. Saturation was performed in 0.3% BSA in PBS for 30 min. Primary antibodies (anti-ERRα from Santa Cruz diluted 1/50; anti-collagen1 from Novotech diluted 1/200) were added or 3 hrs at RT. Secondary antibodies from Jackson (anti-mouse-Alexa488 diluted 1/1000) or Interchim (anti-rabbit-Alexa647 diluted 1/1000) were incubated for 1 hr at RT. Hoescht staining was diluted 1/20,000 and incubated for 10 min. For ALP staining, cells were rinsed with PBS, then fixed with 4% (v/v) formaldehyde for 5 min. After 3 washes with H2O, cells were stained using the alkaline phosphatase fast red violet kit (Sigma) following the indications provided by the manufacturer. Detection of mineralization activity was performed 15 days after the onset of differentiation. To this end cells were washed with PBS, then stained with 5% silver nitrate under UV irradiation for 10 min, then washed and dried.

For lentivirus construction, flagged human-ERRα fragment was inserted into the blunted BamHI site of the pRRL.PPT.SF.i2GFPp plasmid. This plasmid was provided by the Lentivus Production platform (ENS Lyon), which produced the recombinant lentivirus. Virus titers were determined upon infection of 293T cells. Calvarial cells were infected (MOI 5 in PBS) one day after induction of differentiation. Empty virus was used as a control.

Expression Analysis

RNAs were purified using Guanidinium thiocyanate/phenol/chloroforme extraction. Total RNAs were reverse transcribed using iScript retrotranscription kit (Biorad). Quantitative PCR were performed using the iQ SYBR-Green kit (Biorad) in duplicate on a Biorad Cfx1000 apparatus using standard procedures. Results were analysed using the ΔΔCt method normalized to the expression of the 36b4 housekeeping gene.

Sequence of the Primers Used for Real time PCR

36b4:5′-ACCTCCTTCTTCCAGGCTTT-3′ and 5′-CCCACCTTGTCTCCAGTCTTT-3′; ALP: 5′-GCCCTCCA-GATCCTGACCAA-3′ and 5′- GCA-GAGCCTGCTGGTCCTTA-3′;

Col1a: 5′-CTGACGCATGGCCAAGAAGA-3′ and 5′-GCA-TACCTCGGGTTTCCACG-3′; ERRα: 5′-CAAACGCCTCTGCCTGGTCT-3′ and 5′-ACTC-GATGCTCCCCTGGATG-3′; Ocn: 5′-ACCTCACAGATGC-CAAGCCC-3′ and 5′-AGCGCCGGAGTCTGTTCACT-3′; Opn: 5′-TCTCCTTGCGCCACAGAATG-3′ and 5′-TCGTCCATGTGGTCATGGCT-3′; Runx-2:5′-GACGTGCCCAGGCGTATTTC-3′ and 5′-GGAACTGCCTGGGGTCTGAA-3′.

For Western blot analysis, cells were lysed in RIPA buffer. 30 μg proteins were resolved on a 10% SDS-PAGE, blotted onto nitrocellulose membrane (GE-Healthcare) and probed with antibodies (ERRα from Genetex, hsp90 from Santa Cruz) after saturation.

Analysis of Transcriptional Activities

C3H10T1/2 cells were cultured in MEM supplemented with 10% FCS. For transient transfection, 15.10^3 cells were seeded in 96-well plates and transfection using 0.75 ml of ExGen500 (Euromedex), 12.5 ng firefly luciferase reporter plasmid (ERRE-Luc or OSE6-Luc) and the indicated amount of activator-encoding plasmids. 12.5 ng CMV-renilla Luciferase were added to normalize transfection efficiency and pSG5 plasmid was added as a carrier up to 125 ng. Cells were lyzed 48 h after transfection and reporter activities were determined using standard methods. All transfections were performed in triplicate. pSG-ERRα, pSG-ERRγ and ERRE-luc have been described in [36], CMV-Runx2 and 6OSE-Luc (generous gifts of Patricia Ducy) in [31].

Statistical Analysis

Statistical significance was analyzed using one-way ANOVA.

Supporting Information

Movie S1 3D reconstitution of trabecular bone originating from control sham female mice.

Movie S2 3D reconstitution of trabecular bone using control ovx mice.

Movie S3 3D reconstitution of trabecular bone using cKO sham mice.

Movie S4 3D reconstitution of trabecular bone using cKO ovx mice.

Acknowledgments

We acknowledge the contribution of the SFR Biosciences Gerland-Lyon Sud (UMS344/US8) platforms PBES (in particular Nadine Aguilera, for helping in performing animal experimentations) and lentivirus production unit (in particular Els Verhoeven). We thank Irma Machuca-Gayet for critical reading of the manuscript.

Author Contributions

Conceived and designed the experiments: OC MCS JMV. Performed the experiments: MG SS EH JP CM JS JC VT BB CF. Analyzed the data: OC MCS JMV. Contributed reagents/materials/analysis tools: MCB TS. Wrote the paper: OC MCS JMV.

References

1. Manolagas SC, Parfitt AM (2010) What old means to bone. Trends Endocrinol Metab 21: 369–74.
2. Manolagas SC (2010) From estrogen-centric to ageing and oxidative stress: a revised perspective of the pathogenesis of osteoporosis. Endocrine Rev 31: 266–300.
3. Li CI, Malone KE, Porter PL, Weiss NS, Tang MT, et al. (2003) Relationship between long durations and different regimens of hormone therapy and risk of breast cancer. JAMA. 289: 3254–63.
4. Collins JA, Blake JM, Crosignani PG (2005) Breast cancer risk with postmenopausal hormonal treatment. 2005 Hum Reprod Update. 11: 545–60.
5. Horwitz KB (2008) The Year in Basic Science: update of estrogen plus progestin therapy for menopausal hormone replacement implicating stem cells in the increased breast cancer risk. Mol Endocrinol. 22: 2743–50.
6. Marie PJ, Kassem M (2011) Ostoblasts in osteoporosis: past, emerging, and future anabolic targets. Eur J Endrocinol 165: 1–10.
7. Khosla S, Westendorf JJ, Oursler MJ (2008) Building bone to reverse osteoporosis and repair fractures. J Clin Invest 118: 421–8.
8. Komori T (2010) Regulation of bone development and extracellular matrix protein genes by RUNX2 Cell Tissue Res 339: 189–195.
9. Tremblay AM, Giguère V (2007) The NR3B subgroup: an ovERRview. Nucl Recept Signal 5: e009.
10. Willy PJ, Murray IR, Qian J, Busch BB, Stevens WC Jr, et al. (2004) Regulation of PPARgamma coactivator 1alpha (PGC-1alpha) signaling by an estrogen-related receptor alpha (ERRalpha) ligand. Proc Natl Acad Sci U S A. 101: 8912–7.
11. Lanvin O, Bianco S, Kersual N, Chalbos D, Vanacker JM (2007) Potentiation of ICI182,780 (Fulvestrant)-induced estrogen receptor-alpha degradation by the estrogen receptor-related receptor-alpha inverse agonist XCT790. J Biol Chem. 282: 28328–34.
12. Chisamore MJ, Cunningham ME, Flores O, Wilkinson HA, Chen JD (2009) Characterization of a novel small molecule subtype specific estrogen-related receptor alpha antagonist in MCF-7 breast cancer cells. PLoS One. 4: e5624.
13. Duellman SJ, Calaoagan JM, Sato BG, Fine R, Klebansky B, et al. (2010) A novel steroidal inhibitor of estrogen-related receptor alpha (ERR alpha) Biochem Pharmacol 80: 819–26.
14. Ariazi EA, Jordan VC (2006) Estrogen-related receptors as emerging targets in cancer and metabolic disorders. Curr Top Med Chem. 6: 203–15.
15. Stein RA, Gaillard S, McDonnell DP (2009) Estrogen-related receptor alpha induces the expression of vascular endothelial growth factor in breast cancer cells. J Steroid Biochem Mol Biol. 114: 106–12.
16. Bianco S, Lanvin O, Tribollet V, Macari C, North S, et al. (2009) Modulating estrogen receptor-related receptor-alpha activity inhibits cell proliferation. J Biol Chem. 284: 23286–92.
17. Fradet A, Sorel H, Bouazza L, Goehrig D, Dépalle B, et al. (2011) Dual function of ERRα in breast cancer and bone metastasis formation: implication of VEGF and osteoprotegerin. Cancer Res. 71: 5728–38.
18. Bianco S, Sailland J, Vanacker JM (2012) ERRs and cancers: Effects on metabolism and on proliferation and migration capacities J Steroid Biochem Mol Biol. 130: 180–5.
19. Chang CY, Kazmin D, Jasper JS, Kunder R, Zuercher WJ, et al. (2011) The metabolic regulator ERRα, a downstream target of HER2/IGF-1R, as a therapeutic target in breast cancer. Cancer Cell. 20: 500–10.
20. Giguère V (2008) Transcriptional control of energy homeostasis by the estrogen-related receptors. Endocr Rev 29: 677–96.
21. Villena JA, Kralli A (2008) ERRalpha: a metabolic function for the oldest orphan Trends Endocrinol Metab 19: 269–76.
22. Ijichi N, Ikeda K, Horie-Inoue K, Yagi K, Okazaki Y, et al. (2007) Estrogen-related receptor alpha modulates the expression of adipogenesis-related genes during adipocyte differentiation Biochem Biophys Res Commun 358: 813–8.
23. Delhon I, Gutzwiller S, Morvan F, Rangwala S, Wyder L, et al. (2009) Absence of estrogen receptor-related-alpha increases osteoblastic differentiation and cancellous bone mineral density. Endocrinology 150: 4463–72.
24. Teyssier C, Gallet M, Rabier B, Monfoulet L, Dine J, et al. (2009) Absence of ERRalpha in female mice confers resistance to bone loss induced by age or estrogen-deficiency. PLoS One 4: e7942.
25. Auld KL, Berasi SP, Liu Y, Cain M, Zhang Y, et al. (2012) Estrogen-related receptor α regulates osteoblast differentiation via Wnt/β-catenin signaling. J Mol Endocrinol 48: 177–191.
26. Jeong BC, Lee YS, Park YY, Bae IH, Kim DK, et al. (2009) The orphan nuclear receptor estrogen receptor-related receptor gamma negatively regulates BMP2-induced osteoblast differentiation and bone formation. J Biol Chem. 284: 14211–8.
27. Gallet M, Vanacker JM (2010) ERR receptors as potential targets in osteoporosis. Trends Endocrinol Metab 21: 637–41.
28. Dacquin R, Starbuck M, Schinke T, Karsenty G (2002) Mouse alpha1(I)-collagen promoter is the best known promoter to drive efficient Cre recombinase expression in osteoblast. Dev Dyn 224: 245–51.
29. Bonnelye E, Merdad L, Kung V, Aubin JE (2001) The orphan nuclear estrogen receptor-related receptor alpha (ERRalpha) is expressed throughout osteoblast differentiation and regulates bone formation in vitro. J Cell Biol. 153: 971–84.
30. Vanacker JM, Delmarre C, Guo X, Laudet V (1998) Activation of the osteopontin promoter by the orphan nuclear receptor estrogen receptor related alpha. Cell Growth Differ 9: 1007–14.
31. Ducy P, Zhang R, Geoffroy V, Rydall AL, Karsenty G (1997) Osf2/Cbfa1, a transcriptional regulator of osteoblast differentiation. Cell 8: 747–754.
32. Vico L, Vanacker JM (2010) Sex hormones and their receptors in bone homeostasis: insights from genetically modified mouse models. Osteopos Int 21: 365–72.
33. Wei W, Wang X, Yang M, Smith LC, Dechow PC, et al. (2010) PGC1β mediates PPARγ activation of osteoclastogenesis and rosiglitazone-induced bone loss. Cell Metab 11: 503–16.
34. Yoshitake H, Rittling SR, Denhardt DT, Noda M (1999) Osteopontin-deficient mice are resistant to ovariectomy-induced bone resorption. Proc Natl Acad Sci U S A. 96: 8156–60.
35. Macari C, Teyssier C, Tribollet V, Mouzat K, Forcet C, et al. (2010) Estrogens repress PGC1-α expression in the uterus. Mol Cell Endocrinol. 330: 33–40.
36. Vanacker JM, Bonnelye E, Chopin-Delannoy S, Delmarre C, Cavaillès V, et al. (1999) Transcriptional activities of the orphan nuclear receptor ERRα. Mol Endocrinol, 13: 764–773.

14

ERK1 Regulates the Hematopoietic Stem Cell Niches

Nathalie Saulnier[1,2], Soizic Guihard[1,2], Xavier Holy[3], Elodie Decembre[4], Pierre Jurdic[4], Denis Clay[5], Vincent Feuillet[1,2], Gilles Pagès[6], Jacques Pouysségur[6], Françoise Porteu[1,2], Murielle Gaudry[1,2]*

1 Institut Cochin, Université Paris Descartes, Sorbonne Paris Descartes, CNRS (UMR 8104), Paris, France, **2** Inserm U1016, Paris, France, **3** Service histologie et réparation tissulaire, IRBA/IMASSA, Brétigny-sur-Orge, France, **4** Institut de Génomique Fonctionnelle de Lyon, Université de Lyon, Université Lyon 1, CNRS, INRA, Ecole Normale Supérieure de Lyon, Lyon, France, **5** Inserm U972, Institut André Lwoff, Hôpital Paul Brousse, Villejuif, France, **6** Institut de recherche Signalisation, Biologie du Développement et Cancer, Université de Nice, France

Abstract

The mitogen-activated protein kinases (MAPK) ERK1 and ERK2 are among the major signal transduction molecules but little is known about their specific functions *in vivo*. ERK activity is provided by two isoforms, ERK1 and ERK2, which are ubiquitously expressed and share activators and substrates. However, there are not *in vivo* studies which have reported a role for ERK1 or ERK2 in HSCs and the bone marrow microenvironment. The present study shows that the ERK1-deficient mice present a mild osteopetrosis phenotype. The lodging and the homing abilities of the ERK1$^{-/-}$ HSC are impaired, suggesting that the ERK1$^{-/-}$-defective environment may affect the engrafment of HSCs. Serial transplantations demonstrate that ERK1 is involved in the maintenance of an appropriate medullar microenvironment, but that the intrinsic properties of HSCs are not altered by the ERK1$^{-/-}$ defective microenvironment. Deletion of ERK1 impaired *in vitro* and *in vivo* osteoclastogenesis while osteoblasts were unaffected. As osteoclasts derive from precursors of the monocyte/macrophage lineage, investigation of the monocytic compartment was performed. *In vivo* analysis of the myeloid lineage progenitors revealed that the frequency of CMPs increased by approximately 1.3-fold, while the frequency of GMPs significantly decreased by almost 2-fold, compared with the respective WT compartments. The overall mononuclear-phagocyte lineage development was compromised in these mice due to a reduced expression of the M-CSF receptor on myeloid progenitors. These results show that the cellular targets of ERK1 are M-CSFR-responsive cells, upstream to osteoclasts. While ERK1 is well known to be activated by M-CSF, the present results are the first to point out an ERK1-dependent M-CSFR regulation on hematopoietic progenitors. This study reinforces the hypothesis of an active cross-talk between HSCs, their progeny and bone cells in the maintenance of the homeostasis of these compartments.

Editor: Eliana Saul Furquim Werneck Abdelhay, Instituto Nacional de Câncer, Brazil

Funding: NS is a recipient of a fellowship from the Agence Nationale pour la Recherche (ANR-08-BLAN-0332). SG is a recipient of a fellowship from the Ministère de l'Enseignement Supérieur et de la Recherche. This work was supported by Institut National de la sante et de la recherche medicale (INSERM) and grants from the Agence Nationale pour la Recherche (ANR-08-BLAN-0332), the Association pour la Recherche contre le Cancer (SFI20101201698), the Ligue Contre le Cancer, comite d'Ile de France (RS11/75-24) and the Institut National du Cancer (CSHLE 2008 INCa). The funders had no role in study design, data collection and analysis, decision to publish, or preparation of the manuscript.

Competing Interests: The authors have declared that no competing interests exist.

* E-mail: murielle.gaudry@inserm.fr

Introduction

Adult hematopoietic stem cells (HSCs) exist in a relatively quiescent state in the bone marrow (BM) microenvironment to execute long-term self renewal and multilineage differentiation functions [1,2]. The maintenance of HSC quiescence involves both intrinsic and extrinsic mechanisms. HSCs interact with the BM microenvironment in specific anatomical and functional areas, referred as niches, a microenvironment of different cell types and extracellular matrix molecules that dictate stem cell self-renewal and progeny production *in vivo* [3]. Many studies have begun to define the medullar niche but few data are available concerning the cells and factors supporting HSCs in those niches. Likewise, the signaling pathways governing activation of various stromal cells and the specific relationship between this activation state and expansion/maintenance of HSCs are largely unexplored. HSCs reside in medullar niches, mainly localized in the endosteum. The so-called endosteal stem cell niche is a dynamically remodeled tissue that allows interactions between stem cells and their partners, including osteoblasts and stromal cells, which provide HSCs with signals for their homeostatic quiescent state [4,5,6,7]. The architecture of the HSC niche is tightly controlled by a balance between the bone-forming cells (osteoblasts), and the bone-resorbing cells (osteoclasts) [8].

While osteoblasts derive from mesenchymal cells, osteoclasts derive from mononuclear precursors of the monocytic/macrophage lineage [9]. Monocytes develop from hematopoietic stem cells in the bone marrow through several intermediate progenitors that restrict progressively their differentiation potential [10]. The prevalent model for myeloid commitment implicates that progenitors pass through the common myeloid progenitor (CMP), the granulocyte/macrophage progenitor (GMP), and the macrophage/dendritic cell progenitors (MDP) stages [11]. Each of these steps is tightly regulated by the interplay between cytokine-induced signaling pathway and transcription factor activity. Monocyte-colony stimulating factor (M-CSF), through its binding to M-CSFR (CD115, Csf1-R) [12] plays an essential role in both proliferation and differentiation of the myeloid progenitors. M-CSF, and receptor activator of nuclear factor kappa B ligand (RANKL), are essential for osteoclastogenesis [9,13,14,15,16].

Mutational inactivation or genetic ablation of these molecules results in a lack of osteoclast differentiation and consequent defects in BM cavity formation, a condition termed osteopetrosis in which BM cavities are filled with bone [17,18,19]. Accumulating evidence suggests that osteoclasts induce hematopoietic activity by secreting bone-resorbing enzymes which promote the mobilization of HSCs from their quiescent state [7]. However, the influence of HSCs on their microenvironment is not well understood. A recent report demonstrated a cross-talk between HSCs and bone cells in the maintenance of both hematopoietic and bone homeostasis [20].

The ERK MAPK kinases are major signaling actors relaying signals elicited by cytokines, morphogens or integrins. The MAPK pathway exerts pleiotropic effects on cell cycle, apoptosis and differentiation, and has been implicated in the control of many cellular responses. ERK activity is provided by two isoforms, named ERK1 and ERK2, that are highly similar, ubiquitously expressed and that share activators and substrates. We and others have found that the ERK pathway is specifically required for the differentiation of various hematopoietic lineages [21,22,23,24]. However, no studies have reported the role of ERK1 or ERK2 in HSCs *in vivo*. Gene disruption has suggested specific functions for each isoform. Ablation of ERK2 induces embryonic lethality with death of the animals *in utero* at day 7.5, due to defects in the mesoderm and placental development [25]. Conversely, ERK1$^{-/-}$ mice are viable, fertile and present minor defects, showing that ERK1 is dispensable for mouse development and could be compensated by ERK2. So far, ERK1 has been shown to be specifically required for *in vitro* and *in vivo* adipogenesis, terminal differentiation of T lymphocytes, long-term memory and erythropoiesis [26,27,28,29].

The involvement of the MAPK pathway in myeloid maturation has been implicated in several myeloid cell lines [30]. Using ERK chemical inhibitors, Hsu et al. have shown that ERK signaling is involved in the early myeloid commitment of HSCs [31]. On the other hand, ERK inhibitors have been reported to alter osteoclast differentiation and function [32]. Very recently, He Y et al. reported the preponderant role of ERK1 over ERK2 isoform in controlling osteoclast differentiation and bone resorption activity [33]. This suggests that ERKs might have a role in stem cell niche regulation. However, this possibility together with the precise role of the ERK pathway in the regulation of myelopoieseis *in vivo*, to our knowledge, has not been reported.

We show here that ERK1-deficient mice present an alteration of bone density due to impaired osteoclastogenesis. In addition to osteoclasts, the overall mononuclear-phagocyte lineage development was compromised in these mice due to a reduced expression of the M-CSF receptor on myeloid progenitors. Although resting medullar hematopoiesis is normal in the absence of ERK1 [29], serial transplantation experiments revealed that ERK1 deficiency in the microenvironment alters the lodging and the functional activity of normal HSCs. Thus, our findings extend the role of ERK1 *in vivo*, through regulation of M-CSFR, as a key participant in the regulation of the niche size.

Methods

Mice

ERK1$^{-/-}$ mice, backcrossed on C57BL/6 (CD45.2) background, and WT C57BL/6J (CD45.2 and CD45.1) mice (Charles River Laboratories,L'arbresle, France) were housed in a specific pathogen-free environment. All procedures were approved by the Animal Care Committee (registred no. P2.MG.137.10, 2010). Animal studies described herein were reviewed and approved (agreement no. 75-1064) by the Departmental director of veterinary services of Paris, France.

Flow cytometry

For analysis of HSCs, BM cells were first stained with biotinylated-lineage cocktail antibodies (BD Biosciences) with additional biotinylated antibody specific for CD4, CD8, CD19 and NK1.1 (BioLegend), followed by streptavidin-PerCP secondary antibody (BioLegend) and PE-Cy7-conjugated anti-Sca1 (BioLegend), APC-eFluor780-conjugated anti-c-Kit (eBioscience), PE-conjugated anti-CD150 (BioLegend), Pacific Blue-conjugate anti-CD48 (BioLegend), APC-conjugated anti-CD135 (BD Pharmingen) and FITC-conjugated anti-CD34 (eBioscience). To analyze mature lineage cells, freshly isolated BM were immunostained with antibodies for myeloid cells (PE-conjugated anti-CD11b, FITC-conjugated anti-Gr1), B-cells (PE-conjugated anti-B220), T-cells (PE-conjugated anti-CD4, FITC-conjugated anti-CD8) (Biolegend). For analysis of BM monocytes and macrophages (MΦ), cells were preincubated with Fc blocking treatment, and subsequently stained with PE-conjugated anti-Gr1, APC-conjugated anti-CD115, and pacific blue-conjugated anti-F4/80 (MΦ). For phenotypic analysis of myeloid progenitors (CMP, GMP, MEP), cells were stained with the following biotinylated-lineage antibodies B220, CD11b, Gr1, Ter119, CD3ε and Il-7Rα (eBioscience, San Diego, CA). Lineage-positive cells were removed with BD IMag streptavidin particles (BD) and the remaining cells were stained with streptavidin-APC. Cells were incubated with PE/CY7-conjugated anti-Sca-1, PE-conjugated anti-c-Kit, APC-CY7-conjugated anti-FcγRII/III, and FITC-conjugated anti-CD34. The common myeloid progenitors (CMPs) were defined as Lin$^-$Sca-1$^-$IL7R$^-$c-Kit$^+$CD34$^+$FcγRII/III^{lo}, the granulo-macrophage progenitors (GMPs) cells as Lin$^-$Sca-1$^-$IL-7R$^-$c-Kit$^+$CD34$^+$FcγRII/III^{hi}, and the megakaryocyte-erythroid progenitors (MEPs) as Lin$^-$Sca-1$^-$IL-7R$^-$c-Kit$^+$CD34$^-$FcγRII/III^{lo}. All analyses were performed on a FACSCanto (BD Biosciences). Data were processed with the FlowJo software (TreeStar Inc). Myeloid progenitors (CMPs and GMPs) were sorted on the FACS Aria (BD Biosciences).

Histomorphometric analysis

The right femur metaphysis was processed for histomorphometric analysis. The proximal halves of femur were fixed in 10% phosphate-buffered formaldehyde, dehydrated in methanol and embedded in methylmetacrylate resin without decalcification. Undecalcified 5-µm-thick longitudinal sections were prepared using a Leica 2055 microtome (Leica, Rueil-Malmaison, France) equipped with a tungsten carbide blade. Sections were stained with Goldner-Masson stain and histomorphometric indices were measured under blind conditions using a Leitz Aristoplan microscope (Leica) connected to a Sony DXC-930P color video camera. An automatic image analyzer (Microvisions Instruments, Evry, France) was used for bone parameter measurements. The trabecular bone volume (BV/TV), trabecular thickness (Tb.Th), trabecular number (Tb.N), trabecular separation (Tb.Sp) and osteoblast surface (ObS/BS) were measured in the secondary metaphyseal area of the proximal end of the femur in a standardized zone located at 300–500 µm from the growth cartilage and 150–200 µm from the cortices. The cortical thickness was measured at midshaft diaphysis. The left femurs were fixed in 4% paraformaldehyde, decalcified with 5% EDTA for 1 week and embedded in paraffin. Five-µm thick sections were dewaxed and processed for TRAP staining by incubation for 30 mn at 37°C in substrate solutions containing naphthol AS B1 phosphate (20 mg, Sigma), sodium tartrate (460 mg), fast red violet (6 mg) and N,N dimetyl formamide (1 Ml) in 20 ml acetate buffer (pH 5.0). Sections were then rinsed under running tap water for 5 min, counterstained with fast green dye and mounted in coverquick. The surface of TRAP-stained cells was measured for the Oc.S/BS calculation using automatic image analyzer (Microvisions Instruments, Evry, France).

Homing and lodging assays

Total BM cells were isolated from donor animals (ERK1$^{-/-}$ or WT). Cells were labeled with the cytoplasmic dye carboxyfluorescein diacetate succinimidyl diester (CFSE) according to manufacturer's instructions (Molecular Probes, Eugene, OR). In homing assays, lethally irradiated C57BL/6 mice were injected with 15×10^6 ERK1$^{-/-}$ or WT CFSE–stained cells. Three and 24 hours after injection, the percentage of CFSE$^+$ cells in BM was scored by flow cytometry. In lodging assays, 15×10^6 CFSE-labeled BM cells were transplanted into non irradiated mice. Three and 24 hours after injection, the percentage of CFSE$^+$ cells in recipient-derived BM cells was scored by flow cytometry. The frequency of CFSE$^+$ donor cells was determined as previously described [34].

Limiting dilution competitive bone marrow transplantation (BMT) assay

For each BMT experiment, 50, 100 or 250 LSK CD150$^+$CD48$^-$ cells of each genotype were mixed with 25×10^4 CD45.1/CD45.2 competitors, and subsequently transplanted into lethally (9,5 Gy) irradiated recipient mice CD45.1. Peripheral blood in recipient mice was analyzed for the engraftment level of donor cells at 4 and 20 weeks after BM transplantation. Peripheral blood was obtained by retro-orbital punction and blood leukocytes were obtained after hypotonic lysis. Multilineage hematopoietic engraftement was analyzed with FITC-conjugated CD45.1, APC-conjugated CD45.2 and the lineage markers Mac1 (CD11b), B220 and CD4 conjugated to (PE). All antibodies are from BioLegend. Data were analyzed with the FlowJo software (TreeStar Inc). Mice with over 1% donor descent-cells in the peripheral blood were counted as "positive reconstitution". CRU frequencies were calculated using L-Calc software (StemCell Technologies). The data are pooled from 3 independent experiments.

Serial transplantation in WT and ERK1$^{-/-}$ mice

Lethally (9,5 Gy) irradiated 8- to 12-week old ERK1$^{-/-}$ and WT CD45.2 mice were reconstituted with 2000 CD45.1 WT Lin$^-$Sca-1$^+$c-Kit$^+$ (LSK) injected intravenously into the retro-orbital plexus in a total volume of 100 µL. Engraftment of primary recipient mice was analyzed after 20 weeks by flow cytometric analysis of peripheral blood. To test the self-renewal activity of the donor HSCs, bone marrow harvested from WT primary recipients after 20 weeks of engraftment was transplanted into lethally irradiated WT CD45.2 secondary recipients at a dose of 10^6 cells per mouse. BM harvested from ERK1$^{-/-}$ primary recipients was transplanted into lethally irradiated WT or ERK1$^{-/-}$ CD45.2 secondary recipients. Flow cytometric peripheral blood analysis of the secondary recipients was performed 20 weeks after transplantation.

In vitro osteoclastogenesis assays

Bone marrow from 8 week-old mice was flushed and mononuclear cells were purified by centrifugation over lymphocyte separation medium (Eurobio, France). Cells were seeded in 24-well plates at 10^5 cells/well in 1 ml of alpha-MEM supplemented with 10% FBS, 25 ng/ml M-CSF, and 35 ng/ml recombinant RANKL (produced at SFR Biosciences UMS344/US8, PAP facility) [35]. The cultures were maintained for 5 days and re-fed every 2 days. Osteoclasts were identified by staining for TRAP activity, using the leukocyte acid phosphatase kit (Sigma Diagnostics, St. Louis, MO). TRAP-positive multinucleated cells with greater than three nuclei were counted as osteoclasts. RNA was isolated from the cells at day 5 of differentiation with cytokines to measure the expression of osteoclast-associated genes. To assess the osteoclast *in vitro* functionality, bone marrow-derived cells were differentiated *in vitro* for 4 days, and osteoclasts detached by treatment with 0,02% EDTA in PBS and numbered. For resorption test, the same number of osteoclasts from each set were lifted and seeded onto 24-well Osteo Assay dishes (Corning) for an additional 24 h. OsteoAssay wells were subsequently stained with silver nitrate [36]. The surface area was measured with ImageJ software, using an ImageJ plug-in developed by our imaging facility (Platim SFR Biosciences)

Deoxypyridinoline cross-link assays

Bone related degradation products from type 1 collagen, deoxypyridinoline (DPD) cross-links and creatinin were measured in evening urine using the Pyrilinks-D immunoassay and creatinin kit (Quidel Corporation, San Diego, CA), according to the manufacturer's protocols.

Monocyte/macrophage progenitors proliferation

L929-cell conditioned medium (LCCM) was used as a source of macrophage colony stimulating factor (M-CSF). Briefly, BM cells were separated by centrifugation over a Ficoll gradient and further purified by immunomagnetic depletion of CD45R- (B220), Ter119-, and CD3ε-positive cells. Enriched-mouse bone marrow monocytes were grown in DMEM-HG supplemented with 20% fetal calf serum, 30% LCCM, 100 U/ml penicillin, 100 µg/ml streptomycin, and 2 mM L-glutamine, and incubated at 37°C in a 5% CO_2 atmosphere. Cell proliferation was evaluated at days 1, 3, and 7, using Uptiblue viable cell counting reagent (Interchim).

In vitro phagocytic activity assay

Bone marrow-derived macrophages were cultured from WT and ERK1$^{-/-}$ mice. Briefly, marrow was flushed from excised femur and cultured at 37°C in complete medium (DMEM supplemented with 20% FBS, 1% L-glutamine, 100 U/ml penicillin/streptomycin, and 30% LCCM). After 5 days of differentiation, the cells were scraped, and reseeded in 12-well plates at 2×10^5cells/well. For latex bead uptake assay, green-yellow fluorescent latex beads (Molecular probes) were diluted 1:300 with complete culture medium and incubated for 30 minutes at 37°C. Non-adherent latex beads were removed by vigorous washing. Cells were then harvested by treatment with 5 mM EDTA and scraping. The amount of phagocytozed beads was measured by flow cytometry on F4/80+-gated population. The amount of nonspecifically bound beads was determined by incubating macrophages with fluorescent beads on ice. The experiment was done with macrophages cultured from 3 mice for each genotype.

RNA extraction and quantitative real-time PCR (qPCR)

Total RNA was isolated from the various samples using RNeasy mini kit with on-column genomic DNA digestion on column step according to the manufacturer's instructions (Qiagen, Valencia, CA). RNA was then reverse transcribed with random hexamer primers using Superscript II (Invitrogen). qPCR was performed with SYBR Green PCR Master mix on a lightcycler (Roche

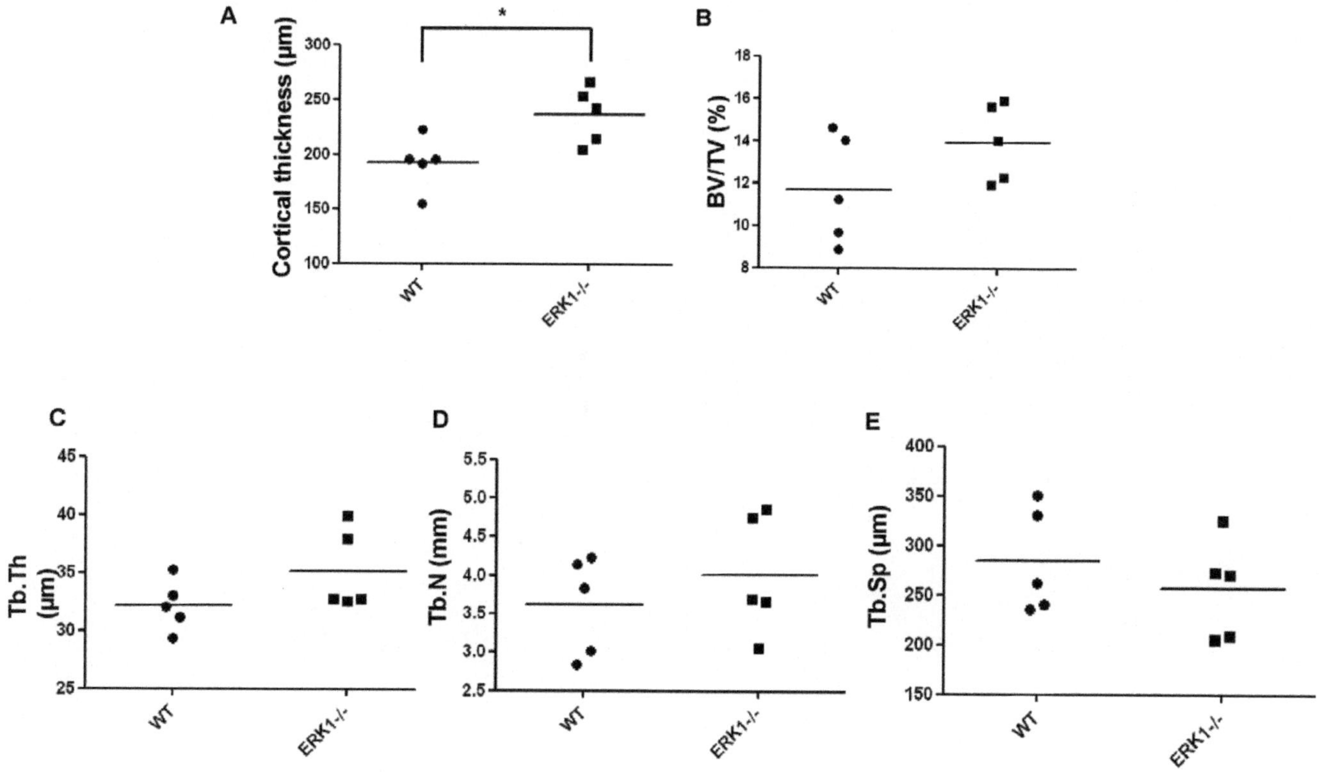

Figure 1. ERK1 loss alters the bone architecture. Cortical and trabecular parameters in WT and ERK1$^{-/-}$ mice (n = 5 for each group). (A) midshaft diaphysis cortical thickness, (B) bone volume/tissue volume (% BV/TV), (C) trabecular thickness (Tb.Th), (D) trabecular number (Tb.N), (E) trabecular separation (Tb.S). The non parametric Mann-Whiney test was used to calculate the *P* value. Horizontal bars show the mean values.

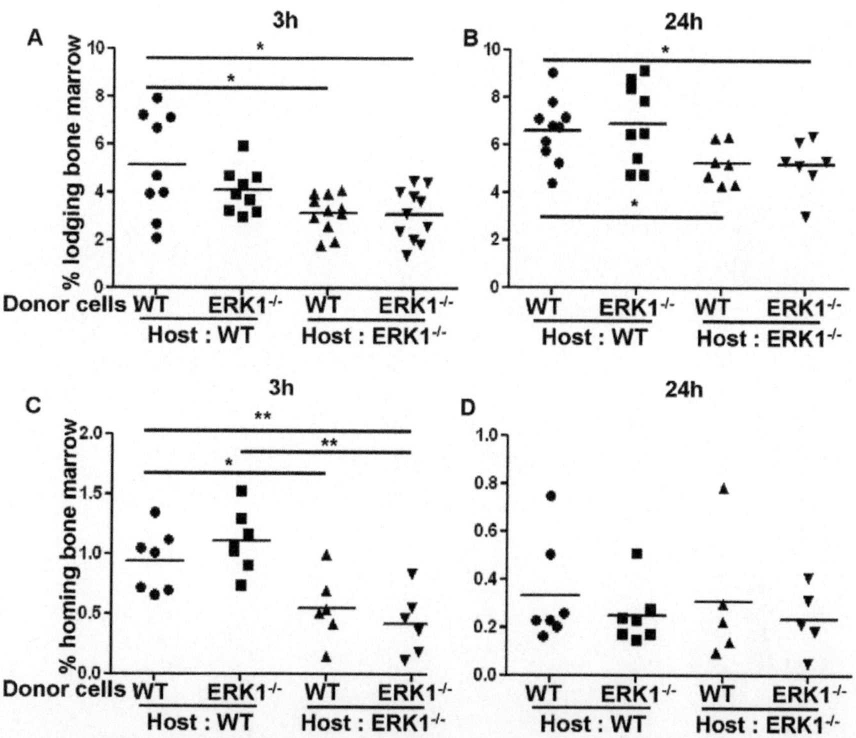

Figure 2. ERK1$^{-/-}$ microenvironment alters the lodging and the homing efficiencies of BM cells. Lodging of the bone marrow cells into a non irradiated host were quantified 3 h (A) and 24 h (B) after injection. Homing of the bone marrow cells into a lethally irradiated host were quantified 3 h (C) and 24 h (D) after injection. Results are presented as scatter plots showing the percentage of recovered CFSE^{+} cells in the BM 3 and 24 hours after transplantation. The non parametric Mann-Whiney test was used to calculate the *P* value. Horizontal bars show the mean values.

Diagnostics, Mannheim, Germany). Sequences of primer pairs used in these qPCR experiments are listed in Table S1. Data were analyzed using the ΔΔ-Ct relative quantification with each duplicate sample normalized to actin.

Statistical analysis

All experimental data were analyzed and compared for statistically significant differences by two-tailed Student's *t* test or the non parametric Mann-Whitney test, as indicated. Data are presented as the averaged values ± standard error of the mean (SEM). All *P* values reported are of comparisons made to results obtained with WT animals. The following values were considered significant: *, $P<0.05$, **, $P<0.01$, and ***, $P<0.001$.

Results

ERK1 deletion increases bone density *in vivo*

Abnormal bone formation was observed in the ERK1$^{-/-}$ mice. Histomorphometric measurements of WT and ERK1$^{-/-}$ mice femurs were applied to analyze the trabecular and cortical microarchitecture. Data indicated that the cortical bone mass of ERK1$^{-/-}$ mice showed a significant increase (Figure 1A). The trabecular bone volume/tissue volume (BV/TV) increased in ERK1$^{-/-}$ mice, though the significance was not reached (Figure 1B). Likewise not statistically significant, the analysis of the main trabecular parameters, including trabecular thickness (Tb.Th, Figure 1C), trabecular number (Tb.N, Figure 1D), and

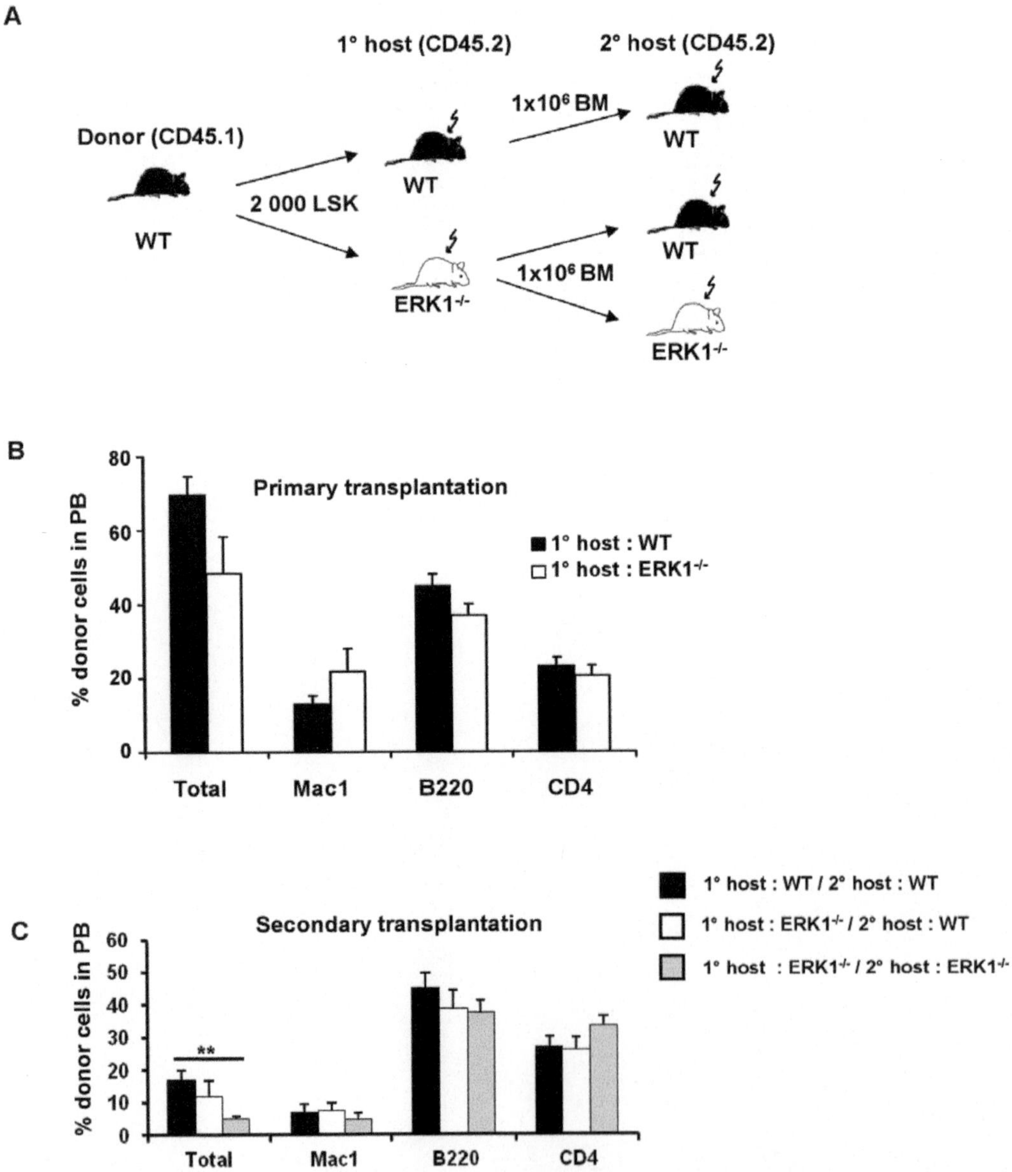

Figure 3. ERK1$^{-/-}$ microenvironment induces a defect in WT HSC activity. (A) Scheme of transplantation assay. (B) Analysis of WT donor cells engraftment in WT (n = 10) and ERK1$^{-/-}$ mice (n = 10) primary recipient 24 weeks after transplantation. (C) Analysis of WT donor cells engraftment in WT (n = 9 per group) and ERK1$^{-/-}$ mice (n = 16) secondary recipient 24 weeks after transplantation. In panels B and C, total donor cells are shown as a percentage of live cells. Individual lineages are shown as a percentage of donor-derived cells. Data represent the mean±SEM, the *t*-test was used to calculate the *P* value.

trabecular separation (Tb.Sp, Figure 1E) showed differences between WT and KO animals in accordance to the increased BV/TV. Though significance was not reached, this finding suggests that bone-remodeling processes are impaired in ERK1$^{-/-}$ mice.

Bone marrow lodging and homing are altered in the absence of ERK1

An abnormal bone formation may have a major impact on the BM microenvironment and, consequently on the lodging and homing abilities of HSCs. In order to study these properties, WT and ERK1$^{-/-}$ BM cells were labelled with CFSE before being transplanted into lethally irradiated (homing) or not irradiated (lodging) WT or ERK1$^{-/-}$ recipients. 15×10^6 BM labelled-cells were injected in non-irradiated recipient mice. WT and ERK1$^{-/-}$ BM cells were found to lodge similarly in WT recipient mice at 3 hours (Figure 2A) or 24 hours (Figure 2B). However WT and ERK1$^{-/-}$ BM cells both presented a striking defect in their ability to lodge in ERK1$^{-/-}$ recipient mice after 3 and 24 hours (Figure 2A and B, respectively). Similarly, a defect in homing of WT and ERK1$^{-/-}$ BM cells in ERK1$^{-/-}$ mice at 3 hours was also observed (Figure 2C) which was not longer seen after 24 hours (Figure 2D). These results indicate that the lodging and the homing abilities of the ERK1$^{-/-}$ HSC are impaired.

The hematopoietic bone marrow microenvironment is defective in the absence of ERK1

The ERK1$^{-/-}$-defective environment may affect the engraftment of HSCs in competitive repopulation assays. Lethally irradiated 8- to 12 week-old ERK1 mutant and littermate control mice (both CD45.2 genotype) were transplanted with 2 000 Lin$^-$Sca1$^+$c-kit$^+$ (LSK) isolated from wild-type CD45.1 mice (Figure 3A). Long term and multilineage engraftment of primary recipients was confirmed by flow cytometry analysis of peripheral blood (Figure 3B). WT donor cells that had been transplanted in ERK1$^{-/-}$ recipients reconstituted hematopoiesis to a lesser extent, even though this was not statistically significant (Figure 3B). In order to test the self-renewal activity of the donor HSCs, BM harvested from WT and ERK1$^{-/-}$ primary recipients after four months of engraftment was transplanted into lethally irradiated WT or ERK1$^{-/-}$ secondary recipients at a dose of 10^6 cells per mouse (Figure 3A). Flow cytometric analysis of PB of the secondary recipients 4 months after transplantation revealed that WT donor cells passaged through a primary mutant microenvironment reconstituted hematopoiesis to a much lower extent when transplanted in a ERK1$^{-/-}$ second recipient (2.9-fold decreased, $P = 0.0005$), compared with WT cells passaged through a primary mutant microenvironment and then transplantated in a secondary WT recipient (Figure 3C). These data strongly support the hypothesis that ERK1 is involved in the maintenance of an appropriate medullar microenvironment, but that the intrinsic properties of HSCs are not altered by the ERK1$^{-/-}$ defective microenvironment. In agreement with that, the frequency of functional ERK1$^{-/-}$ HSCs (CRU) is identical to that of WT HSCs when tested in limiting dilution conditions (Table S2).

Development and maturation of osteoclasts are impaired in the absence of ERK1. Among the cells involved in these specialized microenvironments, osteoclasts and osteoblasts play

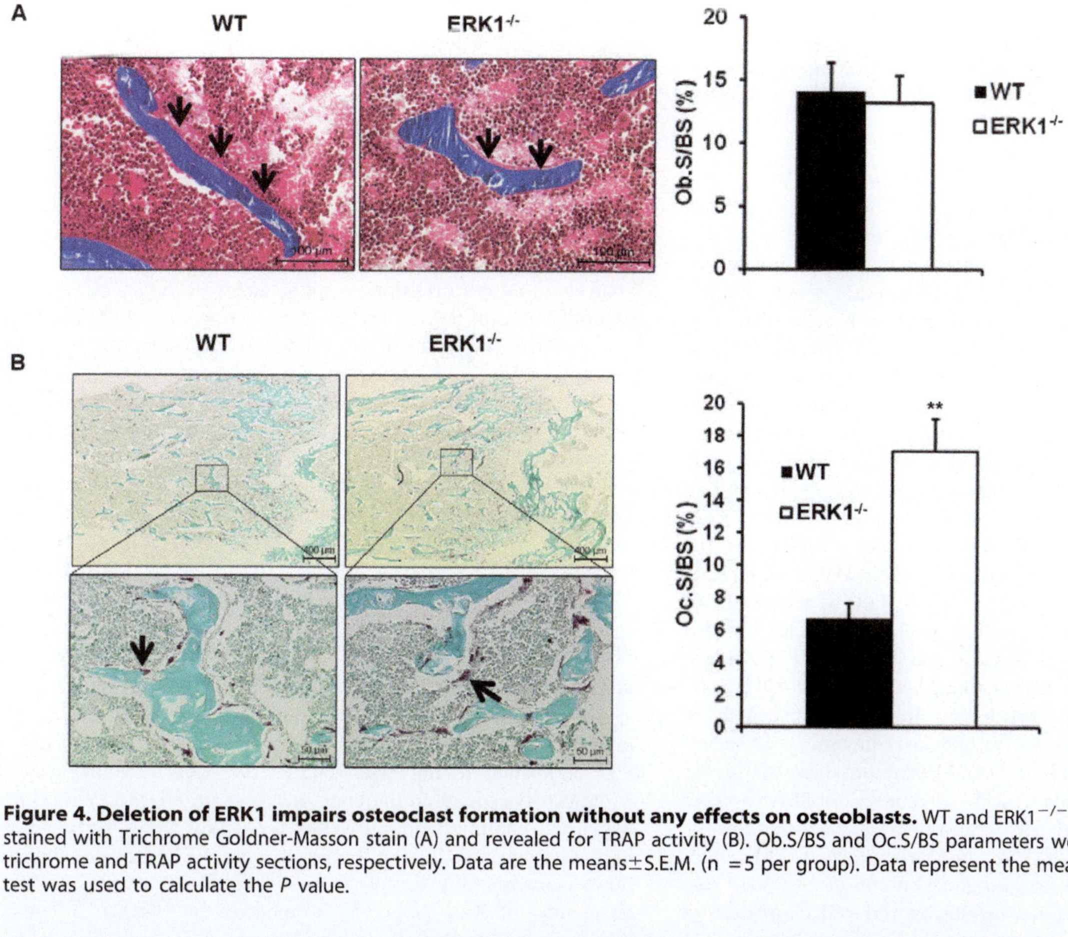

Figure 4. Deletion of ERK1 impairs osteoclast formation without any effects on osteoblasts. WT and ERK1$^{-/-}$ mouse femur sections were stained with Trichrome Goldner-Masson stain (A) and revealed for TRAP activity (B). Ob.S/BS and Oc.S/BS parameters were calculated from Goldner trichrome and TRAP activity sections, respectively. Data are the means±S.E.M. (n = 5 per group). Data represent the mean±SEM, the Mann-Whitney test was used to calculate the *P* value.

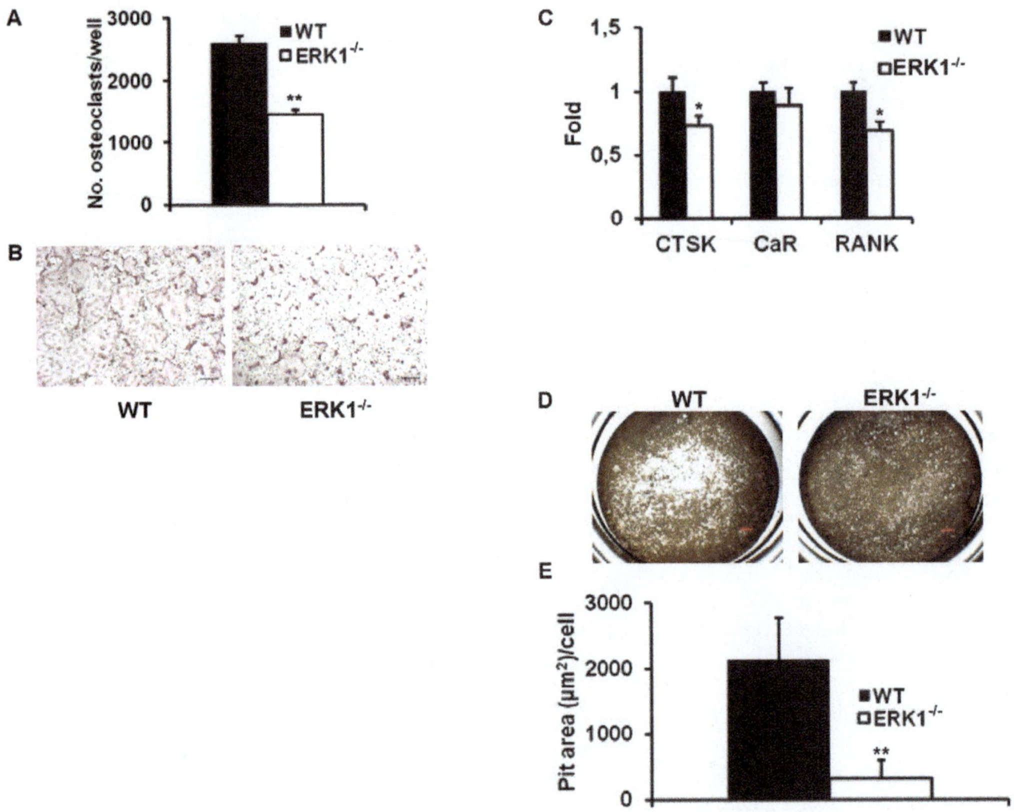

Figure 5. ERK1 deficiency impairs osteoclastogenesis. (A) Total number of osteoclasts per well following 5 days of culture under osteoclastogenic condition (n = 3) (B) Representative picture of TRAP-positive multinucleated osteoclasts generated from BMNCs of WT and ERK1$^{-/-}$ mice. (C) Relative expression of cathepsin K (CTSK), calcitonin receptor (CaR), and receptor activator of nuclear factor *kappa* B (RANK) in WT and ERK1$^{-/-}$ osteoclasts. (D) Representative pictures of the bone resorption pits formed by WT and ERK1$^{-/-}$ derived osteoclasts. (E) Bar graph representing the quantification of the resorptive area per dentin slice for WT and ERK1$^{-/-}$ osteoclasts (n = 3). Data represent the mean± SEM. The *t*-test was used to calculate the *P* value.

major roles. Bone homeostasis is maintained by a tight regulation between bone-forming osteoblasts (OBs), and bone-resorbing osteoclasts (OCs). To address whether the bone phenotype observed in ERK1$^{-/-}$ mice is a consequence of a deregulation of the balance between OBs and OCs, these cells were quantified on bone sections. No difference in OB number between WT and ERK1$^{-/-}$ animals was observed (Figure 4A). Furthermore, the expression of osteoblast-associated genes was similar between the two genotypes (Figure S1). These data suggest that OBs were not altered in ERK1$^{-/-}$ mice. We next determined if increased bone in ERK1$^{-/-}$ mice is a consequence of impaired bone resorption. TRAP staining of bone sections demonstrated a significant increase in the numbers of ERK1$^{-/-}$ TRAP+ cells along the trabecular endosteum, in comparison to their WT counterparts (Figure 4B). To evaluate if ERK1 deletion leads to impaired OC function, we tested the differentiation potential of ERK1$^{-/-}$ and WT BMMCs cultured with M-CSF and RANKL. Following 5 days of differentiation, TRAP staining of WT and ERK1$^{-/-}$ osteoclasts grown *in vitro* revealed a dramatic impairment of osteoclastogenesis in KO cultures with a reduction of osteoclast number by almost 2 fold (Figure 5A). In addition, these ERK1$^{-/-}$ osteoclasts appeared smaller, with a reduced ability to form multinucleated cells (Figure 5B). Transcriptional assessment of the osteoclast-associated genes RANK and cathepsin K (CTSK), after 5 days in culture under osteoclastogenic conditions, revealed that ERK1$^{-/-}$ BM cells exhibited significant reduced expression of these markers of terminal osteoclastic differentiation, while the mRNA levels of the calcitonin receptor (CaR) showed only a modest decrease (Figure 5C). Osteoclast activity was further assessed by analyzing dentin resorption pits after 6 days of culture. Quantification of the resorption areas, normalized to the numbers of osteoclasts, revealed a drastic reduction (~85%) in the resorptive capacity of ERK1$^{-/-}$ osteoclasts as compared to their wild-type counterparts (Figures 5D–E). To address the functionality of OCs *in vivo*, we measured the urinary deoxypyridinoline (DPD) concentration. DPD is the product of the degradation of type I collagen and is a read-out of the ongoing bone resorption process. Urinary excretion of DPD was lower in ERK1$^{-/-}$ mice compared to WT (6.72±0.27 vs 5.52±0.58 nmol/mmol creatinine, $P = 0.06$, n = 8 for each genotype). These results suggest that ERK1 is required for the regulation of normal osteoclast development.

ERK1 loss alters bone marrow monocyte frequency *in vivo* and monocytes progenitors proliferation *in vitro*

As osteoclasts derive from precursors of the monocyte/macrophage lineage, investigation of the monocytic compartment was performed to fully characterize the ERK1 cellular target. Monocytes originate in the bone marrow in a CD115 (M-CSFR)-dependent manner from a myeloid progenitor [37]. We therefore used Gr1 and CD115 antibodies to identify BM monocytes by flow cytometry [38]. Results showed a significant reduction of the frequency of Gr1^{+}/CD115^{+} monocytes in ERK1$^{-/-}$ mice

(Figure 6A, B). Furthermore, the mean fluorescence intensity (MFI) of CD115 was also reduced, indicating that the overall expression of the receptor in this population is decreased (3674±317 for WT vs 3244±234 for ERK1$^{-/-}$). We next investigated if the reduced number of monocytes in the BM may be a consequence of an altered proliferation of monocyte progenitors. BM mononuclear-enriched myeloid cells isolated from WT and ERK1$^{-/-}$ mice were grown in L929-conditioned medium for up to 7 days and tested for their proliferation ability. The results obtained showed that deletion of ERK1 delayed M-CSF-induced monocytes progenitors proliferation (Figure S2). These overall data suggest that ERK1 contribute to the regulation of monocytes progenitors proliferation through the activation of the M-CSF signaling.

ERK1 deletion does not affect macrophage differentiation and functionality

We further investigated if the alteration of the response to M-CSF *in vitro* was correlated with a decrease of mature macrophages number *in vivo*. The splenic macrophages have been characterized as F4/80^{hi}CD11b$^{lo/-}$ cells with strong autofluorescence [39,40]. The WT and the ERK1$^{-/-}$ spleen cells were stained with antibodies to F4/80 and CD11b.The results obtained showed no difference between the ERK1$^{-/-}$ and WT mice (1.18%±0.09% for WT and 1.25%±0.21% for ERK1$^{-/-}$,P = 0.36, n = 6 for both groups). Recently, bone marrow resident macrophages have been described based on differential expression of Gr1, CD115, and F4/80 [38]. According to this labeling, BM macrophages were identified in WT and ERK1$^{-/-}$ mice, and showed no significant difference in their frequency (Figure S3). These data suggest that *in vivo*, mechanisms can compensate for the reduction of monocyte/macrophage progenitors, resulting in a normal distribution of macrophages in the organs under steady-state conditions. In particular, granulocyte-macrophage CSF (GM-CSF) and IL-3 contribute to M-CSF-independent recovery for some macrophages populations in M-CSF-deficient mice [19]. We further investigated the functionality of macrophages from WT and ERK1$^{-/-}$ mice. The phagocytic activity of BM-derived macrophages (BMM) was evaluated by measuring the capacity of the cells to ingest latex beads *in vitro*. The results showed that phagocytosis efficiency was similar in WT and ERK1$^{-/-}$ BMM (Figure S4).

A

B

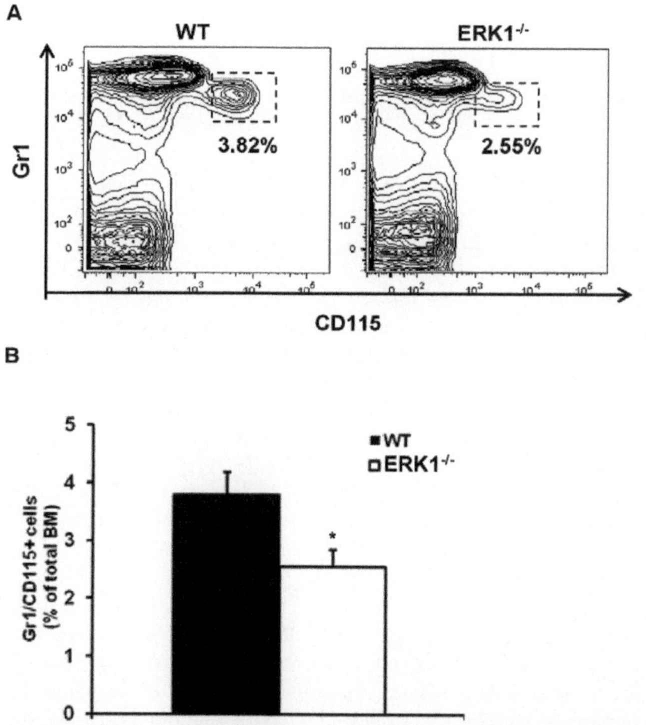

Figure 6. ERK1$^{-/-}$ mice have a reduced fraction of bone marrow monocytes. (A) Representative FACS plot of BM monocytes defined as Gr1$^+$CD115$^+$ cells. (B) Proportion of monocytes as described above in the total BM in WT (n = 11) and ERK1$^{-/-}$ (n = 12). Data represent the mean±SEM. The *t*-test was used to calculate the *P* value.

ERK1 deletion alters the myeloid progenitors compartment

In vivo analysis of the myeloid lineage progenitors, CMP, GMP and MEP subsets revealed a significant phenotypical change in the CMP and GMP subsets in the ERK1$^{-/-}$ mice (Figure 7A). The frequency of CMPs increased by approximately 1.3-fold, while the frequency of GMPs significantly decreased by almost 2-fold, compared with the respective WT compartments (Figure 7A, B). In parallel, the frequency of MEPs showed no change between WT and ERK1$^{-/-}$ mice. These data suggest that ERK1 deletion alters the differentiation of CMPs into GMPs, while it does not affect the MEP commitment and that the CMPs are the cellular targets of ERK1. We have previously shown that ERK1 loss impairs both the osteoclasts and the bone marrow monocytes. As these cells originate in the bone marrow in a CD115 (M-CSFR)-dependent manner from a myeloid progenitor, we next quantified the expression of CD115 in the GMP and CMP subsets. We observed a 2-fold reduction of the GMPs expressing CD115 (14.1%±3% and 6.96%±2.8% for WT and ERK1$^{-/-}$ mice, respectively, P = 0.04; n = 3). Furthermore, the mean fluorescence intensity of CD115 was lower in ERK1$^{-/-}$ GMPs compared to WT (MFI: 2161±190 vs 2550±119; P = 0.04; n = 3). When gated on the CMP subset, the fraction of CD115-positive cells was too low for interpretation. To get insight in the regulation of CD115 expression in myeloid progenitors, we next measured the expression of CD115 mRNA in WT and ERK1$^{-/-}$ GMP-sorted populations. The mRNA expression of CD115 was found to be similar in WT and ERK1$^{-/-}$. No difference in the level of CD115 mRNA was found between WT and ERK1$^{-/-}$ GMP nor CMP, though the level of CD115 gene expression is very low in these latter cells (Figure S5). These results show that the cellular targets of ERK1 are M-CSFR-responsive cells, upstream to osteoclasts.

Discussion

In this study we aimed to decipher the role of ERK1 *in vivo* in the regulation of HSCs. We show that ERK1$^{-/-}$ mice exhibit an overall increase in bone density. These skeletal abnormalities are caused by a deficiency of the osteoclast function. In agreement with these data, mice deficient for ERK1 develop a mild osteopetrosis. Our results provide evidence that ERK1 is involved in the maintenance of an appropriate medullar microenvironment and plays a role in the cells that comprise the hematopoietic microenvironment.

Our results indicate that ERK1 deletion causes defective lodging and homing. This defect results in impaired capacity of WT cells to reconstitute when serially transplanted in ERK1$^{-/-}$ mice. This lower capacity was more pronounced when WT donor cells passaged through a primary mutant microenvironment were transplanted in a ERK1$^{-/-}$ second recipient mice. This result reveals that the negative impact on hematopoietic recovery is

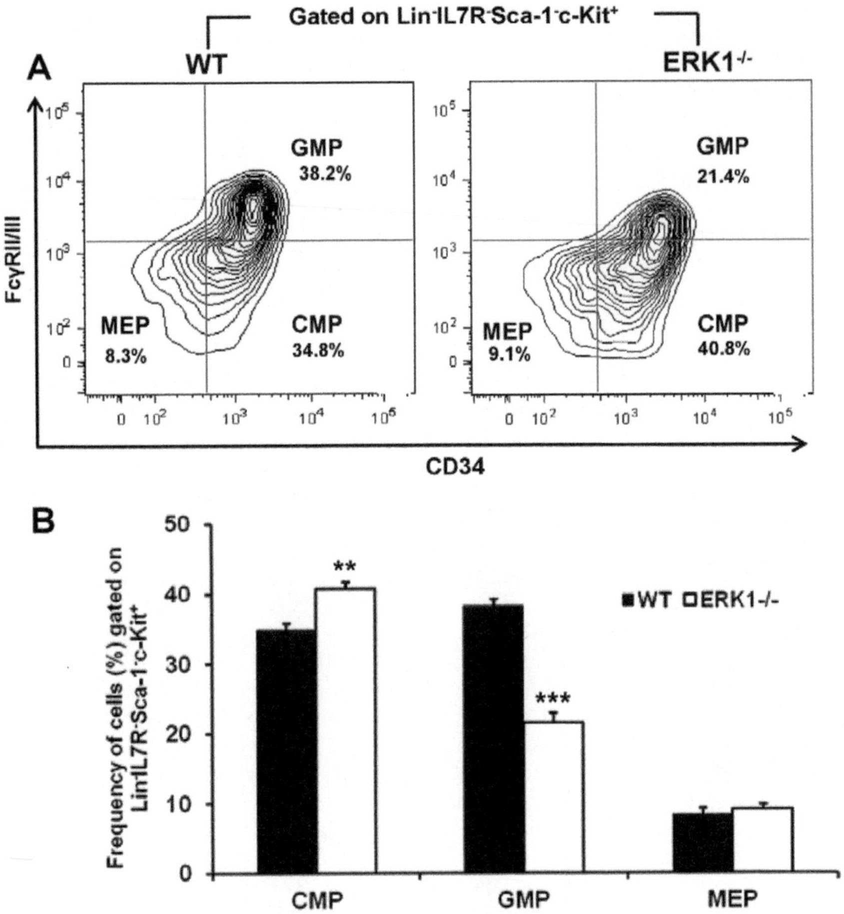

Figure 7. ERK1 deficiency alters the myeloid lineage differentiation. (A) Representative FACS plot of CMP, GMP, and MEP in WT and ERK1$^{-/-}$ mice. (B) Frequency of CMP, GMP, and MEP populations in WT and ERK1$^{-/-}$ mice calculated according to the gating strategy shown in panel A. Values are derived from 6 mice of each genotype. Data represent the mean±SEM. The *t*-test was used to calculate the *P* value.

strictly dependent of the mutant BM microenvironment. By contrast, the deletion of ERK1 was without effect on the functional properties of HSCs. An altered BM niche could explain the defective effects observed. Specifically, ERK1 may be necessary in cell types implicated in the regulation of the niche size. Previous studies have introduced the link between bone remodeling and the regulation of hematopoiesis, suggesting a dynamic nature of the BM stem cell niche [7]. Among the cellular components of the medullar niches, osteoclasts are have been shown to be involved in the hematopoietic niche homeostasis [41,42], controlling both the maintenance and the release of HSC. In the ERK1$^{-/-}$ mice, the major default of *in vitro* osteoclastogenesis contrasts with the *in vivo* increased number of osteoclasts. This could be due to an increased production of osteoclasts to compensate their functional defect. Indeed, similar processes of regulation have been previously described in other osteoclast-defective models [43,44,45]. While this paper was in preparation, Y. He et al. also reported a major defect of bone resorbing activity in ERK1$^{-/-}$ mice [33]. However, they showed that in addition to both *in vitro* and *in vivo* bone-resorbing activity alterations, the number of osteoclasts was markedly reduced in ERK1$^{-/-}$ trabecular area. Variations between these results and ours may reflect differences in the conditions of animal housing and/or ERK1$^{-/-}$ mouse line maintenance, resulting in phenotypes with various degrees of severity. However, although the osteopetrotic phenotype described by He and colleagues was more severe than that we observed, the cellular mechanisms underlying this default are the same.

In addition to the defect in osteoclastogenesis, we report an overall compromised mononuclear-phagocyte lineage development in ERK1$^{-/-}$ mice, through the alteration of M-CSFR expression. Mice defective for M-CSFR (*Csf1r*$^{-}$/*Csf1r*$^{-}$)mice are severely osteopetrotic, with reduced mononuclear phagocyte production, reduced number of macrophages, and development of a splenomegaly [9]. We found similar characteristics in our model, but with a less severe phenotype. This corroborates the reduced expression of M-CSFR^{+} cells in ERK1$^{-/-}$ mice. It is well-known that ERK is a downstream effector of M-CSFR and that it contributes to the regulation of myelopoiesis. However, it is to our knowledge, the first demonstration of a control of M-CSFR expression downstream of ERK1. The loss of ERK1 leads to impaired expression of the M-CSFR in myeloid progenitors and induce a delay in their differentiation program, as shown by the accumulation of CMPs in ERK1$^{-/-}$ bone marrow, while the proportion of GMPs was reduced. The fraction of CD115-positive cells on the CMP subset was too low for interpretation. The CMPs have been shown to be divided into three phenotypically, functionally and developmentally distinct cell subsets [46] that express or not the M-CSFR. In our study we quantified the M-CSFR expression on the overall CMP population. The M-CSFR expression study in the three described subsets in the ERK1$^{-/-}$

mice may allow a quantification of the M-CSFR and explain the increase of the CMP compartment. Furthermore, we reported a decrease in the BM monocytic population ($Gr1^+/CD115^+$) in ERK1$^{-/-}$ mice. Together, these data suggest that ERK1 plays a key role in myelopoiesis by controlling the expression of M-CSFR. This control does not take place at the transcriptional level, as the expression of the M-CSFR mRNA is not different between WT and ERK1$^{-/-}$, in neither GMP or CMP myeloid progenitors. This means that receptor synthesis is more likely to be governed by posttranscriptional regulation as previously suggested [47]. Thus, we can hypothesize that ERK1 is involved in the posttranscriptional mechanisms regulating the expression of the M-CSFR. In line with this hypothesis, it has been shown that the ERK pathway is involved in the mechanisms that control M-CSFR turnover [48].

In summary, our results show that the microenvironmental default observed in ERK1$^{-/-}$ mice is in fact a consequence of an erroneous myeloid lineage commitment. It has been recently published that the inhibitor of differentiation (Id1) gene plays a role in regulation of bone and BM physiology [20]. In Id1$^{-/-}$ mice, the osteoporosis phenotype and increased osteoclasts observed are suggested to be due to a decrease of the CMP population. Likewise, our study suggests that GMPs/CMPs are the ERK1 potential cellular targets. The ERK1-regulated M-CSFR expression characterizes one of the mechanisms involved. While ERK1 is well known to be activated by M-CSF, the present results are the first to point out an ERK1-dependent M-CSFR regulation on hematopoietic progenitors. The observed bone and BM microenvironment phenotypes as well as the decreased osteoclastogenesis in ERK1$^{-/-}$ mice are due to an altered homeostasis of the myeloid precursors cells. This study reinforces the hypothesis of an active cross-talk between HSCs, their progeny and bone cells in the maintenance of the homeostasis of these compartments.

Supporting Information

Figure S1 qPCR analysis of the osteoblast-associated genes RUNX2, alkaline phosphatase (ALP), osteocalcin (OSC), osteopontin (OPN) in WT and ERK1$^{-/-}$ bone samples. Data are presented as the mean ± SEM, n = 3 for each genotype.

Figure S2 M-CSF induced proliferation of BM monocyte/macrophage progenitors. Enriched monocyte/macrophage progenitors were grown *in vitro* in L929-conditioned medium for up to 7 days. Cell proliferation was monitored by means of the fluorimetric metabolic growth indicator Uptiblue (Interchim) at the indicated days. Data show that deletion of ERK1 induces a delay in growth of cells during the first days of culture.

Figure S3 Gating strategy for the BM macrophages. Gated on the $Gr1^-$ population, $F4/80^+CD115^-$ cells were further subdivided on a FSC/SSC plot. $SSC^{int/lo}$ cells are considered as macrophages. Results are representative of 3 independent experiments, for a total of 9 mice for each genotype.

Figure S4 Bead incorporation of BM-derived macrophages. BM-derived macrophages were incubated for 30 minutes with fluorescent latex beads at 37°C. Cells were then detached, and the fluorescence distribution was evaluated by FACS on $F4/80^+$ gated population. No difference was seen between WT and ERK1$^{-/-}$ macrophages. The histograms represent the percentage of macrophages that incorporated the indicated number of beads (n = 3 mice for each genotype).

Figure S5 qPCR analysis of M-CSFR gene expression in WT and ERK1$^{-/-}$ CMPs and GMPs. Data are presented as the mean ± SEM, n = 5 for each genotype.

Table S1 Primer sequence list.

Table S2 CRU frequencies of WT and ERK1$^{-/-}$ HSCs.

Acknowledgments

The authors thank R. Daquin for DPD measurements, M. Theret for LMMC supplying, K. Labrocquère and M. Andrieu for cell sorting assistance.

Author Contributions

Conceived and designed the experiments: NS SG XH PJ VF MG. Performed the experiments: NS SG XH ED DC VF. Analyzed the data: NS SG XH ED PJ DC VF MG. Contributed reagents/materials/analysis tools: JP GP. Wrote the paper: NS FP MG.

References

1. Trumpp A, Essers M, Wilson A (2010) Awakening dormant haematopoietic stem cells. Nat Rev Immunol 10: 201–209.
2. Jones DL, Wagers AJ (2008) No place like home: anatomy and function of the stem cell niche. Nat Rev Mol Cell Biol 9: 11–21.
3. Lo Celso C, Scadden DT (2011) The haematopoietic stem cell niche at a glance. J Cell Sci 124: 3529–3535.
4. Calvi LM, Adams GB, Weibrecht KW, Weber JM, Olson DP, et al. (2003) Osteoblastic cells regulate the haematopoietic stem cell niche. Nature 425: 841–846.
5. Zhang J, Niu C, Ye L, Huang H, He X, et al. (2003) Identification of the haematopoietic stem cell niche and control of the niche size. Nature 425: 836–841.
6. Stier S, Ko Y, Forkert R, Lutz C, Neuhaus T, et al. (2005) Osteopontin is a hematopoietic stem cell niche component that negatively regulates stem cell pool size. J Exp Med 201: 1781–1791.
7. Kollet O, Dar A, Shivtiel S, Kalinkovich A, Lapid K, et al. (2006) Osteoclasts degrade endosteal components and promote mobilization of hematopoietic progenitor cells. Nat Med 12: 657–664.
8. Matsuo K, Irie N (2008) Osteoclast-osteoblast communication. Arch Biochem Biophys 473: 201–209.
9. Dai XM, Ryan GR, Hapel AJ, Dominguez MG, Russell RG, et al. (2002) Targeted disruption of the mouse colony-stimulating factor 1 receptor gene results in osteopetrosis, mononuclear phagocyte deficiency, increased primitive progenitor cell frequencies, and reproductive defects. Blood 99: 111–120.
10. Reya T, Morrison SJ, Clarke MF, Weissman IL (2001) Stem cells, cancer, and cancer stem cells. Nature 414: 105–111.
11. Iwasaki H, Akashi K (2007) Myeloid lineage commitment from the hematopoietic stem cell. Immunity 26: 726–740.
12. Yeung YG, Stanley ER (2003) Proteomic approaches to the analysis of early events in colony-stimulating factor-1 signal transduction. Mol Cell Proteomics 2: 1143–1155.
13. Kodama H, Yamasaki A, Nose M, Niida S, Ohgame Y, et al. (1991) Congenital osteoclast deficiency in osteopetrotic (op/op) mice is cured by injections of macrophage colony-stimulating factor. J Exp Med 173: 269–272.
14. Glantschnig H, Fisher JE, Wesolowski G, Rodan GA, Reszka AA (2003) M-CSF, TNFalpha and RANK ligand promote osteoclast survival by signaling through mTOR/S6 kinase. Cell Death Differ 10: 1165–1177.
15. Hofstetter W, Wetterwald A, Cecchini MC, Felix R, Fleisch H, et al. (1992) Detection of transcripts for the receptor for macrophage colony-stimulating factor, c-fms, in murine osteoclasts. Proc Natl Acad Sci U S A 89: 9637–9641.
16. Sarma U, Flanagan AM (1996) Macrophage colony-stimulating factor induces substantial osteoclast generation and bone resorption in human bone marrow cultures. Blood 88: 2531–2540.

17. Grigoriadis AE, Wang ZQ, Cecchini MG, Hofstetter W, Felix R, et al. (1994) c-Fos: a key regulator of osteoclast-macrophage lineage determination and bone remodeling. Science 266: 443–448.
18. Kong YY, Feige U, Sarosi I, Bolon B, Tafuri A, et al. (1999) Activated T cells regulate bone loss and joint destruction in adjuvant arthritis through osteoprotegerin ligand. Nature 402: 304–309.
19. Wiktor-Jedrzejczak W, Bartocci A, Ferrante Jr. AW, Ahmed-Ansari A, Sell KW, et al. (1990) Total absence of colony-stimulating factor 1 in the macrophage-deficient osteopetrotic (op/op) mouse. Proc Natl Acad Sci U S A 87: 4828–4832.
20. Chan AS, Jensen KK, Skokos D, Doty S, Lederman HK, et al. (2009) Id1 represses osteoclast-dependent transcription and affects bone formation and hematopoiesis. PLoS One 4: e7955.
21. Fichelson S, Freyssinier JM, Picard F, Fontenay-Roupie M, Guesnu M, et al. (1999) Megakaryocyte growth and development factor-induced proliferation and differentiation are regulated by the mitogen-activated protein kinase pathway in primitive cord blood hematopoietic progenitors. Blood 94: 1601–1613.
22. Nagata Y, Takahashi N, Davis RJ, Todokoro K (1998) Activation of p38 MAP kinase and JNK but not ERK is required for erythropoietin-induced erythroid differentiation. Blood 92: 1859–1869.
23. Rouyez MC, Boucheron C, Gisselbrecht S, Dusanter-Fourt I, Porteu F (1997) Control of thrombopoietin-induced megakaryocytic differentiation by the mitogen-activated protein kinase pathway. Mol Cell Biol 17: 4991–5000.
24. Uchida M, Kirito K, Shimizu R, Miura Y, Ozawa K, et al. (2001) A functional role of mitogen-activated protein kinases, erk1 and erk2, in the differentiation of a human leukemia cell line, UT-7/GM: a possible key factor for cell fate determination toward erythroid and megakaryocytic lineages. Int J Hematol 73: 78–83.
25. Yao Y, Li W, Wu J, Germann UA, Su MS, et al. (2003) Extracellular signal-regulated kinase 2 is necessary for mesoderm differentiation. Proc Natl Acad Sci U S A 100: 12759–12764.
26. Bost F, Aouadi M, Caron L, Even P, Belmonte N, et al. (2005) The extracellular signal-regulated kinase isoform ERK1 is specifically required for in vitro and in vivo adipogenesis. Diabetes 54: 402–411.
27. Pages G, Guerin S, Grall D, Bonino F, Smith A, et al. (1999) Defective thymocyte maturation in p44 MAP kinase (Erk 1) knockout mice. Science 286: 1374–1377.
28. Mazzucchelli C, Vantaggiato C, Ciamei A, Fasano S, Pakhotin P, et al. (2002) Knockout of ERK1 MAP kinase enhances synaptic plasticity in the striatum and facilitates striatal-mediated learning and memory. Neuron 34: 807–820.
29. Guihard S, Clay D, Cocault L, Saulnier N, Opolon P, et al. (2010) The MAPK ERK1 is a negative regulator of the adult steady-state splenic erythropoiesis. Blood 115: 3686–3694.
30. Miranda MB, Xu H, Torchia JA, Johnson DE (2005) Cytokine-induced myeloid differentiation is dependent on activation of the MEK/ERK pathway. Leuk Res 29: 1293–1306.
31. Hsu CL, Kikuchi K, Kondo M (2007) Activation of mitogen-activated protein kinase kinase (MEK)/extracellular signal regulated kinase (ERK) signaling pathway is involved in myeloid lineage commitment. Blood 110: 1420–1428.
32. Hodge JM, Collier FM, Pavlos NJ, Kirkland MA, Nicholson GC (2011) M-CSF potently augments RANKL-induced resorption activation in mature human osteoclasts. PLoS One 6: e21462.
33. He Y, Staser K, Rhodes SD, Liu Y, Wu X, et al. (2011) Erk1 positively regulates osteoclast differentiation and bone resorptive activity. PLoS One 6: e24780.
34. Foudi A, Jarrier P, Zhang Y, Wittner M, Geay JF, et al. (2006) Reduced retention of radioprotective hematopoietic cells within the bone marrow microenvironment in CXCR4−/− chimeric mice. Blood 107: 2243–2251.
35. Dacquin R, Domenget C, Kumanogoh A, Kikutani H, Jurdic P, et al. (2011) Control of Bone Resorption by Semaphorin 4D Is Dependent on Ovarian Function. PLoS One 6: e26627.
36. Saltel F, Destaing O, Bard F, Eichert D, Jurdic P (2004) Apatite-mediated actin dynamics in resorbing osteoclasts. Mol Biol Cell 15: 5231–5241.
37. Auffray C, Sieweke MH, Geissmann F (2009) Blood monocytes: development, heterogeneity, and relationship with dendritic cells. Annu Rev Immunol 27: 669–692.
38. Chow A, Lucas D, Hidalgo A, Mendez-Ferrer S, Hashimoto D, et al. (2011) Bone marrow CD169+ macrophages promote the retention of hematopoietic stem and progenitor cells in the mesenchymal stem cell niche. J Exp Med 208: 261–271.
39. Taylor PR, Brown GD, Geldhof AB, Martinez-Pomares L, Gordon S (2003) Pattern recognition receptors and differentiation antigens define murine myeloid cell heterogeneity ex vivo. Eur J Immunol 33: 2090–2097.
40. Kohyama M, Ise W, Edelson BT, Wilker PR, Hildner K, et al. (2009) Role for Spi-C in the development of red pulp macrophages and splenic iron homeostasis. Nature 457: 318–321.
41. Ponomaryov T, Peled A, Petit I, Taichman RS, Habler L, et al. (2000) Induction of the chemokine stromal-derived factor-1 following DNA damage improves human stem cell function. J Clin Invest 106: 1331–1339.
42. Adams GB, Chabner KT, Alley IR, Olson DP, Szczepiorkowski ZM, et al. (2006) Stem cell engraftment at the endosteal niche is specified by the calcium-sensing receptor. Nature 439: 599–603.
43. Shivtiel S, Kollet O, Lapid K, Schajnovitz A, Goichberg P, et al. (2008) CD45 regulates retention, motility, and numbers of hematopoietic progenitors, and affects osteoclast remodeling of metaphyseal trabecules. J Exp Med 205: 2381–2395.
44. Gowen M, Lazner F, Dodds R, Kapadia R, Feild J, et al. (1999) Cathepsin K knockout mice develop osteopetrosis due to a deficit in matrix degradation but not demineralization. J Bone Miner Res 14: 1654–1663.
45. Boyce BF, Yoneda T, Lowe C, Soriano P, Mundy GR (1992) Requirement of pp60c-src expression for osteoclasts to form ruffled borders and resorb bone in mice. J Clin Invest 90: 1622–1627.
46. Nutt SL, Metcalf D, D'Amico A, Polli M, Wu L (2005) Dynamic regulation of PU.1 expression in multipotent hematopoietic progenitors. J Exp Med 201: 221–231.
47. Sherr CJ (1990) Colony-stimulating factor-1 receptor. Blood 75: 1–12.
48. Glenn G, van der Geer P (2008) Toll-like receptors stimulate regulated intramembrane proteolysis of the CSF-1 receptor through Erk activation. FEBS Lett 582: 911–915.

Sensory Neuron Development in Mouse Coccygeal Vertebrae and Its Relationship to Tail Biopsies for Genotyping

Jerald Silverman[1]*, Gregory Hendricks[2]

1 Department of Animal Medicine, University of Massachusetts Medical School, Worcester, Massachusetts, United States of America, 2 Department of Cell Biology, University of Massachusetts Medical School, Worcester, Massachusetts, United States of America

Abstract

A common method of genotyping mice is via tissue obtained from tail biopsies. However, there is no available information on the temporal development of sensory neurons in the tail and how their presence or absence might affect the age for performing tail biopsies. The goals of this study were to determine if afferent sensory neurons, and in particular nociceptive neurons, are present in the coccygeal vertebrae at or near the time of birth and if not, when they first can be visualized on or in those vertebrae. Using toluidine blue neuronal staining, transmission electron microscopy, and calcitonin-related gene peptide immunostaining, we found proximal to distal maturation of coccygeal nerve growth in the C57BL/6J mouse. Single nerve bundles were first seen on postpartum day (PPD) 0. On PPD 3 presumptive nociceptive sensory nerve fibers were seen entering the vertebral perichondrium. Neural development continued through the last time point (PPD 7) but at no time were neural fibers seen entering the body of the vertebrae. The effect of age on the development of pain perception in the neonatal mouse is discussed.

Editor: Izumi Sugihara, Tokyo Medical and Dental University, Japan

Funding: All funding for this study was from internal institutional funds provided to the Department of Animal Medicine by the University of Massachusetts Medical School. The funders had no role in study design, data collection and analysis, decision to publish, or preparation of the manuscript.

Competing Interests: The authors have declared that no competing interests exist.

* E-mail: jerald.silverman@umassmed.edu

Introduction

One of the most common forms of genotyping mice is via tissue obtained from tail biopsy (tailing) [1,2]. However, there is little if any information as to whether the procedure might damage nerves associated with the biopsied areas. More than 150 years ago, researchers identified sensory nerve fibers on and within the long bones of rodents (reviewed in reference [3]). These sensory fibers are essential for an animal's responsiveness to noxious stimuli affecting the bone and periosteum, but also may serve an important role in regulating blood flow and erythrogenesis within the marrow [4] and stimulating osteoblasts and inhibiting osteoclasts [5–7]. In contrast to the long bones, the irregularly shaped coccygeal vertebrae have not been extensively researched relative to the development of their innervation. Perhaps this is because they are no more than "miniature long bones" [8], an observation supported, in part, by the fact that the osseous development of the coccygeal vertebrae is similar to that of long bones [9,10]. Nevertheless, the literature on the coccygeal vertebrae of mice and rats is not entirely barren. For example, the morphology of mouse coccygeal vertebrae has been described [11] as has their general growth and ossification pattern [9,12]. The effects of hypoxia on mouse coccygeal vertebral development [8] and the development of vasomotor innervation in the rat tail [13] also have been studied. But quite unlike long bones, there are no studies addressing the early stages of sensory nerve growth on and within the coccygeal vertebrae of the laboratory mouse.

DNA for genotyping mice can be isolated from tissues such as the animals' tail, ear, blood, or hair. As noted earlier, cutting off a small piece of tail, typically 3–5 mm from animals less than 1 week to more than 4 weeks of age [14], is often the preferred method for obtaining tissue for genotyping; however, that procedure injures all tissues in the path of the cutting blade, including sensory neurons, if present. The degree of pain an animal experiences from tailing is likely to be a function of the tissues injured, the maturation of the animal's peripheral and central nervous systems, and the presence or absence of nociceptive neurons at or near the site of injury. Observations of mice on their day of birth readily demonstrate that these neonates are capable of moving their tails, thereby indicating the presence of functional motor neurons and muscles in the tail. Most likely, this movement is little more than uncontrolled spontaneous twitching. It is not known though, if afferent sensory neurons, and in particular nociceptive neurons, are present in the coccygeal vertebrae at or near the time of birth (as they are with long bones) and if not, when they first can be visualized in those vertebrae. We have answered these questions and extrapolated our findings to their possible impact on pain from tailing.

Materials and Methods

Ethics Statement

This study was performed in accordance with the recommendations of the *Guide for the Care and Use of Laboratory Animals* of the

U.S. Institute for Laboratory Animal Research, National Research Council [15] and carried out under approval A-2301-11 from the Institutional Animal Care and Use Committee of the University of Massachusetts Medical School.

Animals

One timed-pregnant C57BL/6J mouse (The Jackson Laboratory, Bar Harbor, ME) gave birth to 9 pups on postpartum day (PPD) 0. On that day, 3 of the pups were briefly taken from their dam and had the distal 5 mm of their tails removed by a quick cut with a new razor blade. They were then wiped with bedding from their home cage and uneventfully returned to their dam. On PPD 3 the same procedure was performed on 3 different mice from the same litter and on PPD 7 the same procedure was performed on the remaining 3 pups. Externally, the tail of a newborn C57BL/6J mouse is about 1.25 cm in length. We removed 5 mm of the tail as it was the largest section that we were confident could easily and safely be removed from a neonatal mouse [16] and it would allow us to readily integrate our findings with those of a previous study which evaluated the temporal development of mouse coccygeal vertebrae [12].

Each tail tip was cut into 3 approximately equal sections of just under 2 mm in a manner that allowed for the identification of the proximal and distal ends of each section. The middle section shown in Figure 1 was not used in this study but was cut to allow for improved fixation of the proximal and distal segments.

Tissue used for immunohistochemistry to detect calcitonin gene-related peptide (CGRP) was obtained from six C57BL/6J pups born to a second dam. On PPD 0, 3 and 7, two different pups (at each time point) had the distal 5 mm of their tails biopsied as described above.

Epoxy Resin Embedding for Transmission Electron Microscopy (TEM)

Tail segments were fixed by immersion in 2.5% (v/v) glutaraldehyde in 0.5 M Na phosphate buffer (pH 7.2) for 1 hour at room temperature. The fixed samples were washed 3 times in the same buffer. Following the third wash the tail segments were post-fixed for 1 hour in 1% osmium tetroxide (w/v) in the same buffer, washed 3 more times and left overnight at 4°C in fresh buffer. The next morning the samples were dehydrated through a graded series of ethanol to 100% and then transferred into propylene oxide (2 changes) and finally into epoxy resin/propylene oxide and left overnight to complete infiltration. Following infiltration the tissues were transferred through 3 changes of fresh epoxy resin and embedded in flat molds and polymerized at 70°C. The polymerized blocks were then oriented so as to cut cross-sections of the tail segments. One micron sections were taken and stained with 1% toluidine blue and examined by light microscopy for histological appearance and to select areas for correlative TEM. Electron micrographs were collected using a Philips CM 10 transmission electron microscope (Koninklijke Philips, Amsterdam, Netherlands) equipped with a Gatan, Erlangshen 785 digital camera system (Gatan, Pleasanton, CA).

Acrylic Resin Embedding for Immunostaining CGRP

Tail segments were fixed by immersion in 4% paraformaldehyde for 1 hour at room temperature. The segments were then washed overnight in 0.5 M Na phosphate buffer (pH 7.2). Following the overnight wash the tail segments were dehydrated through a graded series of ethanol to 100% (2 changes) and then transferred into a 50:50 (V/V) mixture of LR White acrylic resin and 100% ethanol and left overnight to infiltrate. The following morning the tail segments were transferred through 3 changes of fresh LR White acrylic resin (1 hour each) and then transferred into Beem® capsules, capped, and placed in a 70°C oven to polymerize. One micron sections were cut, stained with 1% toluidine blue, and examined by light microscopy for histological appearance. Consecutive sections were incubated with rabbit anti-CGRP (Sigma-Aldrich #C 8198, St. Louis, MO) for 4 hours at room temperature, washed and incubated with Texas Red®-X goat anti-rabbit IgG (Life Technologies #T6391, Grand Island, NY) in the dark for 1 hour at room temperature. Images were recorded using an Olympus AX90 microscope with an automated stage (Olympus America, Melville, NY) and a Q-Color5 5MP digital camera system (Olympus America, Melville, NY).

Results

PPD 0

Toluidine blue staining on PPD 0 demonstrated single, discrete nerve bundles at the proximal biopsy site (Figure 2). The nerve bundles appeared small and unmyelinated. These results were confirmed by TEM (Figure 3). Toluidine blue staining and TEM of the distal biopsy site displayed a general lack of organization of the developing tissues. CGRP immunostaining indicated that at this age the putative sensory nerves were only along blood vessels, not developing bone (Figure 4).

PPD 3

Toluidine blue staining indicated nerve bundle organization at the proximal biopsy site. TEM at the proximal site revealed a neuromuscular junction in one of the muscle bundles (Figure 5) and numerous nerve fibers going to and through the forming periosteum (Figure 6). None of the fibers seen were myelinated but some had Schwann cells associated with them. The nerves were still single, discrete bundles. At the proximal site CGRP staining revealed immunoreactivity around blood vessels and what appeared to be the first evidence of putative sensory nerve fibers in the periosteum (Figure 7). There also was generalized CGRP staining of the perichondrium, most probably due to the affinity of immunoreactive CGRP with CGRP receptors in osteoclasts and osteoblasts of the mineralizing vertebra [7,17,18]. At the distal biopsy site, CGRP immunostaining of nerve fibers still was present only around blood vessels.

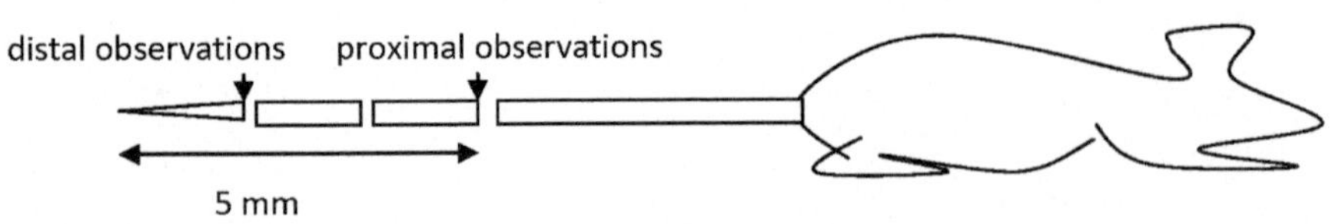

Figure 1. Locations of tail biopsy examination sites. A 5 mm section from the end of the tail was taken from C57BL/6 mice at 0, 3, and 7 days postpartum (PPD). The tissue was cut into 3 pieces and prepared for toluidine blue staining, transmission electron microscopy (TEM), and calcitonin gene-related peptide (CGRP) immunostaining. The arrows indicate the areas examined by TEM and bright field microscopy.

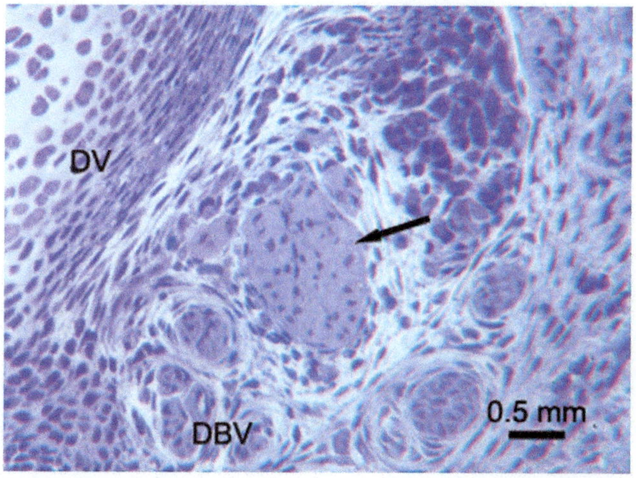

Figure 2. PPD 0, proximal biopsy site. Cross section with toluidine blue staining of a 1 μm epoxy section. An immature nerve bundle (arrow) in the center of the image is clearly visible. DV (developing vertebra), DBV (developing blood vessel).

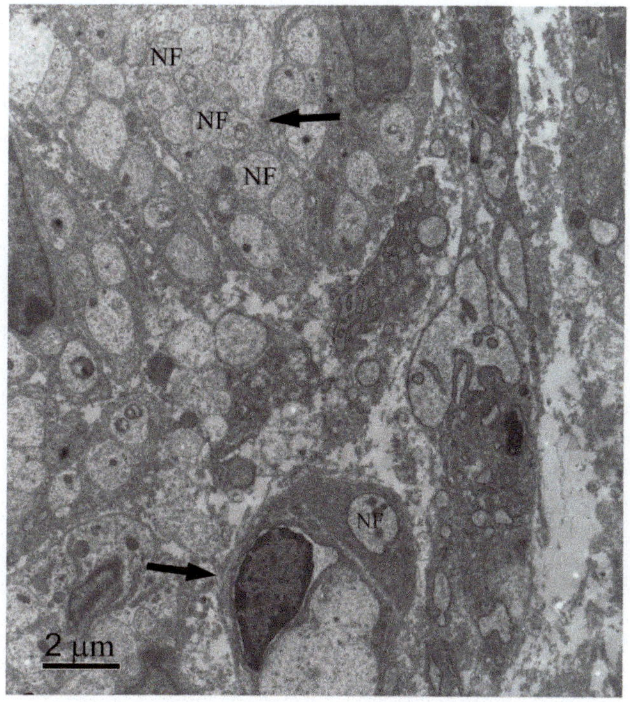

Figure 3. PPD 0, proximal biopsy site, TEM. This thin cross-section shows that individual nerve fibers (NF) within the nerve bundle (upper arrow) on the micrograph appear unmyelinated and no Schwann cells are present. Note the small blood vessel lower center (lower arrow), with what appears to be a small unmyelinated nerve fiber (NF) running next to it surrounded by extracellular matrix.

PPD 7

Toluidine blue staining at the proximal biopsy cut showed that the tissues were well organized, the nerve bundles appeared larger than on previous days, and the bundles contained both myelinated and unmyelinated axons that were found alongside blood vessels and in the developing periosteum. Myelinated individual nerve fibers were readily detected (Figure 8). The toluidine blue observations from the proximal biopsy site were confirmed by TEM examination (Figure 9).

At the distal biopsy site on PPD 7, toluidine blue staining showed that one or more nerves had split into several nerve bundles (not just a single bundle as found at PPD 0 and 3) and they were coursing alongside small blood vessels (Figure 10). With TEM we found nerve fibers in the forming periosteum (Figure 11) and unmyelinated axons were readily detected.

At the proximal biopsy site CGRP immunostaining revealed reactivity around blood vessels and what appears to be the first evidence of a sensory nerve fiber staining in a nerve bundle, along with the immunostaining of the forming periosteum (Figure 12) which we first found on PPD 3. CGRP immunostaining at the distal site was similar to the proximal site.

Discussion

The coccygeal vertebrae of mice and rats increase in number and mature in a proximal to distal direction [9,11,12]. The present data demonstrate that the nerve supply to the coccygeal vertebrae of the C57BL/6J mouse also has proximal to distal maturation. This was anticipated as the sensory nerve supply to mouse and rat long bones exhibits proximal to distal growth and maturation [3,7,19]. Because the proximal biopsy site was about 0.5 cm distal to the base of the animals' tail, it is likely that neural development of the vertebrae closer to the sacrum occurred slightly earlier than our findings from the proximal biopsy site that we used.

With toluidine blue staining, single nerve bundles were first seen on PPD 0 at the proximal biopsy site along with limited CGRP immunoreactivity. By PPD 3 there was continued growth of nerve bundles, nerve fibers were seen in the perichondrium, and there was early CGRP immunoreactivity of the perichondrium, primarily at the proximal biopsy site. By PPD 7 the neural development continued at both the proximal and distal biopsy sites. At the proximal site CGRP immunoreactivity was present in the perichondrium and individual nerves fibers were in nerve bundles; however, even at this age, we did not visualize nerves or nerve fibers entering the vertebral body although fibers may have entered the vertebral body in areas not sectioned for this study.

The neuropeptide CGRP is produced by peripheral and central nervous system neurons, including those of bony tissue. It has been found to participate in the innervation of almost all rat long bones and surrounding soft tissue [5,20] and in rats it has been detected in the lumbar vertebral body [21] and the coccygeal intervertebral disc [22]. Because CGRP can function in the transmission of nociceptive signals, its detection by immunohistochemistry has frequently been used as a marker of the presence of nociceptive nerve fibers [7,22–25].

Using CGRP and Substance P as markers, sensory nerve fibers were visualized in rat long bone periosteum prior to birth [24]. Most of these sensory nerves were located close to blood vessels [20]. They first entered long bone diaphyses and then reached the epiphyses by PPD 7–8 [7,26]. In the present study CGRP immunostaining indicated that presumptive sensory fibers entered the perichondrium of the developing coccygeal vertebra by PPD 7, although weakly staining presumptive sensory fibers were found on and in the perichondrium as early as PPD 3. Myelinated nerve fibers first appear at PPD 14 in the rat femur [3], differing from our finding of 7 days in the proximal coccygeal vertebrae. Todd and Tokito [13], using TEM, identified *vasomotor* innervation of the proximal end of the tail of the rat at PPD 3 but the nerve fibers did not have a Schwann cell covering (i.e., there was no early myelination). In the present study we also found at PPD 3 (using TEM) unmyelinated nerve bundles running alongside coccygeal

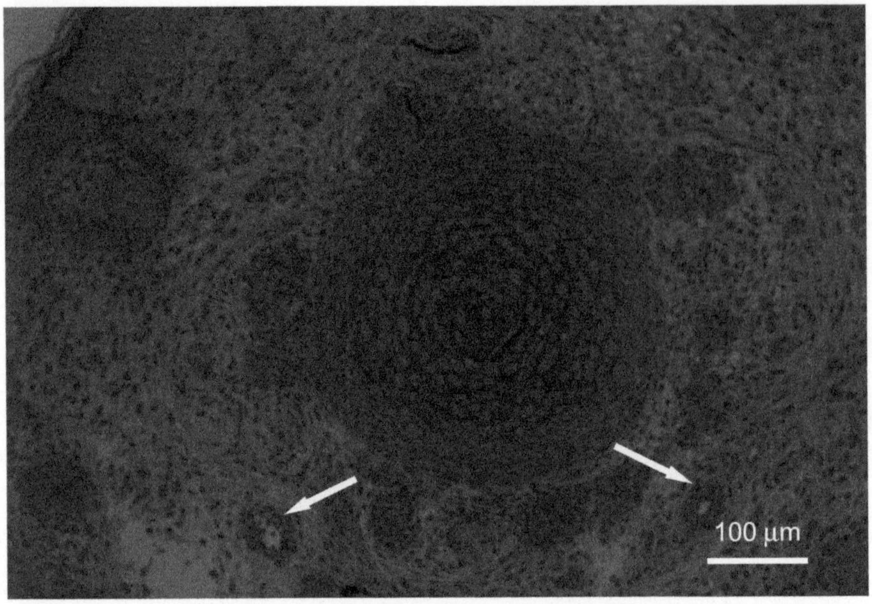

Figure 4. PPD 0. Proximal biopsy site. Adjacent 1 µm LR White acrylic resin sections were merged to show both the Texas Red fluorescent image for CGRP staining and the tissue structure seen with toluidine blue staining. Note that the only evidence of CGRP neural staining is around the small blood vessels (arrows) lower left and right. DV denotes the developing vertebra in the center of the image. The diffuse reddish color is most likely CGRP staining of osteoclasts and possibly osteoblasts, resulting from the early mineralization of the vertebra.

blood vessels and at PPD 7 we found myelinated neural fibers in nerve bundles that were not in proximity to vessels.

The periosteum of the mouse femur is innervated in part by thinly myelinated Aδ-fibers and peptide-rich unmyelinated sensory C-fibers that express CGRP, with the majority of C-fibers likely transmitting noxious stimuli [27,28]. Because of the extensive sensory innervation of the periosteum of long bones [4] it has been

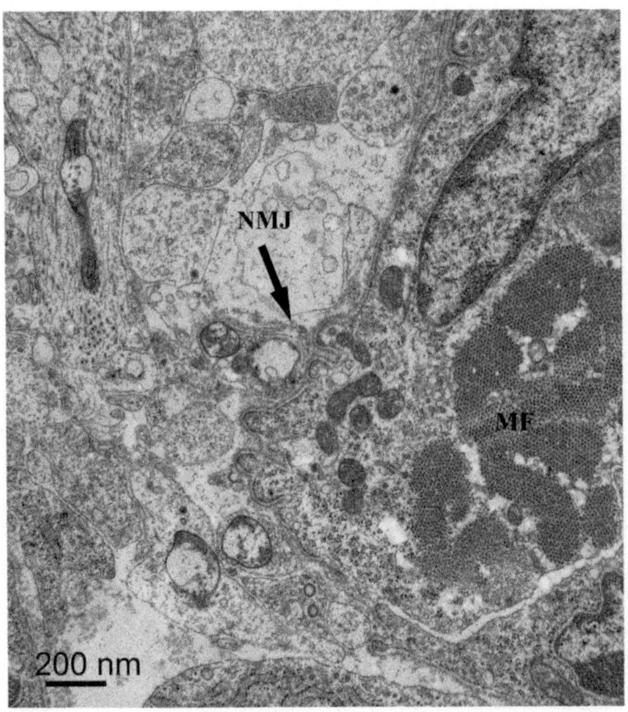

Figure 5. PPD 3, proximal biopsy site, TEM. This thin cross-section shows a neuro-muscular junction (NMJ) below the arrow center of image, on a small muscle cell cross-section (MF).

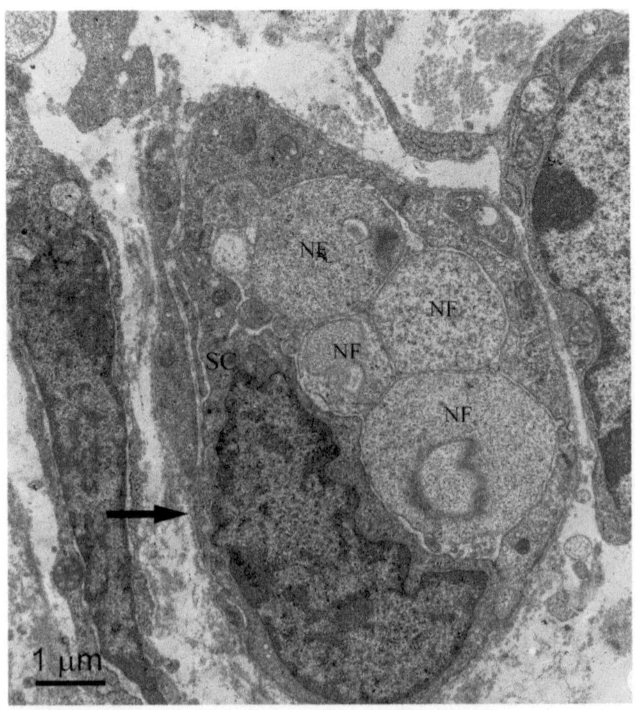

Figure 6. PPD 3, proximal biopsy site, TEM. A thin cross-section shows a nerve fiber in the periosteum with multiple nerve fibers (NF) surrounded by a single Schwann cell (arrow points to the dark nucleus of the Schwann cell).

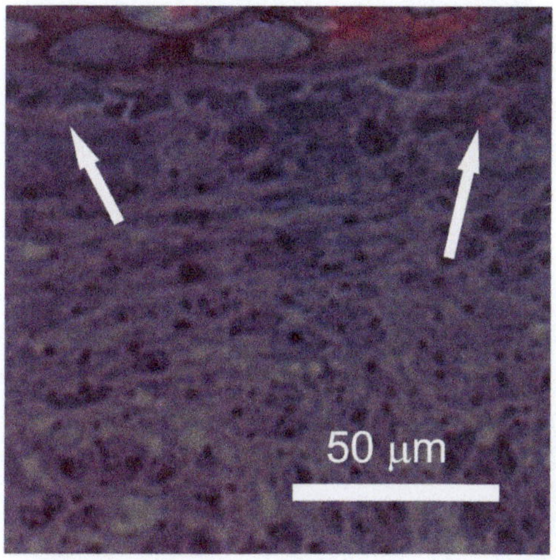

Figure 7. PPD 3, proximal biopsy site. Adjacent 1 μm LR White acrylic resin sections were merged to show both the Texas Red fluorescent image for CGRP staining and the tissue structure seen with toluidine blue staining. Arrows indicate the first faint evidence of CGRP staining in the periosteum. The structure at the top of the image is the developing vertebra and the diffuse reddish color is most likely CGRP staining of osteoclasts and possibly osteoblasts, resulting from the early mineralization of the vertebra.

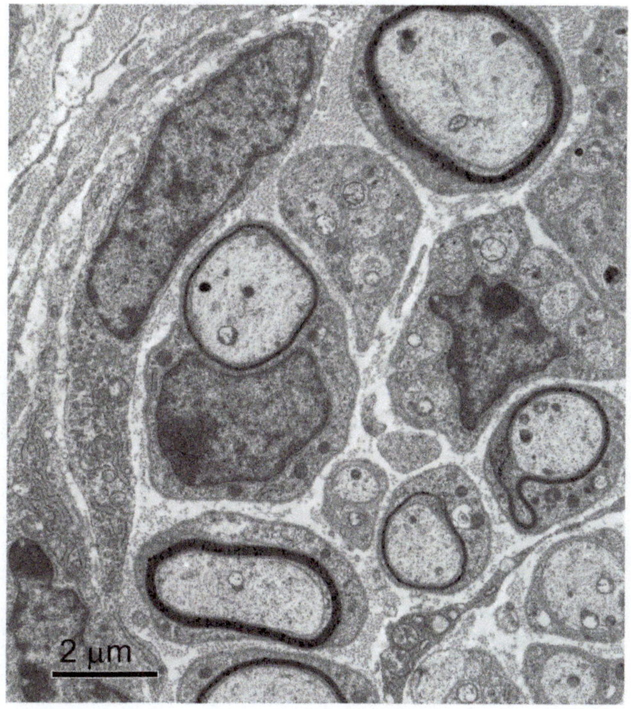

Figure 9. PPD 7, proximal biopsy site, TEM. In this thin cross-section there is a nerve bundle with numerous fiber tracks that are now myelinated to some extent and surrounded by a Schwann cell as indicated by the thick dark staining ring around some cells.

hypothesized that periosteal distortion is painful [4,23]. Whether or not tailing is painful to the mouse, as might occur when the coccygeal periosteum, bone, and soft tissues are cut, has been evaluated and depending on the age of the mouse and the specific experimental conditions (including the strain of mouse studied [12]) different conclusions have been drawn. For example, using 4–6 week old C57BL/6 mice, a 2.5 cm amputation of the tip of the tail resulted in long-lasting hyperalgesia [29]. Using younger C57Bl/6 mice (12 and 20 days of age) and a smaller biopsy sample it was concluded that tail amputation had only minor, short-term negative effects on animal welfare [30].

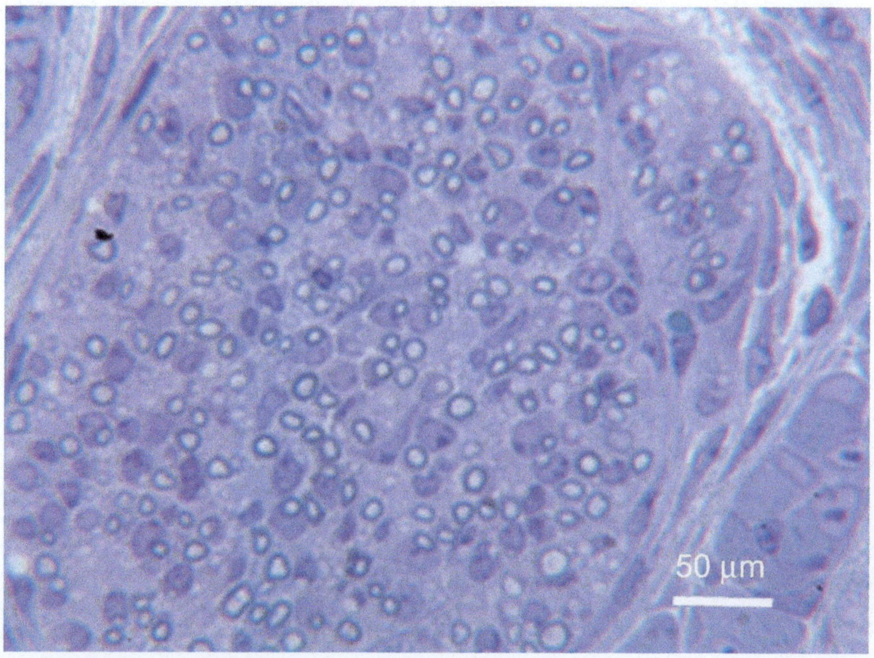

Figure 8. PPD 7, proximal biopsy site, toluidine blue stain. This cross-section shows that many of the nerve fibers are now myelinated (dark rings) and increased in number.

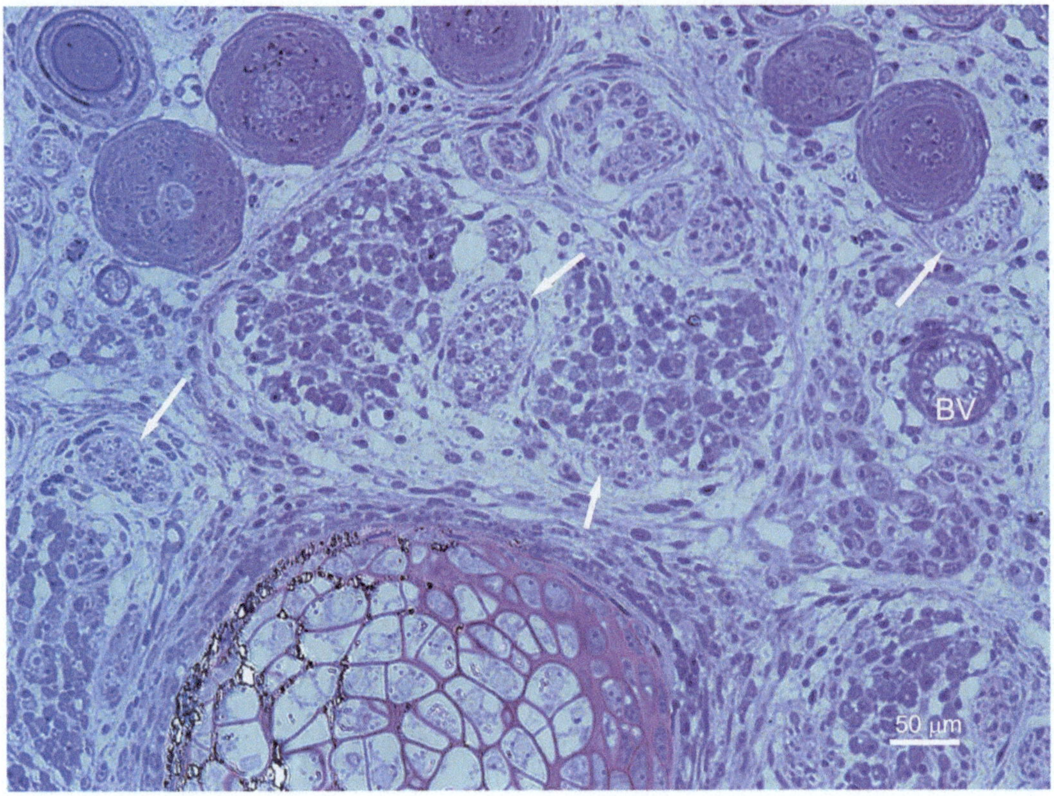

Figure 10. PPD 7, distal biopsy site, toluidine blue stain. In this cross-section the nerve has split into several distinct tracks (arrows).

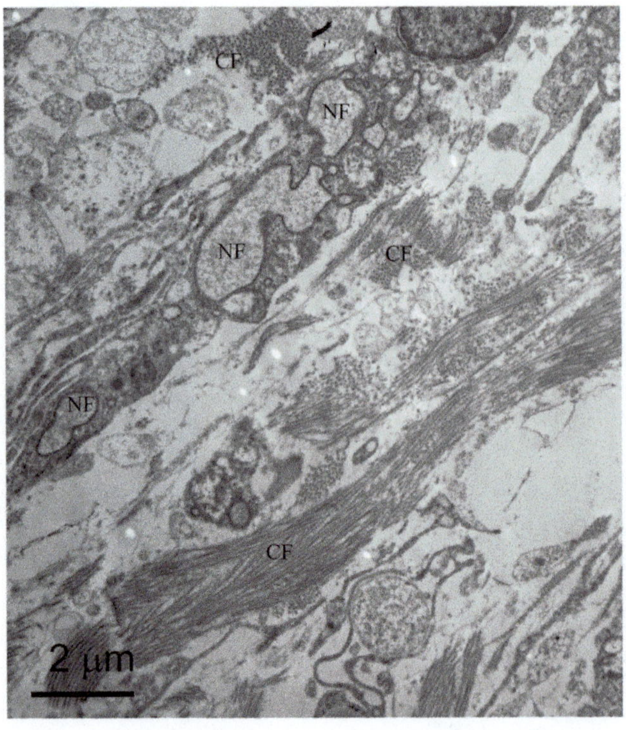

Figure 11. PPD 7, distal biopsy site, TEM. In this thin cross-section there is a nerve fiber (NF) in the periosteum surrounded by collagen filaments (CF).

As noted earlier, although we found nerve fibers in the soft tissues of the tail on the day of birth, it was not until PPD 3 that nerves were clearly identified as entering the vertebral perichondrium, and not until PPD 7 that immunostaining revealed distinct neural CGRP reactivity in the perichondrium rather than only near blood vessels. Using microcomputed tomography, Hankenson and colleagues [12] examined the coccygeal vertebrae of 3 day old C57Bl/6 mice and were unable to visualize immature vertebrae (i.e., those having nonmineralized cartilage or only a primary ossification center) in the severed end of a 2 mm tail biopsy. They did, however, visualize immature vertebrae in the severed end of a 5 mm tail biopsy (i.e., a cut made closer to the animal's body). Correlating the work of Hankenson et al. [12] with the appearance and growth of nerve fibers seen in the current study, it is tempting but nevertheless imprudent to conclude that a 5 mm tail biopsy on PPD 3– with evidence of nerve fibers alongside blood vessels and infiltrating into the vertebral perichondrium – is painful to the animal. This statement is explained further below.

An important corollary question to this study is, "When does the neonatal mouse have sufficient sentience to experience pain if its tail is biopsied?" As stated above, pain cognition is likely to be a function of central and peripheral nervous system maturation. For mice, a species that is moderately neurologically immature at birth, Mellor [31] proposed that they do not exhibit consciousness until at least 4 days of age. This hypothesis was based in part on the work of Diesch et al. [32] who, studying the electroencephalographic responses of rat pups, found pups 5–7 days of age had no electroencephalographic responses to tail clamping and concluded that their pain perception developed gradually from PPD 12 onwards. In contrast, McLaughlin et al. [33] showed that

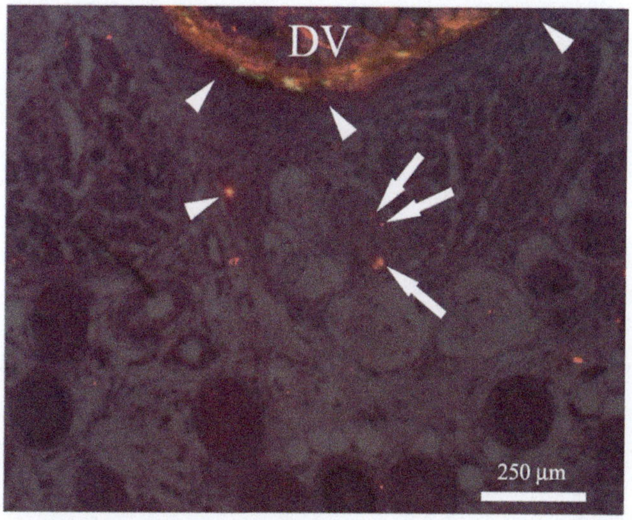

Figure 12. PPD 7, proximal biopsy site. Adjacent 1 μm LR White acrylic resin sections were merged to show both the Texas Red fluorescent image for CGRP staining and the tissue structure seen with toluidine blue staining. Arrows indicate the first evidence of CGRP staining in a nerve bundle. There is significant CGRP staining in the periosteum (arrowheads). The partial ring with diffuse reddish color in the developing vertebra (DV) is most likely CGRP staining of osteoclasts and possibly osteoblasts, resulting from the early mineralization of the vertebra.

3 day old rat pups responded to a tonic pain stimulus (formalin injection into the paw) in a manner similar to that of adult rats and suggested that this response may depend on neurosensory and neuromotor maturation rather than upon experimental conditions. Narsinghani and Anand [34], in a detailed review of pain in neonatal rats as young as PPD 0, concluded that neonates do experience pain. More recently, Fitzgerald [35] reviewed experimental evidence in rats and mice that helps support the views of Mellor [31] and Diesch [32]. She noted that a lower percentage of spinal dorsal horn neurons with nociceptive inputs are observed in the first week of life as compared to adult animals and that electrical stimulation of nociceptive C-fibers at that early age failed to evoke a synchronized spike of postsynaptic currents in the dorsal horn of the spinal cord. C-fiber activation occurs as the animal matures. There are large diameter Aδ fibers present at birth; however, Aδ fibers require a longer postnatal period to acquire their full stimulus-response sensitivity, which corresponds to their developing myelination [35]. Additional pain recognition considerations are that neurotransmitter (such as Substance P) release is not consistent in early age neonates and that certain C-fiber synapses within the spinal cord occur as late as PPD 5 [35]. The last finding suggests that "despite the ability of polymodal nociceptors to signal noxious events in the periphery, central nociceptive processing is immature in the postnatal period" [35]. Recently, Davidson and colleagues [36] demonstrated that the spinothalamic tract axons of CD-1 mice reach the brain before birth and exhibit morphological features of functionality while continuing to increase in diameter until PPD 7. Notwithstanding, central nociceptive processing at the level of the brain may remain immature in the neonatal rodent. For example, the expression of Fos protein, an indicator of nociception, did not increase in the brain of PPD 0 rats after an injection of formalin into the paw. It was not until PPD 14 that thalamic labeling was seen in areas generally considered to be involved with the sensation of pain [37].

Our primary research goal was to determine the age at which nerve fibers, and in particular nociceptive fibers, first entered the developing bones of the mouse coccygeal vertebrae. At the level of the proximal biopsy site we found that this occurs in the developing periosteum between PPD 3 and PPD 7. It seems reasonable that the highly innervated developing bone of the coccygeal vertebrae, even when cartilaginous, could contribute to increased pain when a mouse's tail is injured during the tailing procedure. However, in a neonatal mouse or rat, particularly prior to approximately 12 days of age, a nociceptive stimulus may not result in the conscious perception of pain due to the lack of a competent pain pathway at this age. Using microcomputed tomography on 5 mm tail biopsies from C57BL/6 mice, Hankenson et al. [12] detected immature coccygeal vertebrae at PPD 3 and mature vertebrae at PPD 17 and concluded that tail biopsies for genotyping should preferably be taken at about PPD 14–17. Full neural development in the tail would likely be present at 14–17 days of age but cutting the somewhat less ossified tissue (as compared to after PPD 17) might be less traumatic and subsequently less painful to the animals. Yet, given the potential for true pain perception in rats after PPD 12–14 [32,37] it would be prudent to consider the use of less invasive alternatives than tailing when collecting tissue for the genotyping of mice. [38–40].

Acknowledgments

The authors are grateful to Ms. Michelle Bombard for her technical expertise and Drs. J. Michael Wyss and Lisa G. Barber for their reviews of this manuscript and associated helpful suggestions.

Author Contributions

Conceived and designed the experiments: JS GH. Performed the experiments: GH. Analyzed the data: JS GH. Contributed reagents/materials/analysis tools: JS GH. Wrote the paper: JS GH.

References

1. Morales ME, Gereau RW (2009) The effects of tail biopsy for genotyping on behavioral responses to nociceptive stimuli. PLoS One doi: 10.1371/journal.pone.0006457.
2. Bonaparte (Convenor) D, Cinelli P, Douni E, Hérault Y, Maas A, et al. (2013) FELASA guidelines for the refinement of methods for genotyping genetically-modified rodents. A report of the Federation of European Laboratory Animal Science Associations Working Group. Lab Anim 47: 134–145.
3. Calvo W, Forteza-Vila J (1969) On the development of bone marrow innervation in new-born rats and studied with silver impregnation and electron microscopy. Am J Anat 126: 355–372.
4. Mach DB, Rogers SD, Sabino MC, Luger NM, Schwei MJ, et al. (2002) Origins of skeletal pain: sensory and sympathetic innervation of the mouse femur. Neuroscience 113: 155–156.
5. Hukkanen M, Konttinen YT, Santavirta S, Paavolainen P, Gu XH, et al. (1993) Rapid proliferation of calcitonin gene-related peptide-immunoreactive nerves during healing of rat tibial fracture suggests neural involvement in bone growth and remodeling. Neuroscience 54: 969–979.
6. Spencer GJ, Hitchcock IS, Genever PG (2004) Emerging neuroskeletal signaling pathways: a review. FEBS Lett 559: 6–12.
7. Gajda M, Litwin JA, Cichocki T, Timmermans J-P, Adriaensen D (2005) Development of sensory innervation in rat tibia: co-localization of CGRP and substance P with growth-associated protein 43 (GAP-43). J Anat 207: 135–144.
8. Hunter C, Clegg EJ (1973) The effects of hypoxia on the caudal vertebrae of growing mice and rats. J Anat 116: 227–244.
9. Feik SA, Storey D (1983) Remodelling of bone and bones: growth of normal and transplanted caudal vertebrae. J Anat 136: 1–14.
10. Jerome C, Hoch G (2012) Skeletal System. In: Treuting PM, Dintzis SM, editors. Comparative anatomy and histology: A mouse and human atlas. Amsterdam: Academic Press. 53–70.
11. Shinohara H (1999) The mouse vertebrae: changes in the morphology of mouse vertebrae exhibit specific patterns over limited numbers of vertebral levels. Okajimas Folia Anat Jpn 76(1): 17–31.
12. Hankenson FC, Garzel LM, Fischer DD, Nolan B, Hankenson KD (2008) Evaluation of tail biopsy collection in laboratory nice (*Mus musculus*): vertebral

ossification, DNA quantity, and acute behavioral responses. J Am Assoc Lab Anim Sci 47: 10–18.
13. Todd ME, Tokito MK (1981) An ultrastructural investigation of developing vasomotor innervation in rat peripheral vessels. Am J Anat 160: 195–212.
14. Karas A, Silverman J (2007) Pain and Distress. In: Silverman J, Suckow MA, Murthy S, editors. The IACUC Handbook, 2nd edition. Boca Raton: CRC Press. 241–286.
15. Committee for the Update of the Guide for the Care and Use of Laboratory Animals (2011) Guide for the care and use of laboratory animals, 8th edition. Washington, D.C.: The National Academies Press. 220 p.
16. Henneneberger C, Grantyn R, Rothe T (2000) Rapid genotyping of newborn gene mutant mice. J Neurosci Methods 100: 123–126.
17. Zaidi M, Pazianas M, Shankar V, Bax B, Bax C, et al. (1993) Osteoclast function and its control. Exp Physiol 78: 721–739.
18. Naot D, Cornish J (2008) The role of peptides and receptors of the calcitonin family in the regulation of bone metabolism. Bone 43: 813–818.
19. Patton JT, Kaufman MH (1995) The timing of ossification of the limb bones, and growth rates of various long bones of the fore and hind limbs of the prenatal and early postnatal laboratory mouse. J Anat 186: 175–185.
20. Bjurholm A, Kreicbergs A, Brodin E, Schultzberg M (1988) Substance P- and CGRP-immunorective nerves in bone. Peptides 9: 165–171.
21. Ohtori S, Inoue G, Koshi T, Ito T, Yamashita M, et al. (2007) Characteristics of sensory dorsal root ganglia neurons innervating the lumbar vertebral body in rats. J Pain 8: 483–488.
22. Orita S, Ohtori S, Taniguchi A, Yamashita M, Yamauchi K, et al. (2010) Direct evidence for sensory innervation of the dorsal portion of the Co5/6 coccygeal intervertebral disc in rats. Spine 35: 1346–1352.
23. Martin CD, Jimenez-Andrade JM, Ghilardi JR, Mantyh PW (2007) Organization of a unique net-like meshwork of CGRP+ sensory fibers in the mouse periosteum: implications for the generation and maintenance of bone fracture pain. Neurosci Lett 427: 148–152.
24. Jimenez-Andrade JM, Bloom AP, Mantyh WG, Koewler NJ, Freemen KT, et al. (2009) Capsaicin-sensitive sensory nerve fibers contribute to the generation and maintenance of skeletal fracture pain. Neuroscience 162: 1244–1254.
25. Koshi T, Ohtori S, Inoue G, Ito T, Yamashita M, et al. (2010) Lumbar postereolateral fusion inhibits sensory nerve ingrowth into punctured lumbar intervertebral discs and upregulation of CGRP immunoreactive DRG neuron innervating punctured discs in rats. Eur Spine J 19: 593–600.
26. Sisask G, Bjurholm A, Ahmed M, Kreicbergs A (1995) Ontogeny of sensory nerves in the developing skeleton. Anat Rec 243: 234–240.
27. Julius D, Basbaum A (2001) Molecular mechanisms of nociception. Nature 413: 203–210.
28. Jimenez-Andrade JM, Mantyh W, Bloom AP, Xu H, Ferng AS, et al. (2009) A phenotypically restricted set of primary afferent nerve fibers innervate the bone versus skin: Therapeutic opportunity for treating skeletal pain. Bone 46: 306–313. doi:10.1016/j.bone.2009.09.013.
29. Zhuo M (1998) NMDA receptor-dependent long term hyperalgesia after tail amputation in mice. Eur J Pharma col 349: 211–220.
30. SØrensen DB, Stub C, Jensen HE, Ritskes-Hoitinga M, Hjorth P, et al. (2006) The impact of tail tip amputation and ink tattoo on C567BL/6BomTac mice. Lab Anim 41: 19–29.
31. Mellor DJ (2010) Galloping colts, fetal feelings, and reassuring regulations: Putting animal-welfare science into practice. J Vet Med Educ 37: 94–100.
32. Diesch TJ, Mellor DJ, Johnson CB, Lentle RG (2009) Electroencephalographic responses to tail clamping in anaesthetized rat pups. Lab Anim 43: 224–231.
33. McLaughlin CR, Lichtman AH, Fanselow MS, Cramer CP (1990) Tonic nociception in neonatal rats. Pharmacol Biochem Be 36: 859–862.
34. Narsinghani U, Anand KJS (2000) Developmental neurobiology of pain in neonatal rats. Lab Anim (NY) 29(9): 27–39.
35. Fitzgerald M (2005) The development of nociceptive circuits. Nat Rev Neuroscience 6: 507–520.
36. Davidson S, Truong H, Giesler Jr G (2010) A quantitative analysis of spinothalamic tract neurons in adult and developing mouse. J Comp Neurol 518: 3193–3204.
37. Barr GA (2011) Formalin-induced c-fos expression in the brain of infant rats. J Pain 12: 263–271.
38. Irwin MH, Moffatt RJ, Pinkert CA (1996) Identification of transgenic mice by PCR analysis of saliva. Nat Biotechnol 14: 1146–1148.
39. Schmitteckert EM, Prokop CM, Hedrich HJ (1999) DNA detection in hair of transgenic mice – a simple technique minimizing the distress on the animals. Lab Anim 33: 385–380.
40. Meldgaard M, Bollen PJ, Finsen B (2004) Noninvasive method for sampling and extraction of mouse DNA for PCR. Lab Anim 38: 413–417.

16

Cortical Thickness Mapping to Identify Focal Osteoporosis in Patients with Hip Fracture

Kenneth E. S. Poole[1]*, Graham M. Treece[2], Paul M. Mayhew[1], Jan Vaculík[3], Pavel Dungl[3], Martin Horák[4], Jan J. Štěpán[5], Andrew H. Gee[2]

1 Department of Medicine, University of Cambridge, Cambridge, Cambridgeshire, United Kingdom, **2** Department of Engineering, University of Cambridge, Cambridge, Cambridgeshire, United Kingdom, **3** Department of Orthopaedics, Faculty of Medicine, Charles University Prague and Bulovka Hospital, Prague, Czech Republic, **4** Department of Radiology, Homolka Hospital, Prague, Czech Republic, **5** Department of Rheumatology, Faculty of Medicine 1, Charles University Prague and Institute of Rheumatology, Prague, Czech Republic

Abstract

Background: Individuals with osteoporosis are predisposed to hip fracture during trips, stumbles or falls, but half of all hip fractures occur in those without generalised osteoporosis. By analysing ordinary clinical CT scans using a novel cortical thickness mapping technique, we discovered patches of markedly thinner bone at fracture-prone regions in the femurs of women with acute hip fracture compared with controls.

Methods: We analysed CT scans from 75 female volunteers with acute fracture and 75 age- and sex-matched controls. We classified the fracture location as femoral neck or trochanteric before creating bone thickness maps of the outer 'cortical' shell of the intact contra-lateral hip. After registration of each bone to an average femur shape and statistical parametric mapping, we were able to visualise and quantify statistically significant foci of thinner cortical bone associated with each fracture type, assuming good symmetry of bone structure between the intact and fractured hip. The technique allowed us to pinpoint systematic differences and display the results on a 3D average femur shape model.

Findings: The cortex was generally thinner in femoral neck fracture cases than controls. More striking were several discrete patches of statistically significant thinner bone of up to 30%, which coincided with common sites of fracture initiation (femoral neck or trochanteric).

Interpretation: Femoral neck fracture patients had a thumbnail-sized patch of focal osteoporosis at the upper head-neck junction. This region coincided with a weak part of the femur, prone to both spontaneous 'tensile' fractures of the femoral neck, and as a site of crack initiation when falling sideways. Current hip fracture prevention strategies are based on case finding: they involve clinical risk factor estimation to determine the need for single-plane bone density measurement within a standard region of interest (ROI) of the femoral neck. The precise sites of focal osteoporosis that we have identified are overlooked by current 2D bone densitometry methods.

Editor: Xing-Ming Shi, Georgia Health Sciences University, United States of America

Funding: This analysis was funded by Arthritis Research UK via a Clinician Scientist Fellowship award to KESP. Cambridge National Institute for Health Research Biomedical Research Centre funded PMM. The Evelyn Trust funded GMT. The funders had no role in study design, data collection and analysis, decision to publish, or preparation of the manuscript.

Competing Interests: GMT and KESP are co-inventors on a related GB patent application A method of determining the cortical thickness of a patients bone (GB0917524.1 Accurate cortical thickness measurement from clinical CT data, A method of determining the cortical thickness of a patients bone. International (PCT) Patent Application No PCT/GB2010/051671, CU ref: TRE-2326-09-01, International search ref: PC925159WO. Title: Image data processing systems, Inventors: G.M. Treece & K.E.S Poole). The other authors have declared that no competing interests exist.

* E-mail: kp254@nhs.net

Introduction

The annual incidence of hip fractures is projected to rise fourfold to 6.3 million worldwide by 2050, because of the exponentially increasing risk of fracture as people live longer. Studying femoral neck and trochanteric fractures is therefore a health priority [1]. In older people, the proximal femur breaks when the loads placed on it overcome its strength, with common loading scenarios being sideways falls, stumbles or sudden unusual movements [2]. However, a spontaneous or 'impact-free' mechanism accounts for up to 6% of hip fractures (fig. 1) [3,4]. We know that women with osteoporosis (who have generally thinner and more porous bones) are more likely to suffer hip fracture, but most people who will sustain hip fracture do not have generalised osteoporosis [5]. We also know that the outer 'cortical' bone of the femur where fractures initiate [6] thins rapidly with age [7,8], is a key determinant of bone strength and fracture risk [9–13] and responds well to certain osteoporosis drugs [14,15]. Here we ask; Is there a pattern of femoral bone thinning common to hip fracture patients and, if so, is it generalised or focal? Could focal osteoporosis of the femur be a cause of hip fracture in the elderly? The answer to these questions might illuminate why hip fractures tend to initiate in particular zones (fig. 1).

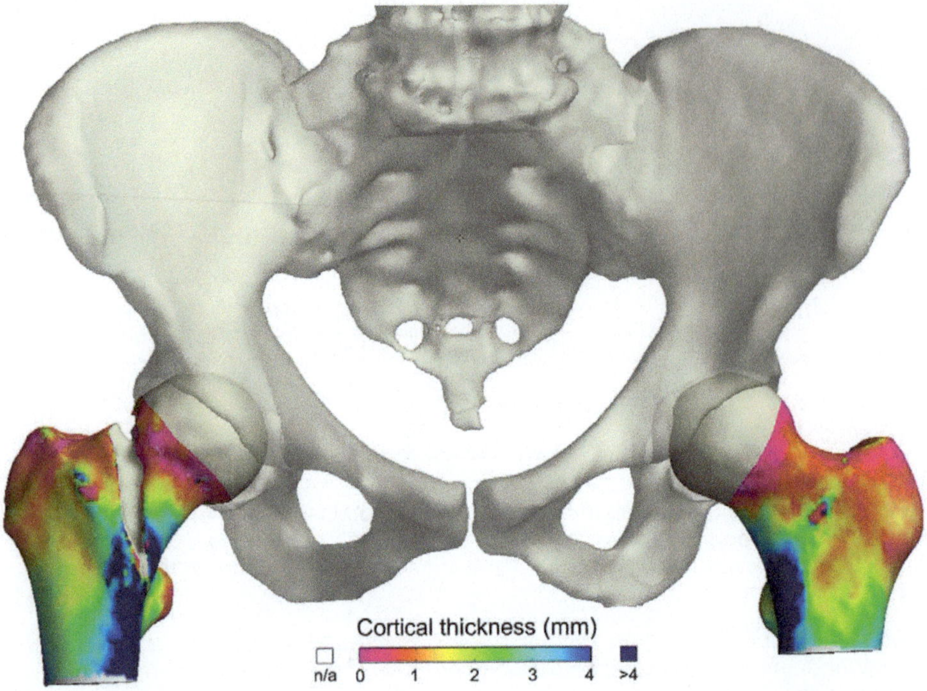

Figure 1. Cortical Thickness Colour Mapping using ordinary clinical CT data. Femora and pelvis from an 84-year-old osteoporotic female who sustained a fracture without falling. She felt her right hip break as she placed her right foot on a low step. Femoral neck BMD was 0.46 g/cm2, T score −3.3. From the Arthritis Research UK FEMCO study (07/H0305/61).

A new CT image processing technique [16] allows us to display cortical thickness as a colour map over the bone surface, with several thousand independent measurements across each proximal femur and sufficient sensitivity to detect even small differences (~30 microns) when expressed systematically by a suitably sized cohort. We use it here to pinpoint differences in bone thickness between women with and without hip fracture. We examined the contra-lateral side as a surrogate for the broken hip in these female fracture patients, having previously identified symmetry in femoral neck cortical thickness [8].

Methods

From 2006 to 2009, women admitted to Bulovka University Hospital, Prague with an acute hip fracture were consented to the pragmatic 'Surgical treatment of the hip joint in trauma' study (PI Professor P Dungl), part of which involved a clinical CT scan of both hips before surgical fixation [17]. Participants were positioned on the Siemens two-compartment Osteo phantom and a single CT scan (either Siemens Sensation 40 or 16 detector, B10/20 kernel, ≤1 mm reconstructed slice thickness) was performed including both hips from above the acetabulum to just below the lesser trochanter. Women were aged over 50, were awaiting surgical repair of a cervical or trochanteric fracture and had sustained a low energy injury. Women were excluded if they had metalwork in either hip, high trauma injury, metastatic cancer, unilateral bone disease, subtrochanteric fracture or terminal illness. Using the same criteria, a convenience control sample of older women without fracture was recruited by invitation at rheumatology clinics and two residential care centres in the same districts of Prague. From 204 invitations, 108 fracture-free women responded of whom 81 were eligible for CT scanning at Homolka hospital, Prague (Siemens Sensation 16 detector B20 kernel, ≤1mm reconstructed slice thickness). At the image quality control step, 6 scans were excluded (due to insufficient scan length or undisclosed metalwork) leaving 75 female controls. One age-matched case was selected for each of the 75 eligible control participants, from the total sample of 242 women with hip fracture. Where precise birth year age matching was not possible, the next nearest matching case was selected up to a maximum 5-year age difference. The final sample taken forward for cortical thickness mapping comprised 150 femurs from 75 women in each group (mean ages of femoral neck fracture cases 78.1+/−7.1 years, trochanteric fracture cases 75.2+/−7.9, controls 76.6+/−7.3 years). There were 36 femoral neck fractures and 39 trochanteric fractures.

The analysis method is illustrated in figure 2. Anonymised axial dicom images were received in Cambridge via the secure DICOM internet connection ePACS (ICZ, Brno, Czech Rep.) where they were reconstructed to classify fracture side and site according to AO criteria. Standard clinical hip bone density (2D areal DXA-equivalent) was measured in the 'total hip' region of interest (ROI) of each femur using QCTpro software (v4.2.3 Mindways, Austin, Texas, USA). The unfractured contralateral hip (or matching side in controls) was segmented semi-automatically in Stradwin v4.2 software (Treece, Gee, Cambridge) before mapping cortical thickness at approximately 6000 surface points per femur. Cortical thickness was estimated from the CT data using the method described by Treece et al. [16]. By making reasonable assumptions about both the anatomy and the imaging blur, thickness can be measured to super-resolution accuracy across the entire proximal femur, apart from at the femoral head where the proximity of the acetabulum is problematic. The methodology has been validated against thickness measurements obtained from high resolution micro-CT scans of cadaveric femurs [16]. Analysis of the 150 thickness maps followed established practice within the neuroimaging community, who have pioneered techniques for statistical inference from dense, spatially correlated data. To account for variations in inter-subject morphology, each map was spatially realigned with a canonical femur surface using a B-spline free-form deformation calculated by the iterative closest point registration algorithm [18]. The spatially normalized maps were then smoothed with a 10 mm full-width-half-maximum filter. We investigated differences in cortical thickness between i) femoral neck fractures (n36) and all controls or ii) trochanteric fractures (n39) and all controls. Formal inference was accomplished by statistical parametric mapping (SPM) [19], as implemented in the SurfStat package [20]. Model effects were group (case*control), age, height and weight. Missing height and weight values (2 fracture cases) were replaced with group mean values. T-statistics were calculated to test the significance of the group term. Random field theory then furnished p-values, corrected for multiple comparisons to control the overall image-wise chance of false positives. Figure 3 shows corrected p maps based on the magnitude of peaks (sensitive to focal effects) and on the extent of connected clusters exceeding an uncorrected p-value threshold of 0.001 (sensitive to distributed effects). All participants with fracture gave written informed consent. Control participants gave verbal consent which was documented in the medical notes as agreed with the Ethics Committee. Ethics committees approved the study in the Czech Republic (Ethical Committee of the Institute of Rheumatology and Ethical Committee of Bulovka Hospital, ref IRB0002384101) and in the UK (Cambridgeshire 4, ref 07/H0305/61).

Results

Percentage differences in cortical thickness between each hip fracture group and the control group were displayed on an average right femur surface map using a colour scale. Views from several anatomical planes were chosen to illustrate the differences (femoral neck fractures vs. controls; fig. 3 *left upper panel* and trochanteric fractures vs controls; fig. 3 *right upper panel*). Similar maps were created to visualise the statistical significance of differences (fig 3. *lower panels*). Several distinct patches of up to 30% thinner cortical bone were identified in fracture cases which coincided with typical sites of hip fracture. No regions of statistically significant thicker bone were seen in fracture cases. WHO-defined osteoporosis (a total hip DXA-equivalent bone mineral density T score <-2.5) was present in less than half of hip fracture patients (31/75, 41.3%) and 9/75 (12%) controls. The age, height and weight adjusted values for the clusters of thinner bone associated with each fracture type are shown in table 1. The mean, unadjusted value of whole proximal femur cortical thickness among femoral neck fracture patients was 1.20 mm$\pm$0.17 mm, compared with a value of 1.25 mm$\pm$0.20 mm among trochanteric fracture patients and 1.30 mm$\pm$0.21 mm among controls (ANOVA $p = 0.0388$). Whole femur cortical thickness was statistically significantly lower in femoral neck fracture compared with control (Dunnett's values* were 0.012 for neck fracture, $p = 0.024$, and -0.04 for trochanteric fracture, $p = 0.34$; *[absolute difference in sample means] - [least significant difference]). The age and weight terms were significant within the 150 femurs (age range 55–98 and weight range 40–89 kg). Significant thinning of approximately 0.02 mm per year from age 55–98 was apparent in the infero-medial region. Significant thickening of approximately 0.02 mm per kilogram was evident in a similar infero-medial region.

Discussion

We used cortical thickness mapping to explore differences between women with and without recent hip fracture and identified generalised thinning of the femoral cortex in fracture patients. We also discovered focal differences manifest as several well-defined patches of markedly thinner femoral cortex in hip fracture patients compared to controls. Since osteoporosis is defined as microarchitectural deterioration of bone tissue, we consider that these areas of focally thinner bone are best described as patches of focal osteoporosis (fig. 4, right panel). The patches were evident at common sites involved in fracture, the most severe being a thumbnail-sized patch of up to 30% thinner bone at the head-neck junction in patients with femoral neck fracture (figs. 3, 4 and 5). Focal osteoporosis at the head-neck junction may play an important role in fractures associated with falls, and might even be involved in 'spontaneous' hip fracture on rare occasions. While the locations of the patches of focal osteoporosis appear to be critical in determining fracture type, we cannot judge whether they are involved in causing hip fracture, which requires prospective research. However it is noteworthy that among all the bone structural parameters measured in the largest prospective study of hip CT in older men and women conducted to date, cortical thickness estimates from a supero-anterior part of the femoral neck were the best predictor of subsequent hip fracture [9].

We assume that a fall onto or near the hip was the principal fracture mechanism in these women, but we did not routinely collect information on how these women fell, a priority for future work. The largest patch of thinner femoral cortex that we identified (fig 3c) appears to correspond to a key site of fracture initiation in a simulation of femoral neck fracture during a sideways fall to the ground [21]. Although the women we studied with trochanteric fracture also had patches of thinner bone in

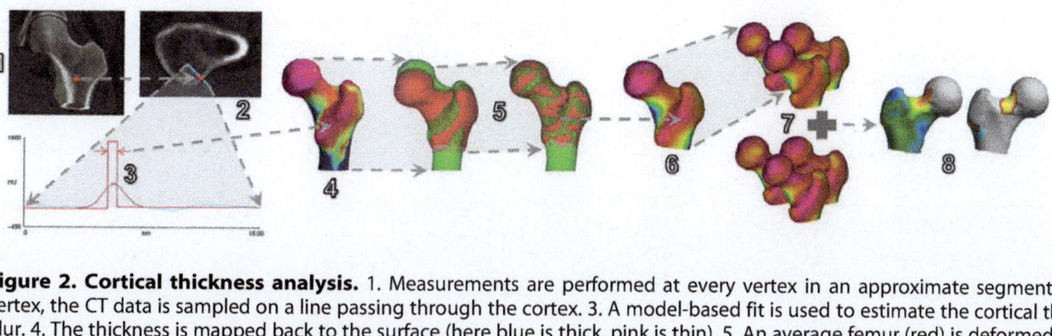

Figure 2. Cortical thickness analysis. 1. Measurements are performed at every vertex in an approximate segmentation of the hip. 2. At each vertex, the CT data is sampled on a line passing through the cortex. 3. A model-based fit is used to estimate the cortical thickness, allowing for image blur. 4. The thickness is mapped back to the surface (here blue is thick, pink is thin). 5. An average femur (red) is deformed to match the current femur (green). 6. Thickness estimates are then transferred to the average femoral surface and smoothed. 7. This process is repeated for all subjects, producing subject-specific thickness estimates all mapped to the same, average surface. 8. The data is analysed using statistical parametric mapping, to obtain mean thickness differences between groups and also the significance of these differences.

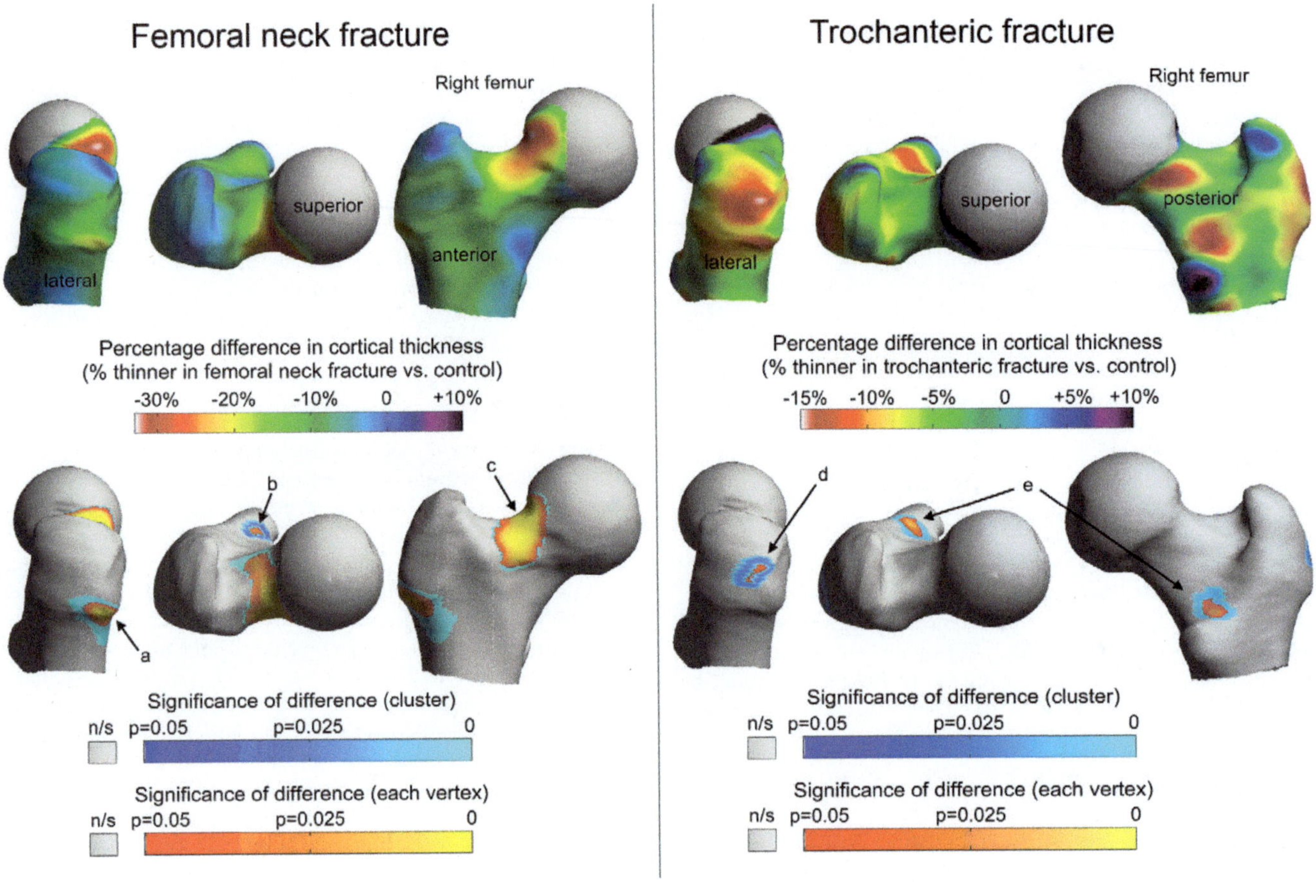

Figure 3. Results for femoral neck fracture (left) and trochanteric fracture (right). Upper colour maps show the average percentage difference in cortical thickness for each fracture type versus control (displayed on an average right femur model). The lower colour maps are the significance of the differences adjusted for age, height and weight, either point by point (vertex) or as a whole patch (blue clusters). Note that all the blue clusters extend uninterrupted beneath their respective orange/yellow vertices. Table 1 gives adjusted thickness values and significance of the clusters a–e.

fracture-relevant zones (fig. 3d and 3e), it is not clear whether they correspond to trochanteric fracture initiation sites in the relevant simulations [21]. Nevertheless, it is interesting to note that the focally thin bone in the lateral facet of the greater trochanter (fig. 3d) in the trochanteric fracture patients coincided with one of the insertion sites of gluteus medius, which receives considerable force during locomotion.

While most hip fractures in the elderly are a result of injurious falls, spontaneous fractures of the femoral neck prior to falls have been implicated in up to 6% of cases, translating to more than

Table 1. Details of thinner patches of femoral cortex in hip fracture.

Hip fracture type	**Location of 'cluster' Patch where bone cortex was thinner in hip fracture cases**	**Mean adjusted cortical thickness in cluster (Cases)**		**Mean adjusted cortical thickness in cluster (Cluster)**		**p value for difference**
		Millimetres	**±SD**	**Millimetres**	**±SD**	
Femoral neck fractures						
Patch a (fig.3a)	Greater trochanter	1.14	0.15	1.34	0.26	0.00407
Patch b (fig.3b)	Lesser trochanter	0.85	0.16	0.98	0.19	0.0319
Patch c (fig.3c)	Head-neck junction	0.62	0.10	0.77	0.14	0.00000350
Trochanteric fractures						
Patch d (fig.3d)	Greater trochanter	1.05	0.25	1.21	0.27	0.0237
Patch e (fig.3e)	Lesser trochanter	0.78	0.15	0.88	0.17	0.0108

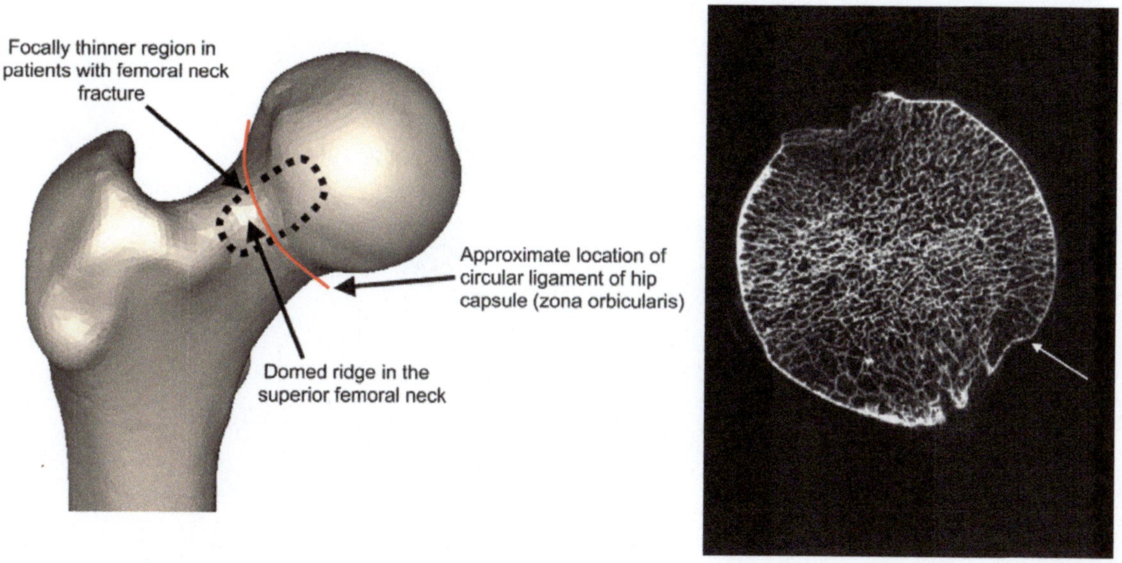

Figure 4. Anatomical context of focal thinning in women with femoral neck fracture. The left pane is a right proximal femur model seen from the front. The thin patch of cortex (fig 3c) in femoral neck fracture patients occurs on the domed ridge called the femoral neck eminence [25]. The right pane is a high resolution CT image through the femoral head of a 90 year old female (aBMD total hip T-score −1.9) which suggests that the patch is osteoporotic with microarchitectural thinning (white arrow). Femur courtesy of the Melbourne Femur Collection, Chairman Professor John Clement (Melbourne Dental School).

4000 hip fractures annually in the UK [22]. Previously, several research groups have reproduced these impact-free hip fractures in cadaveric femurs by simulating either the effects of increasing loads in stance or sudden large hip flexor muscle contractions. In Cristofolini's specimens, increasing the load by simulating one-legged stance (as in fig. 5b), led to crack initiation at the junction between the femoral head and neck, with the subsequent catastrophic failure of the femur closely resembling that observed in our patient with impact-free fracture (fig. 1) [3]. Likewise simulating sudden psoas muscle contraction (as happens when a person attempts to stabilise their trunk on a fixed leg during a slip or stumble) led to subcapital fracture in a similar location [23]. The conserved patch of focal osteoporosis we identified among our femoral neck fracture patients (fig. 3c) appears to correspond with the sites of high tensile stress induced in those simulations. In the light of our findings we wonder what effect osteoporosis medicines might have on the thin patches of bone and in particular if strengthening the thin areas could prevent stumbling-induced or spontaneous hip fractures. Analysis of large clinical trials with serial CT is needed to address this question.

We are currently unable to answer a key question generated by these results; namely how did the focal patches of thin cortex arise? Several intriguing ideas come from histological and macroscopic studies of the head-neck junction in patients with fracture and from cadavers. Freeman et al. discovered that in fracture specimens, the underlying bone from the head-neck junction frequently contains microcallus, considered to be evidence of tensile fatigue damage [24]. Modelling the behaviour of the head-neck junction during habitual locomotion and falls is therefore a priority for biomechanics research. Although there were marked age and weight effects within the women we studied, the decreasing cortical thickness associated with age and increasing thickness associated with weight affected the inferior femur; i.e. on the opposite side of the femoral neck to the patch of focally thin bone. Thus we assume that neither younger nor heavier women were necessarily protected from having a thin cortex at the head-neck junction. The patch of focal osteoporosis in femoral neck fracture patients corresponds macroscopically with the junction between femoral head cartilage and bone, and tracks along the domed ridge running along the top of the femoral neck (called the femoral neck eminentia, or eminence [25], fig. 4). Since the thin cortical bone is so well circumscribed at this site, we concur with Panzer et al. in describing the differences as 'focal osteoporosis', but acknowledge that higher resolution and histological studies would be useful to further characterise the cortical and sub-cortical bone [26]. The circular fibres of the hip capsule (the zona orbicularis) also encircle the femoral neck at the focally thin patch. Pitt and others described a mechanical, abrasive action of the overlying hip capsule, ligaments and psoas muscle at this patch that commonly results in a 'reaction area' with occasional underlying radiolucency. This lucency can be appreciated on plain x-rays and is known to radiologists as 'Pitt's Pit' [27]. Studies of the underlying histology of this zone in femoral neck fracture cases are clearly warranted [28,29], and Pitt suggested that the zone could be involved in hip fracture pathogenesis.

This work has several weaknesses, namely pragmatic case selection, the use of a convenience sample of controls and reliance on the intact hip as a surrogate for the fractured hip. The results need replication in a better-characterised population sample, with particular attention to recalled injury mechanism. Statistical Parametric Mapping does not indicate causality; for instance it is possible (but unlikely) that controls could have substantial thickening of bone at various sites through unknown mechanisms. Finally, although studying the cortex is important in determining bone strength, alternative methods such as finite element (FE) models use whole bone biomechanics, and can therefore be informative in determining how and why individuals fracture their hips (as reviewed recently by Cristofolini et al [30]). In this regard, it is interesting to note that our cortical thickness maps have the potential to be converted into inner and outer surfaces for optimal delineation of cortical and trabecular compartments, which may

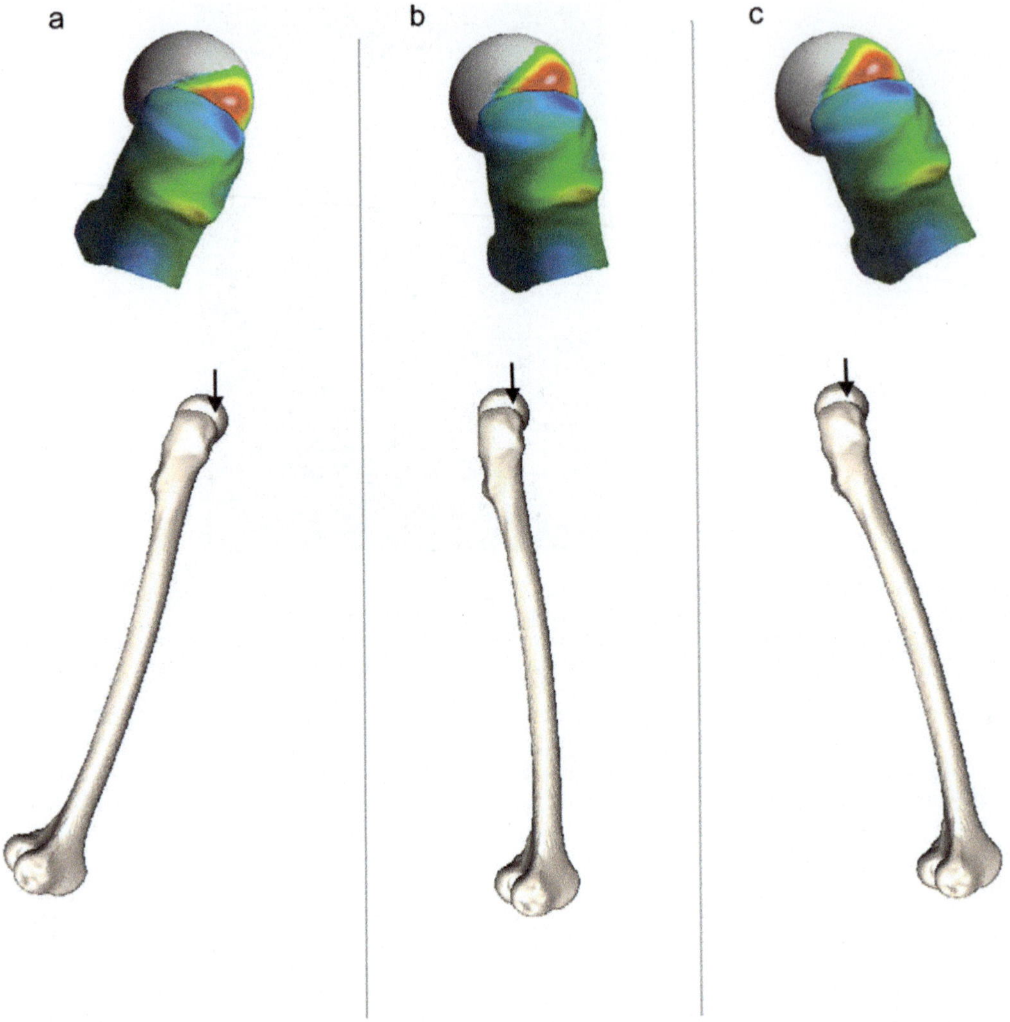

Figure 5. Approximate orientation of the focally thin (red) zone during the different phases of gait. Right femur (a) toe-off, (b) single leg stance and (c) heel strike. A slightly modified stance position (b) conferred the greatest risk of spontaneous femoral neck fracture in the laboratory simulations of Cristofolini et al [3]. The focally thin patch we identified coincides with a region of high tensile stress during simulations of spontaneous fracture.

help to improve the FE methods that currently assume a constant cortical thickness throughout the bone.

In related work, Li et al applied SPM to 3D density maps of femurs and discovered focal regions where clustered voxels of bone density differed significantly between hip fracture cases and controls [31]. In their analysis, several fracture-relevant density ROI's showed promise in defining a hip fracture phenotype. The fact that Li's head-neck junction femoral ROI based on volumetric density appears to coincide with the focally thinner femoral cortex we find at the head-neck junction suggests that having poor quality bone here is particularly concerning for future fracture risk. Previous prospective studies indicated that combining measures (e.g one measure of density, one of cortical thickness and one of bone shape) resulted in the optimum prediction of incident hip fracture [11,32]. However, large prospective studies are necessary to determine what thresholds of cortical thickness or density in these newly discovered zones are predictive of hip fracture and might be a trigger for intervention in an individual. Our work is useful in defining ROI's for cortical bone analysis that can then be taken forward for testing in prospective studies. Current hip fracture prevention strategies are based on case finding: they involve clinical risk factor estimation to determine the need for single plane bone density measurement within a standard femoral neck ROI. The precise sites of focal osteoporosis that we have now identified are overlooked by current 2D bone densitometry methods.

Acknowledgments

We thank Dr Jonathan Reeve, Department of Medicine, University of Cambridge, UK for his help with the Prague-Cambridge collaboration and for guidance on the selection of appropriate control participants.

Author Contributions

Conceived and designed the experiments: KESP PMM JS MH JV PD GMT AHG. Performed the experiments: KESP PMM GMT AHG. Analyzed the data: KESP AHG GMT. Contributed reagents/materials/analysis tools: JS MH JV PD PMM. Wrote the paper: KESP GMT AHG PMM JS MH JV PD. Designed the study to recruit patients with hip fracture in Prague: JV PD. Methods section critical review: JV PD.

References

1. Pulkkinen P, Gluer CC, Jamsa T (2011) Investigation of differences between hip fracture types: a worthy strategy for improved risk assessment and fracture prevention. Bone 49: 600–604.
2. Sievanen H, Kannus P, Jarvinen TL (2007) Bone quality: an empty term. PLoS Med 4: e27.
3. Cristofolini L, Juszczyk M, Martelli S, Taddei F, Viceconti M (2007) In vitro replication of spontaneous fractures of the proximal human femur. J Biomech 40: 2837–2845.
4. Yli-Kyyny T, Tamminen I, Syri J, Venesmaa P, Kröger H (2011) Bilateral hip pain. The Lancet 377: 2248.
5. Wainwright SA, Marshall LM, Ensrud KE, Cauley JA, Black DM, et al. (2005) Hip fracture in women without osteoporosis. J Clin Endocrinol Metab 90: 2787–2793.
6. de Bakker PM, Manske SL, Ebacher V, Oxland TR, Cripton PA, et al. (2009) During sideways falls proximal femur fractures initiate in the superolateral cortex: evidence from high-speed video of simulated fractures. J Biomech 42: 1917–1925.
7. Feik SA, Thomas CD, Clement JG (1997) Age-related changes in cortical porosity of the midshaft of the human femur. J Anat 191 (Pt 3): 407–416.
8. Poole KE, Mayhew PM, Rose CM, Brown JK, Bearcroft PJ, et al. (2010) Changing structure of the femoral neck across the adult female lifespan. J Bone Miner Res 25: 482–491.
9. Johannesdottir F, Poole KE, Reeve J, Siggeirsdottir K, Aspelund T, et al. (2011) Distribution of cortical bone in the femoral neck and hip fracture: a prospective case-control analysis of 143 incident hip fractures; the AGES-REYKJAVIK Study. Bone 48: 1268–1276.
10. Mayhew PM, Thomas CD, Clement JG, Loveridge N, Beck TJ, et al. (2005) Relation between age, femoral neck cortical stability, and hip fracture risk. Lancet 366: 129–135.
11. Gluer CC, Cummings SR, Pressman A, Li J, Gluer K, et al. (1994) Prediction of hip fractures from pelvic radiographs: the study of osteoporotic fractures. The Study of Osteoporotic Fractures Research Group. J Bone Miner Res 9: 671–677.
12. Hansen S, Jensen JE, Ahrberg F, Hauge EM, Brixen K (2011) The combination of structural parameters and areal bone mineral density improves relation to proximal femur strength: an in vitro study with high-resolution peripheral quantitative computed tomography. Calcif Tissue Int 89: 335–346.
13. Holzer G, von Skrbensky G, Holzer LA, Pichl W (2009) Hip fractures and the contribution of cortical versus trabecular bone to femoral neck strength. J Bone Miner Res 24: 468–474.
14. Borggrefe J, Graeff C, Nickelsen TN, Marin F, Gluer CC (2009) Quantitative Computed Tomography Assessment of the Effects of 24 months of Teriparatide Treatment on 3-D Femoral Neck Bone Distribution, Geometry and Bone Strength: Results from the EUROFORS Study. J Bone Miner Res 25: 472–481.
15. Poole KE, Treece GM, Ridgway GR, Mayhew PM, Borggrefe J, et al. (2011) Targeted regeneration of bone in the osteoporotic human femur. PLoS One 6: e16190.
16. Treece GM, Gee AH, Mayhew PM, Poole KE (2010) High resolution cortical bone thickness measurement from clinical CT data. Med Image Anal 14: 276–290.
17. Vaculík J, Malkus T, Majerníček M, Podškubka A, Dungl P (2007) Incidence of proximal femoral fractures. Ortopedie 1: 62–68.
18. Rueckert D, Frangi AF, Schnabel JA (2003) Automatic construction of 3-D statistical deformation models of the brain using nonrigid registration. IEEE Trans Med Imaging 22: 1014–1025.
19. Friston KJ, Holmes AP, Worsley KJ, Poline J-P, Frith CD, et al. (1994) Statistical parametric maps in functional imaging: A general linear approach. Human Brain Mapping 2: 189–210.
20. Worsley K, Taylor J, Carbonell F, Chung M, Duerden E, et al. (2009) SurfStat: A Matlab toolbox for the statistical analysis of univariate and multivariate surface and volumetric data using linear mixed effects models and random field theory. NeuroImage Organization for Human Brain Mapping 2009 Annual Meeting 47: S102.
21. Bessho M, Ohnishi I, Matsumoto T, Ohashi S, Matsuyama J, et al. (2009) Prediction of proximal femur strength using a CT-based nonlinear finite element method: differences in predicted fracture load and site with changing load and boundary conditions. Bone 45: 226–231.
22. Parker MJ, Twemlow TR (1997) Spontaneous hip fractures, 44/872 in a prospective study. Acta Orthop Scand 68: 325–326.
23. Yang KH, Shen KL, Demetropoulos CK, King AI, Kolodziej P, et al. (1996) The relationship between loading conditions and fracture patterns of the proximal femur. Journal of Biomechanical Engineering-Transactions of the Asme 118: 575–578.
24. Freeman MA, Todd RC, Pirie CJ (1974) The role of fatigue in the pathogenesis of senile femoral neck fractures. J Bone Joint Surg Br 56-B: 698–702.
25. Odgers PNB (1931) Two details about the neck of the femur: (1) The eminentia. (2) The empreinte. Journal of Anatomy 65: 352–U321.
26. Panzer S, Esch U, Abdulazim AN, Augat P (2010) Herniation pits and cystic-appearing lesions at the anterior femoral neck: an anatomical study by MSCT and microCT. Skeletal Radiol 39: 645–654.
27. Pitt M, Graham A, Shipman J, Birkby W (1982) Herniation pit of the femoral neck American Journal of Roentgenology 138 1115–1121.
28. Zebaze RM, Ghasem-Zadeh A, Bohte A, Iuliano-Burns S, Mirams M, et al. (2010) Intracortical remodelling and porosity in the distal radius and post-mortem femurs of women: a cross-sectional study. Lancet 375: 1729–1736.
29. Bell KL, Loveridge N, Power J, Garrahan N, Meggitt BF, et al. (1999) Regional differences in cortical porosity in the fractured femoral neck. Bone 24: 57–64.
30. Cristofolini L, Schileo E, Juszczyk M, Taddei F, Martelli S, et al. (2010) Mechanical testing of bones: the positive synergy of finite-element models and in vitro experiments. Philos Transact A Math Phys Eng Sci 368: 2725–2763.
31. Li W, Kornak J, Harris T, Keyak J, Li C, et al. (2009) Identify fracture-critical regions inside the proximal femur using statistical parametric mapping. Bone 44: 596–602.
32. Kaptoge S, Beck TJ, Reeve J, Stone KL, Hillier TA, et al. (2008) Prediction of incident hip fracture risk by femur geometry variables measured by hip structural analysis in the study of osteoporotic fractures. J Bone Miner Res 23: 1892–1904.

17

Delphinidin, One of the Major Anthocyanidins, Prevents Bone Loss through the Inhibition of Excessive Osteoclastogenesis in Osteoporosis Model Mice

Sawako Moriwaki[1,2⁋], Keiko Suzuki[3⁋], Masashi Muramatsu[1¤], Atsushi Nomura[4], Fumihide Inoue[4], Takeshi Into[5], Yuji Yoshiko[6], Shumpei Niida[1,2*]

1 Laboratory of Genomics and Proteomics, National Center for Geriatrics and Gerontology (NCGG), Aichi, Japan, **2** Biobank Omics Unit, National Center for Geriatrics and Gerontology (NCGG), Aichi, Japan, **3** Department of Pharmacology, School of Dentistry, Showa University, Tokyo, Japan, **4** Nihon Seiyaku Kogyo, Co., Ltd., Aichi, Japan, **5** Department of Oral Bacteriology, Division of Oral Infections and Health Sciences, Asahi University School of Dentistry, Gifu, Japan, **6** Department of Oral Growth and Developmental Biology, Hiroshima University Graduate School of Biomedical Sciences, Hiroshima, Japan

Abstract

Anthocyanins, one of the flavonoid subtypes, are a large family of water-soluble phytopigments and have a wide range of health-promoting benefits. Recently, an anthocyanin-rich compound from blueberries was reported to possess protective property against bone loss in ovariectomized (OVX) animal models. However, the active ingredients in the anthocyanin compound have not been identified. Here we show that delphinidin, one of the major anthocyanidins in berries, is a potent active ingredient in anti-osteoporotic bone resorption through the suppression of osteoclast formation. *In vitro* examinations revealed that delphinidin treatment markedly inhibited the differentiation of RAW264.7 cells into osteoclasts compared with other anthocyanidins, cyanidin and peonidin. Oral administration of delphinidin significantly prevented bone loss in both RANKL-induced osteoporosis model mice and OVX model mice. We further provide evidence that delphinidin suppressed the activity of *NF-κB*, *c-fos*, and *Nfatc1*, master transcriptional factors for osteoclastogenesis. These results strongly suggest that delphinidin is the most potent inhibitor of osteoclast differentiation and will be an effective agent for preventing bone loss in postmenopausal osteoporosis.

Editor: Mohan R. Wani, National Center for Cell Science, India

Funding: This work has been supported by Japan Society for the Promotion of Science (KAKENHI Grant No. 20390469 to SN and No. 21791802 to SM) and by Ministry of Health Labour and Welfare (Health Labour Sciences Research Grant No. H24-Choju-007 to SN). The funders had no role in study design, data collection and analysis, decision to publish, or preparation of the manuscript.

Competing Interests: AN and FI are employees of Nihon Seiyaku Kogyo Co., Ltd. Tama Biochemical Co. Ltd., who donated experimental material Cassis-extract-35, also declared that no competing interests exist.

* E-mail: sniida@ncgg.go.jp

¤ Current address: Department of Cancer Genetics, Roswell Park Cancer Institute, Elm and Carlton Streets, Buffalo, New York, United States of America

⁋ These authors contributed equally to this work.

Introduction

Osteoporosis, characterized by low bone mineral density (BMD) and fragility of the bone matrix, is a complex bone disease with various causes, including aging, estrogen deficiency and genetics, and leads to increased fracture risk, especially in the elderly population. Current anti-osteoporosis drugs such as bisphosphonates have been widely used and their bone protective effects are well established. However, many individuals with osteoporosis remain undiagnosed, untreated and at risk of fracture because of the lack of symptoms and public awareness [1]. Hence, a dietary nutritional approach is important for primary prevention of bone loss.

Natural compounds in fruits and vegetables such as polyphenols have a wide range of biological and pharmacological effects [2–5]. Several flavonoids, a subgroup of polyphenols including hesperidin, quercetin and luteolin, have been shown to possess preventive efficacy for bone loss in ovariectomized (OVX) animal models [6–8]. Most showed potent suppressive effects on the differentiation and/or function of osteoclasts, bone resorbing multinucleated giant cells [7–10]. Osteoclasts are formed by the fusion of mononuclear preosteoclasts derived from monocyte-macrophage linage cells. Osteoclast differentiation is tightly regulated by two key molecules, receptor activator of NF-κB ligand (RANKL), a TNF super-family cytokine, produced by osteoblasts, and its receptor RANK, which are expressed on osteoclast precursors [11]. Several flavonoids seem to be inhibitors of RANKL-RANK signaling-related molecules, including NF-κB and nuclear factor for activated T cells (NFATc1), master osteoclastogenic molecules located downstream of NF-κB [7–10].

In this study, we focused on delphinidin, one of the aglycone nuclei of anthocyanins, as an active agent for anti-bone loss *in vivo*. Anthocyanins are a large family of water-soluble red/blue/purple flavonoid pigments in fruits and vegetables, and have a wide range of health-promoting benefits, for example, as anti-oxidants. Many studies have demonstrated the pharmacological effects of anthocyanidins on human diseases, including night blindness, cancer, obesity and heart diseases [12–16]. Recently, a blueberry extract,

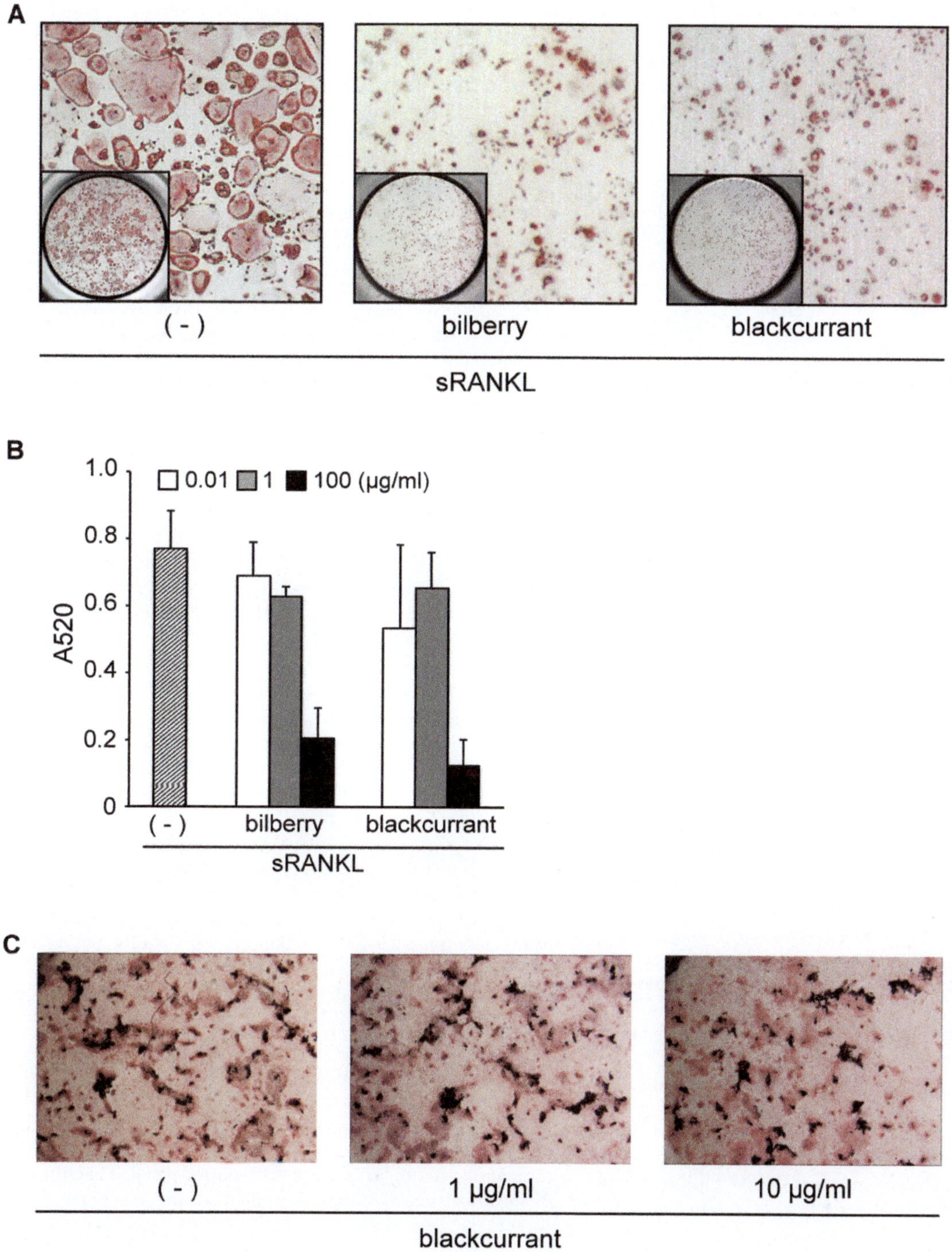

Figure 1. Anthocyanin-rich compounds extracted from bilberry and blackcurrants inhibit *in vitro* osteoclastogenesis, but not osteogenesis. RAW264.7 cells were pre-incubated for 1 h in the presence of various concentrations of anthocyanin compounds, and subsequently cultured for 4 days in the presence of 100 ng/ml RANKL. Cells were fixed and stained with TRAP. A: Numerous TRAP-positive multinucleated giant cells, osteoclasts, were induced by RANKL treatment (left panel). In contrast, large osteoclasts were significantly decreased by addition of anthocyanin compounds (middle and right panels). B: Anti-osteoclastogenic activity of anthocyanin compound was evaluated by the absorption ratio of the red-stained area per well at 520 nm on a spectrometer. C: Primary osteoblastic cells were cultured in the medium containing 50 μg AA, 10 μM Dex and 10 mM β-GP with or without anthocyanin compound for 2 weeks. No significant effect was observed on the osteoblast differentiation and mineral apposition.

an anthocyanin-rich compound, was reported to possess protective properties against bone loss in OVX rats [17]. Moreover, it has been reported that anthocyanins extracted from bilberry and blackcurrant exerted potent inhibitory effects on NF-κB activation in activated monocytes, and consequently led to the downregulation of pro-inflammatory mediators [18]. The NF-κB signaling pathway is well established to be critical for osteoclastogenesis. Commonly, extracted anthocyanin compounds consist of several kinds of anthocyanins derived from plural aglycone bases such as cyanidin, delphinidin and peonidin, major anthocyanidins in extracts of berries, including blueberry. However, to our knowledge, the active ingredients for bone metabolism have not been identified. To address this question is useful for not only developing the high efficient dietary supplements but also finding novel drug seeds. Here we show that delphinidin is the most potent inhibitor of osteoclastogenesis and will be an effective agent for preventing *in vivo* bone degradation.

Materials and Methods

Anthocyanins and Anthocyanidins

Bilberon-25, a concentrated extract of bilberry, was purchased from Tokiwa Phytochemical Co., Ltd. (Chiba, Japan). Cassis extract-35, a concentrated extract of blackcurrant, was generously donated by Tama Biochemical Co., Ltd. (Tokyo, Japan). Cyanidin chloride ($C_{15}H_{11}ClO_6$), delphinidin chloride ($C_{15}H_{11}ClO_7$) and peonidin chloride ($C_{16}H_{13}ClO_6$) were from Extrasynthése (Lyon, France) and Sigma-Aldrich (St Louis, MO, USA), respectively. Epicatechin ($C_{15}H_{14}O_6$) was purchased from Kurita Analysis Service Co., Ltd. (Ibaraki, Japan).

Cell Culture

RAW264.7 cells, a mouse macrophage cell line, were used as osteoclast precursor cells and maintained in α modified essential medium (α-MEM) supplemented with 10% fetal bovine serum (FBS) at 37°C and 5% CO_2. For osteoclast induction, cells were plated in a 96-well plate at a density of 4×10^3 cells/well and stimulated with 100 ng/ml RANKL for 4 days. For the inhibition study, cells were pre-incubated in α-MEM supplemented with vehicle or with various concentrations of anthocyanin-rich extracts and anthocyanidins, 1 h before the addition of RANKL. To confirm multinucleated osteoclast formation, the cultured cells were fixed in 10% formalin for 3 minutes, and then stained with an osteoclast marker enzyme, tartrate-resistant acid phosphatase (TRAP). Effects of anthocyanins and anthocyanidins on osteoclast formation were evaluated by morphological observations and the intensity of TRAP staining was measured at 520 nm using a spectrophotometer (SpectraMax M5; Molecular Devices, Sunnyvale, CA, USA).

Osteoblasts were isolated from newborn calvariae of C57BL/6J mice, as described previously with slight modifications [19]. Briefly, calvariae were minced and sequentially digested with collagenase solution at 37°C. Cells retrieved from the osteogenic cell fractions were separately cultured in α-MEM supplemented with 10% FBS and antibiotics. After 24 h, cells were pooled and grown in multi-well plates in the same medium containing 50 μg/ml of ascorbic acid (AA), 10 μM dexamethasone (Dex) and 10 mM β-glycerophosphate (β-GP) with or without anthocyanin-rich extracts. After two weeks culture, cells were stained with *von* Kossa' s staining to determine the matrix mineralization, as described previously [19].

Animals and Treatments

To assess the protective effect of delphinidin on *in vivo* bone loss, we created soluble RANKL (sRANKL)-induced osteoporosis model mice, which were established by Yasuda and his colleagues [20]. Seven-week-old female C57BL/6 mice (n = 17) were purchased from CLEA Japan (Tokyo, Japan). Mice were divided into three groups: control mice (cont, n = 5), osteoporosis model mice (vehicle, n = 6) and delphinidin-treated osteoporosis mice (Del, n = 6). Twelve mice were intraperitoneally injected with GST-RANKL (1 mg/kg; Oriental Yeast Co., Ltd., Kyoto, Japan) twice at interval of 3 days. First injection was performed at 3 days after starting of delphinidin-treatment. For six mice, delphinidin treatment (10 mg/kg/day) via gavage started 3 days before the first injection of GST-RANKL, and continued for 14 days. Another six mice received the same volume of vehicle, a mixture of dimethyl sulfoxide (DMSO) and water.

We further assessed the effect of delphinidin using OVX mice. Eight-week-old female C57BL/6 mice were purchased from Charles River Laboratory Japan (Kanagawa, Japan). Thirty mice were either sham-operated (n = 6) or OVX (n = 24). OVX mice were divided into four groups (n = 6×4): OVX control, low-dose delphinidin (1 mg/kg), intermediate-dose delphinidin (3 mg/kg), and high-dose delphinidin (10 mg/kg) groups. After OVX, delphinidin was administrated orally, as mentioned above, for 28 days. OVX-control mice received the same volume of vehicle, a mixture of DMSO and water.

All mice were housed in an animal room (temp, 22±2°C; humidity, 50%; light/dark cycle, 12 h) with free access to food and water. At the end of treatment, the mice were sacrificed. Femora were removed and fixed with 3.7% formaldehyde in phosphate-buffered saline solution (pH7.4) for 16 h. After rinsing, bones were immersed in 80% ethanol and stored at 4°C in a refrigerator. These experiments were approved by the Animal Experimental Committees of Showa University and NCGG, respectively.

Microcomputed Tomography

Bone morphometric parameters and microarchitectual properties of the femur were determined using a microcomputed tomography (μCT) system (inspeXio SMX-90CT; Shimadzu Co., Kyoto, Japan) with X-ray tube settings of 90 kV and 108 μA. The femur was placed in a microcentrifuge tube filled with PBS and scanned at a voxel size of 15.0 μm. TRI/3D-BON software (RATOC System Engineering Co., Tokyo, Japan) was used to generate 3D models from 272 2D-transverse slices, and bone morphometry was performed in the distal metaphyseal region (500 μm in length) of femora. For quantitative analysis, BV/TV, trabecular thickness, trabecular number, trabecular separation and trabecular spacing were determined using TRI/3D-BON software.

Histomorphometric Analysis of Bone

Femora were fixed in 70% ethanol and embedded in glycolmethacrylate (GMA) without decalcification. Serial sections were cut and stained with Villanueva bone stain for bone histomorphometry, as previously reported [21]. The histomorphometorical analysis was performed at the Ito Bone Science Institute (Niigata, Japan).

Extraction of Nuclear Protein and Assessment of NF-κB Activation

Nuclear cell lysates were prepared using a Nuclear Extract Kit (Active Motif, Tokyo, Japan) following the manufacturer's instructions. We examined the inhibitory effect of delphinidin on NF-κB activation in RAW264.7 cells. Briefly, cells were pretreated with delphinidin or vehicle for 1 h, and subsequently stimulated with sRANKL. After 3 h of stimulation, cells were washed with ice-cold PBS(−) and hypotonic buffer added from the kit to explore the nucleus. To dissolve the nuclear protein, complete lysis buffer containing 1 mM DTT and protease inhibitor cocktail were added to the cell lysate precipitation and the concentration of protein was measured using Prostain (Active Motif). Cell lysates

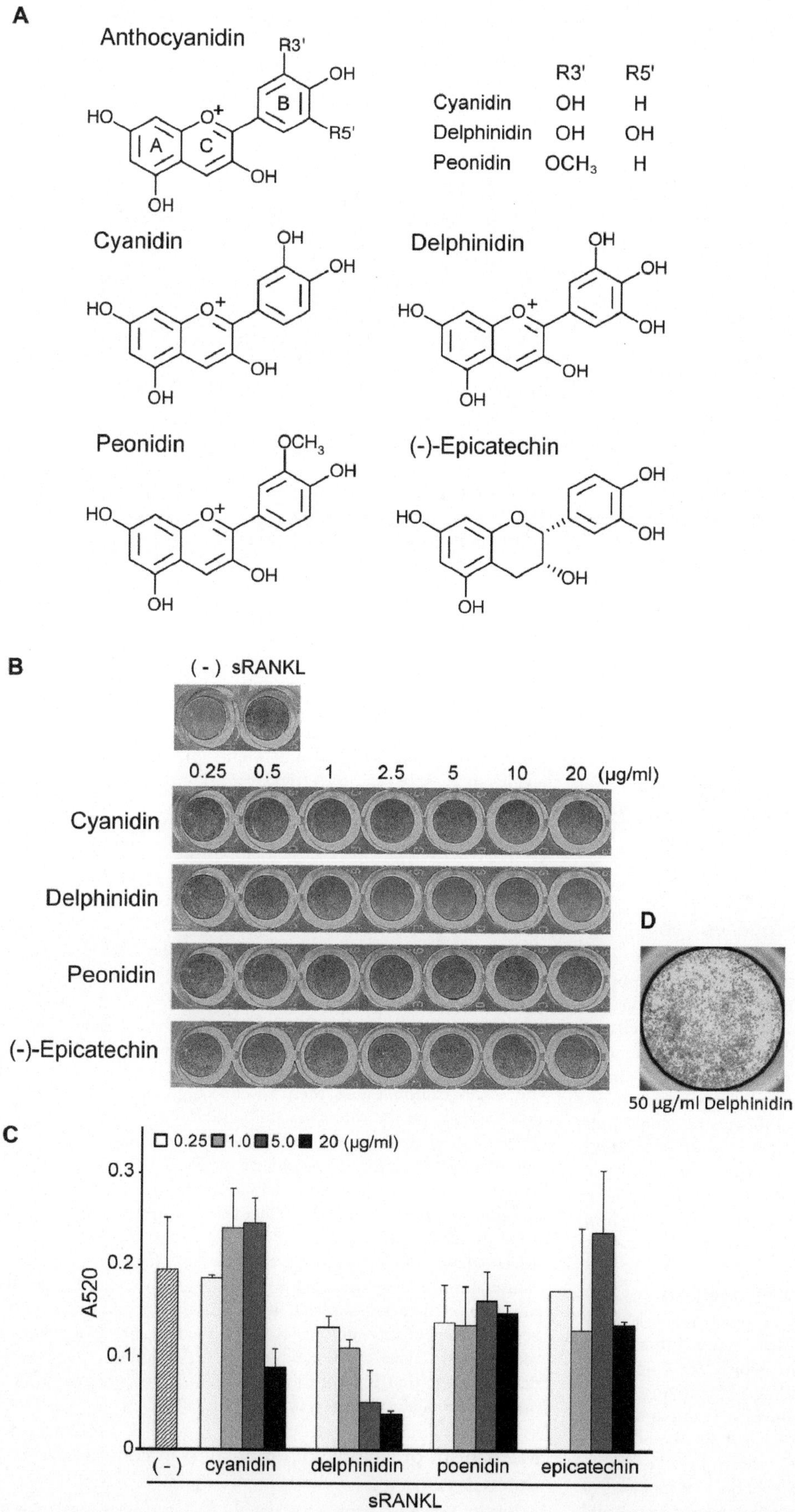
A
Anthocyanidin
R3'
R5'
R3' R5'
Cyanidin OH H
Delphinidin OH OH
Peonidin OCH3 H
Cyanidin
Delphinidin
Peonidin
(-)-Epicatechin
B
(-) sRANKL
0.25 0.5 1 2.5 5 10 20 (µg/ml)
Cyanidin
Delphinidin
Peonidin
(-)-Epicatechin
D
50 µg/ml Delphinidin
C
0.25 1.0 5.0 20 (µg/ml)
A520
0 0.1 0.2 0.3
(-) cyanidin delphinidin poenidin epicatechin
sRANKL

Figure 2. Effects of various anthocyanidins on *in vitro* osteoclastogenesis. A: The structure of tested three anthocyanidins and (−)-epicatechin as a negative control. B: RAW264.7 cells were pretreated for 1 h with increasing concentrations (0.25–20 μg/ml) of three anthocyanidins and epicatechin, and cultured for 4 days in the presence of RANKL (100 ng/ml). Red-stained area in each well indicates osteoclast population. Delphinidin strongly inhibited RANKL-induced osteoclastogenesis at >1 μg/ml. Cyanidin showed moderate inhibition at 20 μg/ml. C: Absorption ratio also supported the results of TRAP-staining observation. D: RAW264.7 cells were cultured with delphinidin alone for 4 days. No cytotoxic effect of delphinidin was found. Cells were stained by crystal violet.

equal to the concentration were measured by TransAM NF-κB p65 Chemiluminescence (Active Motif), which is a high-throughput assay to quantify NF-κB activation, that is, binding activity to DNA-binding fragments fixed to the plate bottom.

Reverse Transcriptase-polymerase Chain Reaction Analysis

For reverse transcriptase-polymerase chain reaction (RT-PCR) assays, total RNA was prepared using an AurumTotal RNA Mini Kit (Bio-Rad, Richmond, CA, USA) according to the manufacturer's instructions. One microgram of total RNA from each sample was reverse-transcribed with Ready-To-Go You-Prime First-Strand Beads (GE Healthcare, Piscataway, NJ, USA). cDNA was amplified by PCR. The PCR products were electrophoresed on a 1.2% agarose gel.

Quantitative Real-time PCR Analysis

Quantitative real-time PCR (qPCR) assays were performed with the CFX96 Real-Time system (Bio-Rad) using the Thunderbird SYBR qPCR Mix (Toyobo, Osaka, Japan). Expression levels were normalized to glyceraldehyde-3-phosphate dehydrogenase (GAPDH).

Statistical Analysis

All data are the mean ± standard deviation (SD). Statistical analyses were performed using unpaired Student t tests. $P<0.05$ was considered significant.

Results

Effects of Anthocyanin on Osteoclastogenesis and Osteogenesis

Initially, we tested the effects of anthocyanin compound extracted from bilberry (*Vaccinium myrtillus* L.) and blackcurrant (*Ribes nigrum*) on osteoclast formation using RAW264.7 cells as osteoclast precursors. The number of TRAP-positive multinucleated giant cells, osteoclasts, differentiated from sRANKL-stimulated RAW246.7 cells, was markedly decreased by pretreatment with both extracts, suggesting that both anthocyanin compounds contain active ingredients to suppress osteoclast formation (Figure 1A and 1B). In contrast, no significant effect of anthocyanin compound (blackcurrant) was found on mineral apposition (Figure 1C). These results indicated that target cell of anthocyanin may be osteoclasts in bone metabolism.

Effects of Anthocyanidins on Osteoclastogenesis

Next, to identify the active ingredients (aglycone bases) as anti-osteoclastogenic factors, we investigated three major anthocyanidins, cyanidin, delphinidin and peonidin, which are commonly contained in many purple berries, including bilberry and blackcurrant (Figure 2A). RAW264.7 cell cultures containing various concentrations of these anthocyanidins were incubated with sRANKL (100 ng/ml) for 4 days. As shown in Figure 2, delphinidin treatment caused a dose-dependent inhibition of osteoclastogenesis. Although cyanidin treatment showed a mild suppressive effect on osteoclastogenesis at a concentration of 20 μg/ml, doses ≤10 μg/ml did not affect osteoclastogenesis. In contrast, peonidin treatment showed no significant effect on osteoclastogenesis, similar to the control compound, (−)-epicatechin. Similar results were also obtained at a higher concentration (50 μg/ml) of anthocyanidins (data not shown). Additionally, we confirmed that delphinidin did not induce cell death in RAW264.7 cell cultures without RANKL (Figure 2D).

Inhibitory Effects of Dietary Delphinidin on Bone Loss *in vivo*

To determine the relevance of our *in vitro* findings of delphinidin bioactivity to the *in vivo* situation, we investigated the anti-osteoporotic effect of delphinidin on sRANKL-induced osteoporosis model mice. 3D-images and morphometric parameters clearly demonstrated that the cancellous bone volume of femoral distal metaphysis was markedly decreased by sRANKL treatment, compared with intact control mice. In contrast, delphinidin treatment significantly inhibited cancellous bone degradation in sRANKL-treated mice (Figure 3A, B).

All animals were weighed daily for 17 days, and there was no significant change among the experimental groups (Figure 3C). Although liver and kidney weights were slightly decreased in sRANKL-treated mice compared with control mice, these differences were not significant (Figure 3D). Also, there was no significance between sRANKL-treated mice and sRANKL/delphinidin-treated mice (Figure 3C).

We further performed histomorphometrical observation of bone tissues. Microscopic observation demonstrated that the number of bone trabeculare obviously decreased in sRANKL-treated osteoporotic mice. In contrast, many bone trabeculae remained in the bones of delphinidin-treated mice (Figure 4A). Despite the limited number of bone trabeulare, osteoclast number was significantly decreased ($p = 0.03$) in delphinidin-treated mice than non-treated osteoporotic mice (Figure 4B). Other major two resorption-parameters were also downregulated in the mice administrated delphinidin, although there were no statistically significant differences between these two groups (Figure 4B). Consistent with the *in vitro* examinations, these results suggested that delphinidin acts, at least, on the osteoclast differentiation directly.

We further assessed the anti-bone resorption effect of delphinidin using OVX mice, a standard model of osteoporosis. OVX mice were orally administered delphinidin at three different doses. A significant anti-osteoporotic effect was confirmed in over half the mice treated with not only high-dose (10 mg/kg) but also intermediate-dose (3 mg/kg) delphinidin (Figure 5). In this examination, uterus weight did not change in delphinidin-treated OVX mice (data not shown), suggesting that delphinidin did not act on the uterus like SERMs (selective estrogen receptor modulators) such as isoflavons [22]. Together, our results demonstrated that ingestion of delphinidin acts as a potent anti-osteoporotic agent for preventing osteoporosis.

Mechanism of Delphinidin-mediated Inhibition of Osteoclastogenesis

Since previous work indicated that anthocyanin extract inhibited NF-κB activation in activated monocytes, we first

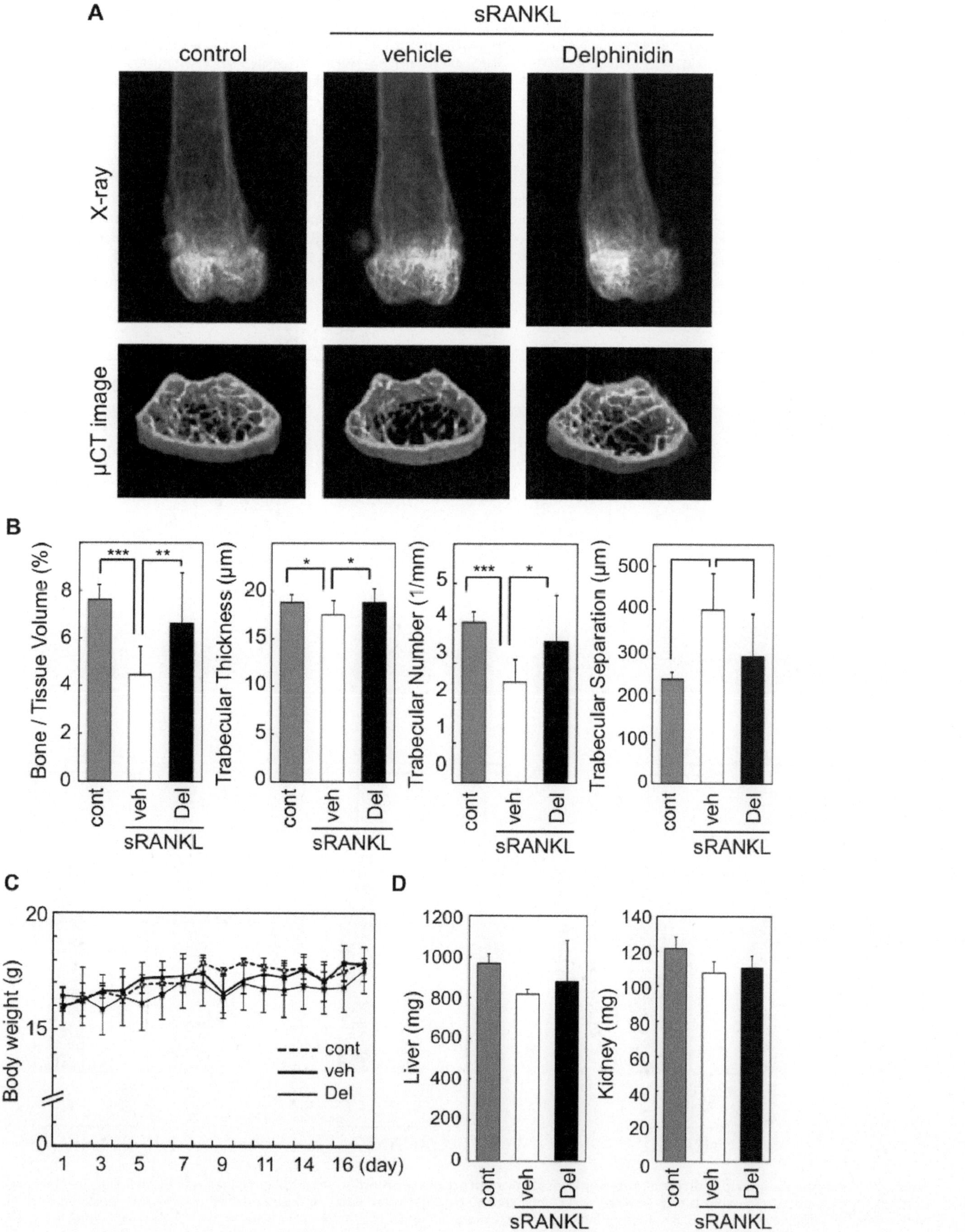
A
sRANKL
control
vehicle
Delphinidin
X-ray
μCT image
B
Bone / Tissue Volume (%)
Trabecular Thickness (μm)
Trabecular Number (1/mm)
Trabecular Separation (μm)
***
**
*
cont
veh
Del
sRANKL
C
Body weight (g)
cont
veh
Del
1 3 5 7 9 11 14 16 (day)
D
Liver (mg)
Kidney (mg)

Figure 3. Effect of delphinidin on bone loss in RANKL-induced osteoporosis mice. A: Representative X-ray and microcomputed tomography images of the distal femurs of intact mice (control), RANKL-induced osteoporosis mice (vehicle), and delphinidin-treated RANKL-induced osteoporosis mice (Delphinidin). B: Effect of RANKL injection and delphinidin treatment on trabecular microarchitectural parameters. Values are expressed as the mean ± SD. *$p<0.05$, **$p<0.01$, ***$p<0.001$. C: Comparison of body weight between each experimental group. Values are expressed as the mean ± SD. D: Comparison of weights of liver and kidney in each experimental group. Values are expressed as the mean ± SD.

examined the activation of NF-κB in RAW264.7 cells using the TransAM assay. When the cells were stimulated by sRANKL, the activation of NF-κB p65 subunit was upregulated promptly. In contrast, RANKL-mediated NF-κB activation was markedly downregulated in cells treated by delphinidin, suggesting its effect at a transcriptional level (Figure 6A).

RANKL-induced *c-fos* activation is another pivotal event in the early phase of osteoclastogenesis [11], [23]. NFATc1 is a master transcriptional factor located at the downstream cross-point of both NF-κB and c-Fos pathways in osteoclastogenesis [11], [23]. We therefore investigated whether delphinidin affects the activation of *c-fos* and *Nfatc1* genes. Additionally, we examined the alteration of the expression levels of osteoclast marker genes in delphinidin-treated RAW264.7 cells. Our results demonstrate that RANKL-induced *c-fos* activation was attenuated by delphinidin treatment. Furthermore, expression levels of the *Nfatc1* gene were

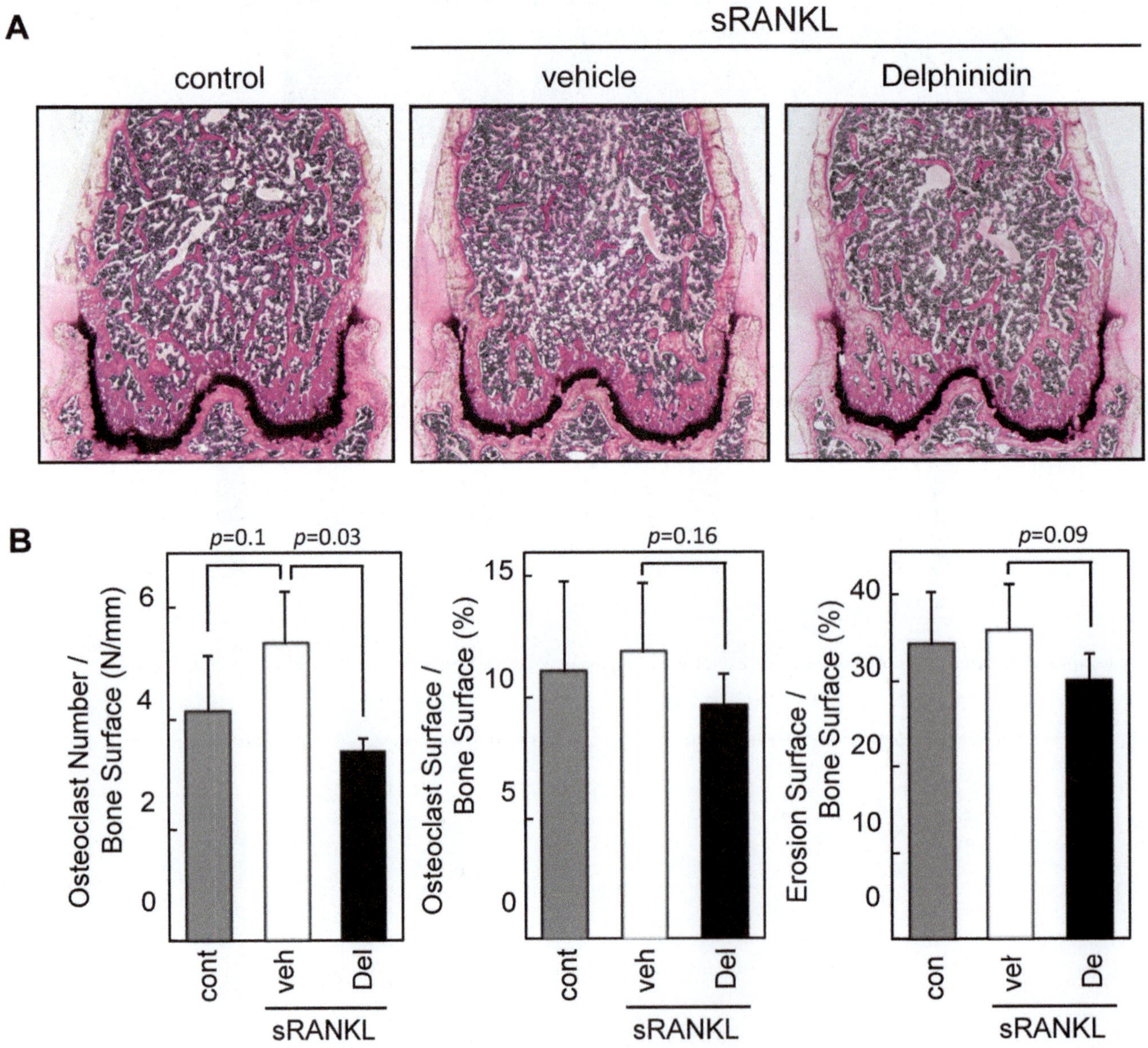

Figure 4. Histomorphometric analysis of anti-bone resorption effect of delphinidin. A: Histological images of distal femurs of intact mice (control), RANKL-induced osteoporosis mice (vehicle), and delphinidin (10 mg/Kg)-treated RANKL-induced osteoporosis mice (Delphinidin). Sections were stained by Villanueva staining. B: Bone-resorption parameters were determined by histomorphometric analysis. Values are expressed as the mean ± SD.

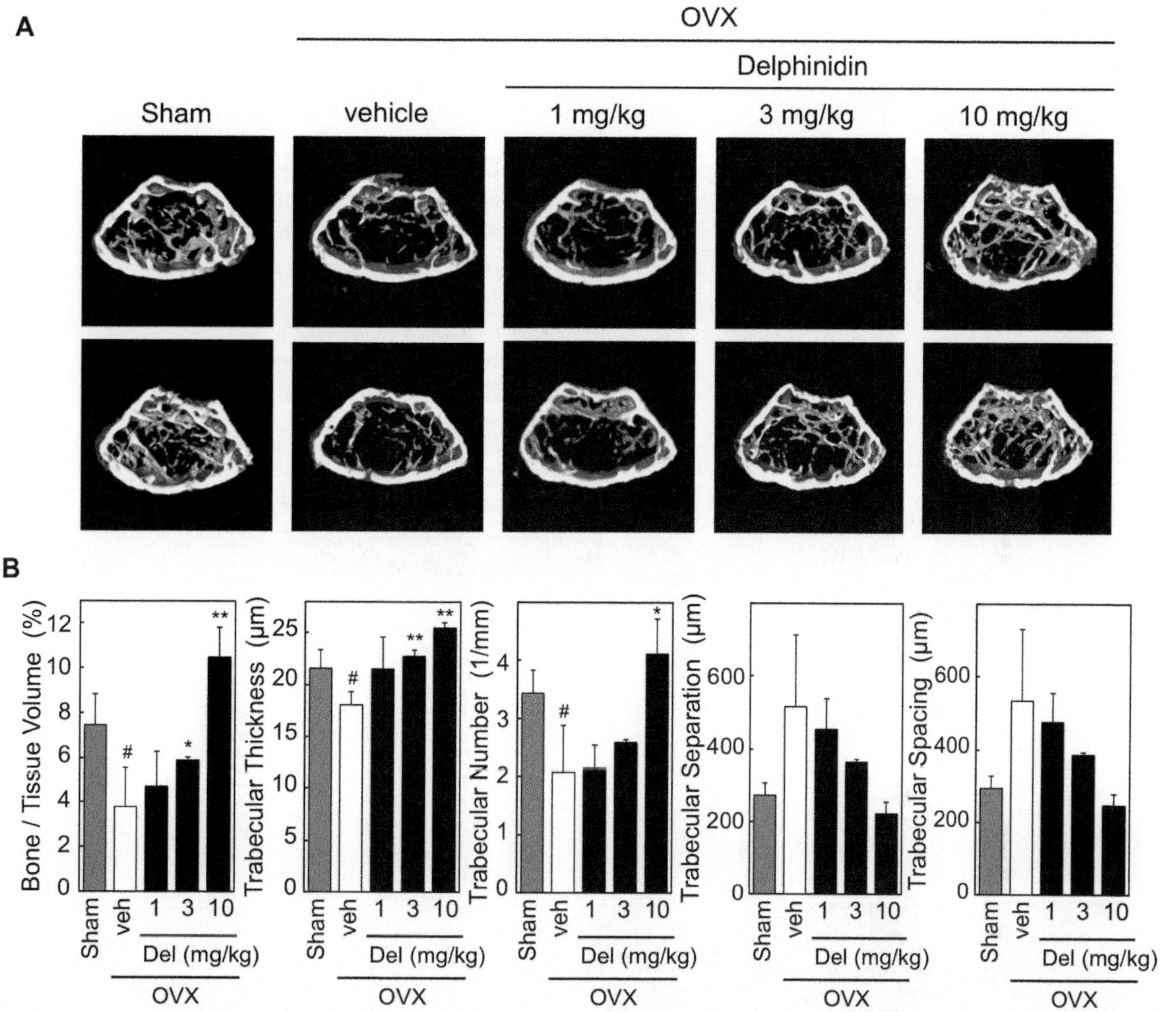

Figure 5. Effect of delphinidin on bone loss in OVX mice. A: Microcomputed tomography images of the distal femurs (axial view of the metaphyseal region) of sham-operated mice, OVX mice (vehicle), and delphinidin-treated OVX mice (Delphinidin). B: Effect of delphinidin on trabecular microarchitectural parameters. Values are expressed as the mean ± SD. **p*<0.05, ***p*<0.01 (vs vehicle), #*p*<0.05 (vs sham).

markedly decreased in delphinidin-treated cells (Figure 6B, C). Consequently, expression levels of osteoclast marker genes, especially *Mmp9* and *Trap*, were reduced by delphinidin treatment (Figure 6B, C). In addition, expression levels of *Dc-stamp*, a fusion protein gene for multinucleation, were significantly decreased in delphinidin-treated cells (Figure 6B, C). Together, these results suggest that the anti-osteoclastogenic effect of delphinidin is clearly associated with alteration of the signaling cascade triggered by RANKL.

Discussion

Last year, an interesting epidemiological report was published in the Journal of Bone Mineral Research. Welch and his colleagues investigated the association between habitual flavonoid intake with bone mineral density in 3,160 women, and concluded that flavonoid intake, especially anthocyanin (median intake: 13.7 mg/day), was beneficial for bone-protective effects in women [24]. Devareddy *et al.* previously reported that the extracted anthocyanin compound showed a protective property against bone loss in OVX rats [17]. However, the active ingredients in the anthocyanin compound still have not been identified. In the present study, we provide evidence that delphinidin, one of the major anthocyanidins, is a potent preventive natural agent for osteoporosis and might support the conclusion of the epidemiological investigation experimentally.

We evaluated the inhibitory effects of three major anthocyanidins contained in berries on *in vitro* osteoclast formation, and consequently identified that delphinidin was the most potent active ingredient. In our preliminary tests using their glycosides, similar results in terms of potency were obtained (data not shown), suggesting that anti-osteoclastogenic activity depends on the structure of aglycone form. Since anthocyanins are much more stable than other hydrophilic flavonoid glycosides, they are rapidly absorbed into blood as glycosides without changing to aglycones after consumption [25], [26]. Then, we directly administrated

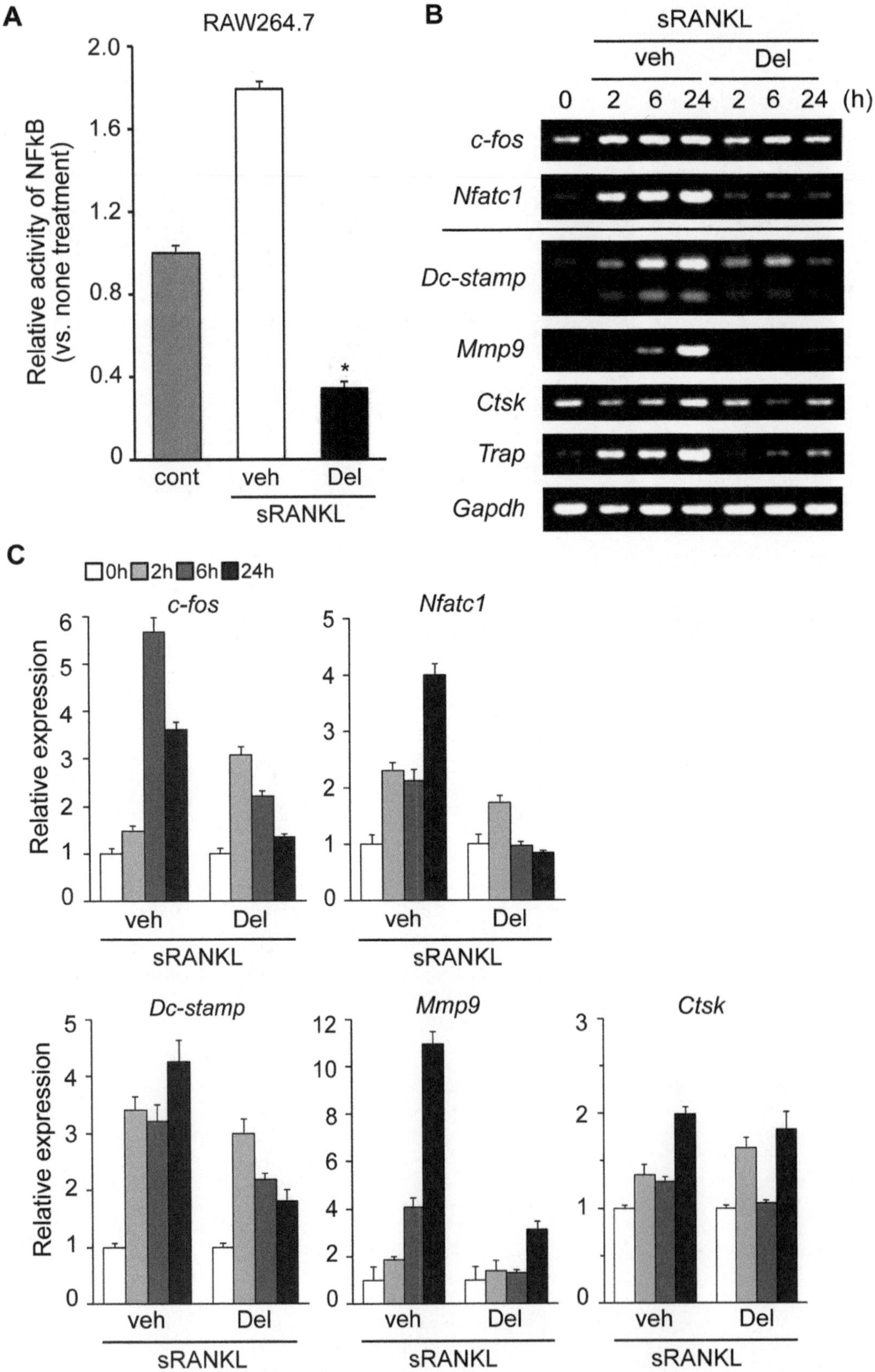

Figure 6. Delphinidin suppresses the expression of major osteoclastogenic molecules in osteoclast precursor cells. (A) Quantification of NF-κB DNA-binding activity in control cells, agent stimulated cells and delphinidin-treated cells. RANKL-stimulated NF-κB DNA-binding activity was significantly inhibited by delphinidin treatment (*$p<0.001$). (B) RT-PCR and (C) qPCR analysis of the expression of osteoclastogenic transcriptional genes, *c-fos* and *Nfatc1*, and osteoclast marker genes, *Dc-stamp*, *Mmp9*, *Ctsk* and *Trap*, in RAW264.7 cells.

delphinidin into the osteoporosis mice, and consequently obtained significant results that delphinidin acts as an inhibitor of bone loss. Generally, aglycones of flavonoids are absorbed more rapidly and in greater amounts than their glycoside forms in human and animals [27], [28]. It is supposed that delphinidin administrated orally was quickly absorbed and delivered to bone tissue. However, *in vivo* kinetics of anthocyanidins (aglycones) have not been much investigated as compared with those of glycosides. To elucidate the mechanisms of absorption and metabolism of the aglycones are important for understanding of bioavailability of anthocyanidins. The results obtained from this study may be useful to investigate the *in vivo* circulation of anthocyanidins in the future.

Consistent with *in vitro* examinations, the increased number of osteoclasts under osteoporotic conditions was significantly decreased by delphinidin treatment, resulting in prevention of bone loss. Delphinidin-mediated suppression of osteoclast formation is likely to be a key event associated with the inhibition of bone resorption in osteoporosis mice, as well as anti-osteoporosis drugs, bisphosphonates. RANK signaling triggered by RANKL modulates the activation of various signal pathways including NF-κB and mitogen-activated protein kinases (MAPKs) via TRAF6, an essential mediator of RANK signaling. Previous studies revealed that anthocyanin compounds or anthocyanidins were involved in several signal pathways in various cell types. Karlsen and his colleagues revealed that anthocyanin inhibited LPS-induced NF-κB activation in monocytes [18]. Hafeez *et al.* indicated that delphinidin inhibited NF-κB signaling at multiple levels in prostate cancer cells, and induced apoptosis [29]. These reports have important implications for our understanding of the mechanism of delphinidin in osteoclastogenesis. Consistent with previous work from other groups, our results demonstrate that delphinidin strongly suppressed the activation of NF-κB in RANKL-stimulated osteoclast precursors, RAW264.7 cells. We also found the downregulation of *c-fos* and *Nfatc1*, pivotal regulators of osteoclastogenesis, in delphinidin-treated cells (Figure 6). It is recognized that the induction of NFATc1 depends on NF-κB and AP-1 containing c-Fos. Karlsen *et al.* further demonstrated that plasma levels of NF-κB-related pro-inflammatory mediators were down-regulated in participants receiving anthocyanin supplementation compared with the placebo group [18]. In this context, it is plausible that delphinidin administration limits the number of osteoclasts through the downregulation of osteoclastogenic genes in osteoporotic mice. However, details of the molecular mechanism whereby delphinidin attenuates the activation of these osteoclastogenic regulators are still unclear. For example, the anti-oxidant property of anthocyanidins including delphinidin is one of the possible mechanisms underlying the limited gene expression, as in other cell types [14–16]. Reactive oxygen species (ROS) act as second messengers in signal transduction and gene expression in various cell types. In osteoclast precursors, intracellular levels of ROS are transiently increased in response to RANKL, and modulate the activity of the RANKL signaling pathway [30,31]. Since NF-κB is an oxidative stress-sensitive molecule [32], downregulation of NF-κB might depend on the anti-oxidant activity of delphinidin.

The finding that peonidin failed to suppress *in vitro* osteoclastogenesis is important to clarify the mechanism. This result suggests that anthocyanidins cannot always inhibit osteoclastogenesis. Peonidin is another representative anthocyanidin and is the principal ingredient in, for example, cranberry anthocyanin extracts. Previous work using mouse epidermal cells (JB6 cells) suggested that peonidin exhibited chemopreventive activity through inhibition of the phosphorylation of extracellular signal-regulated kinases (ERKs) in the cells [33]. If so, peonidin possibly alters the phenotype of osteoclast formation because RANKL-mediated activation of MAPKs, including ERKs, would be implicated in osteoclastogenesis [11], [30], [34]. However, there was no influence of peonidin on osteoclast differentiation in our experiments. Another investigation using JB6 cells also mentioned that peonidin treatment could not attenuate MAPK activity, including ERKs, in activated cells [35]. By contrast, cyanidin exhibited a mild suppressive effect on osteoclastogenesis at high concentration (≥20 μg/ml). Bioactivity of anthocyanidins may be characterized according to different substituent groups on the B-ring. As shown in Figure 2A, the C3′ positions (R3′) of the B-ring of cyanidin and delphinidin are hydroxyl (–OH) groups, while that of peonidin is a methoxy (–OCH_3) group. The ortho-dihydroxyphenyl structure seems to be critical for triggering anti-osteoclastogenic activity among the anthocyanidins. In addition, to clarify the difference whereby delphinidin induces more potent anti-osteoclastogenic activity compared with cyanidin, further studies will be required.

Meanwhile, the bone histomorphometry revealed that delphinidin treatment caused not only decrease of bone resorption but also a slight increase in number of osteoblasts and osteoid volume (no statistical significance). However, in our preliminary tests using the mouse primary osteoblasts, anthocyanin treatment did not stimulate calcification nodule formation (data not shown). Delphinidin consumption may have stimulated concomitantly upregulation of osteogenic potential through the in vivo network. It is desirable that delphinidin induces bone formation simultaneously in osteoporosis. In OVX rats, blueberry diet altered bone formation markers [17]. To investigate regarding the effect of delphinidin on the bone formation may be needed in future.

In summary, this study demonstrated for the first time that delphinidin possesses a potent inhibitory effect against RANKL-mediated osteoclastogenesis via downregulation of osteoclastogenic factors such as *Nfkb*, *c-fos* and *Nfatc1*. Oral administration of delphinidin showed a preventive effect on bone loss in osteoporosis model mice. Our results suggest that dietary delphinidin or anthocyanin supplements containing delphinidin may be useful for the prevention of RANKL-mediated bone loss such as postmenopausal osteoporosis.

Acknowledgments

We are grateful to M. Etoh and T. Ishizuya at Asahi Kasei Phama Corporation for assessment of OVX mice. We thank T. Oki at NARO Kyushu Okinawa Agricultural Research Center for preliminary experiments related to the current study and suggestions, respectively. We also thank S-I. Yasutake for his encouragement of this work. We had native speakers of English (Medical English Service, Kyoto, Japan) proofread our manuscript before resubmission.

Author Contributions

Conceived and designed the experiments: SN. Performed the experiments: SM KS MM YY. Analyzed the data: KS TI YY. Contributed reagents/materials/analysis tools: AN FI. Wrote the paper: SN.

References

1. Gehlbach SH, Fournier M, Bigelow C (2002) Recognition of osteoporosis by primary care physicians. Am J Public Health 92: 271–273.
2. Havsteen B (1983) Flavonoids, a class of natural products of high pharmacological potency. Biochem Pharmacol 32: 1141–1148.

3. Middleton E Jr, Kandaswami C (1992) Effects of flavonoids on immune and inflammatory cell functions. Biochem Pharmacol 43: 1167–1179.
4. Ueda H, Yamazaki C, Yamazaki M (2002) Luteolin as an anti-inflammatory and anti-allergic constituent of Perilla frutescens. Biol Pharm Bull 25: 1197–1202.
5. Gryglewski RJ, Korbut R, Robak J, Swies J (1987) On the mechanism of antithrombotic action of flavonoids. Biochem Pharmacol 36: 317–322.
6. Chiba H, Uehara M, Wu J, Wang X, Masuyama R, et al. (2003) Hesperidin, a citrus flavonoid, inhibits bone loss and decreases serum and hepatic lipids in ovariectomized mice. J Nutr 133: 1892–1897.
7. Tsuji M, Yamamoto H, Sato T, Mizuha Y, Kawai Y, et al. (2009) Dietary quercetin inhibits bone loss without effect on the uterus in ovariectomized mice. J Bone Miner Metab 27: 673–681.
8. Kim TH, Jung JW, Ha BG, Hong JM, Park EK, et al. (2011) The effects of luteolin on osteoclast differentiation, function in vitro and ovariectomy-induced bone loss. J Nutr Biochem 22: 8–15.
9. Wattel A, Kamel S, Prouillet C, Petit JP, Lorget F, et al. (2004) Flavonoid quercetin decreases osteoclastic differentiation induced by RANKL via a mechanism involving NF kappa B and AP-1. J Cell Biochem 92: 285–295.
10. Bu SY, Lerner M, Stoecker BJ, Boldrin E, Brackett DJ, et al. (2008) Dried plum polyphenols inhibit osteoclastogenesis by downregulating NFATc1 and inflammatory mediators. Calcif Tissue Int 82: 475–488.
11. Wada T, Nakashima T, Hiroshi N, Penninger JM (2006) RANKL-RANK signaling in osteoclastogenesis and bone disease. Trends Mol Med 12: 17–25.
12. Matsumoto H, Nakamura Y, Tachibanaki S, Kawamura S, Hirayama M (2003) Stimulatory effect of cyanidin 3-glycosides on the regeneration of rhodopsin. J Agric Food Chem 51: 3560–2563.
13. Einbond LS, Reynertson KA, Luo XD, Basile MJ, Kennelly EJ (2004) Anthocyanin antioxidants from edible fruits. Food Chem 84: 23–28.
14. Mazza G, Kay CD, Cottrell T, Holub BJ (2002) Absorption of anthocyanins from blueberries and serum antioxidant status in human subjects. J Agric Food Chem 50: 7731–7737.
15. Meydani M, Hasan ST (2010) Dietary polyphenols and obesity. Nutrients 2: 737–751.
16. Wallace TC (2011) Anthocyanins in cardiovascular disease. Adv Nutr 2: 1–7.
17. Devareddy L, Hooshmand S, Collins JK, Lucas EA, Chai SC, et al. (2008) Blueberry prevents bone loss in ovariectomized rat model of postmenopausal osteoporosis. J Nutr Biochem 19: 694–699.
18. Karlsen A, Retterstøl L, Laake P, Paur I, Bøhn SK, et al. (2007) Anthocyanins inhibit nuclear factor-kappaB activation in monocytes and reduce plasma concentrations of pro-inflammatory mediators in healthy adults. J Nutr 137: 1951–1954.
19. Yoshiko Y, Maeda N, Aubin JE (2003) Stanniocalcin 1 stimulates osteoblast differentiation in rat calvaria cell cultures. Endocrinology 144: 4134–4143.
20. Tomimori Y, Mori K, Koide M, Nakamichi Y, Ninomiya T, et al. (2009) Evaluation of pharmaceuticals with a novel 50-hour animal model of bone loss. J Bone Miner Res 24: 1194–1205.
21. Kawamori Y, Katayama Y, Asada N, Minagawa K, Sato M, et al. (2010) Role for vitamin D receptor in the neuronal control of the hematopoietic stem cell niche. Blood 116: 5528–5535.
22. Diel P, Geis RB, Caldarelli A, Schmidt S, Leschowsky UL, et al. (2004) The differential ability of the phytoestrogen genistein and of estradiol to induce uterine weight and proliferation in the rat is associated with a substance specific modulation of uterine gene expression. Mol Cell Endocrinol 221: 21–32.
23. Takayanagi H, Kim S, Koga T, Nishina H, Isshiki M, et al. (2002) Induction and activation of the transcription factor NFATc1 (NFAT2) integrate RANKL signaling in terminal differentiation of osteoclasts. Dev Cell 3: 889–901.
24. Welch A, MacGregor A, Jennings A, Fairweather-Tait S, Spector T, et al. (2012) Habitual flavonoid intakes are positively associated with bone mineral density in women. J Bone Miner Res 27: 1872–1878.
25. Matsumoto H, Inaba H, Kishi M, Tominaga S, Hirayama M, et al. (2001) Orally administered delphinidin 3-rutinoside and cyanidin 3-rutinoside are directly absorbed in rats and humans and appear in the blood as the intact forms. J Agric Food Chem 49: 1546–1551.
26. McGhie TK, Walton MC (2007) The bioavailability and absorption of anthocyanins: towards a better understanding. Mol Nutr Food Res 51: 702–713.
27. Manacha C, Moranda C, Demignéa C, Texierb O, Régérat F, et al. (1997) Bioavailability of rutin and quercetin in rats. FEBS Lett 409: 12–16.
28. Hollman PCH (2004) Absorption, bioavailability, and metabolism of flavonoids. Pharm Biol, 42(s1): 74–83.
29. Bin Hafeez B, Asim M, Siddiqui IA, Adhami VM, Murtaza I, et al. (2008) Delphinidin, a dietary anthocyanidin in pigmented fruits and vegetables: a new weapon to blunt prostate cancer growth. Cell Cycle 7: 3320–3326.
30. Lee NK, Choi YG, Baik JY, Han SY, Jeong DW, et al. (2005) A crucial role for reactive oxygen species in RANKL-induced osteoclast differentiation. Blood 106: 852–859.
31. Srinivasan S, Koenigstein A, Joseph J, Sun L, Kalyanaraman B, et al. (2010) Role of mitochondrial reactive oxygen species in osteoclast differentiation. Ann N Y Acad Sci 1192: 245–52.
32. Sen CK, Packer L (1996) Antioxidant and redox regulation of gene transcription. FASEB J 10: 709–20.
33. Kwon JY, Lee KW, Hur HJ, Lee HJ (2007) Peonidin inhibits phorbol-ester-induced COX-2 expression and transformation in JB6 P+ cells by blocking phosphorylation of ERK-1 and -2. Ann NY Acad Sci 1095: 513–520.
34. Inami K, Sawai H, Yakushiji K, Katao Y, Matsumoto N, et al. (2008) Augmentation of TNF-induced osteoclast differentiation by inhibition of ERK and activation of p38: Similar intracellular signaling between RANKL- and TNF-induced osteoclast differentiation. Orthodontic Waves 67: 150–156.
35. Hou DX, Kai K, Li JJ, Lin S, Terahara N, et al. (2004) Anthocyanidins inhibit activator protein 1 activity and cell transformation: structure-activity relationship and molecular mechanisms. Carcinogenesis 25: 29–36.

18

New Insights into Muscle Function during Pivot Feeding in Seahorses

Sam Van Wassenbergh[1,2]*, Billy Dries[1,3], Anthony Herrel[1,2,4]

1 Department of Biology, Universiteit Antwerpen, Antwerpen, Belgium, **2** Department of Biology, Ghent University, Gent, Belgium, **3** Department of Veterinary Medical Imaging and Small Animal Orthopaedics, Ghent University, Merelbeke, Belgium, **4** Département d'Ecologie et de Gestion de la Biodiversité, Centre National de la Recherche Scientifique/Muséum National d'Histoire Naturelle, Paris, France

Abstract

Seahorses, pipefish and their syngnathiform relatives are considered unique amongst fishes in using elastic recoil of post-cranial tendons to pivot the head extremely quickly towards small crustacean prey. It is known that pipefish activate the epaxial muscles for a considerable time before striking, at which rotations of the head and the hyoid are temporarily prevented to allow energy storage in the epaxial tendons. Here, we studied the motor control of this system in seahorses using electromyographic recordings of the epaxial muscles and the sternohyoideus-hypaxial muscles with simultaneous high-speed video recordings of prey capture. In addition we present the results from a stimulation experiment including the muscle hypothesised to be responsible for the locking and triggering of pivot feeding in seahorses (m. adductor arcus palatini). Our data confirmed that the epaxial pre-activation pattern observed previously for pipefish also occurs in seahorses. Similar to the epaxials, the sternohyoideus-hypaxial muscle complex shows prolonged anticipatory activity. Although a considerable variation in displacements of the mouth via head rotation could be observed, it could not be demonstrated that seahorses have control over strike distance. In addition, we could not identify the source of the kinematic variability in the activation patterns of the associated muscles. Finally, the stimulation experiment supported the previously hypothesized role of the m. adductor arcus palatini as the trigger in this elastic recoil system. Our results show that pre-stressing of both the head elevators and the hyoid retractors is taking place. As pre-activation of the main muscles involved in pivot feeding has now been demonstrated for both seahorses and pipefish, this is probably a generalized trait of Syngnathidae.

Editor: Marc H.E. de Lussanet, University of Münster, Germany

Funding: This work was supported by a grant from the Fund for Scientific Research Flanders (G053907; www.fwo.be) and a Fund for Scientific Research Flanders Postdoctoral Fellowship to SVW. The funders had no role in study design, data collection and analysis, decision to publish, or preparation of the manuscript.

Competing Interests: The authors have declared that no competing interests exist.

* Email: sam.vanwassenbergh@ugent.be

Introduction

Constraints on muscular power generation have led to the evolution of mechanisms relying on elastic recoil to perform movements that are fast and powerful enough to capture exceptionally elusive prey. Examples of elastic energy storage and release during prey capture can be found in tongue-projection mechanisms in chameleons [1–3], salamanders [4] and toads [5], hyoid motions during intra-oral prey processing in knifefish [6], raptorial appendage strikes in mantis shrimps [7,8]), carnivorous terrestrial plants employing trap-snapping [9] or tentacle-snapping [10], and aquatic carnivorous plants generating a sudden trap inflation to produce suction [11]. Since these movements rely on the same mechanical principles as catapults (i.e., a slow increase in strain in an elastic material during preparation, followed by a triggered release of the stored elastic energy during the launch), they are sometimes referred to as biological catapults [12].

Syngnathid fishes (pipefishes, seahorses, and seadragons) use movements driven by catapult-like mechanics to rapidly capture elusive prey such as small crustaceans [13–16]. This action involves a very fast dorsal rotation of the head that brings the mouth close to the prey [13,17–19]. Subsequently, suction is produced to draw the prey into the mouth cavity [18]. This dual-phase mechanism (i.e., head rotation followed by suction) is called pivot feeding [17]. Syngnathids can generate very high angular accelerations of the head because this motion is powered by the recoil of the epaxial tendons [14]. The latter study showed that the epaxial muscle of the pipefish *Syngnathus leptorhynchus* is active for at least 200 milliseconds prior to the start of head rotation, allowing the storage of energy by stretching these tendons. Afterwards, the head is suddenly rotated over more than 20 degrees in less than 5 milliseconds, leaving prey almost no chance to react.

Despite the recent advances in our understanding of the feeding mechanics of syngnathid fishes, several hypotheses related to motor control remain untested. Firstly, the timing of activation of the epaxial musculature in syngnathids has only been studied in a single species of pipefish. Still, as considerable variation exists within the Syngnathidae in cranial and post-cranial morphology [20] as well as in the kinematics of head rotation [19], data from sister taxa of this pipefish species are needed to confirm whether the same pattern of epaxial muscle activity is widespread within Syngnathidae. Secondly, while muscle activation patterns have only been measured for the epaxial muscle [14], a similarly long tendon is present on the ventral side of the head: the tendon of the sternohyoideus-hypaxial muscle [14,16] which inserts on the hypohyals and ceratohyals of the hyoid via the urohyal (Figure 1A, B). Consequently, we hypothesised that an activation pattern comparable to that measured for the epaxial muscles may also occur in the sternohyoideus-hypaxials. In addition, two aspects of the prey-capture kinematics suggest a pre-activated state: (1) we argued that the absence of dorsal bending of the trunk during the loading phase suggests that the stress in the epaxial region is countered by forces at the ventral (i.e. hypaxial) side of the vertebral column [14], and (2) the initial angular acceleration of the hyoid is extremely fast compared to other fish [18].

Previous analyses of kinematics showed a considerable amount of variation in the magnitude of head rotation within the seahorse *Hippocampus reidi* [18,21]. We therefore hypothesised that seahorses are capable of active control over the distance they rotate their head as a function of prey distance. If so, this should be reflected in the recruitment and/or activation characteristics of the epaxials (head rotation accelerators) and/or the sternohyoideus-hypaxials (which theoretically can act as head decelerators in the final phase of cranial rotation; [16,17]). Consequently, to increase the magnitude of head rotation, we predict an increased level of epaxial muscle activation and/or a decreased level of sternohyoideus-hypaxial activation.

Finally, the current hypothesis on the triggering mechanism of pivot feeding in syngnathids suggests that the head is prevented from rotating dorsally as long as the hyoid is prevented from rotating ventrally in between the preopercular bones [16,17] (Figure 1C, D). The coupled motion of the hyoid and neurocranium results from a four-bar linkage involving these two elements [13,17,21,22]. Since the preopercula are adducted by the adductor arcus palatini muscle (Figure 1A, B), activation offset in this muscle coupled with activity onset of its antagonist, the levator arcus palatini, may trigger release of the hyoid and neurocranium for rotation. So far, however, no experimental data have been collected to evaluate this hypothesis.

The goal of this study was to test the following hypotheses by means of simultaneous recording of electromyography and high-speed video in the seahorse *Hippocampus kuda*: (1) epaxial pre-activation is not restricted to pipefish; (2) sustained pre-activation is also present in the sternohyoideus-hypaxial muscle complex; (3) seahorses display control of mouth displacement distance in relation to prey distance, and if so (4) this motor control is reflected

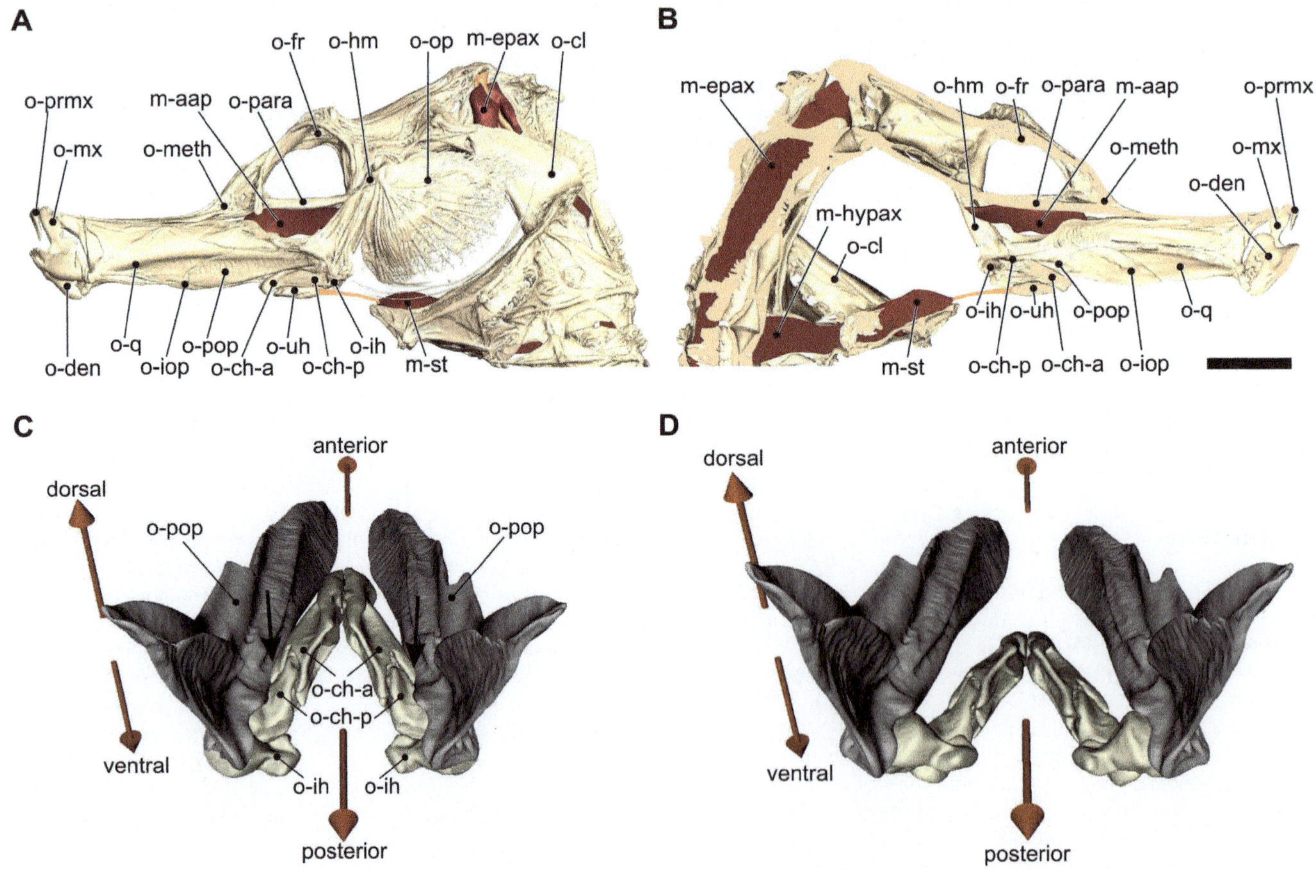

Figure 1. Anatomy of the head and illustration of the hyoid locking hypothesis in *Hippocampus reidi*. Left lateral view of the CT-reconstruction of the cranium with addition of the stimulated muscles based on histological sections (A), a medial view of the left side of the head with the opercular bone removed (B). Below, a detailed view on the hyoid and suspensorium illustrate the morphological configuration hypothesised to be responsible for locking of hyoid and head rotation where the posteriolateral part of the anterior ceratohyals lies dorsally of one of the medial grooves of the adducted preopercular bones (C), and the unlocked configuration where the ceratohyals are free to rotate ventrally after slight abduction of the preopercula (D). Orange lines in (A) and (B) represent tendinous connections. The arrows indicate the most likely contact region between the ceratohyals and the preopercula. Abbreviations: m-aap, adductor arcus palatini; m-epax, epaxial muscle; m-hypax, hypaxial muscle; m-st, sternohyoideus muscle; o-ch-a, anterior ceratohyal bone; o-ch-p, posterior ceratohyal bone; o-cl, cleithrum; o-den, dentary bone; o-fr, frontal bone; o-hm; hyomandibular bone; o-ih, interhyal bone; o-iop, interopercular bone; o-meth, mesethmoid bone; o-mx, maxillary bone; o-op, opercular bone; o-para, parasphenoid bone; o-pop, preopercular bone; o-prmx, premaxillary bone; o-q, quadrate bone; o-uh, urohyal bone. Scale bar, 5 mm.

in the electromyographic patterns of the epaxials and/or the sternohyoideus-hypaxials. Finally, we evaluate the proposed mechanism of the relaxation of preopercular adduction as the trigger of the pivot feeding catapult system via a muscle stimulation experiment in *Hippocampus reidi*.

Materials and Methods

Ethics statement

All experiments were approved by the animal ethics committee at the University of Antwerp (Ethische Commissie Dierproeven, Permit Number: 2011-69, approved 11/2011), under the condition of strictly minimizing the number of individuals used in the experiments.

Study animals

Seahorses of the species *Hippocampus kuda* Bleeker, 1852 (electromyography analysis; 2 individuals) and *Hippocampus reidi* Ginsburg, 1933 (electric stimulation experiment; 2 individuals plus 1 individual for a fatigue test) were used. These species were chosen based on availability in captive-bred stocks of local commercial aquarium trade. The animals were housed in a large aquarium (200l) with a constant temperature (24°C), salinity (35 ppt) and photoperiod (12:12) and were fed daily with freely suspended, defrosted *Neomysis vulgaris*. The *H. kuda* individuals had head lengths (= snout tip to back of the coronet) of 14.1 mm (individual 1) and 15.2 mm (individual 2); head lengths of the *H. reidi* individuals were measured 31.9 mm, 32.4 mm and 34.8 mm.

Electromyography (EMG) and high-speed video recordings

The seahorses were anaesthetized with tricaine methanesulfonate (MS222) prior to insertion of bipolar stainless steel (Advent Research Materials Ltd, Halesworth, England) twisted-hook, quadruple Teflon-insulated electrodes with cross-sectional diameters of 75 μm via hypodermic needles. The approximately 0.5 mm long uncoated tips of the electrodes were inserted into two muscles: the epaxial muscle at the level of the second anterior bony ring of the trunk, and mid-belly in the sternohyoideus-hypaxial muscle (Figure 2). Electrode positions were verified by lateral view radiographs (Ajex 9020H X-ray generator, Ajex Meditech, Seoul, Korea; EVA digital sensor, Imageworks, New York, USA) overlaid on graphical reconstructions of the anatomy (Figure 1A, B). Since no other muscles are present in the close proximity of the insertion positions, correct electrode placement could be safely confirmed. These radiographs also showed that the final pole spacing varied between 0.4 to 0.8 mm (Figure 2). Next, the animal was transferred to a small aquarium (30l), which contained a narrow section to restrict the movement during the recording session (Figure 3A). The electrode signals were amplified by a factor of 10 using Gould Universal preamplifiers (Gould Electronics, Eichstetten, Germany; filter bandpass 1 to 10 000 Hz) and Honeywell Accudata 117DC amplifiers (Honeywell International Inc., Morristown, USA) before being recorded digitally on tape using a TEAC 145 T DAT recorder (TEAC Corporation, Tokyo, Japan). EMG data was monitored and exported to ASCII files using TEAC QuickVu software, and further analyzed in Microsoft Excel. All EMGs were recorded within 36 hours from the start of the anaesthesia.

Dual view high-speed videos were recorded simultaneously with EMG: a Redlake MotionPro HR1000 camera (IDT, Tallahassee, USA) filmed in lateral view at 1000 frames per second, and a Redlake Motionscope M3 camera filmed in frontal view at 500 frames per second (Figure 3A). The camera views were orthogonal and perpendicular to the aquarium walls, which minimizes the distortion of the imaging volume. To allow synchronization between the EMG and the videos, LEDs in view of each camera were powered by a Grass S48 squared wave pulse generator (Grass Technologies, West Warwick, USA), of which the output was connected to an amplifier channel that was recorded on the DAT. Three infrared 140-LED (Scene Electronics, Shenzhen, China) arrays provided the necessary illumination.

Time zero was set as the time of the video image in which the first feeding motion, depression of the hyoid, was visible. Since the signal-to-noise ratios of the EMGs were relatively low due to the small size of the muscles, the following calculation steps had to be performed to determine the onset and offset times of the activity bursts of the muscles. After rectification (Figure 4A), a period of about 1 s only containing noise and occurring well before the strike (>1 s) was selected. Signal threshold was set at the 99% confidence limit (mean +2.576 standard deviations) of the voltage amplitude of this noise period. Next, the EMG amplitudes were averaged for 25 ms intervals. This interval length was selected as shorter intervals regularly yielded multiple crossings of the signal threshold within one burst of EMG. Falsely identified signal or noise intervals were corrected if they were neighbored by two intervals of an opposite result. The onset time then corresponded to the start of the first 25 ms interval value exceeding this noise voltage treshold (Figure 4B). The offset time was the end of the latest 25 ms interval exceeding this treshold (Figure 4B). For the onset-to-offset interval, the following variables were calculated (Figure 4C): duration, mean amplitude, peak amplitude, time of peak amplitude, and time integral. The latter variable was included since the time integral of EMG bursts has shown to correlate particularly well with muscle force during feeding movements [23,24]. EMGs were analysed from 12 successful feeding sequences of individual 1, and 13 successful feeding sequences of individual 2.

Video analysis

To study whether motor patterns are related to prey distance in *Hippocampus kuda*, two variables were quantified based on the dual view high-speed video images: prey distance and mouth travel distance. The three-dimensional prey distances were calculated from video stills at a single frame before the start of the movement (Figure 5). This distance runs from the centre of the mouth (position in between a dorsal and ventral landmark at the mouth in the lateral images; Figure 5) to the centre of the prey (centroid of ten approximately equally spaced landmarks along the contours of both the lateral and frontal view video images). The three-dimensional mouth travel distances were calculated between video stills at one frame before the start of the feeding motion and at one frame after the capture of the prey (Figure 5), using the coordinates of the mouth centre. Two-dimensional landmark coordinates were obtained using Didge (version 2.2.0, A. Cullum, Creighton University, USA) for the lateral view (*xy*-axes) and frontal view (*yz*-axes) to determine 3D coordinates (*xyz*). As the scaling factor increases with the distance of object away from the camera lens, this distance was measured from the other camera view. Next, scale factors were calculated for the front and the back of the camera view, and linear interpolations using the relative position of the mouth and prey in between front and back view planes yielded the scaling factor used in the further analyses. Prey distances could be determined for 9 (individual 1) and 12 (individual 2) prey captures. Mouth travel distances could be determined for 11 (individual 1) and 12 (individual 2) prey captures. All variables (i.e. EMG, prey distance, mouth travel

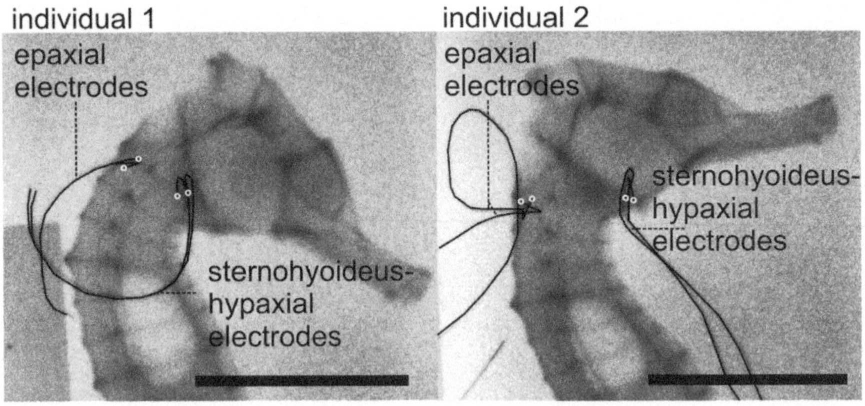

Figure 2. X-ray images showing the placement of the electrodes for both individuals in the electromyography analysis. The uncoated electrode tips are indicated by white circles. Scale bars, 10 mm.

distance) could be gathered for 9 (individual 1) and 10 (individual 2) prey captures.

Stimulation experiment

Three *Hippocampus reidi* specimens were sacrificed using an overdose of MS222 just prior to each stimulation experiment. Nickel-chrome thin wire bipolar electrodes (diameter 50 µm) were implanted in the epaxial, sternohyoideus-hypaxial and adductor arcus palatini muscles (Figure 1A, B) on each side (a total of six electrodes). Single trains of electric pulses were given with a Grass S48 stimulator [25]. Train duration was 0.3 s (corresponding to the minimal burst durations measured in the current study), pulse frequency and duration were respectively 330 Hz and 0.15 ms, and the stimulation voltage was 5 V. Because we wanted to prevent damage to the muscles, we choose a relatively low stimulation voltage. Consequently, it is likely that not all motor unit pools of the muscles under study were maximally activated, resulting in a decreased performance relative to *in vivo* observations. Muscle fatigue was avoided by waiting at least 5 minutes between the stimulation events.

During the stimulation experiments the seahorse was placed in a dissection tray with sea water and positioned on its side, with the trunk touching the bottom of the tray but the head free to move. A Redlake Motionscope M3 camera was used to record the movements of the head in lateral view together with an on- and offset indicator of the stimulator (Figure 6B). Five stimulation events were recorded in two individuals (10 events in total). Next, the electrodes leading to the left and right adductor arcus palatini muscle were cut and an additional five stimulation events for each animal were recorded.

Two video landmarks were digitized frame by frame using Didge: 1) the tip of the snout and 2) transition of the mesethmoid and the frontal bone, located just anterior to the eye. With these two variables, the head angle relative to the horizontal axis was calculated. Since the reference frame of this angle is earthbound, the head angle is expressed as this angle minus the initial head angle.

The third animal was used to validate whether head rotation characteristics remained unaffected by the increasing number of stimulation trials. The six muscles of this animal were stimulated for fifteen consecutive trials using the same stimulation parameters and rest times as described above, while movement of the head was recorded. Regressing (ordinary least squares) the maximal head velocity calculated in each trial to trial number gave a slope of 0.12, and no relation between maximal head velocity and the trial number was observed ($R^2 = 0.002$, $P = 0.87$).

Statistics

To test whether the EMG onset and offset times and durations differ between the two muscles within each individual, two-tailed

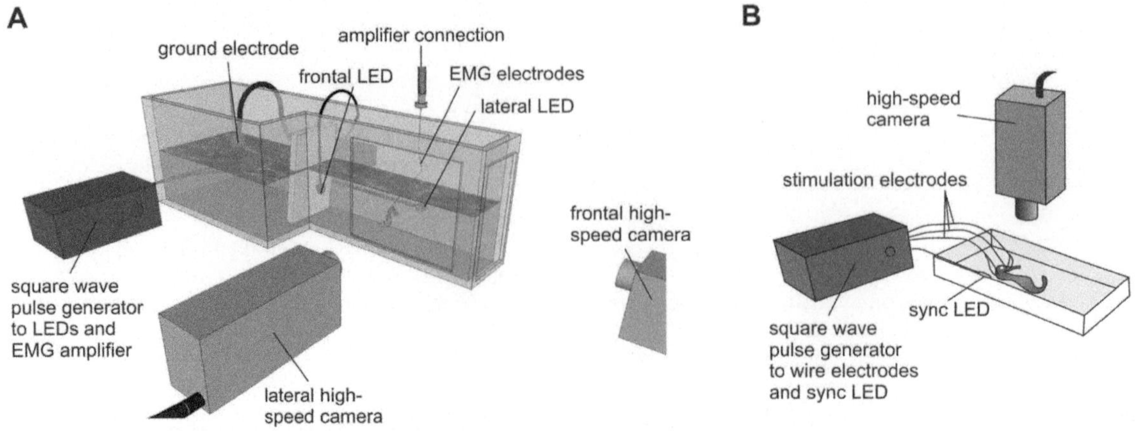

Figure 3. Experimental set-up for electromyography (A) and for the stimulation experiment (B).

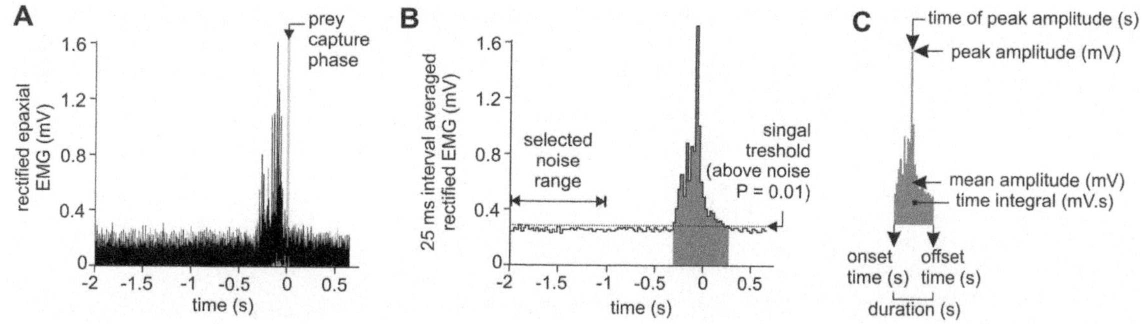

Figure 4. Calculation steps in the analysis of the recorded EMGs. The rectified EMG signal with the duration of the prey capture phase (narrow grey bar) is shown in (A). In (B) noise range selection is illustrated, with determination of the onset and offset times for 25 ms intervals exceeding the signal threshold of the 99% confidence limit of the noise. In (C), the six EMG variables are shown.

paired Student T-tests were performed. Unpaired T-tests are used to test whether there are differences between individuals within muscle. To test whether a correlation exists between prey distance and mouth travel distance, and between prey distance or mouth travel distance and the EMG variables, reduced major axis (RMA) models were used (RMA add-in for Excel; University of Ottawa, LPC Freeware). This type of analysis is recommended when the samples of both co-dependent variables include a comparable

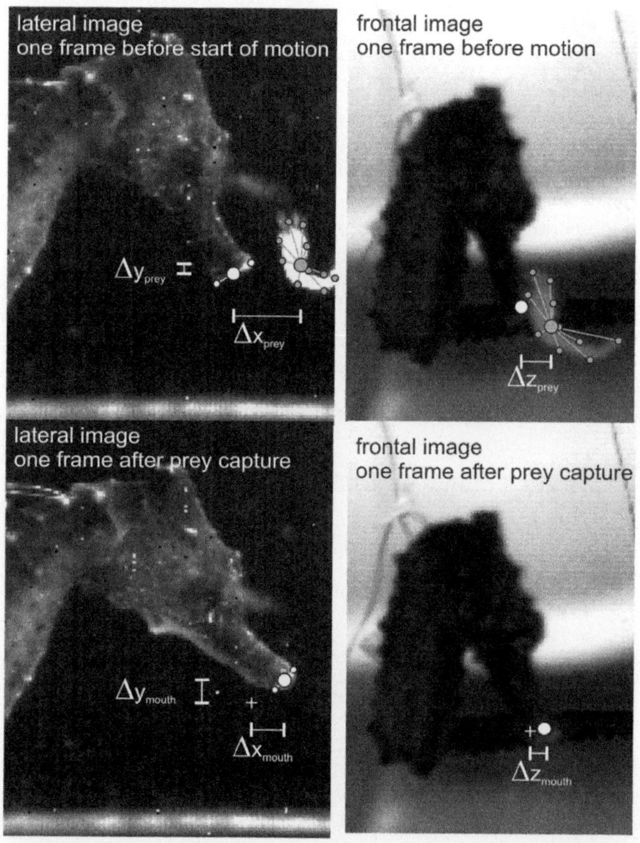

Figure 5. Example of the calculation of prey distance and mouth travel distance. The formulae $\sqrt{\Delta x^2_{prey}+\Delta y^2_{prey}+\Delta z^2_{prey}}$ and $\sqrt{\Delta x^2_{mouth}+\Delta y^2_{mouth}+\Delta z^2_{mouth}}$ were used to calculate these two respective variables via digitization of landmarks at the mouth and at the contours of the prey on video images shot with two perpendicular cameras. In the lower panels, "+" indicates the position of the centre of the mouth at one frame before the start of head rotation. See text for further information.

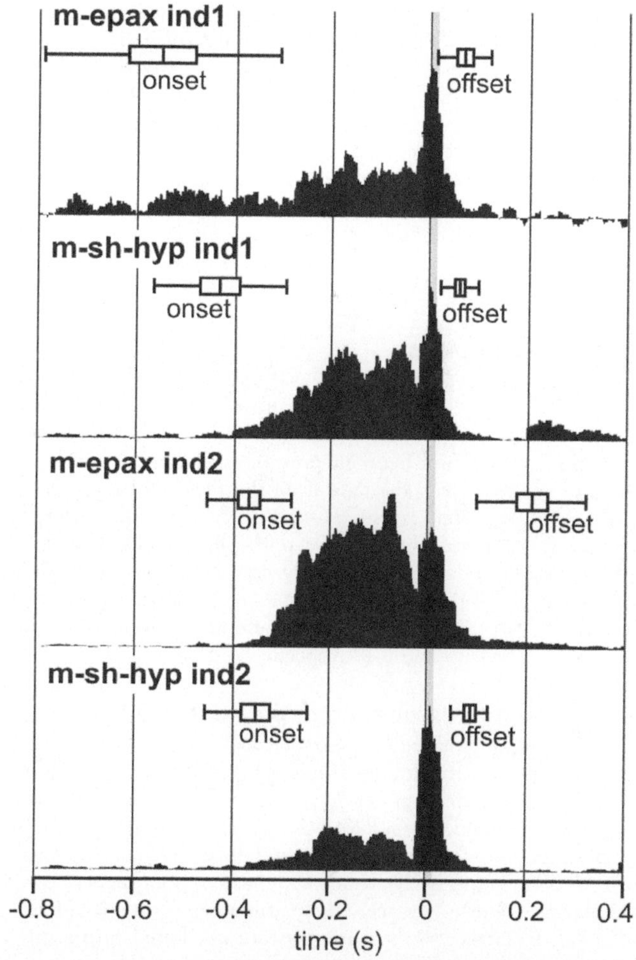

Figure 6. Activation patterns for the epaxial muscle (m-epax) and the sternohyoideus-hypaxial muscle (m-st-hyp). The start of the prey-capture movement equals time = 0 s with a grey bar indicating the duration of the head rotation phase. Boxes (mean±s.e.) and whiskers (mean±s.d) denote the onset and offset times. Black profiles represent the within-individual means of the integrated rectified EMGs above or below the noise level. Mean profile amplitudes are separately scaled to improve clarity.

degree of natural variation, and the *XY* and *YX* line fittings are presumed to display symmetry [26].

Five kinematic variables of the stimulation trials in which the adductor arcus palatini muscles were stimulated, and of the trials in which the adductor arcus palatini muscles were not stimulated, were compared using within each individual using two-tailed T-tests. These variables were (1) the total head rotation, (2) the time between the onset of head rotation and the instant of maximal head rotation, (3) the mean velocity of head rotation, (4) the timing of the instant of maximal velocity, and (5) the time between the first visible movement and the onset of the stimulation.

Results

Onset and offset times

The onset times of the epaxial muscle (m-epax) and sternohyoideus-hypaxial muscles (m-st-hyp) did not differ significantly within each individual (ind.1, $P=0.16$; ind.2, $P=0.63$) (Figure 6). Activation onset of the epaxial muscle preceded the start of head and hyoid rotation by minimally 0.19 s (average±s.d. = −0.55±0.24 s) and 0.23 s (average±s.d. = −0.36±0.24 s) for individual 1 and 2, respectively. Onset of the hypaxial muscle preceded the first motion by a minimum of 0.30 s (average±s.d. = −0.43±0.14 s) and 0.12 s (average±s.d. = −0.35±0.10 s). Activation lasted until shortly after completion of head rotation (Figure 2). Offset times were significantly greater for the m-epax compared to the m-st-hyp for individual 2 ($P=0.005$), but this difference was not detected for individual 1 ($P=0.77$). The second individual showed a later onset and offset time for m-epax only compared to individual 1 ($P=0.016$, onset; $P=0.0005$, offset) suggesting individual differences in electrode position within the muscles or control strategies between individuals.

Kinematic modulation

Prey distance varied between 3.9 mm and 6.1 mm (average±s.d. = 5.3±0.6 mm), and mouth travel distance ranged from 3.2 mm to 4.7 mm (average±s.d. = 4.0±0.4 mm). No significant correlation was found between prey distance and mouth travel distance when pooling the data from the two individuals (RMA regression slope = 0.67±0.14; $R=0.35$; $P=0.14$; data corrected for head length difference between the individuals) (Figure 7). Although both individuals separately showed similar slopes (slope individual 1 = 0.53±0.15, $R=0.48$; slope individual 2 = 0.90±0.28; $R=0.12$), these relationships were also not significant ($P=0.19$ and 0.48 respectively) (Figure 7).

Motor control as a function of prey distance

No significant correlations were detected between prey distance and any of the variables describing the EMG pattern of the m-epax and m-st-hyp within each individual. The only noteworthy trends were a tendency of later onset and longer time to peak m-epax amplitude with more distant prey in individual 1 ($P=0.07$ and 0.053, respectively), and a tendency for higher mean amplitudes of m-st-hyp with more distant prey in individual 2 ($P=0.053$). However, these trends were not found in the other individual.

Variation in mouth travel distance was also not significantly related to the variables describing the EMG pattern of the m-epax and m-st-hyp within each individual. Although the predicted pattern of increased mean EMG amplitude of the m-epax (more powerful dorsal head rotation) combined with a decrease in the mean amplitude of the m-st-hyp (later or less powerful head deceleration) for increased head rotation was indeed observed for both individuals, the correlations were not significant (P always> 0.12). This predicted pattern could not be observed for the EMG time integral.

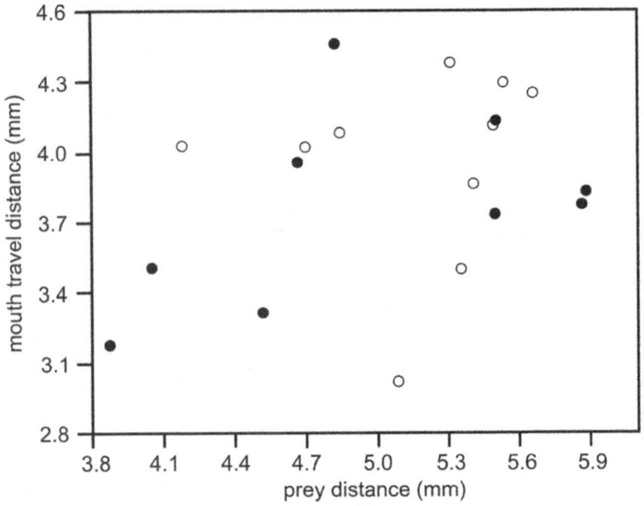

Figure 7. Relationship between prey distance and mouth travel distance. Note that no significant correlations were calculated for each of the individuals (individual 1, filled circles; individual 2, open circles).

Muscle stimulation

A clear difference was observed in the kinematics of head rotation with and without adductor arcus palatini muscle (m-aap) stimulation in *Hippocampus reidi* (Figure 8). The average maximal head angle observed when the m-aap was stimulated in conjunction with the m-epax and m-st-hyp is 34.1±2.8 deg (mean±s.d.). This angle is significantly larger than the angle of 19.1±1.9 deg, observed when the adductor muscles were not activated ($P<0.0001$ for both individuals). However the average time between the onset of head rotation to maximal head rotation did not differ statistically between both treatments ($P>0.05$ for both individuals).

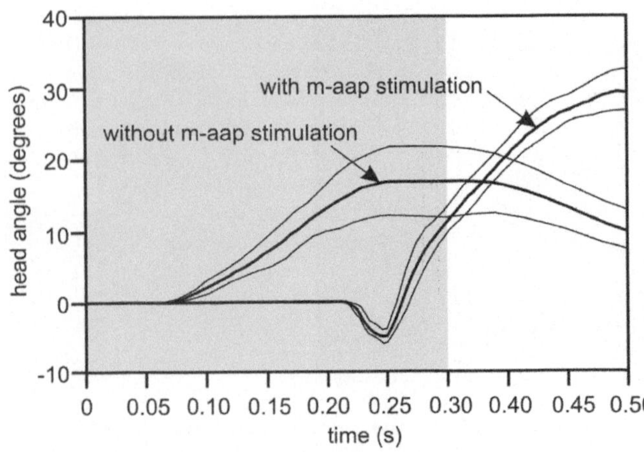

Figure 8. Results of the stimulation experiment. The figure shows the time-dependent kinematic profile of head rotation (mean±s.d.) when the epaxial, hypaxial and adductor arcus palatine muscles are stimulated, and when only the epaxial and hypaxial muscles are stimulated. The grey zone represents the time of stimulation. $N=2$ individuals, five repetitions per individual and stimulation treatment.

After the m-aap were activated the resulting average angular head velocity was 584±40 deg s^{-1}, which was significantly higher than the angular head velocity of 210±24 deg s^{-1} when the adductor muscles were not stimulated ($P<0.00001$ for both individuals). The average timing at which maximal head velocity was reached was also different in both situations ($P<0.0001$). This timing was 0.012±0.003 ms and 0.12±0.03 ms in the stimulated and non-stimulated situation of the m-aap, respectively.

There was a clear difference between stimulation treatments in timing between the first visible movement and the onset of stimulation ($P<0.00001$ for both individuals) (Figure 8). When the m-aap were stimulated, no movement occurred until an average of 48.90±2.11 ms before the end of stimulation. This means that no movement was observed for approximately 250 ms of stimulation. When the adductor arcus palatini muscles are not stimulated, visible movement occurs after 59±17 ms of stimulation.

Discussion

Our results indicate that seahorses activate the epaxial muscles a considerable time before (i.e. >0.3 s) the start of the first visible prey capture movement (Figure 6). This finding matches results from pipefish [14], suggesting that this is a generalized syngnathid trait. Epaxial pre-activation allows the animal to strain the left and right epaxial tendons and store elastic energy which can later be used to power the rotation of the head during pivot feeding. The presence of such a power amplification system in seahorses was already suggested by inverse dynamic modelling in juvenile seahorses, which showed an instantaneous peak power of over 3000 W per kg of epaxial muscle required to accelerate the head as observed on high-speed videos [15]. Such high values of instantaneous power output inevitably call for the use of recoil of pre-stressed elastic tissues, as the maximal instantaneous value reported for vertebrate skeletal muscle is 1120 W per kg [27,28]. The current EMG results confirm the presence of such a mechanism in adults of the species *Hippocampus kuda*.

The hypothesis that the ventral series of muscles inserting on the hyoid (i.e. a complex formed by the sternohyoideus and the hypaxial muscle) would show a sustained pre-activation comparable to that of the epaxial muscles [14] was also confirmed (Figure 6). Since white muscle used for suction feeding in teleost fish (without significant series elastic element) generally need activation times of less than 20 ms to reach half the maximum isometric force upon *in-vitro* tetanus stimulation [29,30], the observed delay between activation onset and the first hyoid motion of generally over 300 ms (Figure 2) means that considerable retraction force will be exerted on the hyoid prior to the start of the strike at the prey. This inevitably implies some stretching of the sternohyoideus tendon, and elastic recoil and power amplification in the ventral muscle-tendons causing the extremely fast rotation of the hyoid [21] seems likely. Yet, empirical evidence for this can only be given by *in-vivo* strain measurements (e.g. wallabee hopping [31]; frog jumping [12]).

The observed activation patterns of the sternohyoideus-hypaxial muscle rule out the option that this muscle would work as the trigger of the pivot-feeding system of Syngnathidae. This triggering function was proposed by [13] by assuming that the line of action of the sternohyoideus muscle differs from the straight line between the ceratohyal symphysis and the pectoral girdle muscle attachment site formed by the urohyal-sternohyoideus compex. A closer morphological inspection of this system in the seahorse *Hippocampus reidi* [21] and the pipefish *Syngnathus acus* [17] failed to reveal such a system: like in other teleosts, the urohyal typically ossifies within the tendon of the sternohyoideus and will therefore be positioned in the working line of sternohyoideus muscle-tendon. The EMG pattern observed here, confirms that the force from the sternohyoideus does not result in a subtle configuration change in the hyoid-neurocranium four-bar linkage causing the "quick-release" of the system. In addition, no correlations between EMG timing and amplitude variables with the motion onset were found.

The presented kinematic data could not prove that a feed-forward control mechanism is involved in *H. kuda* to fine-tune the amount of head rotation to the distance of the prey. Similar to previous studies on other syngnathid fishes [18,19], we have shown that there is a considerable strike-to-strike variation in the magnitude of head rotation, but it could not be confirmed for *H. kuda* that this variation is related to the distance from the mouth to the prey at the onset of the strike (Figure 7). Yet, as suction is only effective to draw prey into the mouth from a relatively short distance in stationary predators (e.g. [32]), an accurate positioning of the mouth close to the prey is critical to improve prey capture success. Alternatively, being able to modulate head rotation magnitude would reduce the time and energy spent in pursuing the prey by broadening the range head positions with respect to the prey from which successful strikes can be initiated. Motor control to adjust the degree of head rotation during suction feeding has been shown previously for catfish [33]. The reason why we assume that this would require a feed-forward mechanism in sygnathids, rather than feed-back control as described for other fishes [34,35], is the extremely short time (generally <5 ms) between the onset of the movement and the actual ingestion of the prey. This time is shorter than the range of reaction latencies measured for fish, which vary from 5 to 40 ms among different species as illustrated for escape responses by Eaton and Hackett [36]. However, our data were not conclusive on the existence of such a feed-forward mechanism during pivot-feeding in *H. cuda*.

In addition, no indication of an active control of the epaxial and sternohyoideus-hypaxial muscles in function of prey distance or mouth travel distance was detected in our EMG data. In other words, it remains unclear how syngnathids manage to vary their head rotation amplitude. We hypothesised that either an increased activation of the epaxials for farther-reaching strikes would occur, or that that tension would build faster in the ventral series of muscles, tendons and ligaments by altered activation patterns of the sternohyoideus-hypaxial muscles. Neither of these hypotheses could be confirmed with our data. However, the signal-to-noise ratio of our measurements may have been too low due to the relatively small size of the muscles (Figure 4A). This may have introduced error in the electromyographic variables preventing us from detecting correlations between muscle activation patterns and the relatively small kinematic changes. Alternatively, control may be manifested in other regions of these muscles (only a single electrode per muscle was used), or in other muscles (e.g., protractor hyoidei, adductor arcus palatini).

The results from the stimulation experiment are in line with the current hypothesis [17] that the main muscle responsible for locking and triggering the release of the hyoid is the adductor arcus palatini muscle (m-aap). Activation of the m-aap blocks the hyoid from moving ventrally for a considerable time, which upon release increased the acceleration, peak velocity and head rotation magnitude (Figure 8). Although the precise *in-vivo* behaviour could not be reproduced in this artificial stimulation experiment, it clearly points to an important role of suspensorium abduction in the locking and triggering process. Electromyographic data of the m-aap during prey capture would be extremely informative in this respect, but the small size of this muscle and its position medial of the suspensorium make this measurement untractable. Previous work has shown that the mass of the m-aap is considerably higher than needed if its role during feeding would be limited to reposition the abducted suspensorium by compressing the buccal cavity to its resting state after feeding [37]. Combined with this observation, our stimulation experiments support the role of the m-aap as the lock and trigger of the elastic recoil mechanism during pivot feeding in seahorses.

In conclusion, the hypothesis that fast head rotation during pivot feeding is driven by catapult-like mechanics of the musculoskeletal system [13] was confirmed for seahorses. The pre-activated state of the head-rotator muscles for generally more than 0.3 s prior to the onset of the strike allows storage of energy in the epaxial tendons (Figure 6). As this is similar to previous results on pipefish [14], this suggests that this type of feeding mechanics is probably widespread among syngnathid species. The present study is the first to show that a pre-activated state is also present in the hyoid-retractor muscles at the ventral side of the head (Figure 6). As long as the rotation of the hyoid is prevented by suspensorium adduction (Figure 1C, D) while experiencing retraction force, the dorsal and ventral pre-activated muscles will work antagonistically, the head remains static, and elastic elements in series with these muscles can be strained. The adductor arcus palatini muscles are probably of crucial importance in locking and release triggering of this mechanism, as shown by our stimulation experiment (Figure 8). After the release of the hyoid, quick dorsal rotation of the head will bring the mouth close to the prey. The present study could not demonstrate that prey located farther away from the mouth elucidated a higher magnitude of head rotation (Figure 7), and neither did our data show altered muscle activity patterns that could be causing the observed kinematic variation.

Acknowledgments

Gert Roos and Peter Aerts are acknowledged for their help with the stimulation experiments. We thank Heleen Leysen for providing images for Figure 1. Also thanks to Dominique Adriaens, Nicolai Konow, and four anonymous reviewers for comments on earlier versions of this manuscript.

Author Contributions

Conceived and designed the experiments: SVW AH. Performed the experiments: SVW BD. Analyzed the data: SVW BD. Contributed reagents/materials/analysis tools: AH. Wrote the paper: SVW BD AH.

References

1. Herrel A, Meyers JJ, Aerts P, Nishikawa KC (2000) The mechanics of prey prehension in chameleons. J Exp Biol 203: 3255–3263.
2. De Groot JH, van Leeuwen JL (2004) Evidence for an elastic projection mechanism in the chameleon tongue. Proc R Soc B 271: 761–770. doi:10.1098/rspb.2003.2637.
3. Anderson CV, Deban SM (2012) Thermal effects on motor control and in vitro muscle dynamics of the ballistic tongue apparatus in chameleons. J Exp Biol 215: 4345–4357. doi:10.1242/jeb.078881.
4. Deban SM, O'Reilly JC, Dicke U, van Leeuwen JL (2007) Extremely high-power tongue projection in plethodontid salamanders. J Exp Biol 210: 655–667. doi:10.1242/jeb.02664.
5. Lappin AK, Monroy JA, Pilarski JQ, Zepnewski ED, Pierotti DJ, et al. (2006) Storage and recovery of elastic potential energy powers ballistic prey capture in toads. J Exp Biol 209: 2535–2553. doi:10.1242/jeb.02276.
6. Konow N, Camp AL, Sanford CPJ (2008) Congruence between muscle activity and kinematics in a convergently derived prey-processing behavior. Int Comp Biol 48: 246–260. doi:10.1093/icb/icn045.
7. Patek SN, Nowroozi BN, Baio JE, Caldwell RL, Summers AP (2007) Linkage mechanics and power amplification of the mantis shrimp's strike. J Exp Biol 210: 3677–3688. doi:10.1242/jeb.006486.
8. McHenry MJ, Claverie T, Rosario MV, Patek SN (2012) Gearing for speed slows the predatory strike of a mantis shrimp. J Exp Biol 215: 1231–1245. doi:10.1242/jeb.061465.
9. Forterre Y, Skotheim JM, Dumais J, Mahadevan L (2005) How the Venus flytrap snaps. Nature 433: 421–425. doi:10.1038/nature03185.
10. Poppinga S, Hartmeyer SRH, Seidel R, Masselter T, Hartmeyer I, et al. (2012) Catapulting tentacles in a sticky carnivorous plant. PLoS ONE 7: e45735. doi:10.1371/journal.pone.0045735.
11. Singh AK, Prabhakar S, Sane SP (2011) The biomechanics of fast prey capture in aquatic bladderworts. Biol Lett 7: 547–550. doi:10.1098/rsbl.2011.0057.
12. Astley HC, Roberts TJ (2012) Evidence for a vertebrate catapult: elastic energy storage in the plantaris tendon during frog jumping. Biol Lett 8: 386–389. doi:10.1098/rsbl.2011.0982.
13. Muller M (1987) Optimization principles applied to the mechanism of neurocranial levation and mouth bottom depression in bony fishes (Halecostomi). J Theor Biol 126: 343–368. doi:10.1016/S0022-5193(87)80241-2.
14. Van Wassenbergh S, Strother JA, Flammang BE, Ferry-Graham LA, Aerts P (2008) Extremely fast prey capture in pipefish is powered by elastic recoil. J R Soc Interface 5: 285–296. doi:10.1098/rsif.2007.1124.
15. Van Wassenbergh S, Roos G, Genbrugge A, Leysen H, Aerts P, et al. (2009) Suction is kids play: extremely fast suction in newborn seahorses. Biol Lett 5: 200–203. doi:10.1098/rsbl.2008.0765.
16. Van Wassenbergh S, Leysen H, Adriaens D, Aerts P (2013) Mechanics of snout expansion in suction-feeding seahorses: musculoskeletal force transmission. J Exp Biol 216: 407–417. doi:10.1242/jeb.074658.
17. de Lussanet MHE, Muller M (2007) The smaller your mouth, the longer your snout: predicting the snout length of *Syngnathus acus*, *Centriscus scutatus* and other pipette feeders. J R Soc Interface 4: 561–573. doi:10.1098/rsif.2006.0201.
18. Roos G, Van Wassenbergh S, Herrel A, Aerts P (2009) Kinematics of suction feeding in the seahorse *Hippocampus reidi*. J Exp Biol 212: 3490–3498. doi:10.1242/jeb.033050.
19. Van Wassenbergh S, Roos G, Ferry L (2011) An adaptive explanation for the horse-like shape of seahorses. Nat Comm 2: 164. doi:10.1038/ncomms1168.
20. Leysen H, Roos G, Adriaens D (2011) Morphological variation in pipefish and seahorse head shape in relation to snout length and developmental growth. J Morphol 272: 1259–1270. doi:10.1002/jmor.10982.
21. Roos G, Leysen H, Van Wassenbergh S, Herrel A, Jacobs P, et al. (2009) Linking morphology and motion: a test of a four-bar mechanism in seahorses. Physiol Biochem Zool 82: 7–19. doi:10.1086/589838.
22. Flammang BE, Ferry-Graham LA, Rinewalt C, Ardizzone D, Davis C, et al. (2009) Prey capture kinematics and four-bar linkages in the bay pipefish, *Syngnathus leptorhynchus*. Zoology 112: 86–96. doi:10.1016/j.zool.2008.04.003.
23. Hylander WL, Johnson KR (1989) The relationship between masseter force and masseter electromyogram during mastication in the monkey *Macaca fascicularis*. Arch Oral Biol 34: 713–722. doi:10.1016/0003-9969(89)90078-2.
24. Ottenhoff FA, van der Bilt A, van der Glas HW, Bosman F, Abbink JH (1996) The relationship between jaw elevator muscle surface electromyogram and simulated food resistance during dynamic condition in humans. J Oral Rehabil 23: 270–279. doi:10.1111/j.1365-2842.1996.tb00852.x.
25. Aerts P, De Vree F (1993) Feeding performance and muscular constraints in fish. J Exp Biol 177: 129–147.
26. Smith RJ (2009) Use and misuse of the reduced major axis for line-fitting. Am J Phys Anthropol 140: 476–486. doi:10.1002/ajpa.21090.
27. Askew GN, Marsh RL (2001) The mechanical power output of the pectoralis muscle of blue-breasted quail (*Coturnix chinensis*): the in vivo length cycle and its implications for muscle performance. J Exp Biol 204: 3587–3600.
28. Curtin NA, Woledge RC, Aerts P (2005) Muscle directly meets the vast power demands in agile lizards. Proc R Soc B 272: 581–584. doi:10.1098/rspb.2004.2982.
29. Coughlin DJ, Carroll AM (2006) *In vitro* estimates of power output by epaxial muscle during feeding in largemouth bass. Comp Biochem Phys A 145: 533–539. doi:10.1016/j.cbpa.2006.08.026.
30. Van Wassenbergh S, Herrel A, James RS, Aerts P (2007) Scaling of contractile properties of catfish feeding muscles. J Exp Biol 210: 1183–1193. doi:10.1242/jeb.000109.
31. Biewener AA, Baudinette RV (1995) In vivo muscle force and elastic energy storage during steady-speed hopping of tammar wallabies (*Macropus eugenii*). J Exp Biol 198: 1829–1841.
32. Higham TE, Day SW, Wainwright PC (2006) Multidimensional analysis of suction feeding performance in fishes: fluid speed, acceleration, strike accuracy and the ingested volume of water. J Exp Biol 209: 2713–2725. doi:10.1242/jeb.02315.
33. Van Wassenbergh S, Herrel A, Adriaens D, Aerts P (2006) Modulation and variability of prey capture kinematics in clariid catfishes. J Exp Zool 305A: 559–569. doi:10.1002/jez.a.293.
34. Aerts P (1990) Variability of the fast suction feeding process in *Astatotilapia elegans* (Teleostei: Cichlidae): a hypothesis of peripheral feedback control. J Zool Lond 220: 653–678. doi:10.1111/j.1469-7998.1990.tb04741.x.
35. Van Wassenbergh S, De Rechter D (2011) Piscivorous cyprinid fish modulates suction feeding kinematics to capture elusive prey. Zoology 114: 46–52. doi:10.1016/j.zool.2010.10.001.

36. Eaton RC, Hackett JT (1984) The role of Mauthner cells in fast-starts involving escape in teleost fish. In: Eaton RC, editor. Neural Mechanisms of startle behavior. New York: Plenum Press. 213–266.
37. Roos G (2010) Specialization of extreme head morphology: a detailed functional morphological study of feeding in seahorses and pipefishes (Syngnathidae). PhD thesis. Universiteit Antwerpen, Department of Biology.

19

MCP/CCR2 Signaling Is Essential for Recruitment of Mesenchymal Progenitor Cells during the Early Phase of Fracture Healing

Masahiro Ishikawa[1,2], Hiromu Ito[1]*, Toshiyuki Kitaori[1], Koichi Murata[1], Hideyuki Shibuya[1], Moritoshi Furu[1,2], Hiroyuki Yoshitomi[3], Takayuki Fujii[1], Koji Yamamoto[4], Shuichi Matsuda[1]

1 Department of Orthopaedic Surgery, Kyoto University Graduate School of Medicine, Kyoto, Japan, **2** Department of the Control for Rheumatic Disease, Kyoto University Graduate School of Medicine, Kyoto, Japan, **3** The Center for Innovation in Immunoregulative Technology and Therapeutics, Kyoto University Graduate School of Medicine, Kyoto, Japan, **4** Center for the Promotion of Interdisciplinary Education and Research, Kyoto University, Kyoto, Japan

Abstract

Objective: The purpose of this study was to investigate chemokine profiles and their functional roles in the early phase of fracture healing in mouse models.

Methods: The expression profiles of chemokines were examined during fracture healing in wild-type (WT) mice using a polymerase chain reaction array and histological staining. The functional effect of monocyte chemotactic protein-1 (MCP-1) on primary mouse bone marrow stromal cells (mBMSCs) was evaluated using an *in vitro* migration assay. MCP-1$^{-/-}$ and C-C chemokine receptor 2 (CCR2)$^{-/-}$ mice were fractured and evaluated by histological staining and micro-computed tomography (micro-CT). RS102895, an antagonist of CCR2, was continuously administered in WT mice before or after rib fracture and evaluated by histological staining and micro-CT. Bone graft exchange models were created in WT and MCP-1$^{-/-}$ mice and were evaluated by histological staining and micro-CT.

Results: *MCP-1* and *MCP-3* expression in the early phase of fracture healing were up-regulated, and high levels of MCP-1 and MCP-3 protein expression observed in the periosteum and endosteum in the same period. MCP-1, but not MCP-3, increased migration of mBMSCs in a dose-dependent manner. Fracture healing in MCP-1$^{-/-}$ and CCR2$^{-/-}$ mice was delayed compared with WT mice on day 21. Administration of RS102895 in the early, but not in the late phase, caused delayed fracture healing. Transplantation of WT-derived graft into host MCP-1$^{-/-}$ mice significantly increased new bone formation in the bone graft exchange models. Furthermore, marked induction of MCP-1 expression in the periosteum and endosteum was observed around the WT-derived graft in the host MCP-1$^{-/-}$ mouse. Conversely, transplantation of MCP-1$^{-/-}$ mouse-derived grafts into host WT mice markedly decreased new bone formation.

Conclusions: MCP-1/CCR2 signaling in the periosteum and endosteum is essential for the recruitment of mesenchymal progenitor cells in the early phase of fracture healing.

Editor: Federico Quaini, University-Hospital of Parma, Italy

Funding: This work was supported by Grant-in-Aids from the Ministry of Education of Japan (No. 19591756, 21591942). The funders had no role in study design, data collection and analysis, decision to publish, or preparation of the manuscript.

Competing Interests: The authors have declared that no competing interests exist.

* Email: hiromu@kuhp.kyoto-u.ac.jp

Introduction

The prevalence of osteoporosis is increasing with the aging of society. In particular, osteoporotic fractures are a major public health problem with a low one-year patient's survival rate [1,2]. Management of the fracture is difficult because of poor bone quality, and there is a high risk of fixation failure and nonunion. To avoid these difficulties, numerous attempts have been made to develop techniques to improve fracture healing, including addition or injection of bone-forming factors or cells such as mesenchymal stem/progenitor cells [3,4]. However, treatment options remain below expectations despite vigorous attempts to find new useful therapies. One major reason is that the mechanisms responsible for fracture healing are complex and not fully understood. Hence, elucidating the mechanisms involved in fracture healing is fundamental to developing novel therapeutic strategies to improve fracture healing.

Normal fracture healing follows a unique, distinct healing process, which can be divided into three overlapping phases: inflammation, repair and remodeling [5]. Among these three phases, the repair and remodeling phases largely recapitulate the process of normal bone development [6]. In contrast, the inflammation phase is a unique process that is not observed in the organogenesis of bone and develops after birth to induce bone repair. Previous studies have shown that inflammation plays a pivotal role in fracture healing [7,8] and that mesenchymal stem/progenitor cells are systemically or locally recruited to the fracture site in the early inflammatory phase [5,9]. Many proinflammatory cytokines and chemokines are released from the fracture site in the early inflammatory phase [9,10]. Chemokines are small, chemoattractant cytokines that play key roles in the recruitment of leukocytes to sites of inflammation and injury. Studies have shown that stem/progenitor cell migration and organ-specific recruitment are regulated by chemokines and their receptors [11–13]. In addition, mesenchymal stem/progenitor cells express a variety of chemokine receptors [14], and chemokine-mediated mesenchymal stem/progenitor cell migration has been shown *in vitro* and *in vivo* [15,16].

Over the past decade, attention has focused on stem/progenitor cells because of their pivotal role in tissue regeneration. Mesenchymal stem/progenitor cells exhibit extensive tropism for tissue injury sites [17]. These cells differentiate into mesenchymal lineage cells when exposed to appropriate environmental cues and can promote tissue repair of many organs, including bone. In addition, mesenchymal stem/progenitor cells appear to exist in almost all tissues, including bone marrow, muscle and the periosteum, and if not present, can reach tissues via the blood circulation [18]. Therefore, mesenchymal stem/progenitor cells can be recruited from the circulation or surrounding tissues and participate in the repair of the injured organs [12,19].

Several studies have shown that systemically infused mesenchymal stem/progenitor cells can migrate to, and participate in, the repair of injured tissue [20–22]. We have previously demonstrated in a bone graft model that stromal cell-derived factor-1 (SDF-1) is induced in the periosteum of fracture sites and promotes endochondral bone repair by recruiting C-X-C chemokine receptor 4 (CXCR4)-expressing mesenchymal stem/progenitor cells [23]. Thus, mesenchymal stem/progenitor cell therapy may be a novel therapeutic strategy to improve fracture healing. To develop an efficient therapy, it is crucial to elucidate the precise mechanisms for recruitment of mesenchymal stem/progenitor cells to the fracture site. However, these mechanisms, especially during the early inflammatory phase, are largely unknown.

To identify the factor(s) essential for normal fracture healing, we used a polymerase chain reaction (PCR) array and mouse rib fracture model in which cell potential is non-impaired by surgical intramedullary fixation. We also used an exchange-graft model to show gain- or loss-of-function. We demonstrate herein that the expression level of monocyte chemotactic protein-1 (MCP-1) is up-regulated exclusively in the early fracture phase and that MCP-1 is expressed at the periosteum and endosteum of the fractured bones. Gain- and loss-of-function studies showed that the MCP-1/C-C chemokine receptor 2 (CCR2) axis is crucial in the early phase of fracture healing. In summary, these results indicate that the MCP-1/CCR2 axis provides essential signaling for normal bone healing and may be a novel, potent therapeutic target for fracture healing.

Materials and Methods

Reagents

Recombinant mouse MCP-1 and MCP-3 were purchased from Abcam (Cambridge, MA, USA). CCR2 antagonist (RS102895) was purchased from Sigma (St. Luis, MO, USA).

Mouse rib fracture model

All animal studies were conducted in accordance with principles and procedures approved by the Kyoto University Committee of Animal Resources. Surgeries were undergone under anesthesia with diethylether, and mice were euthanatized with cervical dislocation upon sacrifice. Mouse rib fracture models were created using 6-week-old C57BL/6 wild-type (WT), MCP-$1^{-/-}$ and CCR$2^{-/-}$ mice, as described previously [24]. Five mice from each fracture group were sacrificed 0, 1, 2, 3, 5, 7, 10, 14, 21, and 25 days after fracture. To evaluate the inhibitory effect of the receptor antagonist, the mice received continuous administration of the selective CCR2 antagonist, RS102895. RS102895 was dissolved in dimethyl sulfoxide (DMSO) and via an osmotic pump (model 1002; Durect, Cupertino, CA, USA), was delivered to a total of 10 mg/kg/day, beginning 2 days before or 4 days after rib fracture, and until day 12. In the control group, DMSO alone was administered for 14 days.

Femoral segmental bone graft transplantation model

A mouse segmental bone graft model was created using 6-week-old C57BL/6 WT and MCP-$1^{-/-}$ mice as described previously [25]. Briefly, 4-mm of mid-diaphyseal segmental bone was removed from the femur of the donor mouse. The graft was dissected carefully to remove the muscle and bone marrow without compromising the periosteum, and segmental bone derived from a WT or MCP-$1^{-/-}$ mouse was transplanted immediately into a 4-mm segmental defect in a host WT or MCP-$1^{-/-}$ mouse. Four groups of segmental bone graft models were used: MCP-$1^{-/-}$ donor to MCP-$1^{-/-}$ host [knockout (KO)-to-KO], WT donor to MCP-$1^{-/-}$ host (WT-to-KO), WT donor to WT host (WT-to-WT), and MCP-$1^{-/-}$ donor to WT host (KO-to-WT). The bone graft was stabilized using a 25 G stainless pin placed through the intramedullary marrow cavity, and the mice were sacrificed on day 21 after the surgery for RNA extraction and histological analysis.

Micro-CT analysis

Mice were sacrificed postoperatively for micro-computed tomography (micro-CT) imaging on days 7 (femoral bone graft model) and 21 (rib fracture model). The rib and femur were scanned using a micro-CT system (SMX-100CT-SV3; Shimadzu, Tokyo, Japan) at 2400 views, five frames per view, 40 kV, and 40 μA. Three-dimensional (3D) images were rendered and evaluated using VG Studio MAX (Nihon Visual Science Software, Tokyo, Japan). The newly formed callus was spatially segmented from the native cortical bone in the two-dimensional (2D) tomograms, the 3D images of the callus were rendered, and the total volume was measured on the digitally extracted callus tissue. The newly formed calluses in a region of interest covering the entire length of the bone graft, including 1 mm of the host bone at both proximal and distal bone graft junctions, were analyzed to determine bone graft healing.

RNA extraction, quantitative real-time PCR and PCR array

Total RNA was extracted from mouse rib and femoral bone graft specimens as described previously [26]. A PCR array was performed to measure mRNA levels for chemokines during the fracture healing process. Two micrograms of RNA was processed using an RT2 First Strand Kit (SA Biosciences, Frederick, MD, USA) according to the manufacturer's specifications. Quantitative PCR analysis for chemokines and receptors was assessed using a chemokine array (Chemokines & Receptors PCR Array, Mouse, PAMM-022, SA Biosciences). We analyzed the data using the RT2 profiler PCR Array Data Analysis software (SA Biosciences). The change in gene expression level determined by PCR array analysis was confirmed by quantitative real-time PCR. All gene

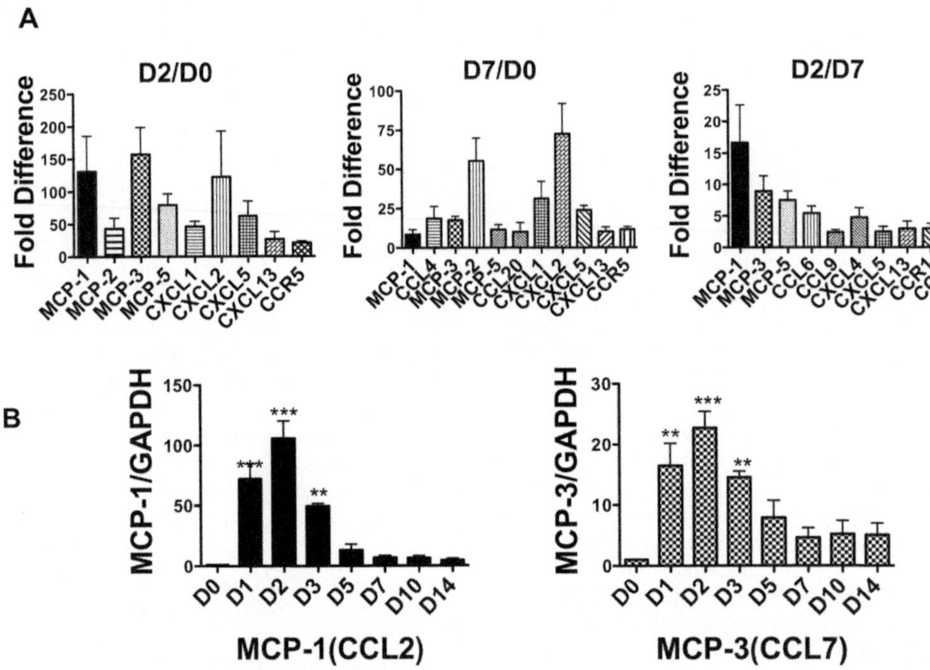

Figure 1. The expression profiles of chemokines and their receptors during fracture healing. Expression levels during fracture healing were examined using a rib fracture model. **A**: PCR array data for up-regulated chemokines and their receptors during fracture healing are shown. Expression levels were compared between days 0 and 2, days 0 and 7, and days 2 and 7. **B**: Time course of *MCP-1* and *MCP-3* mRNA expression in a rib fracture model, as analyzed by real-time PCR. Expression levels are the fold change from day 0 levels. Values are means ± SEM of more than four separate experiments. $^{**}P<0.01$ $^{***}P<0.001$ compared with the day 0 group.

expression data were normalized against glyceraldehyde phosphate dehydrogenase (GAPDH).

Histological analysis

Rib and femur specimens were processed as paraffin-embedded sections and stained with hematoxylin and eosin and were subjected to immunohistochemical analyses as described previously [23,24].

In vitro chemotaxis assay

In vitro cell migration of primary mouse bone marrow stromal cells (mBMSCs) (1.0×10^5 cells/100 µl) was assessed using Transwell inserts with an 8-µm pore membrane, as described previously [23]. For the chemotaxis assay, different concentrations of MCP-1 or MCP-3 (0, 10, or 100 ng/ml) in 500 µl of medium were applied to the lower chambers. For the inhibition assay, RS102895 (400 nM) was also applied to the lower chambers. After 24 h of incubation, the migrated cells were counted under light microscopy.

Primary cell culture, cell line, osteogenesis and chondrogenesis assay

For the osteogenesis assay, mBMSCs were harvested and cultured as described previously [23]. mBMSCs were cultured with osteogenic base media (R&D Systems, Minneapolis, MN, USA) for 2 days. On reaching 70% confluence, the medium was replaced with osteogenic differentiation medium and was changed every 3 days thereafter. In some experiments, recombinant mouse MCP-1 (200 ng/ml) was added every 3 days with each medium change. On day 14 after plating, cells were harvested for alizarin red staining and gene expression analysis. For the chondrogenesis assay, ATDC5 cells were cultured and maintained in Dulbecco's Modified Eagles Medium (DMEM) and Ham's F-12 at a 1:1 ratio with 5% fetal bovine serum (FBS) supplemented with insulin (10 mg/mL, Sigma), transferrin (5.5 mg/mL, Sigma), and sodium selenite (5 ng/mL, Sigma) to induce chondrocyte differentiation as described previously [27]. The medium was changed every 2 days thereafter. In some experiments, MCP-1 (0, 20, 100 or 200 ng/ml) was simultaneously added every 2 days with the medium change. On day 28 after plating, cells were harvested for gene expression analysis.

Statistical analysis

Data are presented as means ± standard error of the mean (SEM). We analyzed the data using GraphPad Prism Version 5.00 (GraphPad software). Statistical comparisons between two groups were performed using a Student's two-tailed t test. Differences between three groups were analyzed using the Bonferroni method. P values <0.05 were considered significant.

Results

Chemokine expression profile in the early phase of fracture healing

We first used PCR array to investigate the expression profile of chemokines during fracture healing in the WT mouse rib fracture model. The PCR array analysis showed that the expression levels of *MCP-1* and *MCP-3* were significantly higher on day 2 compared with days 0 and 7 (Figure 1A). *MCP-1* and *MCP-3* expression levels were more than 100 times higher on day 2 than on day 0. *MCP-1* and *MCP-3* expression levels on day 2 were five times higher than those on day 7. To confirm the PCR array data, we next examined the gene expression levels for *MCP-1* and

MCP-3 during the fracture healing process. Consistent with the PCR array analysis, the expression of *MCP-1* and *MCP-3* increased during the early phase of fracture healing (Figure 1B). *MCP-1* and *MCP-3* were expressed on day 1 and their expression peaked on day 2. By day 7, expression of both genes had declined markedly.

In vivo expression of MCP-1 during the early inflammatory phase of fracture healing

Because CCR2 is the major and common receptor for MCP-1 and MCP-3, we focused on the expression of MCP-1, MCP-3 and CCR2 in fracture healing, especially during the early inflammatory phase. To confirm the localization of MCP-1, MCP-3 and CCR2 expression during the early inflammatory phase of fracture healing, we used immunohistochemistry to examine rib fracture healing in WT mice. Low expression levels of MCP-1 and MCP-3 were observed at the periosteum in the unfractured rib, (Figures S1A, B) and high levels of MCP-1 and MCP-3 protein were observed at the periosteum and endosteum on day 3 in the fractured rib (Figure 2A, B). Conversely, little or no CCR2 staining was detected in the unfractured rib (Figure S1C), and on day 3, CCR2-positive cells were found predominantly within the bone marrow and surrounding tissues (Figure 2C).

MCP-1 induces mBMSCs migration *in vitro*

To examine the functional roles of MCP-1 and MCP-3 signaling in fracture healing, we first examined whether MCP-1 and MCP-3 could induce the migration of mBMSCs. MCP-1 significantly increased mBMSC migration in a dose-dependent manner, whereas MCP-3 did not (Figure 3A). Because MCP-1 and MCP-3 act through their receptor CCR2, we examined the expression of CCR2 in these cells. Consistent with a previous report [30], RT-PCR analysis showed that CCR2 was expressed in mBMSCs (Figure 3B). We also examined whether CCR2 mediates MCP-1-induced migration of mBMSCs. RS102895 (400 nM) effectively inhibited the MCP-1-induced migration of mBMSCs (Figure 3A). Because MCP-3 did not affect migration of the cells, we therefore focused on MCP-1. To further investigate possible roles of MCP-1, we next examined osteogenic differentiation of mBMSCs in response to MCP-1. Isolated mBMSCs were capable of spontaneously differentiating into alizarin red-positive cells and showed increased levels of *Runx2*, *osterix* and *alkaline phosphatase (ALP)* in the osteoinduction media on day 14. However, alizarin red staining revealed no difference between osteoinduced mBMSCs with or without MCP-1 (Figure S2A). Similarly, no difference in the gene expression of *Runx2, osterix, or ALP* was observed in cells treated with or without MCP-1 (Figure S2A). Because MCP-1 did not affect the osteogenic differentiation of mBMSCs, we also examined whether MCP-1 affects chondrogenic differentiation using ATDC5 cells *in vitro*. Alcian blue staining showed that the presence of MCP-1 was not associated with any obvious differences in cells treated with or without MCP-1 on day 28. Moreover, *SOX9, Col-2* and *Col-10* showed similar expression patterns in cells treated with or without MCP-1 (Figure S2B).

In vivo roles of MCP-1 and CCR2 during the early inflammatory phase of fracture healing

To investigate the functional roles of MCP-1 and CCR2 in fracture healing, rib fracture healing was assessed in WT and KO mice. Fracture calluses were examined by micro-CT and histological analysis. Histological analyses showed a smaller proportion of cartilage in the callus in MCP-1$^{-/-}$ mice compared with WT mice on day 7 (Figure S3A). By day 21, fractures had healed in the WT mice and cartilage was almost completely replaced by bone in the callus (Figure 4A). Conversely, the healing processes progressed incompletely in MCP-1$^{-/-}$ and CCR2$^{-/-}$ mice by day 21, and the central area of the cartilaginous callus remained (Figure 4A). By day 25, a bridging callus was apparent in MCP-1$^{-/-}$ and CCR2$^{-/-}$ mice, and was similar in appearance to that observed in WT mice on 21 day (Figure S3B). The callus volume was significantly smaller in both MCP-1$^{-/-}$ and CCR2$^{-/-}$ mice than in WT mice on day 21 (Figure 4B, C).

Next, to elucidate whether the MCP-1/CCR2 axis is involved during the early phase of fracture healing, we continuously administered RS102895 before (pre-treatment) or after (post-treatment) rib fracture. Micro-CT analysis showed delayed fracture healing in the pre-treatment group compared with both the control and post-treatment groups. On day 21, the callus volume was significantly smaller in the pre-treatment group than in the control and post-treatment groups (Figures 5A, B). Histological analysis showed that fractures in both the control and post-treatment groups had healed by day 21 and that cartilaginous tissue was absent in the callus. Conversely, less cartilaginous tissue was observed in the callus in the pre-treatment group on day 7 (Figure 5C), and cartilaginous tissue in a central area of the callus was observed on day 21 (Figure S3C). These results indicate that the MCP-1/CCR2 axis is an essential component during the early phase of fracture healing.

Periosteal bone formation in grafts from WT mice implanted into MCP-1-deficient mice: gain-of-function

To examine the roles of MCP-1 at the periosteum and endosteum during fracture healing, we performed gain-of-function studies using a segmental bone graft transplantation model. A segmental bone graft was transplanted from an MCP-1$^{-/-}$ mouse to another MCP-1$^{-/-}$ mouse (KO-to-KO). Micro-CT and histological analysis were used to quantify new bone formation on day 21. Radiologic and micro-CT analyses showed that KO-to-KO transplantation caused a delay in fracture healing on day 21 (Figure 6A). Minimal periosteal bone formation was observed along the surface of the bone graft because of the lack of periosteal bone formation. We next created bone graft exchanging models between MCP-1$^{-/-}$ and WT mice, in which a segmental bone derived from a WT mouse was transplanted into a host MCP-1$^{-/-}$ mouse (WT-to-KO). In contrast to KO-to-KO bone graft transplantation, transplantation of the WT-derived graft into the host KO mouse significantly increased new bone formation and led to marked recovery of periosteal bone formation on day 21 (Figures 6A, B). Histological analysis further revealed marked and localized induction of MCP-1 expression in the callus and endosteum around the WT-derived graft in the host MCP-1$^{-/-}$ mouse (Figure 6C). By contrast, no MCP-1 expression was observed in the callus and endosteum of the host bone in the same section.

Reduction in periosteal bone formation in grafts from MCP-1-deficient mice implanted into WT mice: loss-of-function

To confirm whether MCP-1 is a crucial chemokine in the fracture healing process, we performed loss-of-function studies using WT-to-WT and KO-to-WT bone graft models. Transplantation of a WT donor graft into a WT host mouse led to abundant new bone formation and a bridging callus around the WT-derived graft on day 21 (Figures 6D, E). By contrast, transplantation of a KO-derived graft into a WT host markedly reduced the amount of periosteal bone formation in the donor graft.

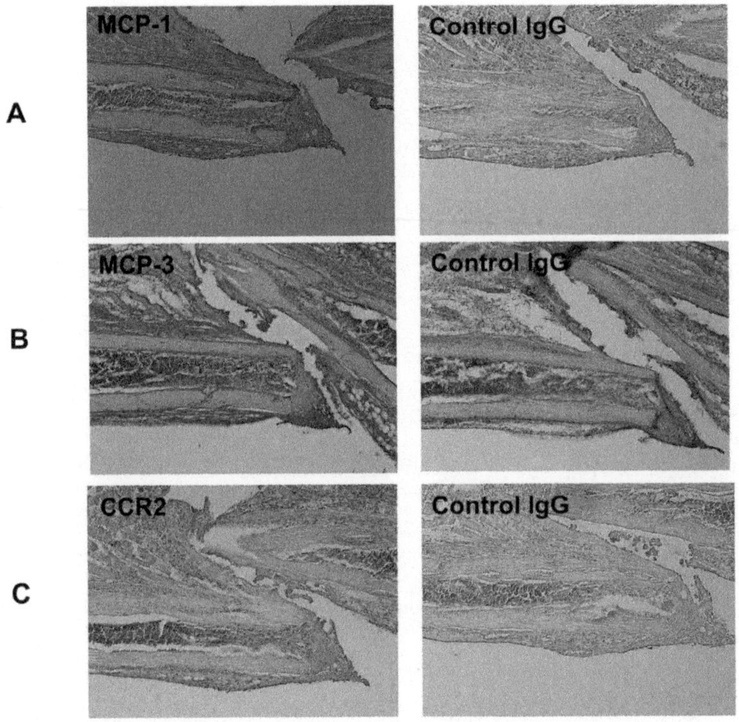

Figure 2. Immunohistochemical analysis of WT rib fracture on day 3. A, B, Protein expression levels of MCP-1 (**A**) and MCP-3 (**B**) were identified at the periosteum and endosteum on day 3. **C**, CCR2-positive cells were predominantly found within the bone marrow and surrounding tissues on day 3. Original magnification, 40×. Middle panel, high-magnification views (original magnification, 200×). The result is representative of three separate experiments.

Discussion

Our data highlight crucial roles of the MCP-1/CCR2 axis in the early phase of fracture healing. Compared with no fracture, the expression levels of many inflammatory chemokines increased on day 3 after fracture. In particular, *MCP-1* and *MCP-3* expression were temporarily up-regulated in the early phase of fracture healing (Figure 1). Then, we found that deletion of either MCP-1 or CCR2 caused delayed fracture healing (Figure 4), and that, blockade of CCR2 only in the early phase of healing caused delayed fracture healing (Figure 5). Taken together, these results

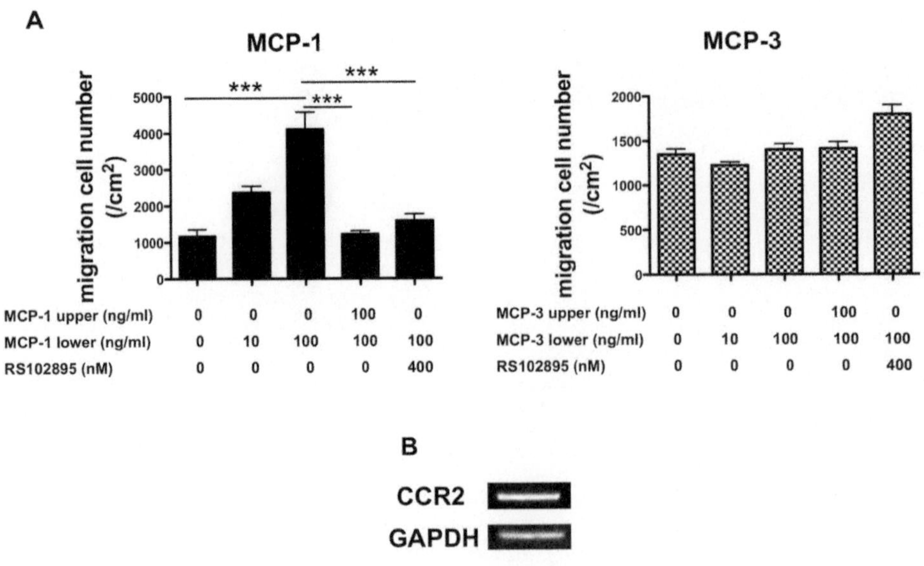

Figure 3. Effect of MCP-1 on cell migration. A: *In vitro* migration assay. mBMSCs were stimulated by MCP-1 or MCP-3 at indicated doses and RS102895 at 400 nM. Cells that migrated to the undersurface of the membrane were counted. Numbers of cells are represented as cell number per cm^2. Values are means ± SEM ($n = 5$, respectively). **B**: Expression of *CCR2* mRNA in mBMSCs. Data are shown as means ± SEM. *$P < 0.05$.

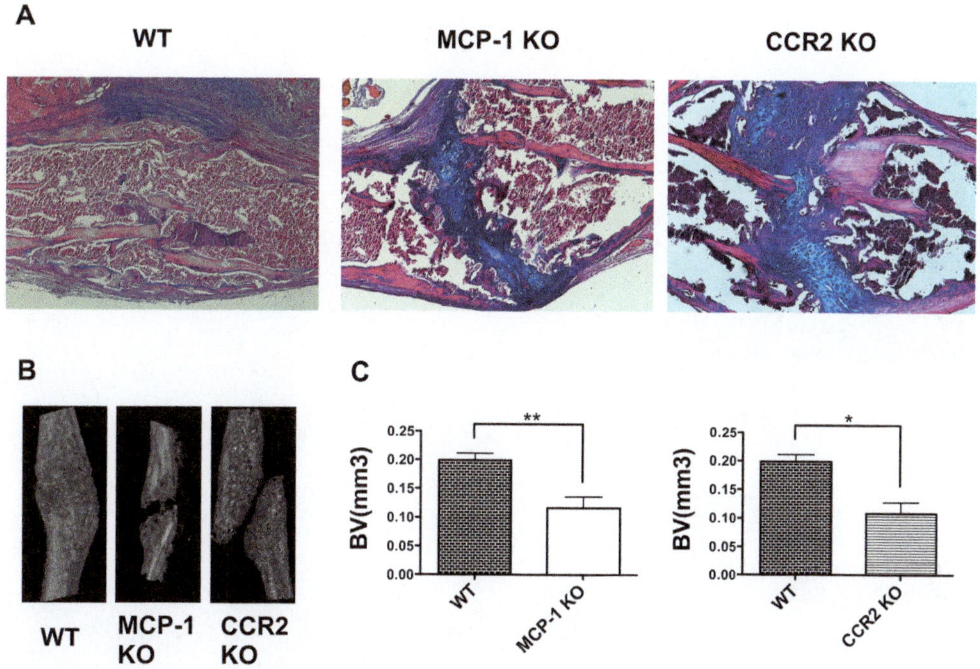

Figure 4. MCP-1$^{-/-}$ and CCR2$^{-/-}$ mice displayed delayed fracture healing *in vivo*. A: Histology of the fracture callus stained by hematoxylin-eosin/alcian-blue staining on day 21. **B**: Representative 3D micro-CT image of a fractured rib on day 21. **C**: Newly formed callus volume in the MCP-1$^{-/-}$ and CCR2$^{-/-}$ mice on day 21 was quantified using micro-CT.

suggest that the temporary increase of MCP-1, MCP-3 and CCR2 expression in the early inflammatory phase may play a pivotal role for successful fracture healing. A recent study reported that deletion of CCR2 induces delayed fracture healing because of a decreased ability to resorb bone by osteoclasts in the remodeling phase [28]. The persistent cartilage fracture healing phenotype

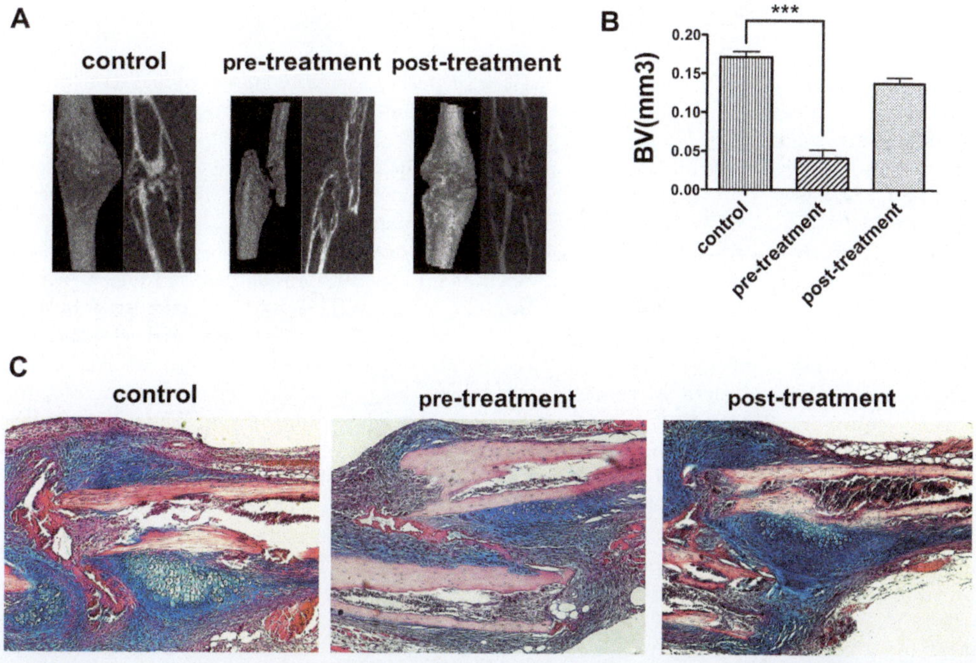

Figure 5. Blockade of CCR2 in the early phase displayed delayed fracture healing *in vivo*. A: WT mice received continuous administration of CCR2 antagonist, RS102895, or DMSO (controls) until day 12, beginning 2 days before or 4 days after rib fracture. In the control group, DMSO was administered as a control for 14 days. Representative micro-CT image of a fractured rib on day 21. **B**: Newly formed callus volume on day 21 in the pre-treatment or post-treatment group was quantified using micro-CT. **C**: Histology of the fracture callus stained by hematoxylin-eosin/alcian-blue staining on day 7.

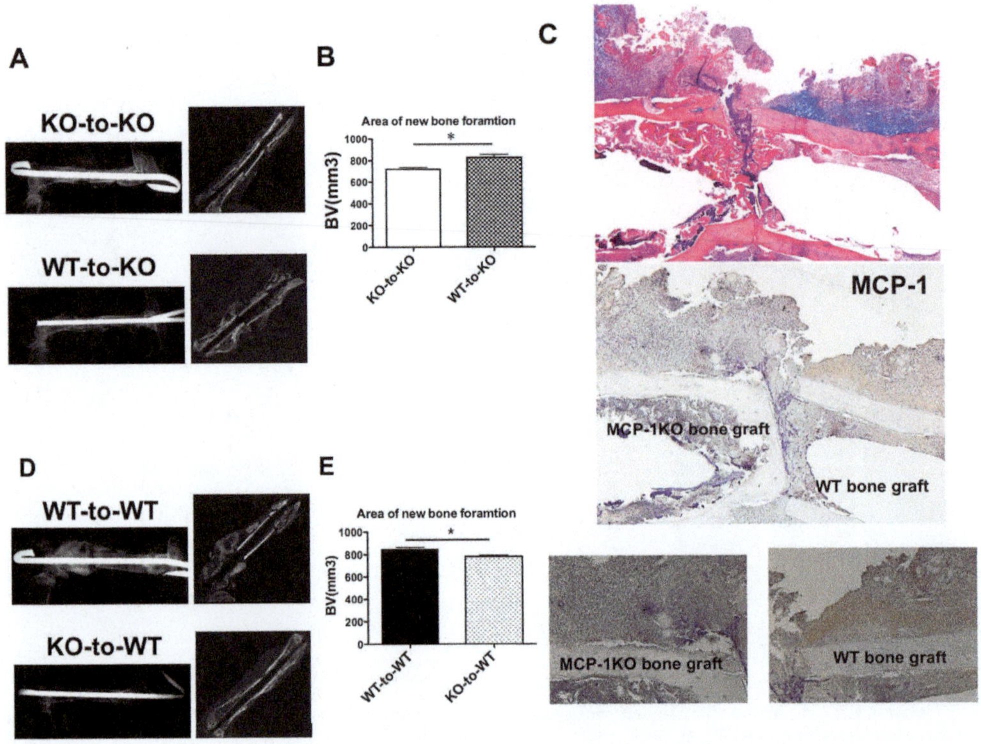

Figure 6. Femoral segmental bone graft exchanging model. Bone exchange surgeries were performed between WT and MCP-1$^{-/-}$ mice as described in the Methods section. Samples were harvested on day 21 for micro-CT and histological analyses. **A and B**, Representative micro-CT images and quantitative analyses demonstrate that WT mouse-derived bone graft caused a significant increase of new bone formation compared with KO mouse-derived bone graft. **C**, Immunohistochemical staining for MCP-1 in MCP-1$^{-/-}$ mice is shown. Pronounced MCP-1 expression at the periosteum and endosteum in the WT graft was observed in the host MCP-1$^{-/-}$ mouse. **D**, Representative micro-CT images and quantitative analyses demonstrate that MCP-1$^{-/-}$ mouse-derived bone graft caused a significant decrease of new bone formation compared with WT mouse-derived bone graft. Values are means ± SEM of more than three separate experiments. *$P<0.05$.

could be caused by defects in chondroclast/osteoclast chemotaxis that delays vascular invasion, calcification and/or remodeling. However, MCP-1 expression is known to induce the early inflammatory phase [29], when osteoclasts do not play major roles in fracture healing. Consistent with the findings of previous studies, our data show that *MCP-1* and *MCP-3* mRNA were up-regulated on day 3 (Figure 1) and that localized MCP-1 and MCP-3 expression were increased in the periosteum and endosteum in the early phase of fracture healing (Figure 2A). This suggests that increased MCP-1 and MCP-3 expression in the early inflammatory phase may be essential for normal fracture healing.

MCP-1 and its receptor CCR2 are involved in recruitment of various cells, including leukocytes, BMSCs and hematopoietic stem cells [30–33], and in the regeneration of damaged tissues [34,35]. As established in earlier developmental studies, CCR2 is necessary for organ-specific homing of bone marrow-derived pluripotent mesenchymal stem cells into damaged tissues [36,37]. Consistent with this finding, our data showed that *CCR2* mRNA was induced in the mBMSCs derived from WT mice (Figure 3B). We also found that MCP-1, but not MCP-3, induced the migration of mBMSCs in a dose-dependent manner and that *in vitro* migration was markedly inhibited by a CCR2 antagonist (Figure 3A). Therefore, this axis may be a potent candidate in the development of stem/progenitor cell-based therapy for improving fracture healing.

We have previously demonstrated that SDF-1 is induced in the periosteum during bone injury and promotes endochondral bone repair by recruiting mesenchymal stem/progenitor cells to the site of injury. In the PCR array, an increased level of SDF-1 was not observed during fracture healing in this current study, especially in the early inflammatory phase. This inconsistency may be explained partly by the differences between the presence of the unimpaired bone marrow in simple fracture healing and bone graft healing with an intramedullary nail. Moreover, the previous study investigated allograft healing, in which the surgical site is greatly avascular, and under hypoxia this induces hypoxia-inducible factor-1 activation and subsequent SDF-1 up-regulation. Hence, we consider that the MCP-1/CCR2 axis is a crucial signaling pathway during the normal fracture healing process.

Previous studies have demonstrated that damage to the periosteum and bone marrow leads to impaired osteogenesis and chondrogenesis, and delays bone healing [38,39]. Thus, the periosteum and bone marrow seem to be important sources for recruiting mesenchymal stem/progenitor cells or osteogenic progenitor cells for promoting osteogenesis and chondrogenesis. In this study, we found that the expression of CCR2 increased transiently in the bone marrow in the early inflammatory phase and that the expression of MCP-1 also increased transiently in the periosteum and endosteum during the same period (Figure 2). We also found that WT mouse-derived bone graft markedly increased new bone formation and promoted successful fracture healing, whereas the MCP-1$^{-/-}$ mouse-derived bone graft caused less new bone formation and delayed fracture healing (Figure 6). Importantly, although other osteogenic factors were present at the fracture site, they could not compensate for the lack of MCP-1. Collectively, these findings indicate clearly that increased MCP-1 expression in the periosteum and endosteum recruits CCR2-expressing cells and is essential for successful fracture healing.

This study has several limitations. First, we did not fully analyze the functions of other ligands for CCR2, such as MCP-3 and MCP-5, which may have roles different from those of MCP-1 in fracture healing. However, CCR2 KO mice showed similar impairment of bone healing compared with MCP-1$^{-/-}$ mice. Therefore, it is reasonable to consider that other ligands may also have similar functions. Second, the MCP-1/CCR2 axis may have a function other than the recruitment of progenitor cells in the early phase of fracture healing, such as promoting angiogenesis. Several studies report the role of the MCP-1/CCR2 axis in angiogenesis, but not in fracture healing. This point should be clarified in the future. Lastly, we did not elucidate the cell source(s) of mesenchymal stem/progenitor cells for fracture healing in this study. Recent reports, including ours, indicate the periosteum is the key source of potent cells [19,40], but this requires further investigation.

In conclusion, we have shown that increased expression of MCP-1 in the early phase plays a pivotal role in fracture healing by recruiting CCR2-expressing cells derived from surrounding tissues. The MCP-1/CCR2 axis is a potential target for achieving successful fracture healing. Further studies are needed to understand the functional relevance of the MCP-1/CCR2 axis in fracture healing.

Supporting Information

Figure S1 Immunohistochemical analysis of WT unfractured rib. A, B, C, Low expression levels of MCP-1, MCP-3 and CCR2 were observed at the periosteum in the unfractured rib.

Figure S2 Effects of MCP-1 on osteogenesis, and chondrogenesis. A: mBMSCs were cultured in osteoinduction media with or without MCP-1 for 14 days and stained with alizarin red S. The expression of each gene was analyzed by quantitative RT-PCR. ($n = 5$, respectively). **B**: ATDC5 cells were induced chondrocyte differentiation. MCP-1 (0, 20, 100 or 200 ng/ml) was simultaneously added every 2 days with the medium change. On days 28 after plating, cells were harvested, and the expression of each gene was analyzed by quantitative RT-PCR. ($n = 6$, respectively).

Figure S3 A, C: Histology of the fracture callus stained by hematoxylin-eosin/alcian-blue staining on day 7 (A) or day 21(C). B: Histology of the fracture in MCP-1 or CCR2 KO stained by hematoxylin-eosin on day 25 (left panel) or 23 (right panel).

Acknowledgments

We are grateful to Drs. R. Tsutsumi, S. Tanida and K. Nishitani (Kyoto University Graduate School of Medicine) for their valuable technical assistance.

Author Contributions

Conceived and designed the experiments: MI HI SM. Performed the experiments: MI TK KM HS KY TF. Analyzed the data: MI HI HY MF Contributed reagents/materials/analysis tools: MI TK. Contributed to the writing of the manuscript: MI HI TK.

References

1. Tsuboi M, Hasegawa Y, Suzuki S, Wingstrand H, Thorngren KG (2007) Mortality and mobility after hip fracture in Japan: a ten-year follow-up. J Bone Joint Surg Br 89: 461–466.
2. Bliuc D, Nguyen ND, Milch VE, Nguyen TV, Eisman JA, et al. (2009) Mortality risk associated with low-trauma osteoporotic fracture and subsequent fracture in men and women. JAMA 301: 513–521.
3. Griffin M, Iqbal SA, Bayat A (2011) Exploring the application of mesenchymal stem cells in bone repair and regeneration. J Bone Joint Surg Br 93: 427–434.
4. Hernigou P, Poignard A, Manicom O, Mathieu G, Rouard H (2005) The use of percutaneous autologous bone marrow transplantation in nonunion and avascular necrosis of bone. J Bone Joint Surg Br 87: 896–902.
5. Claes L, Recknagel S, Ignatius A (2012) Fracture healing under healthy and inflammatory conditions. Nat Rev Rheumatol 8: 133–143.
6. Vortkamp A, Pathi S, Peretti GM, Caruso EM, Zaleske DJ, et al. (1998) Recapitulation of signals regulating embryonic bone formation during postnatal growth and in fracture repair. Mech Dev 71: 65–76.
7. Glass GE, Chan JK, Freidin A, Feldmann M, Horwood NJ, et al. (2011) TNF-alpha promotes fracture repair by augmenting the recruitment and differentiation of muscle-derived stromal cells. Proc Natl Acad Sci U S A 108: 1585–1590.
8. Lange J, Sapozhnikova A, Lu C, Hu D, Li X, et al. (2010) Action of IL-1 beta during fracture healing. J Orthop Res 28: 778–784.
9. Dimitriou R, Tsiridis E, Giannoudis PV (2005) Current concepts of molecular aspects of bone healing. Injury 36: 1392–1404.
10. Mountziaris PM, Mikos AG (2008) Modulation of the inflammatory response for enhanced bone tissue regeneration. Tissue Eng Part B Rev 14: 179–186.
11. Sasaki M, Abe R, Fujita Y (2008) Mesenchymal stem cells are recruited into wounded skin and contribute to wound repair by transdifferentiation into multiple skin cell type. J Immunol 180: 2581–2587.
12. Schenk S, Mal N, Finan A, Zhang M, Kiedrowski M, et al. (2007) Monocyte chemotactic protein-3 is a myocardial mesenchymal stem cell homing factor. Stem Cells 25: 245–251.
13. Si Y, Tsou C, Croft K, Charo I (2010) CCR2 mediates hematopoietic stem and progenitor cell trafficking to sites of inflammation in mice. J Clin Invest 120: 1192–1203.
14. Docheva D, Haasters F, Schieker M (2008) Mesenchymal stem cells and their cell surface receptors. Curr Rheumatol Rev 4: 155–160.
15. Bielby R, Jones E, McGonagle D (2007) The role of mesenchymal stem cells in maintenance and repair of bone. Injury 38 Suppl 1: S26–32.
16. Augello A, Kurth TB, De Bari C (2010) Mesenchymal stem cells: a perspective from in vitro cultures to in vivo migration and niches. Eur Cell Mater 20: 121–133.
17. Caplan A (2009) Why are MSCs therapeutic? New data: new insight. J Pathol 217(2): 318–324.
18. Jones E, Yang X (2011) Mesenchymal stem cells and bone regeneration: current status. Injury 42: 562–568.
19. Ito H (2011) Chemokines in mesenchymal stem cell therapy for bone repair: a novel concept of recruiting mesenchymal stem cells and the possible cell sources. Mod Rheumatol 21: 113–121.
20. Granero-Moltó F, Weis JA, Miga MI, Landis B, Myers TJ, et al. (2009) Regenerative effects of transplanted mesenchymal stem cells in fracture healing. Stem Cells 27: 1887–1898.
21. Khosla S, Westendorf JJ, Mödder UI (2010) Concise review: Insights from normal bone remodeling and stem cell-based therapies for bone repair. Stem Cells 28: 2124–2128.
22. Kumar S, Wan C, Ramaswamy G, Clemens TL, Ponnazhagan S (2010) Mesenchymal stem cells expressing osteogenic and angiogenic factors synergistically enhance bone formation in a mouse model of segmental bone defect. Mol Ther 18: 1026–1034.
23. Kitaori T, Ito H, Schwarz EM, Tsutsumi R, Yoshitomi H, et al. (2009) Stromal cell-derived factor 1/CXCR4 signaling is critical for the recruitment of mesenchymal stem cells to the fracture site during skeletal repair in a mouse model. Arthritis Rheum 60: 813–823.
24. Ito H, Akiyama H, Shigeno C, Iyama K, Matsuoka H, et al. (1999) Hedgehog signaling molecules in bone marrow cells at the initial stage of fracture repair. Biochem Biophys Res Commun 262: 443–451.
25. Ito H, Koefoed M, Tiyapatanaputi P, Gromov K, Goater JJ, et al. (2005) Remodeling of cortical bone allografts mediated by adherent rAAV-RANKL and VEGF gene therapy. Nat Med 11: 291–297.
26. Murata K, Kitaori T, Oishi S, Watanabe N, Yoshitomi H, et al. (2012) Stromal cell-derived factor 1 regulates the actin organization of chondrocytes and chondrocyte hypertrophy. PLoS One 7: e37163.
27. Murata K, Ito H, Yoshitomi H, Yamamoto K, Fukuda A, et al. (2014) Inhibition of miR-92a enhances fracture healing via promoting angiogenesis in a model of stabilized fracture in young mice. J Bone Miner Res 29: 316–326.

28. Xing Z, Lu C, Hu D, Yu Y, Wang X, et al. (2010) Multiple roles for CCR2 during fracture healing. Dis Model Mech 3: 451–458.
29. Shireman PK, Contreras-Shannon V, Reyes-Reyna SM, Robinson SC, McManus LM (2006) MCP-1 parallels inflammatory and regenerative responses in ischemic muscle. J Surg Res 134: 145–157.
30. Qian BZ, Li J, Zhang H, Kitamura T, Zhang J, et al. (2011) CCL2 recruits inflammatory monocytes to facilitate breast-tumour metastasis. Nature 475: 222–225.
31. Zhang F, Tsai S, Kato K, Yamanouchi D, Wang C, et al. (2009) Transforming growth factor-beta promotes recruitment of bone marrow cells and bone marrow-derived mesenchymal stem cells through stimulation of MCP-1 production in vascular smooth muscle cells. J Biol Chem 284: 17564–17574.
32. Tsou C, Peters W, Si Y (2007) Critical roles for CCR2 and MCP-3 in monocyte mobilization from bone marrow and recruitment to inflammatory sites. J Clin Inv 117: 2–9.
33. Serbina NV, Pamer EG (2006) Monocyte emigration from bone marrow during bacterial infection requires signals mediated by chemokine receptor CCR2. Nat Immunol 7: 311–317.
34. Lu H, Huang D, Saederup N, Charo IF, Ransohoff RM, et al. (2011) Macrophages recruited via CCR2 produce insulin-like growth factor-1 to repair acute skeletal muscle injury. FASEB J 25: 358–369.
35. Shireman PK, Contreras-Shannon V, Ochoa O, Karia BP, Michalek JE, et al. (2007) MCP-1 deficiency causes altered inflammation with impaired skeletal muscle regeneration. J Leukoc Biol 81: 775–785.
36. Belema-Bedada F, Uchida S, Martire A, Kostin S, Braun T (2008) Efficient homing of multipotent adult mesenchymal stem cells depends on FROUNT-mediated clustering of CCR2. Cell Stem Cell 2: 566–575.
37. Van Linthout S, Stamm C, Schultheiss H-P, Tschöpe C (2011) Mesenchymal stem cells and inflammatory cardiomyopathy: cardiac homing and beyond. Cardiol Res Pract: ID 757154. DOI:10.4061/2011/757154
38. Colnot C (2009) Skeletal cell fate decisions within periosteum and bone marrow during bone regeneration. J Bone Miner Res 24: 274–282.
39. Utvåg SE, Grundnes O, Reikeraos O (1996) Effects of periosteal stripping on healing of segmental fractures in rats. J Orthop Trauma 10: 279–284.
40. Murao H, Yamamoto K, Matsuda S, Akiyama H (2013) Periosteal cells are a major source of soft callus in bone fracture. J Bone Miner Metab 31: 390–398.

20

An NMR Metabolomic Study on the Effect of Alendronate in Ovariectomized Mice

Shin-Yu Chen[1,2,3], Hui-Tzu Yu[1], Ju-Po Kao[4], Chung-Chun Yang[4], Shen-Shih Chiang[1,2], Darya O. Mishchuk[5], Jeng-Leun Mau[1,2]*, Carolyn M. Slupsky[5,6]*

1 Department of Food Science and Biotechnology, National Chung Hsing University (NCHU), Taiwan, R.O.C., 2 NCHU-UCD Plant and Food Biotechnology Center, NCHU, Taiwan, R.O.C., 3 Agricultural Biotechnology Center, NCHU, Taiwan, R.O.C., 4 Veterinary Medical Teaching Hospital, College of Veterinary Medicine, NCHU, Taiwan, R.O.C., 5 Department of Food Science and Technology, University of California Davis, Davis, California, United States of America, 6 Department of Nutrition, University of California Davis, Davis, California, United States of America

Abstract

Alendronate sodium (Fosamax) is most widely used for the prevention and treatment of osteoporosis. It is a type of anti-resorptive agent that reduces the risk of fractures by changing bone turnover and bone mineral density. We investigated the effect of Fosamax on a mouse model of osteoporosis. Twenty-seven female C57BL/6JNarl mice were divided into three groups: sham, ovariectomized (OVX) and OVX + Fosamax (Fosamax). After 23 weeks, bone density of femurs was analyzed using microcomputed tomography (micro-CT), and serum was analyzed for osteoblast and osteoclast activity, as well as metabolites using nuclear magnetic resonance (NMR) spectroscopy. Fosamax increased bone mineral density and cortical bone thickness, and decreased osteoblast activity slightly. Fosamax did not significantly change osteoclast activity. Serum metabolomics revealed that Fosamax had profound effects on overall metabolism, as significantly higher concentrations of metabolites associated with energy metabolism (including TCA-cycle intermediates and glucose), 3-hydroxybutyrate, taurine, allantoin, acetate, and ethanol, as well as lower concentrations of aspartate were observed in the Fosamax-treated mice compared with the OVX mice. These results suggest that alendronate may work by increasing bone density through altered metabolic activity.

Editor: Daniel Monleon, Instituto de Investigación Sanitaria INCLIVA, Spain

Funding: This study was supported by the National Science Council, Republic of China (NSC-101-2911-I-005-301, NSC-102-2911-I-005-301, NSC 100-2313-B-005-022-MY3) and the Ministry of Education, Taiwan, R.O.C., under the ATU plan. The funders had no role in study design, data collection and analysis, decision to publish, or preparation of the manuscript.

Competing Interests: The authors have declared that no competing interests exist.

* Email: cslupsky@ucdavis.edu (CMS); jlmau@dragon.nchu.edu.tw (JLM)

Introduction

Osteoporosis is a major public health issue. It is a skeletal disease that is defined by decreased bone mass combined with microarchitectural deterioration of bone tissue resulting in a consequent increase in bone fragility and susceptibility to fracture. Osteoporosis typically presents later in life, particularly in postmenopausal women, and its prevalence is expected to increase dramatically in the coming decades due to an ageing population [1,2,3]. The reason postmenopausal women are more susceptible to osteoporosis is due to reduced ovarian function resulting in decreased estrogen. Estrogen directly affects bone turnover by stimulating osteoblast activity (which forms bone) through increasing osteoblast formation, differentiation, proliferation, and function, and inhibiting osteoclast activity (which resorbs bone) through inducing osteoclast apoptosis, and inhibiting osteoclast formation [4,5]. Thus, estrogen deficiency is directly related with bone loss, and postmenopausal estrogen deficiency causes accelerated bone loss. Postmenopausal osteoporosis affects 20% of women aged 60–69 years, and in the UK it was found that out of the 60,000 people who suffer osteoporotic hip fractures each year, 15–20% die from complications within a year [6].

Alendronate sodium (Fosamax), a nitrogen-containing bisphosphonate, is most widely used for the prevention and treatment of osteoporosis. Bisphosphonates accumulate in the mineral phase of bone and inhibit bone resorption through inhibition of osteoclast activity. The degree to which bone turnover and bone mineral density change upon treatment with anti-resorptive agents is directly correlated with a reduction in the risk of fractures [4,7–10]. However, many side effects of bisphosphonate medications, including severe suppression of bone turnover that may develop during long-term therapy, actually increase the risk of fracture [11,12]. Bisphosphonates can also cause osteonecrosis of the jaw (ONJ), with higher risk in oncology patients treated with high dose bisphosphonate therapy [13–15]. Other relevant possible side effects include gastrointestinal (GI) upset, musculoskeletal pain, atrial fibrillation, and esophageal cancer [16,17].

There are few reports on the relationship between postmenopausal osteoporosis treatment with Fosamax and overall metabolism. To understand the global changes associated with Fosamax use, we investigated ovariectomized mice treated with Fosamax to determine its effects on serum metabolites using NMR spectroscopy. These results are compared with bone density using micro-CT as well as indicators of osteoblast and osteoclast activity using ELISA.

Materials and Methods

Ethics statement

This study was performed in strict accordance with animal use protocols approved by National Chung Hsing University Institutional Animal Care and Use Committee (IACUC, approval number: 99–62). All surgery was performed under anesthesia, and all efforts were made to minimize suffering.

Animals and design

Twenty-seven female C57BL/6JNarl mice aged 7 weeks were purchased from the National Laboratory Animal Center (Taipei, Taiwan) and acclimated to conditions for 5 weeks before the start of the experiment. Animals were housed in an air-conditioned room in autoclavable cages (4–5 mice per cage) with ventilating tops and stainless steel lips (BioLASCO, Taipei, Taiwan) with 12 h light/dark illumination cycles at a constant temperature of 25±2°C and humidity of 65±5%. Tapvei aspen bedding was purchased from Young Li (New Taipei, Taiwan) and changed every week. Drinking water and food (basal diet Lab 5001 (Purina Mills, St. Louis, MO, USA)) were supplied *ad libitum*. The mice were weighed on a weekly basis during the experimental period, and food intake was measured from week 8 until the end of the experiment by subtracting the weight of the leftover food from the weight of the food provided on a weekly basis, and averaging across all mice.

Bilateral ovariectomy (OVX) was performed on 19 twelve weeks old mice after intramuscular injection of an anesthetic cocktail composed of 0.03 mL Zoletil 50 and 0.01 mL 0.2% Xylazine, as described by Lasota [18]. Another eight mice were given sham surgery. At 2 weeks post-surgery (week 0), 9 of the 19 ovariectomized mice were randomly assigned to the OVX (no treatment) group, and 10 to the Fosamax (treatment) group. The Fosamax group was then fed Fosamax plus (Merck, Whitehouse Station, NJ, USA) once a week based on the human equivalent dose [19], and contained 70 mg alendronic acid and 2800 IU of cholecalciferol. Blood was collected from the cheeks of mice after 12 weeks of treatment to measure osteocalcin and alkaline phosphatase (ALP). After 23 weeks, mice were sacrificed by CO_2 asphyxiation, and blood was collected by cardiac puncture. Tissue was removed from each femur, and the bone was placed in ethanol until analysis. For serum, blood was allowed to clot for 15 minutes on ice, centrifuged at 5,000 rpm for 15 min, and the top layer was collected and stored at −80°C until ready for analysis.

Histomorphometric analysis using microcomputed tomography

To perform qualitative and quantitative analysis of bone, the right femurs were analyzed using a high performance *in vivo* micro-CT Skyscan 1076 (Skyscan, Kontich, Belgium), with image field at pixel size 9 μm. Three-dimensional images were reconstructed using CTVol (Skyscan). The distal femoral metaphysis was analyzed from a region that was 1.0 mm below the growth plate and 1.5 mm in length. For quantitative analysis, the software CTAn (Skyscan) was used to obtain the following parameters within the region of interest (ROI): bone volume/tissue volume (BV/TV), bone surface/bone volume (BS/BV), bone surface/tissue volume (BS/TV), trabecular thickness (Tb.Th), trabecular separation (Tb.Sp), trabecular number (Tb.N), trabecular pattern factor (Tb.Pf), structure model index (SMI), connectivity density (Conn.Dn) and trabecular bone mineral density (Tb.BMD). The SMI quantifies the plate-rod characteristics of the 3D trabecular structure [20]. The Conn.Dn was calculated using the Euler method [21]. Cortical bone parameters (including cortical bone shell thickness, cortical BMD, endosteal circumference (EC), periosteal circumference (PC) and cross-sectional area) were analyzed in the middle of the diaphysis of the femur.

Measurement of serum indicators of osteoblast and osteoclast activity, and serum concentrations of calcium and phosphate

We determined the activity of osteoblast and osteoclast cells using serum indicators rather than histomorphometry. Serum concentrations of alkaline phosphatase (ALP), osteocalcin, procollagen I C-terminal propeptide (PICP), pyridinoline (PYD), cross-linked N-telopeptide of type I collagen (NTXI) were all measured using commercial kits according to manufacturer's instructions. (ALP: Alkaline phosphatase activity fluorometric assay kit (Biovision, Mountain View, CA, USA); osteocalcin: Mouse osteocalcin EIA kit (Biomedical Technologies, Stoughton, MA, USA); PICP: ELISA kit for mouse PICP (USCN Life Science, Wuhan, Hubei, China); PYD: Mouse pyridinoline ELISA kit (CUSABIO, Wuhan, Hubei, China); NTXI: ELISA kit for mouse NTXI (USCN Life Science, Wuhan, Hubei, China)). Calcium was determined with a calcium colorimetric assay kit (Biovision, Mountain View, CA, USA), and phosphate was measured with a phosphate colorimetric assay kit (Biovision, Mountain View, CA, USA).

Serum Metabolomics

For serum metabolomics measurement, serum samples were prepared by thawing and centrifuging at maximum speed for 20 min and 4°C to remove particulate matter. The serum supernatant was subsequently filtered through Amicon 3,000 molecular weight (MW) cutoff filters to remove protein and lipid particles. If needed, the serum filtrates were diluted with deionized water to a total volume of 207 μL and 23 μL of an internal standard (Chenomx Inc., Edmonton, Alberta, Canada) containing 4.8566 mM 3-(trimethylsilyl)-1-propanesulfonic acid-d 6 (DSS-d6) and 0.2% NaN_3 in 98% D_2O was added. The pH value was adjusted to 6.8 for each sample by adding small amounts of 1 N HCl or NaOH. 180 μL of each sample was transferred into a 3 mm NMR tube, and samples were stored at 4°C until NMR data acquisition (within 24 h of sample preparation).

NMR spectra were acquired using the Bruker noesypr1d experiment on a Bruker Avance 600 MHz NMR spectrometer equipped with a SampleJet as previously described [22]. Identification and quantification of metabolites were accomplished using Chenomx NMRSuite 7.6 (Chenomx Inc., Edmonton, Canada) [23]. For each mouse, 55 metabolites were measured and quantified from the serum which included 2-hydroxybutyrate, 2-oxoglutarate, 2-oxoisocaproate, 3-hydroxybutyrate, acetate, acetoacetate, acetone, alanine, allantoin, arginine, ascorbate, asparagine, aspartate, betaine, carnitine, choline, citrate, creatine, creatinine, dimethylamine (DMA), ethanol, formate, fumarate, glucose, glutamate, glutamine, glycerol, glycine, histidine, isoleucine, lactate, leucine, lysine, malate, mannose, methanol, methionine, N,N-dimethylglycine (DMG), acetylcarnitine, ornithine, phenylalanine, proline, pyruvate, serine, serotonin, succinate, taurine, threonine, trimethylamine (TMA), tryptophan, tyrosine, uracil, urea, uridine and valine. Samples were corrected for dilution by multiplying by a correction factor calculated by the ratio of the final sample volume divided by the initial volume of serum. Those samples for which there was limited volume were excluded from NMR analysis.

Statistics

Unless otherwise indicated, all comparisons between the Fosamax group and either the sham or OVX group regarding bone measurements were made using Student's *t*-test, and comparison between multiple groups were made using ANOVA followed by Bonferroni's multiple *t* test. For metabolite data, all comparisons were made using Kruskal-Wallis non-parametric analysis followed by Dunn's multiple comparison test. For time-course data (body weight), analysis was accomplished using repeated measures two-way ANOVA. Statistical significance was defined as $p<0.05$. All data are expressed as mean ± standard error (SEM) or mean ± standard deviation (SD). Data sets were analyzed for statistical significance using Prism GraphPad 6 software (GraphPad Software Inc., San Diego, CA). Multivariate data analysis (Principal Component Analysis (PCA) and Partial Least Squares-Discriminant Analysis (PLS-DA)) was performed on $\log_{10}$ - transformed metabolite concentrations using SIMCA-P (version 13.0, Umetrics, Umeå, Sweden) as described in Slupsky [24]. The number of components was chosen using a 7-fold cross validation rule. The quality of the models were judged by the goodness-of-fit parameter (R^2X), and the predictive ability parameter (Q^2), as well as permutation testing (for the PLS-DA model), where each data point was randomly assigned a class 100 times, and the corresponding R^2 and Q^2 calculated and compared with the original model.

Results

Total body weight

Average body weight for each group of mice over 23 weeks after surgery is shown in Figure 1. Analysis by repeated measures 2-way ANOVA revealed a significant effect of time ($p<0.0001$) and treatment ($p = 0.0011$) on each group, and a significant interaction effect ($p<0.0001$). Calculation of the % increase in body weights of each of the groups at week 22 revealed an increase of 23% (sham), 36% (OVX) and 47% (Fosamax), compared with the starting weight. Analysis of the rate of weight gain over 23 weeks revealed significantly different slopes ($p<0.0001$), with sham mice gaining: 0.15±0.01 g/w ($R^2 = 0.48$); OVX mice gaining: 0.24±0.02 g/w ($R^2 = 0.56$); and Fosamax mice gaining: 0.32±0.02 g/w ($R^2 = 0.56$). Interestingly, average food intake per week per mouse from week 8 until the end of the experiment revealed OVX and sham mice had similar food intakes, Fosamax and OVX had similar food intakes, but Fosamax mice had significantly higher food intake compared with sham mice (Figure 2).

Micro-computed tomography analysis

After 23 weeks of treatment, the trabecular bone parameters in the distal femur were analyzed by micro-CT and are shown in Figure 3. No significant difference was observed between sham and OVX mice for any of the parameters; however, Tb.BMD, BV/TV, BS/TV, Tb.Th, Tb.N and Conn.Dn were significantly higher, and BS/BV, Tb.Sp, Tb.Pf, and SMI were significantly lower in Fosamax-treated mice compared with OVX mice. Measurement of the cortical bone in the middle of the femur revealed that Fosamax-treated mice had significantly thicker cortical bone compared with sham and OVX mice suggesting increased bone strength. However, Fosamax-treated mice did not show significantly different cortical BMD, EC, PC and cross-sectional area compared with OVX mice. Three-dimensional (3D) micro-CT images of the middle diaphysis of the distal femur with trabecula are shown in Figure 4. A larger trabecular network was observed in the Fosamax treated mice compared with sham or OVX mice.

Serum osteoblast and osteoclast activity, and calcium and phosphate concentrations

Activity of osteoblasts and osteoclasts were measured indirectly through a series of markers (Figure 5). For osteoblasts, elevated concentrations of osteocalcin, ALP, and PICP indicate elevated osteoblast activity, whereas elevated osteoclast activity is indicated through higher levels of PYD and NTXI. The serum osteocalcin concentration of Fosamax-treated mice was significantly higher than sham and OVX at week 12, but no difference was observed at week 23. Serum ALP showed no significant difference among three treatments at week 12, but Fosamax-treated mice had significantly lower levels than sham and OVX at week 23. Sham mice showed higher PICP levels than Fosamax and OVX at week 23. These results suggest little negative effect of Fosamax or ovariectomy on the indicators of osteoblast activity. In terms of the indicators of osteoclast activity, no significant difference between Fosamax treated mice and sham or OVX mice was observed. Sham mice showed lower PYD and NTXI than OVX, but the difference was not considered significant ($p = 0.070$ and 0.057, respectively) (Figure 5). Additionally, Fosamax treatment did not affect the serum concentration of calcium or phosphate significantly (Figure 5).

Serum Metabolomics

PCA of metabolite concentrations obtained from the analysis of mouse serum after 23 weeks is shown in Figure 6A. Fosamax-treated mice were observed to have a completely different serum metabolite profile in comparison with the OVX and sham mice. To maximize the separation between sham, OVX, and Fosamax, PLS-DA was employed and is shown in Figure 6B. The largest difference was between the Fosamax-treated mice and the sham or OVX mice as shown by separation in the first component, whereas a smaller difference between sham and OVX mice was observed in the second component. Twelve metabolites were primarily responsible for the difference between OVX and Fosamax-treated mice after 23 weeks of treatment, and are summarized in Table 1. TCA-cycle intermediates (citrate, 2-oxoglutarate, malate, fumarate, and succinate), amino acids (taurine), glucose, 3-hydroxybutyrate (a ketone), and others (acetate, allantoin, and ethanol) were significantly higher in Fosamax-treated mice compared with OVX, while aspartate was significantly lower.

Comparison of sham and OVX mice after 23 weeks revealed four metabolites that were significantly different (Table 1). Glycine, DMA, ethanol and allantoin were all significantly higher in sham mice compared with OVX mice.

Discussion

Type 1 (postmenopausal) osteoporosis is characterized by hormonal deprivation resulting in accelerated bone turnover and bone loss [25]. The OVX rat and mouse are classic models used to study postmenopausal bone loss since removal of the ovaries mimics postmenopausal hormonal changes that occur in humans, including decreases in estrogen and progesterone [26]. In this study, OVX mice were compared with OVX mice treated with Fosamax, as well as mice that received sham surgery. Interestingly, weight gain of OVX mice over 23 weeks was higher than sham mice, even though their food intake was similar. It has previously been shown that estrogen deficiency can cause higher body weight and body fat deposition [27,28], which may partially explain our results.

Metabolomics can measure changes in the levels of metabolites found in biological fluids and tissues, which can produce a

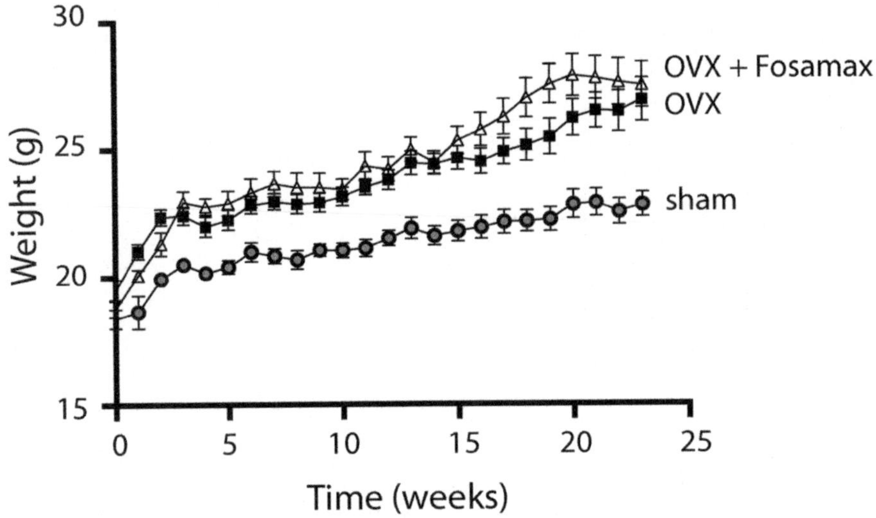

Figure 1. Body weight of mice over 23 weeks. Body weight of sham (circle), OVX (square), and OVX + Fosamax (triangle) C57BL/6 mice over 23 weeks. Time 0 represents the time of surgery. Analyzed by 2-way analysis of variance (ANOVA). Each value is expressed as mean ± SEM.

quantitative and comprehensive indication of metabolic pathway activity. It can offer information to understand the effect of diet, drugs and disease, and assessment of a disease state [29,30]. Few metabolic differences between OVX and sham mice were observed. One interesting difference was the significantly lower glycine concentration in OVX mice compared with sham. Glycine has been shown to be inversely associated with cholesterol, phospholipid, free fatty acid, and triglyceride accumulation [31], which may indicate changes in fat metabolism. Lower dimethylamine, and ethanol may be related to changes in gut microbial metabolism, and lower allantoin may indicate lower oxidative stress [32] in mice with ovariectomy compared with sham.

Despite the minor metabolic changes that occurred in the OVX mice, they were similar to sham mice with respect to bone-related measurements. We speculate that the age of the mice may have been a factor. Indeed, a report evaluating age-related changes in trabecular architecture in C57BL/6J mice showed that the trabecular bone volume (BV/TV) is greatest at 6–8 weeks of age, and declines steadily thereafter. Moreover, trabecular bone loss, as measured by trabecular number (Tb.N), is most rapid between 2–6 months of age, with a more gradual decline thereafter [33]. Our study commenced when the mice were 3 months of age (12 weeks), and continued until the mice were ~9 months of age (35 weeks).

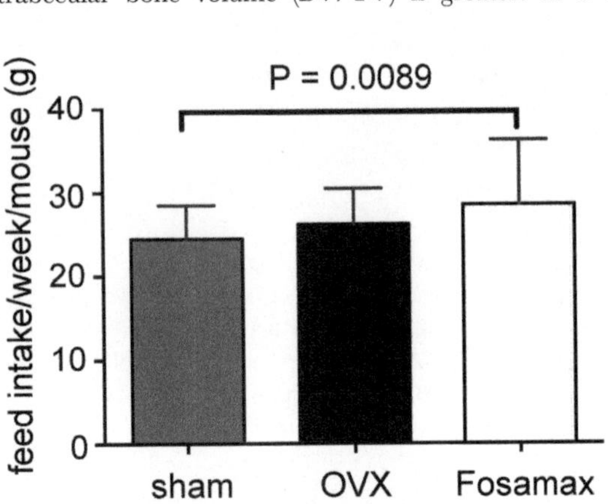

Figure 2. Weekly food intake. Average weekly food intake of sham C57BL/6 female mice compared with ovariectomized mice with and without Fosamax treatment during weeks 8–23. Analyzed by analysis of variance (ANOVA) followed by Bonferroni's multiple *t* test. Statistical significance is defined as $p<0.05$. Each value is expressed as mean ± SD.

Fosamax-treated ovariectomized mice revealed increased Tb.BMD, BV/TV, Tb.Th, Tb.N, and cortical bone thickness as well as decreased Tb.Sp, and SMI compared with both OVX and sham, which demonstrates that Fosamax appears to increase bone mass and strength as has been previously reported [34–36]. Furthermore, some reports indicate that bisphosphonates suppress the resorption and formation of bones, thereby decreasing bone turnover and lowering bone loss [37,38]. Several serum indicators of osteoblast and osteoclast activity, indicators of bone turnover, were examined. Indicators of osteoblast activity included ALP, osteocalcin, and PICP. Fosamax-treated mice exhibited lower ALP, but no significant difference in osteocalcin or PICP at week 23 compared with the OVX mice. Various studies have shown that alendronate treatment either decreases serum osteocalcin significantly, or brings about no significant change in osteoblast activity [34,37,39], which supports the observations presented here. Interestingly, osteocalcin levels in Fosamax-treated mice at week 12 were higher than sham or OVX mice, and higher than all three groups of mice at 23 weeks. We speculate that the cholecalciferol found in Fosamax may be responsible for the initial increase of osteocalcin observed at 12 weeks [40]. No significant difference in either of the osteoclast activity indicators (PYD and NTXI) after Fosamax treatment for 12 or 23 weeks was observed.

Administration of Fosamax for 23 weeks to OVX mice resulted in a significantly higher rate of weight gain over the course of the experiment compared with both sham and OVX mice. While the OVX mice receiving Fosamax treatment had a slightly elevated intake of chow compared with sham, intake was not significantly different between OVX and Fosamax-treated mice, suggesting that other factors may be responsible for the increased rate of weight gain of Fosamax mice. Interestingly, other studies in rats have shown that alendronate treatment results in higher body weight compared with OVX [28]. One possibility of the increased

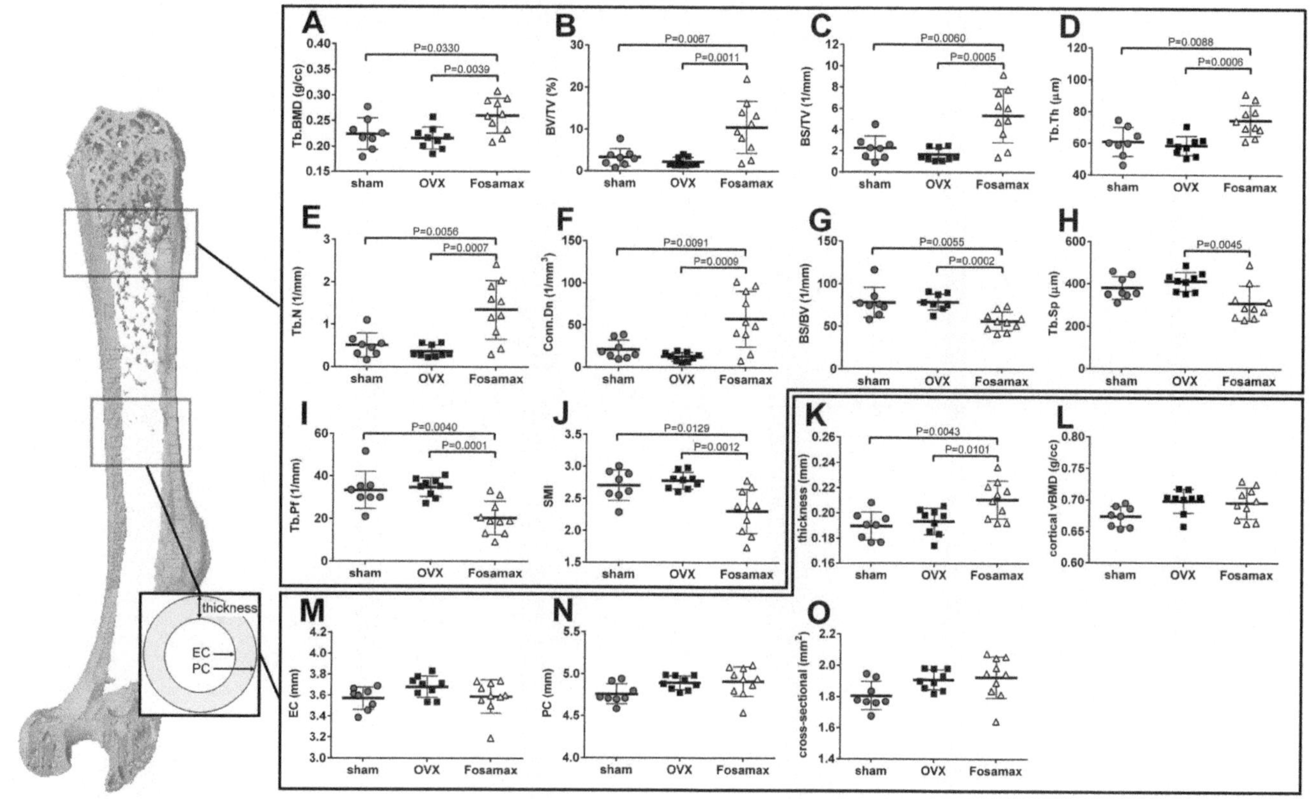

Figure 3. Micro-CT femur parameters. Bone characteristics of sham C57BL/6 female mice compared with ovariectomized mice with and without Fosamax treatment for 23 weeks. (A-J) Bone parameters of the distal femur analyzed by micro-CT. (A) Tb.BMD, trabecular bone mineral density; (B) BV/TV, bone volume/tissue volume; (C) BS/TV, bone surface/tissue volume; (D) Tb.Th, trabecular thickness; (E) Tb.N, trabecular number; (F) Conn.Dn, connectivity density; (G) BS/BV, bone surface/bone volume; (H) Tb.Sp, trabecular separation; (I) Tb.Pf, trabecular pattern factor; (J) SMI, structure model index. (K-O) Cortical bone parameters of the middle diaphysis analyzed by micro-CT. (K) Thickness, cortical bone shell thickness; (L) cortical BMD, cortical bone mineral density; (M) EC, endosteal circumference; (N) PC, periosteal circumference; (O) cross-sectional, cross-sectional area. Analyzed by analysis of variance (ANOVA) followed by Bonferroni's multiple *t* test. Statistical significance is defined as $p<0.05$. Each value is expressed as mean ± SD.

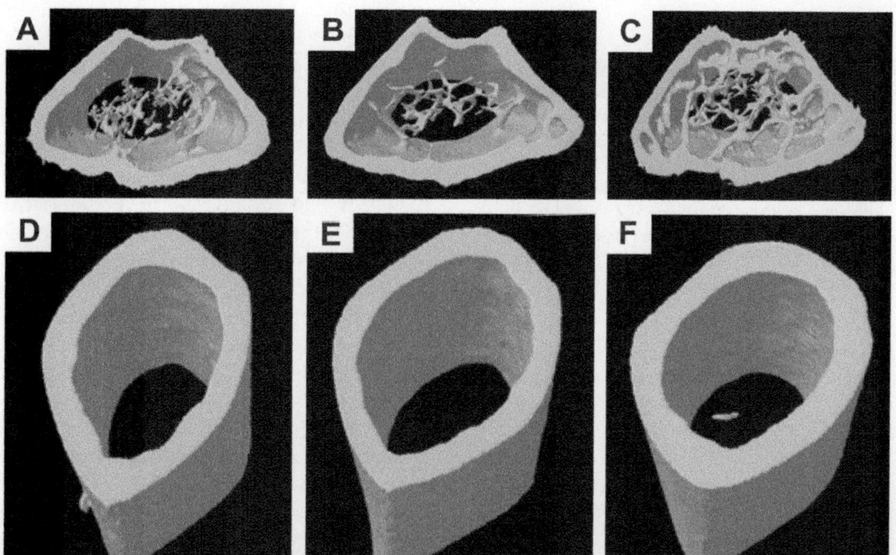

Figure 4. Micro-CT three-dimensional images. Femur images of sham, OVX and OVX + Fosamax C57BL/6 female mice treatment for 23 weeks. The distal femur region of: (A) sham mice, (B) OVX mice, and (C) Fosamax-treated mice. Femoral mid-diaphysis of: (D) sham mice (E) OVX mice, and (F) Fosamax-treated mice.

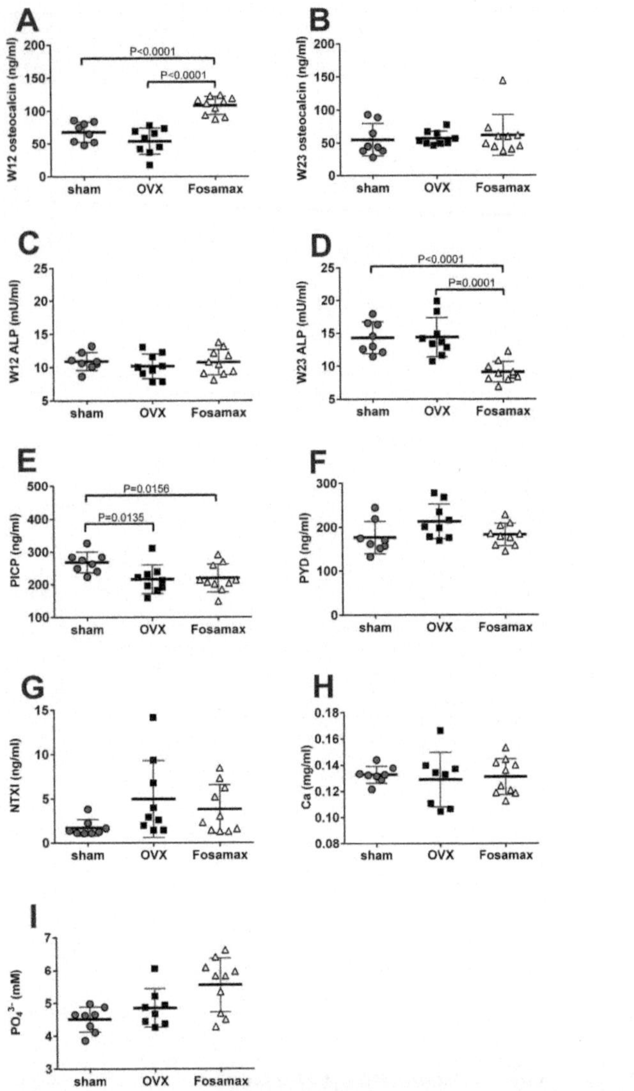

Figure 5. The concentrations of osteoblast and osteoclast indicators, calcium and phosphate in serum. Effects on serum osteoblast and osteoclast indicators, calcium and phosphate concentration of sham C57BL/6 female mice compared with ovariectomized mice with and without Fosamax treatment for 12 (W12) or 23 (W23) weeks. (A-E) Osteoblast indicators. (A) W12 osteocalcin; (B) W23 osteocalcin; (C) W12 ALP, alkaline phosphatase; (D) W23 ALP; (E) PICP, procollagen I C-terminal propeptide after 23 weeks treatment. (F.G) Osteoclast indicators. (F) PYD, pyridinoline after 23 weeks treatment. (G) NTXI, cross-linked N-telopeptide of type I collagen after 23 weeks treatment. Serum concentration of: (H) calcium after 23 weeks treatment, and (I) phosphate after 23 weeks treatment. Analyzed by analysis of variance (ANOVA) followed by Bonferroni's multiple *t* test. Statistical significance is defined as $p<0.05$. Each value is expressed as mean ± SD.

weight gain could be the neo-formation of bone tissue [41]. However, other factors may also affect body weight, including changes in global metabolism through changes in adiponectin, leptin and energy metabolism (glucose, 3-hydroxybutyrate and taurine), as well as activity of osteoblast cells. Interestingly, adiponectin and leptin, the main circulating peptides secreted by adipose tissue, have been shown to be involved with regulation of bone metabolism [42,43], and treatment with alendronate for 12 months has been shown to slightly decrease serum leptin [44].

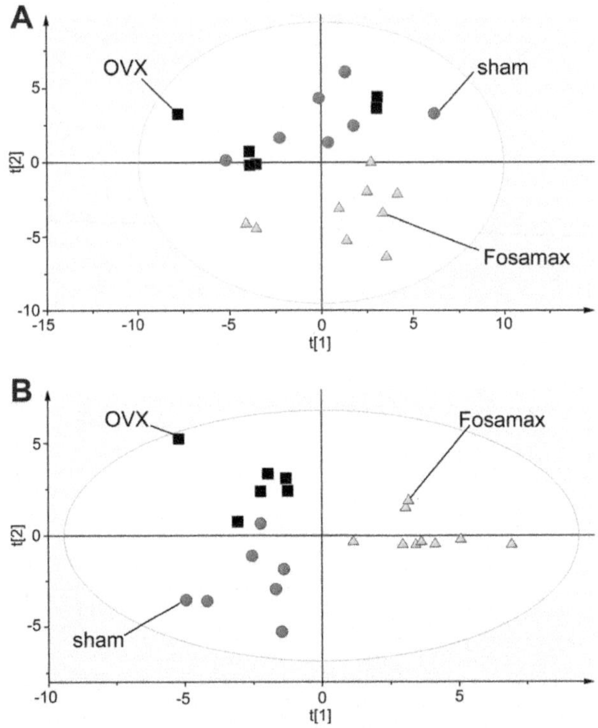

Figure 6. Comparison of metabolic composition of serum. (A) PCA ($R^2X=0.642$, $Q^2=0.178$) and (B) PLS-DA ($R^2Y=0.915$, $Q^2=0.700$) models of serum metabolite concentrations of sham C57BL/6 female mice compared with ovariectomized mice with and without Fosamax treatment for 23 weeks. Permutation testing revealed that the model was valid, with all values of the permuted R^2Y and Q^2 data being significantly less than the original model ($p<0.001$).

One interesting observation was a decrease in osteocalcin at week 23 compared with week 12 in Fosamax-treated mice. Osteoblasts are known to secrete hormones that affect energy metabolism. Indeed, mice deficient in osteocalcin are obese, having decreased β-cell proliferation and secretion, greater insulin resistance, and decreased energy expenditure [45–47]. Insulin is an important molecule associated with bone remodeling and energy metabolism [48]. While insulin was not directly measured in this study, serum metabolites of Fosamax-treated mice were compared with OVX mice, revealing higher serum glucose and higher 3-hydroxybutyrate in Fosamax-treated mice compared with OVX mice. Hyperglycemia has been correlated with diabetic ketoacidosis, which can result in stimulation of lipolytic pathways, resulting in free fatty acids and ketone bodies in the blood [49].

However, it is puzzling that there is an almost 2-fold higher concentration of osteocalcin in Fosamax-treated mice at week 12, which then appears to return to levels similar to OVX and sham mice at week 23. It is tempting to speculate that this change in osteocalcin levels may lead to insulin resistance and lipolysis [48], followed by increased weight gain and risk of diabetes [39,45,47]. Indeed, most of the increased weight gain of the Fosamax treated mice was in the later part of the experiment, and these results could suggest that prolonged use of the drug may have negative consequences. However, this will need to be elucidated in a further study. Indeed, there is much controversy in the literature on the correlation of bisphosphonate therapy with glycemia, diabetes and body weight [50–52], and whether these observations are restricted to mice or may be extended to humans remains to be clarified.

Table 1. Comparison of serum metabolite concentrations after 23 weeks.

Metabolite[a] (μM)		Sham	OVX	Fosamax	*p*-value	Adjusted *p*-value OVX vs Fosamax	Adjusted *p*-value Sham vs OVX
TCA cycle	Citrate	293.1±24.6	263.5±38.2	365.2±37.6	<0.0001	0.0020	>0.99
	2-Oxoglutarate	32.3±12.0	35.3±2.7	49.7±9.8	0.0010	0.0202	>0.99
	Malate	106.4±26.6	93.0±38.4	176.4±47.4	0.0010	0.0055	>0.99
	Fumarate	10.9±5.0	13.0±5.0	19.6±5.1	0.0067	0.0693	>0.99
	Succinate	436.8±139.9	389.7±138.3	679.8±187.3	0.0165	0.0341	>0.99
Amino acids	Aspartate	39.1±10.3	38.2±9.0	23.8±7.2	0.0020	0.0325	>0.99
	Taurine	460.8±95.1	467.6±116.0	669.2±127.6	0.0040	0.0341	>0.99
	Glycine	313.8±41.1	249.8±42.5	289.5±38.5	0.0482	0.5338	0.0468
Energy metabolism	Glucose	13188.6±2517.5	14309.8±1897.3	18547.8±2747.4	0.0007	0.0468	>0.99
Ketones	3-Hydroxybutyrate	110.8±44.8	76.2±17.9	168.5±63.8	0.0052	0.0081	0.6103
Others	Acetate	65.1±19.2	44.6±16.1	78.7±14.9	0.0095	0.0110	0.2787
	Allantoin	165.6±50.3	100.4±12.2	138.7±32.8	0.0047	0.0609	0.0089
	Ethanol	188.4±81.4	85.1±35.5	300.1±233.9	0.0025	0.0062	0.0397
	Dimethylamine	4.1±1.5	1.9±0.7	2.7±0.6	0.0015	0.4062	0.0012

[a]Significantly different metabolites between OVX and Fosamax-treated mice or Sham and OVX mice. Each value is expressed as mean ± SD. *P*-values were calculated using the Kruskal-Wallis test, and adjusted *p*-values were calculated using Dunn's multiple comparison test. Alpha was set to 0.05.

Other metabolites that may be connected with osteoporosis include 3-hydroxybutyrate and taurine [53-56]. 3-hydroxybutyrate has been shown to reduce bone absorption, maintain normal bone function and femur bone mineral density, thus reducing osteoporosis [53]. We observed higher 3-hydroxybutyrate in Fosamax-treated mice. Our results also showed taurine was higher in Fosamax-treated mice. Interestingly, taurine supplementation has been shown to increase bone mineral density in rats [54,55]. It can bind divalent cations, including Mg^{2+}, and has an important role in bone remodeling and skeletal development [56].

Our results showed that while Fosamax increased bone mineral density and lowered bone loss, it only decreased serum osteoblast activity slightly, and did not affect osteoclast activity. Serum metabolomics revealed that Fosamax primarily affected energy metabolism. Specifically, Fosamax increased the concentrations of serum glucose, 3-hydroxybutyrate and taurine, which have been shown to be positivity related to bone health, but also significantly increased the concentrations of TCA cycle intermediates, suggesting that mitochondrial function may also be affected by Fosamax treatment. Significantly increased weight gain of Fosamax-treated mice, particularly in the later weeks of treatment, suggest that long-term Fosamax use appears to impact metabolism, but it is unclear at this stage how these metabolic changes may lead to complications observed with long-term use of bisphosphonates. Future studies will explore changes in serum insulin, adiponectin, and leptin with treatment, as well as determine global metabolic changes at 12 weeks to compare with 24 weeks to determine the length of time of maximum benefit.

Acknowledgments

We would like to thank the National Laboratory Animal Center of Taiwan for technical support in Micro-CT experiment.

Author Contributions

Conceived and designed the experiments: SYC JPK CCY SSC JLM CMS. Performed the experiments: SYC HTY DOM. Analyzed the data: SYC CMS. Contributed reagents/materials/analysis tools: JPK CCY SSC JLM CMS. Contributed to the writing of the manuscript: SYC CMS JLM.

References

1. Burge R, Dawson-Hughes B, Solomon DH, Wong JB, King A, et al. (2007) Incidence and economic burden of osteoporosis-related fractures in the United States, 2005–2025. J Bone Miner Res 22: 465–475.
2. Chang KL, Hu YC, Hsieh BS, Cheng HL, Hsu HW, et al. (2013) Combined effect of soy isoflavones and vitamin D_3 on bone loss in ovariectomized rats. Nutrition 29: 250–257.
3. Kanis JA, the WHO Study Group (1994) Assessment of fracture risk and its application to screening for postmenopausal osteoporosis: synopsis of a WHO report. Osteoporos Int 4: 368–381.
4. Faienza MF, Ventura A, Marzano F, Cavallo L (2013) Postmenopausal osteoporosis: the role of immune system cells. Clin Dev Immunol 2013: 1–6.
5. Riggs BL, Khosla S, Melton III LJ (2002) Sex steroids and the construction and conservation of the adult skeleton. Endocr Rev 23: 279–302.
6. Talaulikar VS, Chambers T, Manyonda I (2012) Exploiting the antioxidant potential of a common vitamin: could vitamin C prevent postmenopausal osteoporosis? J Obstet Gynaecol Res 38: 253–257.
7. Sambrook PN, Geusens P, Ribot C, Solimano JA, Ferrer-Barriendos J, et al. (2004) Alendronate produces greater effects than raloxifene on bone density and bone turnover in postmenopausal women with low bone density: results of EFFECT (Efficacy of FOSAMAX versus EVISTA Comparison Trial) International. J Intern Med 255: 503–511.
8. Russell RGG, Watts NB, Ebetino FH, Rogers MJ (2008) Mechanisms of action of bisphosphonates: similarities and differences and their potential influence on clinical efficacy. Osteoporos Int 19: 733–759.
9. Kendler DL, Roux C, Benhamou CL, Brown JP, Lillestol M, et al. (2010) Effects of denosumab on bone mineral density and bone turnover in postmenopausal women transitioning from alendronate therapy. J Bone Miner Res 25: 72–81.
10. Delmas PD, Seeman E (2004) Changes in bone mineral density explain little of the reduction in vertebral or nonvertebral fracture risk with anti-resorptive therapy. Bone 34: 599–604.
11. Odvina CV, Zerwekh JE, Rao DS, Maalouf N, Gottschalk FA, et al. (2005) Severely suppressed bone turnover: a potential complication of alendronate therapy. J Clin Endocrinol Metab 90: 1294–1301.
12. Neustadt J, Pieczenik S (2012) Osteoporosis: beyond bone mineral density. A special report on the state of osteoporosis research. NBI Health website. Available: http://www.nbihealth.com/supporting/osteoporosisreport.pdf. Accessed 2014 Jun 7.
13. Varun B, Sivakumar T, Nair BJ, Joseph AP (2012) Bisphosphonate induced osteonecrosis of jaw in breast cancer patients: A systematic review. J Oral Maxillofac Pathol 16: 210–214.
14. Yamazaki T, Yamori M, Tanaka S, Yamamoto K, Sumi E, et al. (2013) Risk factors and indices of osteomyelitis of the jaw in osteoporosis patients: results from a hospital-based cohort study in Japan. PLoS One 8: e79376.
15. Khan AA, Sándor GK, Dore E, Morrison AD, Alsahli M, et al. (2009) Bisphosphonate associated osteonecrosis of the jaw. J Rheumatol 36: 478–490.
16. Watts NB, Diab DL (2010) Long-term use of bisphosphonates in osteoporosis. J Clin Endocrinol Metab 95: 1555–1565.
17. Sener G, Kapucu C, Cetinel S, Cikler E, Ayanoğlu-Dülger G (2005) Gastroprotective effect of leukotriene receptor blocker montelukast in alendronat-induced lesions of the rat gastric mucosa. Prostaglandins Leukot Essent Fatty Acids 72: 1–11.
18. Lasota A, Danowska-Klonowska D (2004) Experimental osteoporosis- different methods of ovariectomy in female white rats. Rocz Akad Med Bialymst 49 Suppl 1: 129–131.
19. U.S. Department of Health and Human Services Food and Drug Administration (2002) Estimating the safe starting dose in clinical trials for therapeutics in adult healthy volunteers. FDA website. Available: http://www.fda.gov/OHRMS/DOCKETS/98fr/02d-0492-gdl0001-vol1.pdf. Accessed 2014 Jun 7.
20. Hildebrand T, Rüegsegger P (1997) Quantification of bone microarchitecture with the structure model index. Comput Methods Biomech Biomed Engin 1: 15–23.
21. Odgaard A, Gundersen HJ (1993) Quantification of connectivity in cancellous bone, with special emphasis on 3-D reconstructions. Bone 14: 173–182.
22. O'Sullivan A, Willoughby RE, Mishchuk D, Alcarraz B, Cabezas-Sanchez C, et al. (2013) Metabolomics of cerebrospinal fluid from humans treated for rabies. J Proteome Res 12: 481–490.
23. Weljie AM, Newton J, Mercier P, Carlson E, Slupsky CM (2006) Targeted profiling: quantitative analysis of ^1H NMR metabolomics data. Anal Chem 78: 4430–4442.
24. Slupsky CM, Rankin KN, Wagner J, Fu H, Chang D, et al. (2007) Investigations of the effects of gender, diurnal variation, and age in human urinary metabolomic profiles. Anal Chem 79: 6995–7004.
25. Vs K, K P, Ramesh M, Venkatesan V (2013) The association of serum osteocalcin with the bone mineral density in post menopausal women. J Clin Diagn Res 7: 814–816.
26. Rendina E, Hembree KD, Davis MR, Marlow D, Clarke SL, et al. (2013) Dried plum's unique capacity to reverse bone loss and alter bone metabolism in postmenopausal osteoporosis model. PLoS One 8: e60569.
27. Zhao X, Wu ZX, Zhang Y, Yan YB, He Q, et al. (2011) Anti-osteoporosis activity of *Cibotium barometz* extract on ovariectomy-induced bone loss in rats. J Ethnopharmacol 137: 1083–1088.
28. Abdel-Sater KA, Mansour H (2012) Effects of leptin on metabolic bone turnover in ovariectomy rats. Acta Endocrinol 8: 189–198.
29. Nicholson JK, Lindon JC (2008) Systems biology: Metabonomics. Nature 455: 1054–1056.
30. DeBerardinis RJ, Thompson CB (2012) Cellular metabolism and disease: what do metabolic outliers teach us? Cell 148: 1132–1144.
31. Senthilkumar R, Viswanathan P, Nalini N (2003) Glycine modulates hepatic lipid accumulation in alcohol-induced liver injury. Pol J Pharmacol 55: 603–611.
32. Dryland PA, Love DR, Walker MF, Dommels Y, Butts C, et al. (2008) Allantoin as a biomarker of inflammation in an inflammatory bowel disease mouse model: NMR analysis of urine. Open Bioact Compd J, 1, 1–6.
33. Glatt V, Canalis E, Stadmeyer L, Bouxsein ML (2007) Age-related changes in trabecular architecture differ in female and male C57BL/6J mice. J Bone Miner Res 22: 1197–1207.
34. Cho DC, Kim KT, Jeon Y, Sung JK (2012) A synergistic bone sparing effect of curcumin and alendronate in ovariectomized rat. Acta Neurochir 154: 2215–2223.
35. Yamane H, Sakai A, Mori T, Tanaka S, Moridera K, et al. (2009) The anabolic action of intermittent PTH in combination with cathepsin K inhibitor or alendronate differs depending on the remodeling status in bone in ovariectomized mice. Bone 44: 1055–1062.
36. Davison KS, Siminoski K, Adachi JD, Hanley DA, Goltzman D, et al. (2006) Bone strength: the whole is greater than the sum of its parts. Semin Arthritis Rheum 36: 22–31.

37. Seo SK, Yang HI, Lim KJ, Jeon YE, Choi YS, et al. (2012) Changes in serum levels of cartilage oligomeric matrix protein after estrogen and alendronate therapy in postmenopausal women. Gynecol Obstet Invest 74: 143–150.
38. Iwamoto J, Seki A, Takeda T, Sato Y, Yamada H, et al. (2006) Comparative effects of alendronate and alfacalcidol on cancellous and cortical bone mass and bone mechanical properties in ovariectomized rats. Exp Anim 55: 357–367.
39. Lacombe J, Karsenty G, Ferron M (2013) In vivo analysis of the contribution of bone resorption to the control of glucose metabolism in mice. Mol Metab 2: 498–504.
40. Clemens TL, Tang H, Maeda S, Kesterson RA, Demayo F, et al. (1997) Analysis of osteocalcin expression in transgenic mice reveals a species difference in vitamin D regulation of mouse and human osteocalcin genes. J Bone Miner Res 12: 1570–1576.
41. Notomi T, Okimoto N, Okazaki Y, Nakamura T, Suzuki M (2003) Tower climbing exercise started 3 months after ovariectomy recovers bone strength of the femur and lumbar vertebrae in aged osteopenic rats. J Bone Min Res 18: 140–149.
42. Wu N, Wang QP, Li H, Wu XP, Sun ZQ, et al. (2010) Relationships between serum adiponectin, leptin concentrations and bone mineral density, and bone biochemical markers in Chinese women. Clin Chim Acta 411: 771–775.
43. Legiran S, Brandi ML (2012) Bone mass regulation of leptin and postmenopausal osteoporosis with obesity. Clin Cases Miner Bone Metab 9: 145–149.
44. Sebastián-Ochoa A, Fernández-García D, Reyes-García R, Mezquita-Raya P, Rozas-Moreno P, et al. (2012) Adiponectin and leptin serum levels in osteoporotic postmenopausal women treated with raloxifene or alendronate. Menopause 19: 172–177.
45. Clemens TL, Karsenty G (2011) The osteoblast: an insulin target cell controlling glucose homeostasis. J Bone Miner Res 26: 677–680.
46. Lee NK, Sowa H, Hinoi E, Ferron M, Ahn JD, et al. (2007) Endocrine regulation of energy metabolism by the skeleton. Cell 130: 456–469.
47. Semenkovich CF, Teitelbaum SL (2007) Bone weighs in on obesity. Cell 130: 409–411.
48. Ng KW (2011) Regulation of glucose metabolism and the skeleton. Clin Endocrinol 75: 147–155.
49. Van Ness-Otunnu R, Hack JB (2013) Hyperglycemic crisis. J Emerg Med 45: 797–805.
50. Kaji H, Hisa I, Inoue Y, Naito J, Sugimoto T, et al. (2009) Analysis of factors affecting increase in bone mineral density at lumbar spine by bisphosphonate treatment in postmenopausal osteoporosis. J Bone Miner Metab 27: 76–82.
51. Schwartz AV, Schafer AL, Grey A, Vittinghoff E, Palermo L, et al. (2013) Effects of antiresorptive therapies on glucose metabolism: results from the FIT, HORIZON-PFT, and FREEDOM trials. J Bone Miner Res 28: 1348–1354.
52. Hong SH, Koo JW, Hwang JK, Hwang YC, Jeong IK, et al. (2013) Changes in serum osteocalcin are not associated with changes in glucose or insulin for osteoporotic patients treated with bisphosphonate. J Bone Metab 20: 37–41.
53. Zhao Y, Zou B, Shi Z, Wu Q, Chen GQ (2007) The effect of 3-hydroxybutyrate on the *in vitro* differentiation of murine osteoblast MC3T3-E1 and *in vivo* bone formation in ovariectomized rats. Biomaterials 28: 3063–3073.
54. Choi MJ, DiMarco NM (2009) The effects of dietary taurine supplementation on bone mineral density in ovariectomized rats. Adv Exp Med Biol 643: 341–349.
55. Choi MJ, Chang KJ (2013) Effect of dietary taurine and arginine supplementation on bone mineral density in growing female rats. Adv Exp Med Biol 776: 335–345.
56. Jeon SH, Lee MY, Kim SJ, Joe SG, Kim GB, et al. (2007) Taurine increases cell proliferation and generates an increase in $[Mg^{2+}]i$ accompanied by ERK 1/2 activation in human osteoblast cells. FEBS Lett 581: 5929–5934.

21

Radiological Assessment of Bioengineered Bone in a Muscle Flap for the Reconstruction of Critical-Size Mandibular Defect

Randa Al-Fotawei[1], Ashraf F. Ayoub[1]*, Neil Heath[2], Kurt B. Naudi[3], K. Elizabeth Tanner[4], Matthew J. Dalby[5], Jeremy McMahon[6]

1 University of Glasgow, Glasgow, United Kingdom, **2** Oral & Maxillofacial Radiology, Glasgow University Dental Hospital & School, Glasgow, United Kingdom, **3** Oral Surgery, Glasgow University Dental Hospital & School, Glasgow, United Kingdom, **4** Biomedical Materials, School of Engineering, University of Glasgow, Glasgow, United Kingdom, **5** Centre for Cell Engineering, University of Glasgow, Glasgow, United Kingdom, **6** Oral & Maxillofacial Surgery, Southern General Hospital, Glasgow, United Kingdom

Abstract

This study presents a comprehensive radiographic evaluation of bone regeneration within a pedicled muscle flap for the reconstruction of critical size mandibular defect. The surgical defect (20 mm×15 mm) was created in the mandible of ten experimental rabbits. The masseter muscle was adapted to fill the surgical defect, a combination of calcium sulphate/ hydroxyapatite cement (CERAMENT™ |SPINE SUPPORT), BMP-7 and rabbit mesenchymal stromal cells (rMSCs) was injected inside the muscle tissue. Radiographic assessment was carried out on the day of surgery and at 4, 8, and 12 weeks postoperatively. At 12 weeks, the animals were sacrificed and cone beam computerized tomography (CBCT) scanning and micro-computed tomography (µ-CT) were carried out. Clinically, a clear layer of bone tissue was identified closely adherent to the border of the surgical defect. Sporadic radio-opaque areas within the surgical defect were detected radiographically. In comparison with the opposite non operated control side, the estimated quantitative scoring of the radio-opacity was 46.6% ±15, the mean volume of the radio-opaque areas was 63.4% ±20. Areas of a bone density higher than that of the mandibular bone (+35% ±25%) were detected at the borders of the surgical defect. The micro-CT analysis revealed thinner trabeculae of the regenerated bone with a more condensed trabecular pattern than the surrounding native bone. These findings suggest a rapid deposition rate of the mineralised tissue and an active remodelling process of the newly regenerated bone within the muscle flap. The novel surgical model of this study has potential clinical application; the assessment of bone regeneration using the presented radiolographic protocol is descriptive and comprehensive. The findings of this research confirm the remarkable potential of local muscle flaps as local bioreactors to induce bone formation for reconstruction of maxillofacial bony defects.

Editor: Gwendolen Reilly, University of Sheffield, United Kingdom

Funding: The authors have no support or funding to report.

Competing Interests: The authors have declared that no competing interests exist.

* Email: Ashraf.Ayoub@glasgow.ac.uk

Introduction

Loss of bone due to trauma, infection or resection of pathological lesions results in large, osseous, segmental defects of the facial skeleton which are difficult to reconstruct. Even in the best hands, inadequate vascularisation at the site of the bone defect (recipient site) has been the main obstacle for successful reconstruction with bone grafting [1]. Many strategies have been proposed for the management of mandibular surgical defects following bone loss, vascularized autogenous bone grafts are considered the most reliable method for reconstruction. However, this type of graft is not suitable if the patient has been subjected to radiotherapy or is suffering from peripheral vascular disease which compromises the blood supply to the surgical site. The harvesting of vascularised bone graft is associated with well documented morbidities [2]. Bone bioengineering using biomaterial, bioactive molecules and autogenous stem cells have been studied extensively and variable rates of success are reported [3–5]. Other studies have investigated various ways to induce angiogensesis and arteriogenesis which are essential for the bone regeneration process [6,7]. The applications of vascular endothelial growth factors (VEGF), angiogenic proteins and hypoxia induced factor-1α to improve vascularity at the surgical site have also been reported [8–10].

More advanced surgical techniques were advocated to overcome the problems of the limited vascularity at the surgical defects "the recipient site" by utilizing local skeletal muscle flap to induce bone formation due to its reliable source of adequate blood supply [11–13]. The muscle has the propensity to induce bone formation because of its intrinsic osteogenic potential when exposed to osteogenic stimuli including bone matrix substitutes and bone morphgenic proteins (BMP) [14].

In clinical practice, plain radiographs are the most common method for the evaluation of bone regeneration [15]. However, this type of radiograph provides two diminsional (2D) representation of three diminsional (3D) structures, the superimposition of

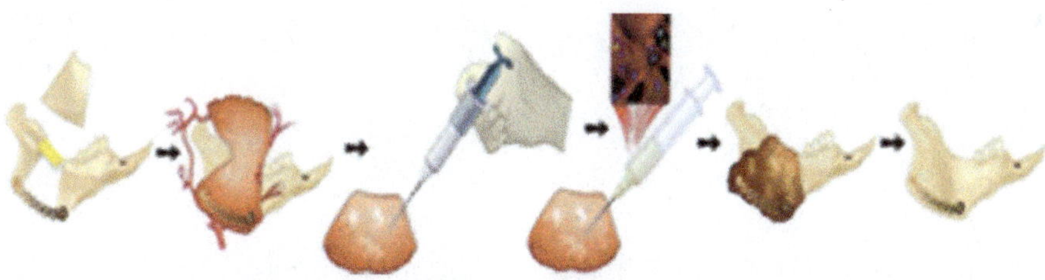

Figure 1. Diagrammatic illustation of the surgically created defect at the ramus of the mandible, fixation of the titanium plate, adaptation of the deep layer of masseter muscle into the defect followed by injection of Cerement^{TM}, BMP-7, and rMSc.

the medial and lateral surfaces confuses the analysis of bone regeneration. On the other hand the objective evaluation of radiographs and the application of a comprehensive scoring system are mandatory for the assessment of the quality and magnitude of the bioengineered bone. Radiographic assessment of bone regeneration should be comprehensive enough to record the dynamics of bone formation and the rate of degradation of bio-scaffold [16–19]. It has been recognized that cone beam computerized tomography (CBCT) is a reliable imaging modality for the 3D assessment of bioengineered bone [20]. The main advantage of this radiographic method is the reduction of radiation dose in comparison with conventional CT scanning [21].

Micro-computed tomography (μ-CT) is a sophisticated radiographic technique that permits quantitative morphometry of the bone structure in three dimensions [22]. The method produces high resolution images for accurate assessments of the micro-architecture of the bone tissue [23]. It allows the volumetric assessment of complex structures which consists of materials and tissues of variable densities which is the case of bone regeneration within radio-opaque biphasic calcium phosphate cement [24].

This study evaluated the reconstruction of critical size mandibular defects in rabbits using a pedicled masseter muscle flap which was injected with calcium sulphate/hydroxyapatite cement (CERAMENT^{TM}|SPINE SUPPORT), BMP-7 and rabbit mesenchymal stromal cells (rMSCs). Bone regeneration within the muscle tissue was monitored using plain extra-oral lateral oblique radiographs at three time points; 4, 8, 12 weeks post-operatively. CBCT, and Micro-CT assessments were carried out at 12 weeks following surgery. This article provides a comprehensive protocol for the assessment of bone regeneration process and highlights the importance of the objective 3D radiographic analysis and the assessment of the micro-structural details of the regenerated bone tissue.

Materials and Methods

Surgical procedure

Approval was obtained from the Home Office of the United Kingdom under the Animals (Scientific Procedures) Act 1986 to carry out regulated procedures on living animals. Rabbit bone marrow aspiration, rMSCs isolation, culture, characterization, and assessment of cells to cement interactions were carried out by our team as reported previously [25]. The cement used in this study was injectable and commercially available (CERAMENT^{TM}|SPINE SUPPORT, Bone Support AB, Sweden) which consisted of 60% calcium sulphate, 40% hydroxyapatite powder, and a liquid phase made of water and pacifier (iohexol). This study was carried out on ten New Zealand rabbits weighing 3.5–4.0 kg. The animals were obtained from a designated farm and kept in a dedicated animal house under veterinary supervision in the small animal research facilities. Each case was premedicated with 12.5 μg Fentanyl transdermal patch applied the afternoon prior to surgery. Fentanyl citrate & Fluanisone (Hypnorm, 0.5 ml/kg) was given intramuscularly 30 minutes before surgery and Midazolam (2 mg/kg) was administered intravenously at induction. The animals received endotracheal intubation and were given Insflurane, nitrous oxide, and oxygen. Oxygen saturation was monitored throughout the surgical procedure. A 2 cm right submandibular skin incision was performed to expose the angle of the mandible. This region was cut about 3–5 millimeters posterior to the last molar tooth, and the second cut was made 10 mm posterior to the first cut across the ascending part of the ramus of the mandible to create a surgical defect of 20 mm×15 mm. The upper border of

Table 1. Grading system for the quality and quantity of radiographic bone regeneration.

Extent of bone formation	Description
Grade 0	No change compared to the immediate post-operative appearance regarding the size and the shape of the surgical defect
Grade 1	Traces of radio-dense materials in the surgical defect
Grade 2	Flocculent radio-density with flecks of calcification
Grade 3	Defect is bridged at least at one point with radio-dense material
Grade 4	Defect is bridged on both medial and lateral sides with material of a uniform radio-density, the ends of the cortices remains visible.
Grade 5	Same as Grade 3; at least one of the cortices is obscured by the new formed radio-opaque tissue.
Grade 6	Surgical defect is bridged by uniform radio-opaque tissue; which is completely indistinguishable from the surrounding bony edge.

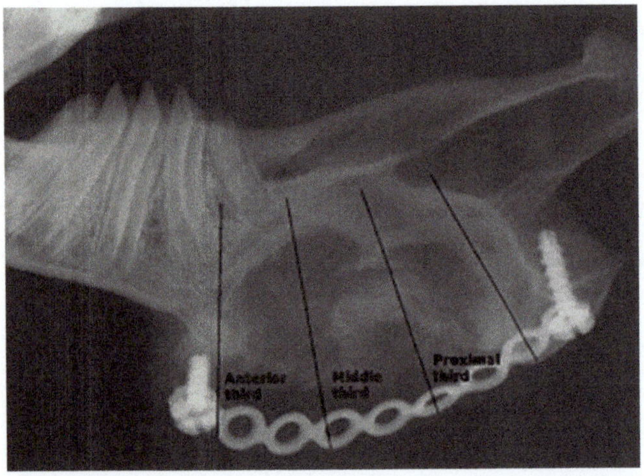

Figure 2. Radiographic image of the ramus of the mandible three months following surgery, showing the anatomical subdivision of the radiograph into anterior, middle, and posterior thirds for qualitative assessment.

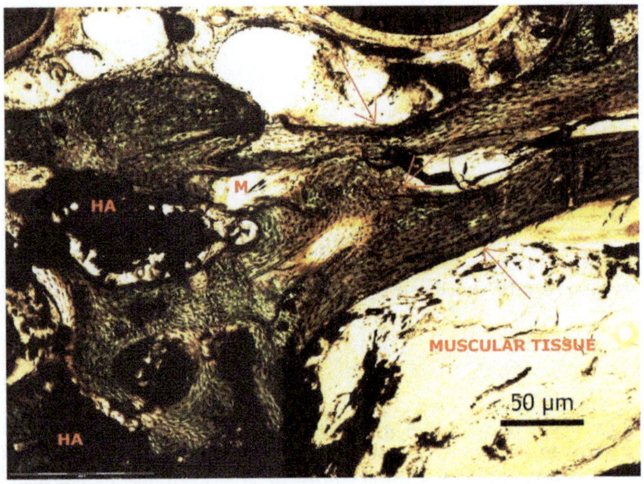

Figure 3. Histological picture of the regenerated tissue showing the pattern of newly formed bone (red arrows) within the muscle tissue (M) around the residual component of the cement (Hydroxyapatite) "HA".

the mandible was kept intact. To maintain the stability of the mandible a titanium plate was applied at the inferior border and secured in place by two screws, one on each side of the created defect. The deep layer of masseter muscle was dissected, reflected from its insertion and adapted into the created defect in the ramus of the mandible. The cement, 1.5 ml CERAMENT^{TM}|SPINE SUPPORT was mixed with 0.4 mg/ml BMP-7 (Op-1 Osigraft, Stryker Biotech, Ireland) and the mixture was injected into the masseter muscle flap. Once the material set, which took about 10 minutes, the prepared rMSCs suspension which contained three and half million cells was injected around the cement (Figure 1). This two injections protocol was based on our previous laboratory studies [25]. The surgical site was sutured in layers, the animals followed a standard postoperative protocol to minimize infection and to reduce postoperative pain. The surgical site was inspected and cleaned daily. Animals were kept on soft food for 3–4 days following surgery. Postoperative analgesic Meloxicam (NSAID) 0.2 mg/kg subcutaneous was given and prophylactic antibiotics cover using Oxytetracyclin 10% injection of 0.2 ml/kg. After full recovery, the rabbit was transferred to the normal holding cage and 10 ml saline was given S/C to avoid dehydration. The activity of the rabbit was monitored on a daily basis, as was the site of the operation for any bleeding or signs of infection. A mushy diet was offered to the animals, 0.16 ml Metacam (NSAID) was given S/C during the first 24 hours following surgery and on the 2nd post-operative day.

The rabbits were euthanatized three months following surgery by an overdose of IV sodium pentobarbitone (140 mg/kg). The mandibles were explanted and the surgical sites were examined. Samples were subjected to a comprehensive radiological evaluation as explained below. Histological assessments were carried out, the details are beyond the scope of this article.

Plain radiographic assessment - oblique extra-oral film

Assessment during the lifetime of the animals was carried out by taking extr-oral lateral radiograph using dental occlusal films (Kodak Ultra-speed DF-50, Eastman Kodak Company, 3 NY,

Table 2. Scale used in calculating quantitative score (ΣQS) and its interpretation.

Grade	∑QS	Interpretation
0	0	0% radio-opacity
1–2	25%	25% radio-opacity
3–4	50%	50% radio-opacity
4–5	75%	75% radio-opacity
6	100%	100% radio-opacity

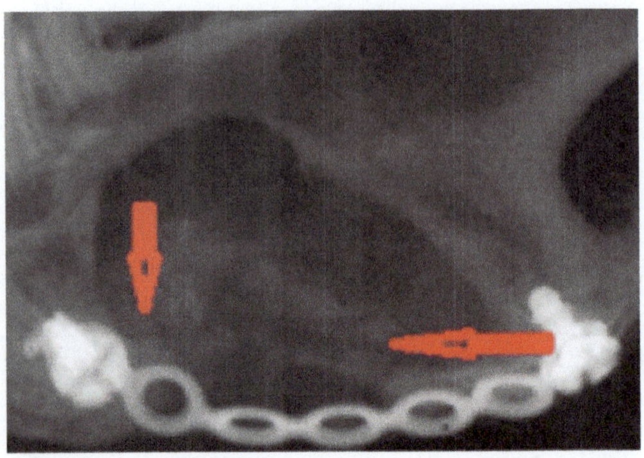

Figure 4. Micro CT scanning for one of the samples showing the Field of Vision (FOV) that was selected for all the samples; blue arrows indicate the boundaries of FOV, the anterior arrow (A) refers to area of the last premolar tooth; the last proximal screw represents the posterior limit (P) of the FOV, vertically the FOV extended 1 cm above the ramus notch denoted with yellow arrow.

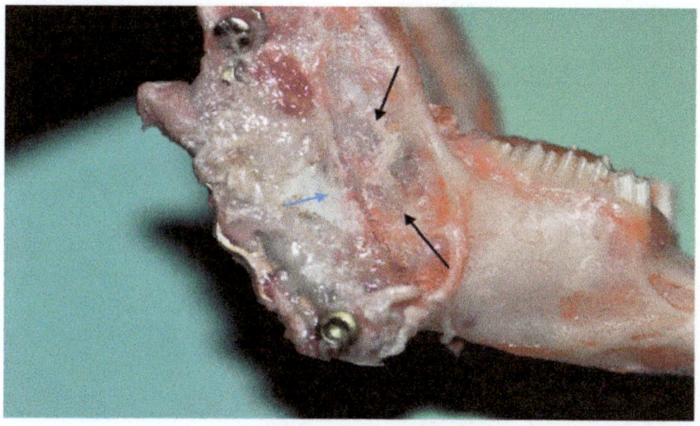

Figure 5. Clinical picture for the operated side of a harvested mandible, showing the muscle tissue occupying most of the area of the created defect. The figure shows the fixation screw and the titanium plate (red arrows) across the inferior border of the defect. The blue arrows denote an area of residual cement, and areas of calcified tissue at the superior border of the defect (black arrows).

USA) on day 0 (day of operation) and at 4, 8, 12 weeks after surgery; the rabbits were sedated with IV Hypnorm 0.16 ml 30 minutes before taking the radiographs.

The rabbits were rolled and placed on their sides with the heads stretched backwards. The occlusal radiographs were placed against the surgical side of mandibular ramus. The X-ray tube was positioned 30 cm from and perpendicular to the radiographs. The tube was directed from the submandibular region of the opposite side. The X-ray machine was adjusted to 70 kV for 0.32 seconds and 10 mA. The quantity of bone formation was assessed using a validated scoring system [18], as shown in Table 2.1. Similar radiographes were taken for the contra-lateral control side.

Table 3. Shows the estimated quantitative scoring of different anatomical sections of the defect taken from the radiographs, ∑QS represents the percentage of the regenerated tissue for all the radiographs that were analyzed for each rabbit (Rb).

Rabbit no.	Radiographic examined sections grading and the total quantitative scoring using average percentage			
	Proximal	Middle	Anterior	Total ∑QS
Rb1 (151)	5	3	5	66.6±8.4
Rb2 (152)	5	4	3	58.3±12.7
Rb3 (214)	3	1	0	25±20
Rb (215)	2	1	1	25±19
Rb5 (218)	4	3	4	66.6±8.9
Rb (217)	4	2	2	41.6±13.8
Rb (216)	5	4	5	66.6±7.9
Rb (239)	4	2	5	50±20
Rb (240)	0	0	4	25±20.9
Rb (241)	1	3	4	41.6±17.6

The mean ∑QS reading was 46.6% (25–66.6).

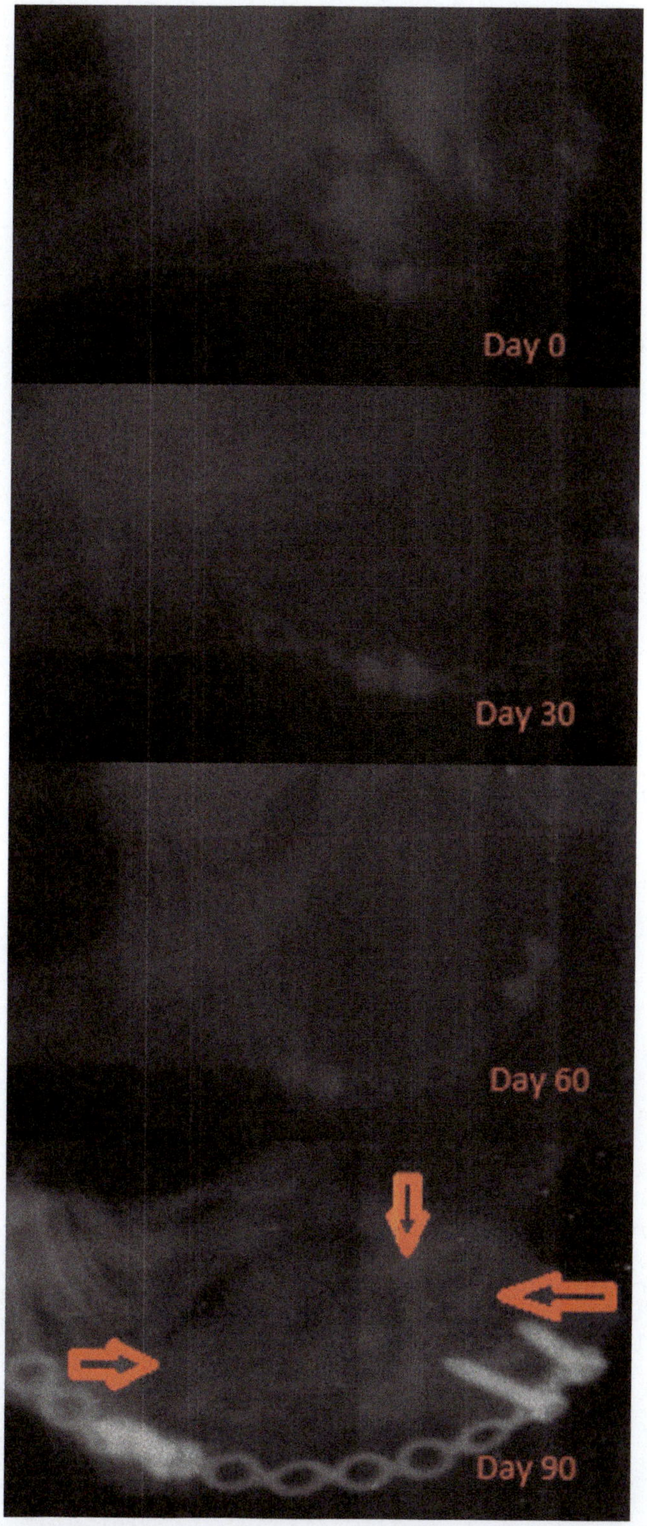

Figure 6. Radiographic images taken at different time points. A) immediately after surgery which shows the injected cement as radio-opaque patches, B) One month after surgery showing the disappearance of radio-opaque patches of cement, C) Two months following surgery, the radiograph shows homogeneous radio-opaque shadow, D) Three months postoperative radiograph showing radio-opaque mass occupying the area of the created defect.

Table 4. Data from CBCT analysis, showing the estimated volume of radio-opaque tissues present at the defect & the mineralized density at the centre and the borders of the defect for all the rabbits (Rb).

Rabbit no.	CBCT examination				
	Average volume of the radio-dense tissue/mm^3	Percentage of radio-dense mass in relation to ROD/%	HU of the Regenerated tissue	HU at the control side	% of border tissue density in relation to the host bone/%
Rb1 (151)	871±13	160±11	748±285	761±250	+130
Rb2 (152)	2365±9	70±15	528±127	706±345	+25
Rb3 (214)	181±13	41±13	576±165	1003±242	+23
Rb (215)	315±19	67±5	666±160	931±233	+70
Rb5 (218)	196±20	39±8	918±234	824±268.8	+42
Rb (217)	456±27	120±14	1056±223	968±285	+75
Rb (216)	486±23	98±10	1470±234	836±300	−4
Rb (239)	656±17	122±6.7	1412±267	990±325	+9
Rb (240)	686±10	139±6	1390±241	1153±281.6	+45
Rb (241)	400±22	68±5	1294±253	1066±321	+38

To assess the pattern, radio-density, and quantity of the regenerated mineralised tissue (bone) in the created surgical defect, the radiographs were subdivided into thirds: anterior, middle, and posterior (Figure 2). The extent of bone formation was expressed in terms of the clinical qualitative score (CQS) and quantitative radiographic score (∑QS) which were developed by our research group [26]. This clinical qualitative score (CQS) represented the lowest score of each third of the examined region according to the described criteria in Table 1.

The quantitative scoring (∑QS) was calculated for the overall bone formation in each surgical defect. ∑QS is the average percentage of the three grades of bone formation in each surgical defect. This was calculated according to the following equation: ∑QS = {% GRADE anterior + %GRADE middle + %GRADE posterior}/3 (table 2).

Cone beam computerised tomography (CBCT)

CBCT machine (i-CAT, Imaging Sciences International, Hatfield, UK) was adjusted at the following settings: 6 cm field of vision (FOV) scan, 120 kV at 20 sec, 0.3 mm pixel/voxel size, for radiographic image capture [27]. The explanted jaws were kept on a stable plastic mounting table, the fixation plate and the screws were left in place during image capture. Data was stored on optical discs to assess the cross-sectional of bone tissue and the volume of the regenerated bone.

The histological assessment of the decalcified and undecalcified sections of the regenerated tissue confirmed bone formation within the muscle tissue (Figure 3), the details of the histology assessment are beyond the scope of this article.

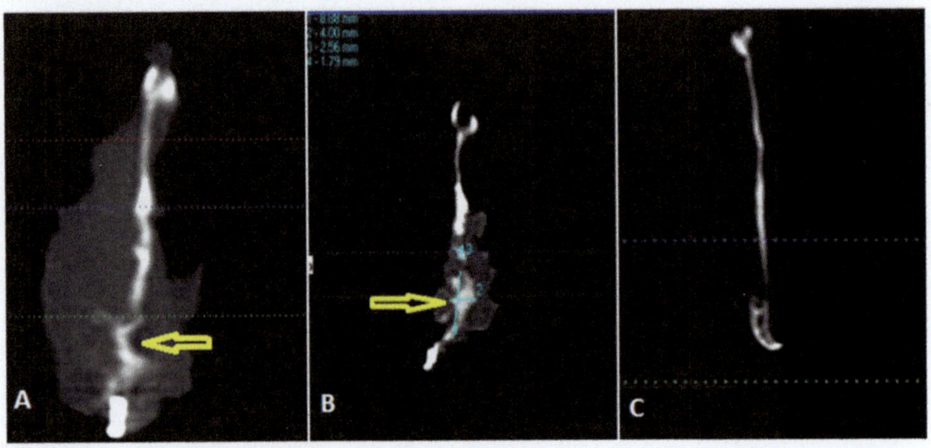

Figure 7. Coronal radiographic scan through the ramus of the mandible; the thickness of the slice is 1.6 mm. A, shows the bone regeneration area (yellow arrow). B, shows linear measurement of the newly formed bone. C shows coronal section of the bone of the contra-lateral side.

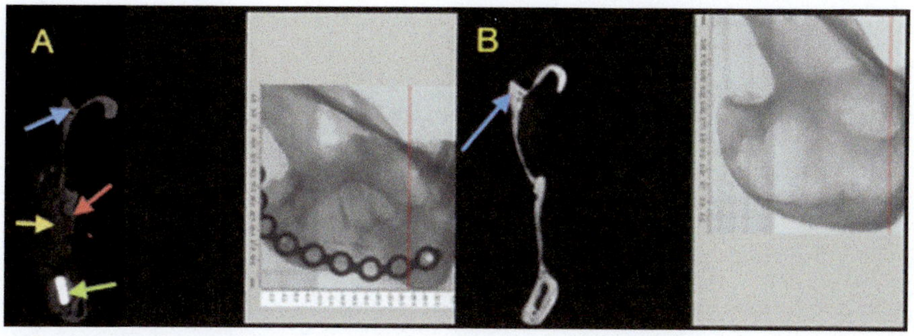

Figure 8. Micro-CT screen of the coronal section at the anterior third of the defect showing an area of tissue regeneration. A, shows an area of bone bridging the surgical defect, red arrows is pointed medially toward the native bone, the yellow arrow refers to the radio-opacity of the newly generated tissue that is indistinguishable from the native bone, the green arrow is marking the titanium plate. B shows the corresponding anatomical region of the contra lateral non-operated side.

Assessment of bone volume and density

The volume of the regenerated bone was calculated from the coronal CBCT scans taken in contiguous 1.6 mm radiographic sections; a total of 10 coronal sections were retrieved and examined. The volume in cubic centimetres was calculated by multiplying the measured surface area of the radio-opaque mass of each section by 1.6 "the thickness of each section" and by the number of examined sections. The mean value and the standard deviation "SD" of all the specimens were calculated for statistical analysis. Means and SD of the bone mineral density were also estimated from the radiographic grayscale value of the Hounsfield unites "HU" [28]

Micro-CT analysis

This was carried out using a micro-CT system (Skyscan 1172 HR; Skyscan, Aartselaar, Belgium). One non-operated hemi-mandible was scanned as a control. The following micro-CT settings were applied: X-ray energy levels at 100 kV, electric current at 167 μA, and integration time of 120 ms with 17 μm voxel size, and 360° rotation. The captured and reconstructed images were segmented using a threshold algorithm [29]. Thresholding was applied to separate the regenerated bone or the remaining cement from the surrounding soft tissue, this process was based on subjective matching of images followed by objective global thresholding which was optimized for the used cement "biphasic calcium phosphate cement" [30] (Figure 4). To determine the field of view (FOV) from the sagittal micro-CT images the following reference points were placed; anterior point marked 5 mm posterior to the last molar, and a posterior point at the angle of the mandible tangent with the ramus notch (Figure 5). Three-dimensional analysis was performed, bone volume (BV) was measured, bone volume fraction was calculated as the ratio of BV to the total volume (TV), and the remaining cement volume (CV) was calculated using Image J software (version 10.3) [6]. This was achieved by calibrating the scale bar of the software, changing the image into gray scale at 8 bit, followed by selection of the field of view. The image was processed in a binary format; the areas of

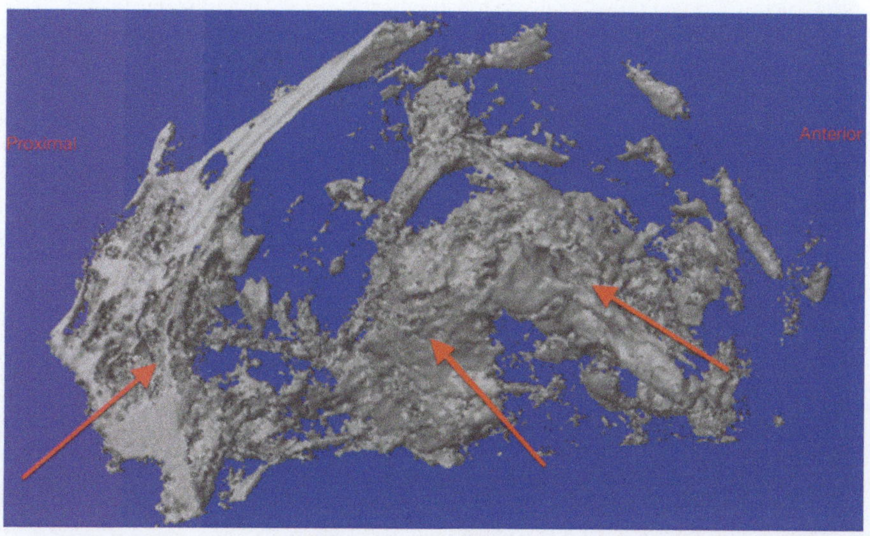

Figure 9. Sagittal section of the 3D model of one of the cases showing the surgical defect filled with a radio-dense mass which appears irregular in shape (red arrows).

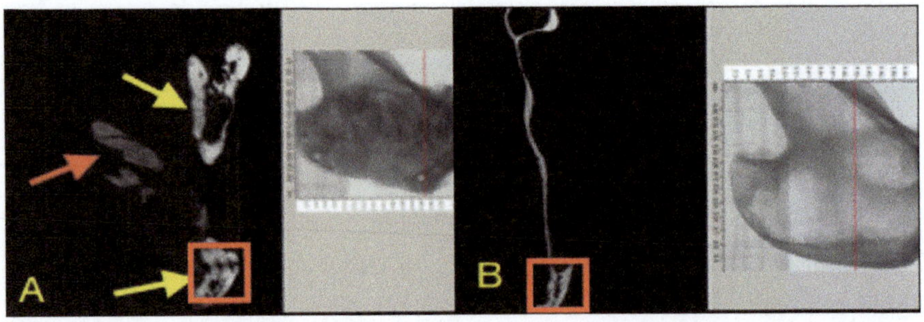

Figure 10. Micro-CT screen image of a coronal slice through the area of the defect showing bone bridging the gap (red box). A: Red arrow represents area of bone regeneration located lateral to the defect, the red box represents areas of bone overgrowth (yellow arrows) at the interface between the newly generated bone and the native bone. B: The contra-lateral non-operated side of the mandible, the red box represents the corresponding region as seen in figure A (Field of view = 10.0×7.0×4.0).

interest were measured by counting the number of pixels/µm of the selected region. The interface between the newly generated radio-opaque calcified tissue and the surrounding bone was examined. Trabecular thickness (TbTh) (or pore wall) and trabecular separation (TbSp) (or pore diameter), trabecular number (TbN), degree of anisotropy and bone mineral densities were calculated by direct measurements.

Results

The rabbits completed the course of the study without significant adverse effects. Clinically, a thin layer of hard tissue regenerate appeared between the muscle tissues that emerged from the most inferior side of the graft. Fibrous tissue was found around the titanium plate. Bone overgrowth was observed at the area around the proximal (posterior) screw in most of the cases. An area of white rubbery mass was observed between muscle fibers which was the un-degraded remaining of the injected cement (Figure 5).

Plain radiographic assessment "oblique extra-oral film"

At day 0 (immediately following surgery) the injected cement appeared as bright radio-opaque patches covering the surgical defect. Radiographs taken at 1 month post-surgery showed complete disappearance of the bright radio-opaque patches (Grade 1). This was due to the rapid absorption of the iohexol, the pacifier of the liquid phase of the cement. This image was considered the baseline for radiographic analysis. The radiographs taken 2 months following surgery showed sporadic radio-opaque areas in close approximation with the defect's borders attempting to bridge the gap of the surgical defect (Grade 2). Areas of mixed radio-opacity and radiolucency were present at the centre of the defect. At 3 months post-surgery, the centre of the defect was occupied with a heterogeneous radio-opaque masses (Grade 3) extending from the centre of the defect. A more homogenous radio-dense mass appeared at the proximal end of the surgical defect (Figure 6). In one case complete bridging of the surgical defect with the radio-dense structure was noted (Grade 4). Table 3

Table 5. Summary of the micro-CT quantitative analysis (mean percentages±SD) and trabecular characteristics of the newly regenerated tissue in comparison with the bone of control sides at three months following surgery (n = 3).

Structural index		*Rb 151*	*Rb152*	*Rb 216*	*Rb 239*	*Control*
BV mm^3 (inside ROD)		0.60±0.20	0.48±0.14	0.44±0.05	0.37±0.03	0.99±1.40
BV mm^3 (outside ROD)		84.9±13.4	26.9±7.0	320.7±23.0	249.1±29.9	
CV		8.6±0.6	7.6±2 3	0.07±0.06	0	-
% BV/TV in ROD		1.45±5.9	1.17±4.8	0.16±.02	0.16±0.08	1.00±0.58
% BV/TV at area of interface		1.2±0.4	1.78±1.39	1.8±0.20	1.29±7.0	1.00±0.07
Bone Surface area (BS)/Total surface area (BS/TS)*		0.51	0.52	0.99	0.59	1.00
	Tb Th (mm)	0.21±0.04	0.42±0.06	0.48±0.20	0.34±0.10	0.56±0.14
	Tb N (mm^{-1})	1.21±0.9	0.75±0.20	0.57±0.02	0.87±0.22	0.32±0.20
Trabecular analysis	Tb Sp (mm)	0.7±0.1	1.19±0.5	1±0.2	0.9±0.2	1.4±0.1
	DA	1.63±0.90	1.72±0.34	1.78±0.33	1.79±0.4	2.24±0.51
	Bone density g/cm^2	0.59±0.20	0.58±0.05	0.97±0.24	0.56±0.07	0.99±0.09

*Image analysis using ImageJ (ImageJ, 1.46 h, Wayne Rasband, National Institutes of Health, USA).
BV = Bone Volume, CV = Cement Volume, ROD = Region of the defect, BV/TV = Bone Volume fraction, TV = Tissue volume, BS = Bone surface area, BS/TS = Bone surface area fraction, TbTh = Trabecular thickness, Tb N = Trabecular number.
Tb Sp = Trabecular separation, DA = degree of anisotropy.

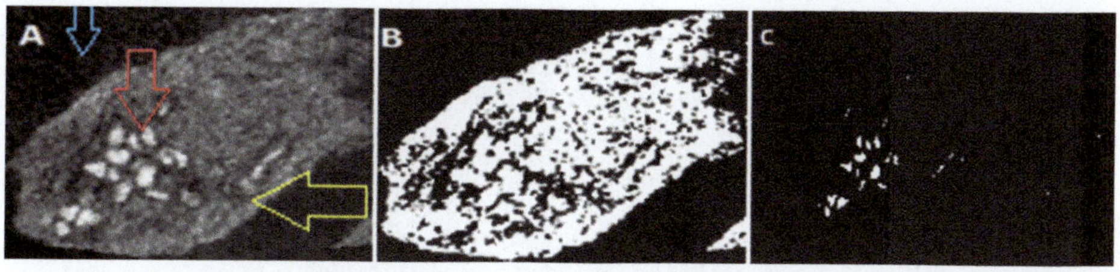

Figure 11. Axial view of micro-CT indicates an area of bone formation which appears gray (yellow arrow), the surrounding soft tissue appears black (blue arrow) and area of the remaining cement in white color (red arrow). B: Binary picture of the threshold of the same image. C: The white particles of the remaining cement analyzed by Sky scan image analysis software.

summarizes the estimated quantitative scoring of the regenerated tissue for all the examined case. The mean percentage of radio-opaque tissue present in the created defect was 46.6%±15%.

CBCT for volumetric bone assessment & evaluation of bone density

CBCT assessment and evaluation of 3D radiographic image revealed the presence of notable calcified tissue of a heterogeneous nature inside the masseter muscle at the site of the created defect (Figure 7). Areas of hypo-calcification were readily detectable within the muscle tissue. More cases showed calcified radio-opaque areas at the proximal third of the defect with no clear demarcation between the regenerated tissue and the surrounding native bone. The assessment confirmed that the volume of the radio-opaque tissue within the muscle flap was more than of the original bone at the region of the defect (ROD). In 4 cases there was an increase in volume of calcified tissue by 35%±15% compared to the volume of the ROD. However, this has to be interpreted carefully due to the fact that large areas of radio-opacities were detected around the periphery rather than in the centre of the defect. In the other six rabbits the mean estimated volume of regenerated bone was 302 mm^3±120 mm^3 which constituted 63.85%±20% of the volume of ROD (Table 4). The radio-opacity of the thickened bone at the margin of the defect was 35%±25% and was denser than the contra-lateral non-operated control side.

Micro-CT analysis

The boundary between the regenerated tissue and the surrounding native bone was indistinguishable (Figure 8). The regenerated bone tissue at the defect site was either medial or lateral to the surrounding native bone. The surface morphology of the regenerated tissue was rough in comparison with the surrounding bone which is suggestive of an active remodeling process. The presence of hydroxyapatite crystal remnants of the injected cement may have contributed to the apparent surface roughness (Figure 9).

The coronal cross-sections confirmed that the regenerated tissue has a trabecular pattern and were thicker medio-laterally than the contra-lateral non-operated side (Figure 10). The average bone volume fraction (BV/TV) of the regenerated bone within the ROD was 36.2%±14%. However, the mean volume of the new bone formed outside the ROD was 237.8 mm^3±50.9 mm^3 which was 5 times the volume of the bone within the ROD, and the percentage of the remaining cement was 15.9% ±10% (Figure 11). At the area of interface between the regenerated and native surrounding bone, the mean bone volume fraction was 28.8 mm^3 which was double the volume of bone on the same representative anatomical region at the non-operated side (Table 5).

With regard to bone architecture for the same regions, the average TbN/mm^3 of the newly regenerated bone was double that of the contra-lateral non-operated side. TbTh, and TbSp were 63.3%±4.6%, and 73%±7.6% respectively in comparison with the contra-lateral (Figure 12). The degree of anisotropy (DA) was close to the contra-lateral side, and bone density was 85% ±50 of that of the contra-lateral non-operating side (Figure 13a, 13b).

The newly formed bone attained more volume than the ROD; the bone also showed a thinner but more condensed trabecular pattern with a lower degree of anisotropy which suggests that the bone had a fast deposition rate and had undergone an active remodeling process.

On the other hand, 2D analysis of the sagittal micro CT images using image analysis software (Image J, version 10.1) revealed that 65.4%±14% of the ROD was occupied by calcified regenerated tissues. The latter was almost consistent with plain radiographic quantitative assessment of bone formation with a mean score of 60.4%±9% (Figure 14).

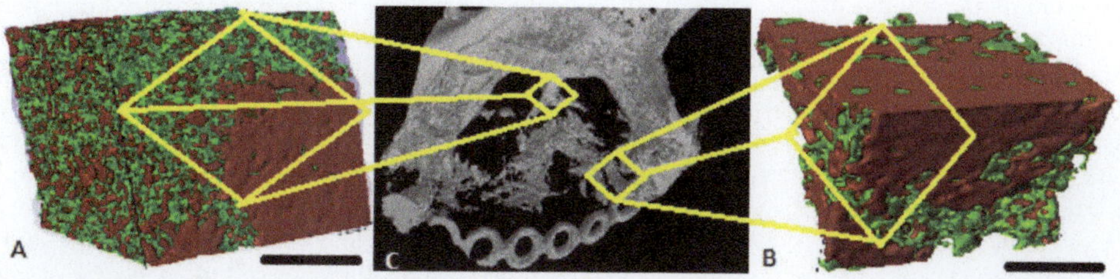

Figure 12. Micro-computed tomographic images. A illustrates bone generation at the superior margin of the surgical defect as shown in C. B is for the regenerated bone at the anterior border of the defect as shown in C. The red areas represent a mixture of a radio-dense tissue of bone and cement, the green areas represent the muscle tissue (marker bars = 1 mm).

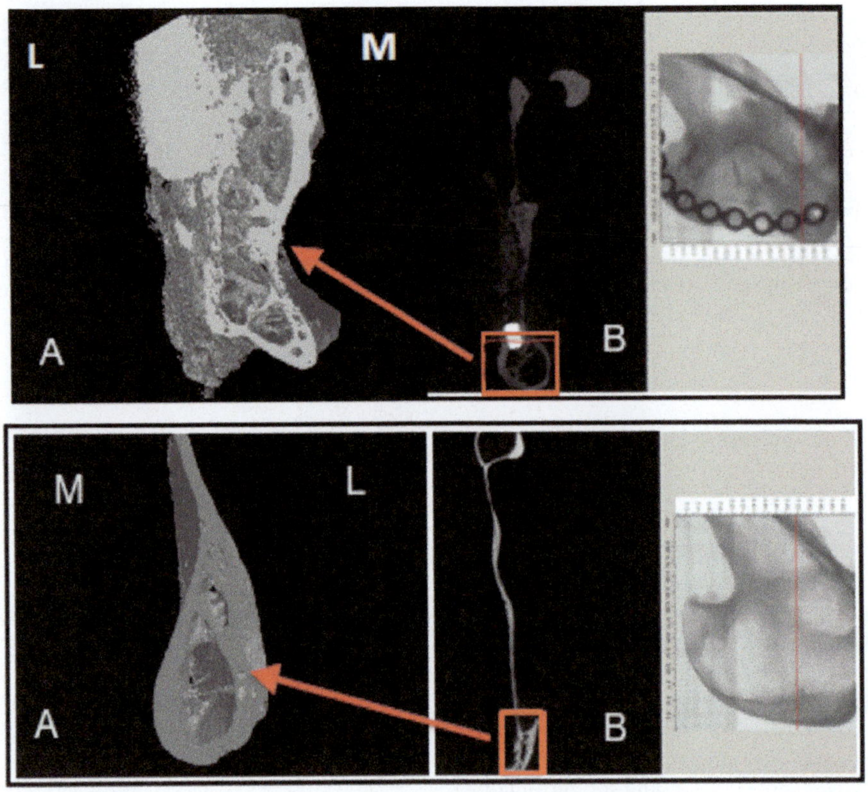

Figure 13. a: 3D model of the micro CT scan of an area of bone regeneration at the anterior region of the surgical defect demonstrating the enlargement of trabecular bone in the medio-lateral direction (M-L), B shows the coronal section through the same area (red box) of the regenerated bone. **b:** The corresponding 3D micro-CT scan of the same region of the contra-lateral non-operated side.

More bone formation was observed at the borders and lateral to ROD. Figure 12 shows a schematic representation of the pattern of bone regeneration at the border, the centre, medial side and at the lateral side of the ROD.

Discussion

This study demonstrates the remarkable potential for the use of muscle flap, injectable cement, BMP-7 and rMSC to induce bone formation. The muscle flap provided the required blood supply for bone bioengineering and acted as a bioreactor for bone formation. On average, more bone formation was detected within the muscle flap in comparison to the contra-lateral side, but the defect was not fully reconstructed with the regenerated bone due to the difficulty of injecting the cement at the centre of the defect.

The most widely available diagnostic tool for bone assessment is plain X-ray; despite its shortcomings it allowed assessment of bone regeneration during the life of the animal in this study. Cook's scoring system [18] combined with the quantitative scoring system ∑QS provided a comprehensive measurement of the quantity of bone formation at the surgical bone defect, which was consistent with the morphometeric analysis of the micro-CT images. In this experimental model the application of a radio-dense material, the ceramic cement, which had a similar radio-opacity to that of bone, added to the complexity of studying the pattern of bone regeneration.

CBCT provided more precise information about the actual bone formation in comparison with 2D radiographs [31,32]. In this study, the radio-opaque mass of the regenerated tissue had a large bucco-lingual dimension as shown in the coronal section. The volume of regenerated bone at the ROD was on average 35%±15% in comparison to the bone of the contra-lateral non-operated side. This finding was due to the fact that the injection of the cement included the entire mass of the muscle flap within the defect. Micro-CT was an essential tool to investigate the nature of the interface between the regenerated calcified tissue and the surrounding native bone and to explore the trabecular pattern of the regenerated bone [33,24]. Micro-CT facilitated the differentiation between the structure of the remaining cement and the regenerated calcified tissue, this was achieved by adjusting the thresholding of the radiographic images manually. The global thresholding for biophasic calcium phosphate cement has been documented [24]. The estimated average new bone was 36.2% inside the region of the defect in all assessed cases. The mean volume of the newly formed bone outside the ROD was $237.8\ mm^3 \pm 50.9\ mm^3$ which was 5 times the bone volume inside the ROD. The magnitude of the remaining cement was variable among the examined samples, the average percentage was 15.9% ±1%0. This was expected as the resorption rate of calcium sulphate component of CERAMENT™ |SPINE SUPPORT is faster than the hydroxyapatite part which takes longer to dissolve; a similar finding was reported when the cement was implanted in the abdominal muscle of rats [34]. The thin trabecular pattern and the increased number of the trabeculae of the newly formed bone suggest that it had a fast deposition rate and active remodelling process [35]. The observed lower degree of anistropy of the newly formed bone compared to the non-operated side is most probably due to the reduced extra cellular mineral deposition of the regenerated tissue [36]. The reduced anisotropy is due to the presence of HA crystals attached to the bony trabeculae.

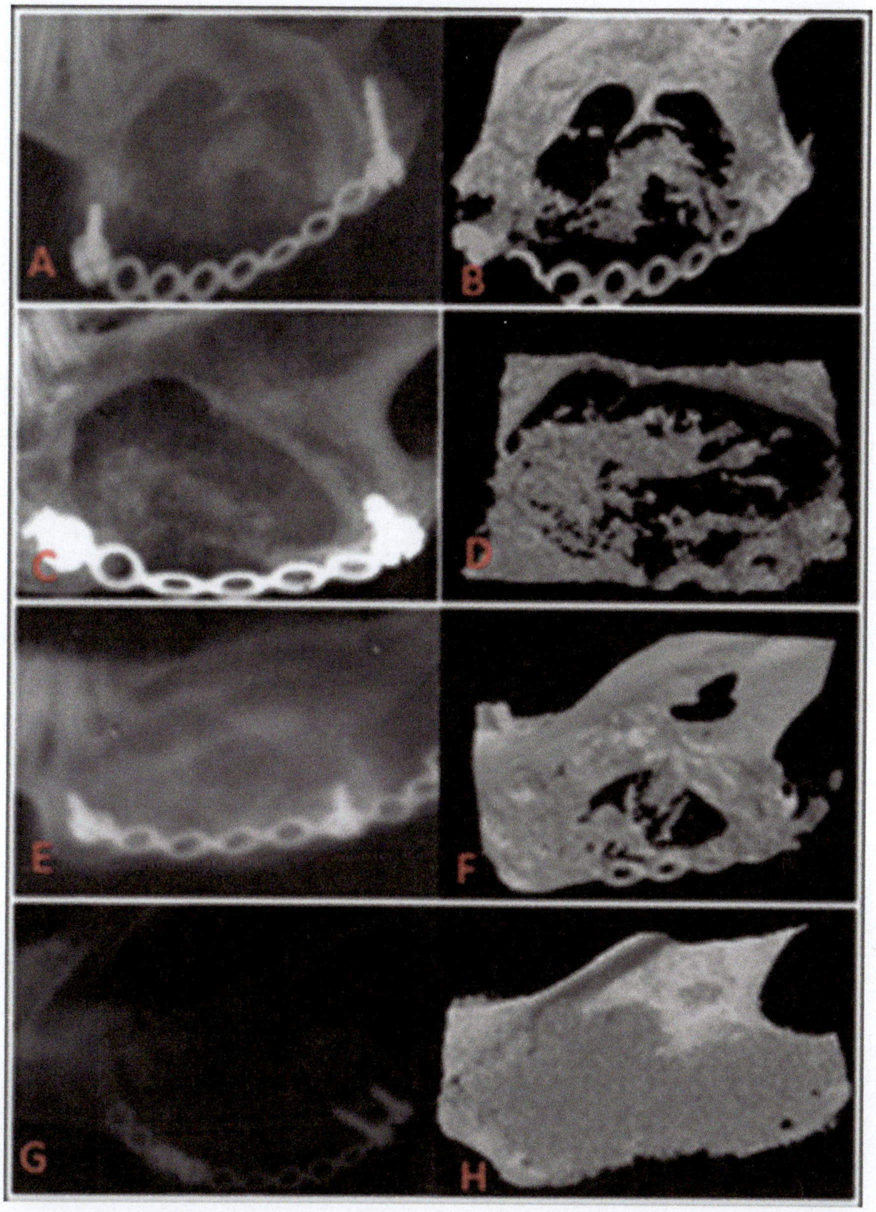

Figure 14. A comparison between the plain radiographs (A, C, E, G) and the corresponding micro-CT images (B, D, F, H). Analysis on the micro-CT scans using image analysis software revealed that 65.4%±14% of the ROD was occupied by calcified tissues which was consistent with plain radiographic quantitative assessment of bone formation.

This study demonstrated the value of the comprehensive radiographic assessment using various imaging modalities and highlighted the importance of various scoring systems to quantify bone formation for better understanding of the pattern of calcified tissue regeneration. It provides the first comprehensive radiology based 3D investigation to assess bone regeneration within muscle flaps in the oro-facial region. The findings confirm the ability of injectable cement loaded with BMP-7 and seeded with MSCs to stimulate bone regeneration and restore the trabecular bone structure within three months of injection inside a local muscle flap in the maxillofacial region. Nevertheless, complete conversion of the muscle into bone and full reconstruction of the defect was not achieved. This was partially due to the physical nature of the injected cement that prevented the diffusion of the material at a micro level between the fibres of the muscle tissue. The muscle flap obliterated the surgical defect making it clinically difficult to insure that the injected cement had uniformly reached the desirable location within the ROD. This may have been achieved with a thinner pedicled muscle that could be fully enclosed within the ROD. On the other hand one could argue that use of full thickness muscle flap is essential to maintain the integrity of the blood supply which is essential for bone regeneration. It has been reported that muscle volume and surface area are detrimental factors that govern the amount of bone regeneration [14].

Conclusions

This study provided the proof of the concept that bone formation could be induced within a pedicled muscle flap in the maxillofacial region using an injectable cement loaded with BMP and seeded with rMSCs which has clear potential clinical applications. Further development and refinements of this approach are required before the clinical use in maxillofacial bone reconstruction.

Author Contributions

Conceived and designed the experiments: RA NH KN ET JM MD AA. Performed the experiments: RA AA KN MD JM. Analyzed the data: RA AA KN NH ET MD. Contributed reagents/materials/analysis tools: MD NH. Wrote the paper: RA NH KN ET JM MD AA. Designed the study: RA AA KN JM MD LT. Carried out the lab work: RA MD. Carried out the surgery: RA KN JM AA. Analyzed the results: ET MD RA AA. Radiographic assessment: NH AA RA KN.

References

1. Cancedda R, Giannoni P, Mastrogiacomo M (2007) A tissue engineering approach to bone repair in large animal models and in clinical practice. Biomaterials 28: 4240–4250.
2. Gimbel M, Ashley RK, Sisodia M, Gabbay JS, Wasson KL, et al. (2007) Repair of alveolar cleft defects; Reduced morbidity with bone marrow stem cells in a resorbable matrix. J Craniofac Surg 18: 895–901.
3. Kim BC, Yoon JH, Choi B, Lee J (2013) Mandibular reconstruction with autologous human bone marrow stem cells and autogenous bone graft in a patient with plexiform ameloblastoma. J Craniofac Surg 24: e409–e411.
4. Su J, Xu H, Sun J, Gong X, Zhao H (2013) Dual delivery of BMP-2 and bFGF from a new nano-composite scaffold loaded with vascular stents for large-size mandibular defect regeneration. Int J Molecular Sci 14: 12714–12728.
5. Alfotawi R, Naudi KB, Lappin D, Barbenel J, Di Silvio L, et al. (In press) The use of Tri-Calcium Phosphate (TCP) and stem cells for the regeneration of osteoperiosteal critical-size mandibular bony defects, an in vitro and preclinical study. J Cranio-maxillofac Surg.
6. Das A, Segar CE, Hughley BB, Bowers DT, Botchwey EA (2013) The promotion of mandibular defect healing by the targeting of S1P receptors and the recruitment of alternatively activated macrophages. Biomaterials 34: 9853–9862.
7. Berglund JD, Galis ZS (2003) Designer blood vessels and therapeutic revascularization. Brit J Pharmacol 140: 627–636.
8. Da Silva Meirelles L, Sand TT, Harman RJ, Lennon DP, Caplan AI (2009) MSC frequency correlates with blood vessel density in equine adipose tissue. Tissue Engineering 15: 221–229.
9. Griffith LG (2002) Emerging design principles in biomaterials and scaffolds for tissue engineering. NY Academy Science 961: 83–95.
10. Meijer GJ, de Bruijn JD, Koole R, van Blitterswijk CA (2008) Cell based bone tissue engineering in jaw defects. Biomaterials 29: 3053–3061.
11. Ayoub A, Challa S, Abu-Serriah M, McMahon J, Moos K, et al. (2007) Use of a composite pedicled muscle flap and rhBMP-7 for mandibular reconstruction. Int J Oral Maxillofac Surg 36: 1183–119.
12. Warnke PH, Wiltfang J, Springer I, Acil Y, Bolte H, et al. (2006). Man as living bioreactor: Fate of an exogenously prepared customized tissue-engineered mandible. Biomaterials 27: 3163–3167.
13. Heliotis M, Lavery KM, Ripamonti U, Tsiridis E, di Silvio L (2006) Transformation of a prefabricated hydroxyapatite/osteogenic protein-1 implant into a vascularised pedicled bone flap in the human chest. Int J Oral Maxillofac Surg 35: 265–269.
14. Liu F, Porter RM, Wells J, Glatt V, Pilapil C, et al. (2012) Evaluation of BMP-2 gene-activated muscle grafts for cranial defect repair. J Orthopaed Res 30: 1095–1102.
15. Lu M, Zhou YX, Du H, Zhang J, Liu J (2013) Reliability and validity of measuring acetabular component orientation by plain anteroposterior radiographs. Clinical Orthopaedics and Related Research 471: 2987–2994.
16. Mulconrey DS, Bridwell KH, Flynn J, Cronen GA, Rose PS (2008) Bone morphogenetic protein (RhBMP-2) as a substitute for iliac crest bone graft in multilevel adult spinal deformity surgery. Spine 33: 2153–2159.
17. Eck KR, Lenke LG, Bridwell KH, Gilula LA, Lashgari CJ, et al. (2000) Radiographic assessment of anterior titanium mesh cages. J Spinal Disorder 13: 501–509.
18. Cook SD, Salkeld SL, Patron LP (2005) Bone defect healing with an osteogenic protein-1 device combined with carboxymethylcellulose. J Biomed Mat Res 75B: 137–145.
19. Jeffcoat MK, Lewis CE, Reddy MS, Wang CY, Redford M (2000) Post-menopausal bone loss and its relationship to oral bone loss. Periodont 23: 94–102.
20. Burkus JK, Dorchak JD, Sanders DL (2003) Radiographic assessment of interbody fusion using recombinant human bone morphogenetic protein type 2. Spine 28: 372–377.
21. Ito K, Gomi Y, Sato S, Arai Y, Shinoda K (2001) Clinical application of a new compact CT system to assess 3-D images for the preoperative treatment planning of implants in the posterior mandible - A case report. Clin Oral Implantol Res 12: 539–542.
22. Kinney JH, Lane NE, Haupt DL (1995) In-Vivo, 3-Dimensional microscopy of trabecular bone. J Bone Min Res 10: 264–270.
23. Kothari M, Keaveny TM, Lin JC, Newitt DC, Genant HK, et al. (1998) Impact of spatial resolution on the prediction of trabecular architecture parameters. Bone 22: 437–443.
24. Muller R, Ruegsegger P (1997) Micro-tomographic imaging for the nondestructive evaluation of trabecular bone architecture. Stud Health Technol Inform 40: 61–79.
25. Alfotawi R, Naudi K, Dalby MJ, Tanner KE, McMahon JD, et al. (2013) Assessment of cellular viability on calcium sulphate/hydroxyapatite injectable scaffolds. J Tissue Eng 4, 2041731413509645.
26. Abu Serriah M, Ayoub A, Wray D, Milne N, Carmicheal S, et al. (2006) Contour and volume assessment of repairing mandibular osteopriosteal continuity defects in sheep using recombinant human osteogenic protein 1. J Cranio Maxillofac Surg 34: 62–167.
27. Weldon E, Brockelbank I, Narin N, Naudi K, Ayoub A (2008) Cone beam CT for in vitro research: A practical approch for using the i-CAT radiography-Glasgow Dental School& Hospital, The University of Glasgow, the UK.
28. Lagravere M, Fang Y, Carey J, Toogood R, Packota GV, et al. (2006) Density conversion factor determined using a cone-beam computed tomography unit NewTom QR-DVT 9000. Dentomaxillofac Radiolo 35: 407–409.
29. Lu M, Rabie AB (2003) Microarchitecture of rabbit mandibular defects grafted with intramembranous or endochondral bone shown by micro-computed tomography. Brit J Oral Maxillofac Surg 41: 385–391.
30. Gauthier O, Khairoun I, Bosco J, Obadia L, Bourges X, et al. (2003) Noninvasive bone replacement with a new injectable calcium phosphate biomaterial. J Biomed Mat Res 66: 47–54.
31. Oberoi S, Chigurupati R, Gill P, Hoffman WY, Vargervik K (2009) Volumetric assessment of secondary alveolar bone grafting using cone beam computed tomography. Cleft Palate Craniofac J 46: 503–511.
32. HamadaY, Kondoh T, Noguchi K, Iino M, Isono H, et al. (2005) Application of limited cone beam computed tomography to clinical assessment of alveolar bone grafting: A preliminary report. Cleft Palate Craniofac J 42: 128–137.
33. Muller R, Van Campenhout H, Van Damme B, Van Der Perre G, Dequeker J, et al. (1998) Morphometric analysis of human bone biopsies: A quantitative structural comparison of histological sections and micro-computed tomography. Bone 23: 59–66.
34. Nilsson M (2003) Injectable Calcium Sulphate and Calcium Phosphate Bone Substitutes. PhD Lund University, Faculty of Medicine, Lund, Sweden.
35. Frost HM (1999) On the trabecular "thickness" - Number problem. J Bone Min Res 14: 1816–1821.
36. Turner CH, Chandran A, Pidaparti RMV (1995) The anisotropy of osteonal bone and its ultrastructural implications. Bone 17: 85–89.

22

EPO Promotes Bone Repair through Enhanced Cartilaginous Callus Formation and Angiogenesis

Lin Wan[1], Fengjie Zhang[1,2], Qiling He[3], Wing Pui Tsang[1,2], Li Lu[1,4], Qingnan Li[4], Zhihong Wu[5], Guixing Qiu[5], Guangqian Zhou[6], Chao Wan[1,2]*

1 Ministry of Education Key Laboratory for Regenerative Medicine, School of Biomedical Sciences, Faculty of Medicine, The Chinese University of Hong Kong, Hong Kong SAR, China, **2** School of Biomedical Sciences Core Laboratory, Shenzhen Research Institute, The Chinese University of Hong Kong, Shenzhen, China, **3** Departments of Microbiology and Pathology, University of Alabama at Birmingham, Birmingham, Alabama, United States of America, **4** Guangdong Key Laboratory of Pharmaceutical Bioactive Substances, New Drug Function Research Center, School of Life Science and Biopharmacy, Guangdong Pharmaceutical University, Guangzhou, China, **5** Department of Orthopaedics, Peking Union Medical College Hospital, Peking Union Medical College and Chinese Academy of Medical Sciences, Beijing, China, **6** The Center for Anti-Ageing and Regenerative Medicine, Medical School, Shenzhen University, Shenzhen, China

Abstract

Erythropoietin (EPO)/erythropoietin receptor (EPOR) signaling is involved in the development and regeneration of several non-hematopoietic tissues including the skeleton. EPO is identified as a downstream target of the hypoxia inducible factor-α (HIF-α) pathway. It is shown that EPO exerts a positive role in bone repair, however, the underlying cellular and molecular mechanisms remain unclear. In the present study we show that EPO and EPOR are expressed in the proliferating, pre-hypertrophic and hypertrophic zone of the developing mouse growth plates as well as in the cartilaginous callus of the healing bone. The proliferation rate of chondrocytes is increased under EPO treatment, while this effect is decreased following siRNA mediated knockdown of EPOR in chondrocytes. EPO treatment increases biosynthesis of proteoglycan, accompanied by up-regulation of chondrogenic marker genes including SOX9, SOX5, SOX6, collagen type 2, and aggrecan. The effects are inhibited by knockdown of EPOR. Blockage of the endogenous EPO in chondrocytes also impaired the chondrogenic differentiation. In addition, EPO promotes metatarsal endothelial sprouting *in vitro*. This coincides with the *in vivo* data that local delivery of EPO increases vascularity at the mid-stage of bone healing (day 14). In a mouse femoral fracture model, EPO promotes cartilaginous callus formation at days 7 and 14, and enhances bone healing at day 28 indexed by improved X-ray score and micro-CT analysis of microstructure of new bone regenerates, which results in improved biomechanical properties. Our results indicate that EPO enhances chondrogenic and angiogenic responses during bone repair. EPO's function on chondrocyte proliferation and differentiation is at least partially mediated by its receptor EPOR. EPO may serve as a therapeutic agent to facilitate skeletal regeneration.

Editor: Domenico Ribatti, University of Bari Medical School, Italy

Funding: This work was supported by Hong Kong Research Grant Council General Research Fund (RGC GRF 475910), National Natural Science Foundation of China (NSFC 81130034), and NSFC-RGC Joint Research Scheme (CUHK445/10) to CW. The funders had no role in study design, data collection and analysis, decision to publish, or preparation of the manuscript.

Competing Interests: The authors have declared that no competing interests exist.

* Email: cwan@cuhk.edu.hk

Introduction

Impaired bone regeneration following injury or under pathological conditions causes severe pain to the patients and considerable financial burden to the society [1,2]. These conditions include delayed fracture union or non-union, osteoporotic fracture healing, impaired bone repair associated with diabetes, and large bone defects caused by trauma or surgical treatments [3,4,5,6]. Hallmarks of impaired bone repair in patients and animal models include the deficiency in vascular supply and cartilaginous callus formation at the site of injury, suggesting that impaired angiogenic and chondrogenic responses are major contributors to the pathology [7,8].

Bone regeneration is a complex process in which the recovery of skeletal tissue integrity relies upon close temporal and spatial coordination of molecular and cellular events involving resident bone cells, inflammatory cells, marrow stromal elements, and associated vascular structures [9,10,11,12] to achieve structural reconstitution and bone remodeling. The regeneration process has generally been characterized by four steps including inflammation phase with hematoma, cartilage callus formation, bony callus formation and bone remodeling [13,14]. During bone regeneration, angiogenesis is essential and depends on hypoxic stimuli and production of proangiogenic factors such as vascular endothelial growth factor (VEGF) [7], Erythropoietin (EPO) [15], fibroblast growth factor (FGF) [16], transforming growth factor-beta (TGF-beta) [17] and insulin like growth factor (IGF-1) [18].

The bone cells are readily located in a hypoxic microenvironment during development and regeneration. Hypoxia inducible factor-α (HIF-α) is identified as key mediator for cell adaptation to low oxygen tension. VEGF and EPO are established downstream targets of HIF-α. It is well established that VEGF is expressed in osteoblasts [19,20] and the HIF-α/VEGF pathway couples angiogenesis and osteogenesis during bone development and regeneration [7,21,22] while the study on the involvement of EPO in bone regeneration is just emerging.

EPO is a 34 kD circulating glycoprotein hormone which is initially recognized as the crucial growth factor that controls red blood cell development in bone marrow through binding to its high affinity receptor (EPOR) expressed on erythroid progenitor cells [23,24,25]. EPO is predominantly produced by the interstitial fibroblasts of the renal cortex and outer medulla in adult animals, and by Kuffer's cells in the liver during embryonic development [26,27,28,29], under the control of oxygen sensing HIF pathway [30]. In addition to its principal function in erythropoiesis, nonehematopoietic functions of EPO such as angiogenic [25], cardioprotective [31], neuroprotctive and neurotrophic [32,33] effects have raised great interest and been extensively studied, due to the findings that EPO is also produced in non-renal tissues such as brain [34], and that EPOR is present in a variety of non-hematopoietic cell types such as brain capillary endothelial cells [35], vascular smooth muscle cells [36], myocardial cells [37], neurons [38] and astrocytes [39]. The potential physiological effects of EPO on skeletal tissue were suggested by both clinical and animal studies that bone modulation was associated with erythropoiesis stimulation by systemic administration of EPO [40,41,42]. However, the underlying mechanism is largely unknown. It was reported that EPO activated JAK/STAT signaling in hematopoietic stem cells (HSCs) to produce bone morphogenetic proteins (BMPs) and thus exerted indirect function in bone formation [43]. Although there is one study showing that EPO indirectly increased bone turnover rate and induced trabecular bone loss [42], several other studies demonstrated that EPO improved bone healing [44,45,46], possibly through the proposed direct interaction between EPO with EPOR-expressed hypertrophic chondrocytes to promote endochondral ossification [45] or with EPOR-expressed bone marrow stromal cells to induce osteoblastic differentiation [43]. In addition, significant vascular expansion was also noted during bone healing when EPO was applied [44,46]. It is known that EPO and EPOR are expressed in the vasculature during embryogenesis, and exert a critical role for angiogenesis [25]. Therefore the improved bone healing may also be attributed to a better angiogenesis caused by EPO.

In the present study, we systemically examined the roles of EPO in regulating chondrogenesis and angiogenesis *in vitro* and *in vivo*. The promotive effects of EPO during the chondrogenic and angiogenic phases of femur fracture repair highlight its therapeutic potential in skeletal regenerative medicine.

Materials and Methods

Animals

C57BL/6 mice at age of three-days, fourteen-days and twelve-weeks were used in this study. Mice were housed in the controlled conditions with room temperature of 22±1°C and a light-dark cycle of 12:12 hour, and were fed with standard mouse chow and water ad libitum. Experimental procedures were carried out in accordance with the protocols approved by Animal Experimentation Ethics Committee from the Chinese University of Hong Kong and Animal (Control of Experiments) Ordinance from Department of Health, Hong Kong SAR.

Culture of primary chondrocytes from neonatal mice

The primary chondrocytes were isolated from growth plates following previous procedures [47]. Cells were cultured in minimum essential medium alpha (αMEM) supplemented with 10% fetal bovine serum (FBS), 2 mM L-glutamine and 100 U/ml penicillin and 100 μg/ml streptomycin (all from Gibco). The 1st and 2nd passage cells were processed in the below experiments.

Knockdown of EPOR in chondrocytes

Knockdown of EPOR in chondrocytes was performed by siRNA (Santa Cruz) method using lipofectamine2000 (Invitrogen) following standard protocol. 24 hours after transfection, cells were collected for real-time PCR and Western blot analysis to examine the efficiency of gene knockdown.

Bromodeoxyuridine (BrdU) incorporation assay

Chondrocytes were treated with 40 ng/ml or 80 ng/ml EPO (Sigma-Aldrich) for 2 days and compared with that without EPO treatment. The proliferation rate of chondrocytes was analyzed using the cell proliferation ELISA BrdU assay (Roche).

Cell mass culture

Cells were plated at density of 1×10^5 cells/10 μl and cultured for 3 hours to form the cell masses. Cell masses were then treated with no EPO, 40 ng/ml EPO or EPO block peptide (500 ng/ml, Santa Cruz) in chondrogenic medium supplemented with dexamethasone (100 nM, Sigma-Aldrich), ascorbic acid (50 μg/ml, Sigma-Aldrich), sodium pyruvate (100 μg/ml, Gibco), ITS+ Premix (50 mg/ml, BD) for 7 days following previous procedures [48].

Alcian blue staining

The Alcian blue staining was performed to examine proteoglycan synthesis during chondrocytes differentiation as previously described [49]. Briefly, the cell masses were rinsed with PBS after 7 days of culture, and stained with 1% acidic Alcian blue for 2 hours, followed by 5 times washing using 70% ethanol to remove the residual dyes. The proteoglycan was stained blue.

Quantitation of sulfated glycosaminoglycan (sGAG)

sGAG was quantitated using a dimethylmethylene blue colourimetric assay following established protocol (Blyscan sulfated glycosaminoglycan assay) [50,51]. DMB dye (1, 9-Dimethyl-Methylene Blue zinc chloride double salt) was added to measure the sGAG content in the digested substances.

RT PCR and real-time PCR

Total mRNA was extracted from primary chondrocytes using the TRIzol reagent (Life Technologies) following the manufacturer's instructions. First strand cDNA was synthesized from 1 μg of total RNA in the presence of oligo-dT_{12-18} primer (Invitrogen) and MMLV reverse transcriptase according to manufacturer's instructions (Promega). Quantitative real-time PCR was performed with SYBR Premix Ex Taq (Takara) in ABI Fast Real-time PCR 7900HT System (Applied Biosystems). All samples were performed in triplicates. Primer sequences used for RT-PCR include: EPO-F, 5′-GCTGCTTTTACTCTCCTTGC-3′, EPO-R, 5′-C-TGTTCTTCCACCTCCATTC-3′; EPOR-F, 5′-CTCACCT-TCCAGCTTT-GAGT-3′, EPOR-R, 5′-TTCTCATAGGGGT-GGGAGTA-3′; β-actin-F, 5′-GTCCCT-CACCCTCCCAAA-AG-3′, β-actin-R, 5′-GCTGCCTCAACACCTCAACCC-3′. Primer sequences used for real-time PCR are: SOX9-F, 5′-AGGA-AGCTGGCAGACCAGTA-3′, SOX9-R, 5′-TCCAC-GAAGGGTCTCTTCTC; SOX5-F, 5′-CCAGGAGCTTG-TCTTTCCAG-3′, SOX5-R, 5′-CCCTGAAGCAGAGGAA-GATG-3′; SOX6-F, 5′-CTTCCTCTCCATC-CGCTGTA-3′, SOX6-R, 5′-ACCAGTGACTTCTGGGTGCT-3′; aggrecan-F,

5′-CTG-AAGTTCTTGGAGGAGCG-3′, aggrecan-R, 5′-CGC-TCAGTGAGTTG-TCATGG-3′; Col2α1-F, 5′-CTACGGTGT-CAGGGCCAG-3′, Col2α1-R, 5′-GCAAGA-TGAGGGCTTC-CATA-3′; EPOR-F, 5′-AAACTCAGGGTGCCCCTCTGGC-CT-3′, EPOR-R, 5′-GATGCGGTGATAGCGAGGAGAACC-3′; β-actin-F, 5′-CCCAGAGC-AAGAGAGG-3′, β-actin-R, 5′-GTCCAGACGCAGGATG-3′.

Western blot analysis

Cells were lysed and homogenized in RIPA lyses buffer with protease inhibitors (Gibco). Aliquots of protein extracts were separated by SDS-PAGE, and blotted on PVDF membrane (Millipore). The membrane was blocked by TBS-0.1% Tween 20 (TBST) containing 5% skim milk at room temperature for 1 hour, probed with anti-EPOR (Santa Cruz) primary antibody at 4°C overnight, washed in TBST, and then incubated with the appropriate horseradish peroxidase (HRP)-conjugated secondary antibody at room temperature for 1 hour. After intensive washing with TBST, immunoblots were developed using the ECL detection system.

In vitro fetal mouse metatarsal angiogenesis assay

The assay was performed according to established procedure [52,53]. Briefly, metatarsal bones were dissected from E17.5 embryos, cultured in 24-well plates in 150 μl αMEM containing 10% fetal calf serum, L-glutamine (2 mM) and penicillin (100 U/ml)/streptomycin (100 μg/ml) for 72 hours, and then changed to 250 μl of fresh medium. Medium was then replaced every two days. After 14 days, the explants were fixed in zinc formalin for 15 minutes and subsequently immunostained for endothelial marker CD31 using a rat polyclonal antiserum (BD Pharmingen).

Femur fracture model in mice

12-week-old mice were anesthetized by intraperitoneal injection of 0.1 ml xylene (2.6 mg/ml) and ketamine (17.4 mg/ml) cocktail. A 2 cm incision was performed between the greater trochanter and the knee joint. The quadriceps femoris muscles were mobilized anteriorly towards the knee and the hip. A hole was drilled on the intracondylar notch using a 21 gauge needle which was inserted into the intramedullary canal, and then pulled out. Subsequently, an osteotomy of the mid-shaft of the femur was made by a surgical saw and the fracture was stabilized by a needle inserting into the intramedullary cavity. The muscles and skin were closed with interrupted sutures. EPO (40 ng/mouse) was administered every other day directly at the fracture site from day 4 to day 12 post-surgery, with saline as non-treatment control.

Histology, histochemistry and immunohistochemistry

Paraffin sections of the long bones were dewaxed and processed for Safranin O staining. Briefly, the sections were stained with Weigert's iron hematoxylin working solution for 5 min, washed in running tap water for 10 min, and then stained with 0.05% fast green solution for 5 min. After quick rinse with 0.1% acetic acid solution for 2 min, the sections were stained in 0.1% Safranin O solution for 5 min (materials are all from Sigma-Aldrich) followed by rapid dehydration in graded ethanol, clearness and mounting in Permount mounting medium (SP15-100, Fisher Scientific). For preparation of cryosections, the femurs were fixed in 4% paraformaldhyde for 3 days at 4°C, and decalcified in 10% EDTA for 14 days at 4°Cwith gentle agitation followed by dehydration for cryoprotection in graded concentrations (15% and then 30%) of sucrose at 4°C until the femurs were fully sank in the sucrose. The femurs were then embedded in optimal cutting temperature (OCT) compound (Tissue-Tek, Sakura Finetek USA) and flash frozen in liquid nitrogen. 5 μm thick sections were cut on a cryostat. Immunostaining for EPO and EPOR was performed following established protocols.

MicroCT angiography analysis

At 14 days post-fracture, mice were anesthetized following above procedures. The abdominal cavity and heart were exposed. After opening the hepatic portal vein, the entire vascular system was completely flushed through injection of heparinized saline (20 U/ml, Sigma-Aldrich) into the left ventricle. Microfil (Flow Tech) was prepared immediately and injected into left ventricle. The specimens were then placed at 4°C overnight before the fractured femurs were harvested. The femurs were fixed in 10% formalin for 7 days, decalcified in 10% EDTA for 14 days with gentle agitation and were then processed for micro-CT scanning. Histomorphometric parameters of blood vessels including vessel volume (VV), total volume (TV), VV/TV, vessel surface (VS), vessel thickness (VTh), vessel separation (VSp), and vessel number (VN) were analyzed.

Radiological analysis of bone

The healing bones are examined by bench top digital X-ray system at day 28 post-surgery. The bone union at fracture site was quantified according to the X-ray scoring system described by Lane and Sandhu with modifications [54]. For analysis of the 3D microarchitecture of the healing bone, the femurs were scanned by the Scanco μCT40 desktop cone-beam micro-CT scanner [55]. In brief, the femurs were placed vertically in the scanning holder with diameter of 12 μm. The scans were performed at the following settings: 12 mm resolution, 55 kvp, 145 μA with an integration time of 200 ms. Images were automatically reconstructed into 2-D slices, and region of interest was outlined in every slice via micro-μCT Evaluation Program (v5.0A, Scanco Medical). Direct calculation of bone histomorphometric parameters is performed including bone volume (BV), total volume (TV), BV/TV, bone surface (BS), trabecular thickness (TbTh), trabecular separation (TbSp) and trabecular number (TbN).

Biomechanical test

Femurs were collected at 28 days post-fracture and fresh frozen. Specimens were thawed in PBS at room temperature for 3 h before mechanical testing. Specimens were tested to failure by three-point bending using the LR10K Plus Extended machine (Lloyd Instruments Ltd). Briefly, femurs were placed horizontally on two support rollers with a span of 7 mm while a vertical load was applied to the center of the diaphysis using a material testing apparatus until failure. Biomechanical parameters including peak load, elastic modulus, bend strain at maximum and bend strength at maximum were calculated from the force displacement data.

Statistics

For the quantitative real-time PCR, cell proliferation and colony formation assays, all the experiments were repeated at least three times unless otherwise stated. Data was presented as mean ± standard deviation (SD). Statistical analysis was performed using SPSS software. Two-tailed Student's *t* test, one-way ANOVA or two-way ANOVA were employed according to the experimental design. $P<0.05$ was considered as statistical significance.

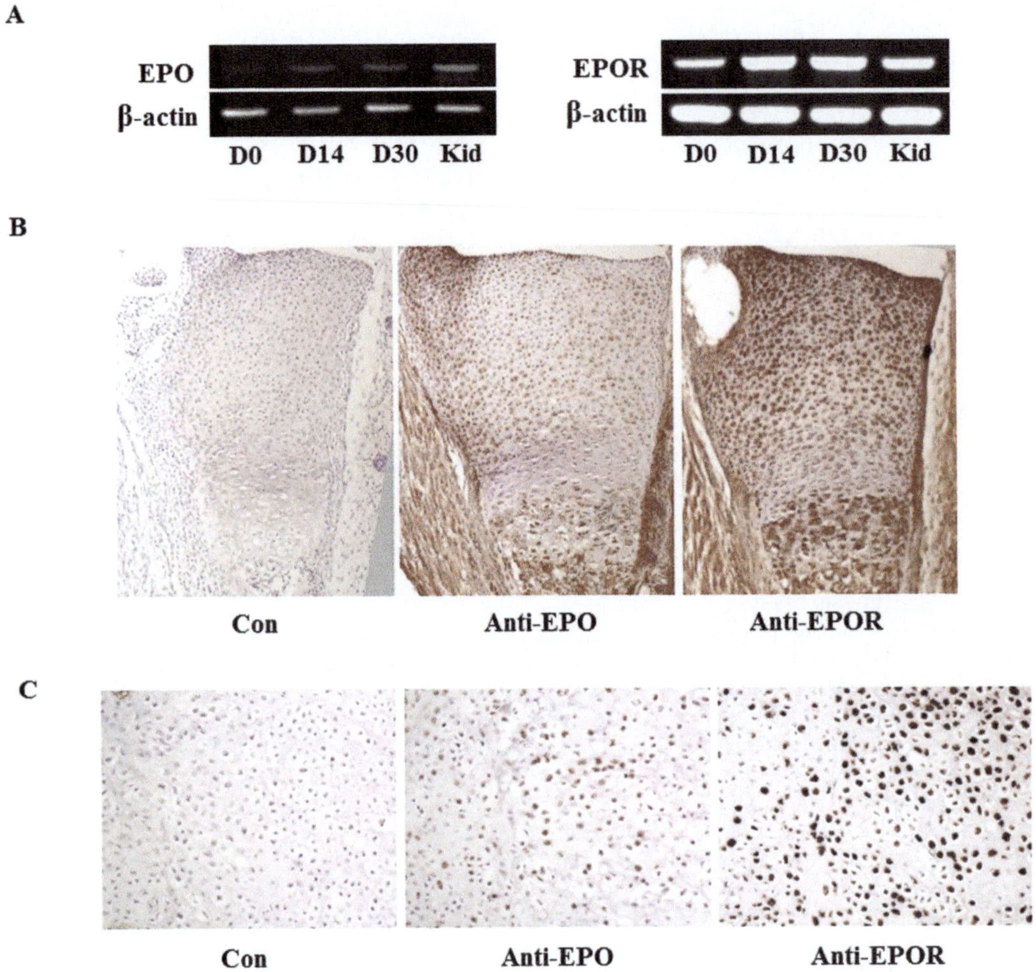

Figure 1. The expression and localization of EPO and EPOR in the developing bones. (A) mRNA expression of EPO and EPOR in the developing growth plates of tibiae by RT-PCR at indicated postnatal days. Tissues from kidney (Kid) of new born mice were used as positive control. (B) Immunohistochemistry for EPO and EPOR in growth plates of tibiae from new born mice. Con, non-primary antibody control. Magnification: 40×. (C) Immunohistochemistry for EPO and EPOR in cartilaginous callus of the bone healing in femoral fracture model of mouse. Con, non-primary antibody control. Magnification: 100×.

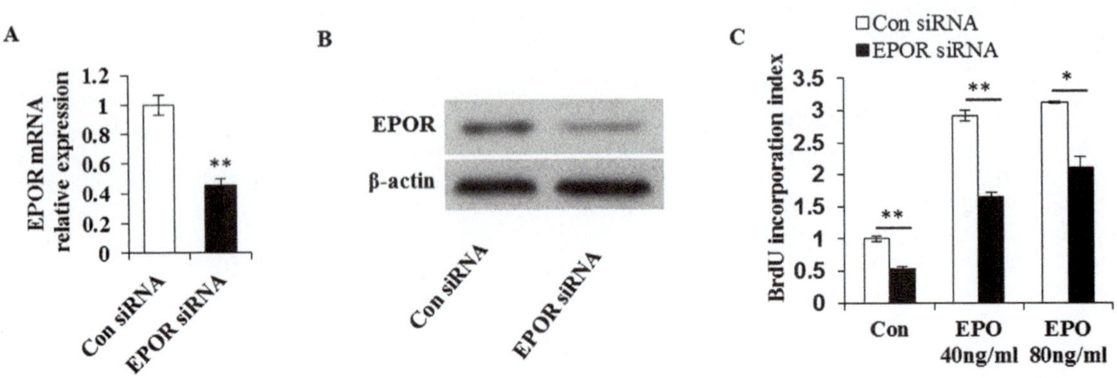

Figure 2. EPO promotes the proliferation of primary chondrocytes. (A) Examination of mRNA expression of EPOR in chondrocytes by real-time PCR after siRNA mediated knockdown of EPOR. (B) Western blot analysis of EPOR expression in primary chondrocytes with or without siRNA mediated knockdown of EPOR. (C) BrdU incorporation assay in primary chondrocytes with or without siRNA mediated knockdown of EPOR after 48 hours of EPO exposure. Con, non-treatment control. *$P<0.05$; **$P<0.01$; $n=3$.

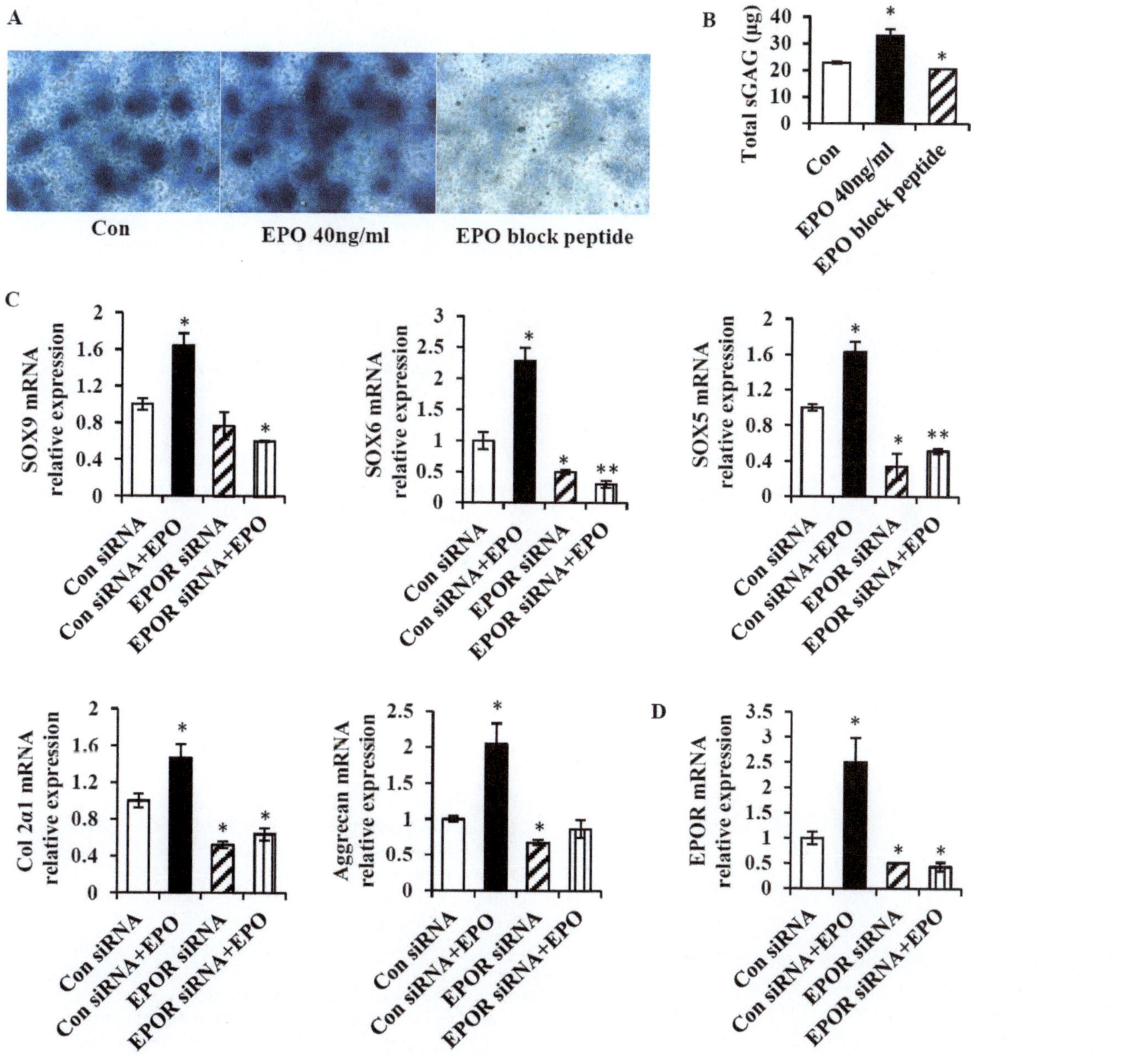

Figure 3. EPO increases biosynthesis of proteoglycan and upregulates chondrogenic marker genes expression during chondrogenic differentiation. (A) Alcian blue staining for preoteoglycan synthesis in the chondrogenic micromass culture supplemented with EPO, and with or without EPO block peptide for 7 days. Con, non-treatment control. Magnification: 10×. (B) Quantitation of total sGAG in the micromass culture by dimethylmethylene blue assay. (C) Detection of mRNA expression of chondrogenic marker genes including SOX9, SOX5, SOX6, Col2α1 and aggrecan by real-time PCR in chondrocytes in response to EPO treatment following siRNA mediated EPOR knockdown. (D) Real-time PCR quantification of EPOR mRNA expression in chondrocytes in response to EPO treatment following siRNA mediated EPOR knockdown. Con siRNA, control siRNA. **P*<0.05; ***P*<0.01, *n* = 3.

Results

The expression and localization of EPO and EPOR in the developing growth plate and the cartilaginous callus of healing bone

To examine the expression of EPO and EPOR in chondrocytes of the developing growth plates, we performed RT-PCR for EPO and EPOR using tissues obtained from the developing long bone growth plates of new born mice. EPO and EPOR mRNA was expressed in the growth plates derived from new born mice. Both of their expression in the growth plates was also detected at ages of day 14 and 30 (Fig. 1A). To identify the localization of EPO and EPOR in the growth plates, immunostaining for EPO and EPOR was performed in new borne mice. Our results showed that EPO and EPOR were abundantly present in proliferating, pre-hypertrophic and hypertrophic zones of growth plates of the developing bones (Fig. 1B). We next examined the localization of EPO and EPOR in the cartilaginous callus in the middle stage of bone healing. It showed that Both EPO and EPOR were localized in the proliferating, pre-hypertrophic and hypertrophic chondrocytes of the cartilaginous callus (Fig. 1C). These results suggested

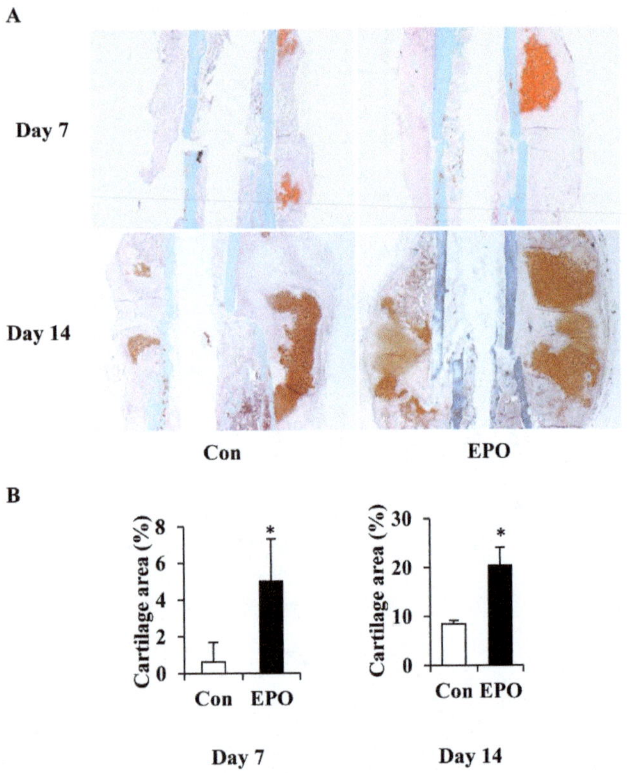

Figure 4. EPO enhances cartilaginous callus formation during bone healing. (A) Safranin O staining of the cartilaginous callus at days 7 and 14 post-surgery. Con, non-treatment control. Magnification: 2.5×. (B) Quantitation of the volume of cartilaginous callus formation at days 7 and 14 post-surgery. *$P<0.05$, $n=5$.

that EPO and EPOR might play an important role in the physiological development of the growth plate and cartilaginous formation during bone healing.

EPO increases the proliferation of primary chondrocytes

To elucidate EPO function in the development of growth plate, we first determined the effect of EPO treatment on the proliferation of primary chondrocytes with or without knockdown of EPOR. Using siRNA method, we achieved approximately 60% knockdown efficiency in the EPOR transcription level as shown by quantitative real-time PCR (Fig. 2A). Western blot verified the dramatically down-regulated EPOR protein level in chondrocytes following EPOR-siRNA transfection (Fig. 2B). We then added varied doses of EPO into the cultures of the primary chondrocytes transfected with control-siRNA or EPOR-siRNA, and cultured for two days followed by 6 hours of BrdU pulse labeling. In the cultures of the control-siRNA transfected chondrocytes, the BrdU incorporation index (indicating the numbers of BrdU incorporated cells) increased by (1.91±0.04) units in the 40 ng/ml EPO treatment group compared with that in the untreated group, and further increased by (2.12±0.02) units when 80 ng/ml EPO was applied (Fig. 2C), indicating that EPO may serve as a mitogenic factor for primary chondrocytes. We next asked whether the EPO-induced increase in the chondrocyte proliferation was EPOR dependent by looking at the effect of EPO on the chondrocytes following EPOR knockdown. Indeed, EPO's mitogenic effect on primary chondrocytes significantly decreased following siRNA mediated knockdown of EPOR. The increase of BrdU incorporation index induced by 40 ng/ml EPO and 80 ng/ml EPO dropped to (1.11±0.11) units and (1.57±0.08) units respectively in the chondrocytes transfected with EPOR-siRNA, which was significantly lower than what was observed in the control-siRNA groups (1.11 vs 1.91 and 1.57 vs 2.12; $P<0.05$). These results suggested that at least part of the proliferative effect of EPO on chondrocyte was mediated by its cognate receptor EPOR. Whether the elevation in BrdU incorporation index in EPOR-knockdown groups induced by the addition of EPO was caused by the interaction of EPO with the remaining EPOR, or by EPOR-independent function of EPO remains to be defined. Of interest, after knockdown of EPOR, the number of BrdU incorporated chondrocytes was significantly reduced when the cells were cultured in basal medium without exogenous EPO (Fig. 2C), suggesting that EPOR may be involved in the chondrocyte proliferation either independently or through its interaction with the endogenous EPO present in the chondrocytes.

EPO promotes chondrogenic differentiation *in vitro*

We then examined whether EPO also regulates chondrogenic differentiation by monitoring the proteoglycan biosynthesis in the extracellular matrix of chondrocyte micromass cultures following chondrogenic induction. After 7 days of chondrogenic induction. EPO (40 ng/ml) administration group showed more intense Alcian blue staining of chondrogenic nodules than the control group without EPO treatment (Fig. 3A), indicating increased amount of proteoglycan production. However, there appeared fewer and smaller Alcian blue stained nodules in the group where endogenous EPO was blocked by using EPO block peptide (Fig. 3A). The total amount of sGAG in chondrocytes was increased by 40% under EPO administration compared with the control group without EPO treatment, while there was a 20% decrease in the group treated with EPO block peptide (Fig. 3B). The reduction in proteoglycan levels after blockage of endogenous EPO and the increase of them following the addition of exogenous EPO implied the significance of both endogenous and exogenous EPO in chondrogenic differentiation.

To further understand the function of EPO in chondrogenic differentiation, mRNA expression of chondrogenic marker genes including SOX9, SOX5, SOX6, aggrecan, and Col2α1 was evaluated by quantitative real-time PCR in the micromass cultures of the EPOR-knockdown and control chondrocytes following 7 days of EPO treatment. The SOX family members SOX9, SOX5 and SOX6 have been demonstrated to be key transcription factors for chondrocyte specification [56,57]. EPO administration significantly up-regulated the above chondrogenic marker genes in the control chondrocytes by 1.5 to 2.5-fold while dramatic down-regulation of these marker genes was observed in EPOR-knockdown chondrocytes without EPO treatment (Fig. 3C), moreover, addition of EPO to the EPOR-knockdown chondrocyte cultures did not increase the expression of these genes to the levels that were comparable to what was achieved in the control chondrocytes treated with EPO (Fig. 3C). In addition, exogenous EPO significantly up-regulated EPOR mRNA level in chondrocytes (Fig. 3D). These results clearly demonstrated that EPO exerted a positive effect on chondrogenic differentiation, and this effect was mediated at least partially by EPOR.

EPO enhances cartilaginous callus formation during bone healing

We next determined the role of EPO in chondrogenesis *in vivo* using a femur fracture model in mouse. Direct delivery of EPO at

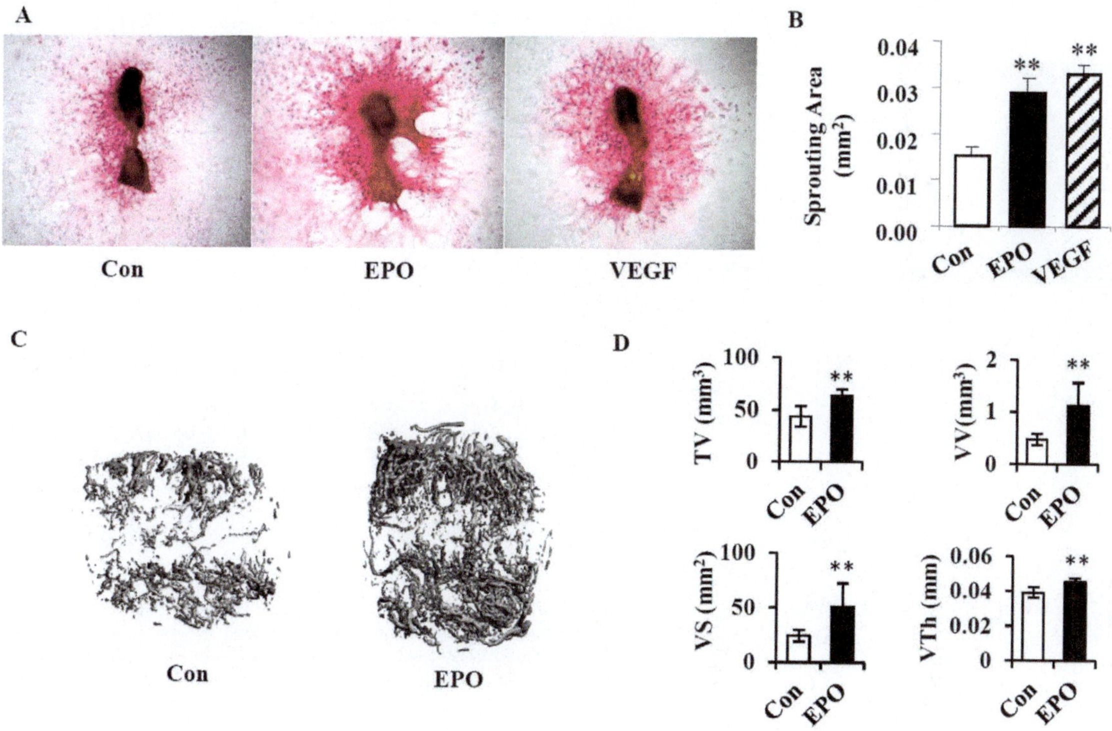

Figure 5. EPO stimulates angiogenesis *in vitro* and *in vivo*. (A) Representative images of endothelial sprouting from metatarsal bones of E17.5 embryos which were treated with different conditions as indicated. The endothelial sprouting was visualized by immunostaining for CD31. VEGF was used as positive control. Con, non-treatment control. Magnification: 2.5×. (B) Quantitation of the endothelial sprouting area for each group. (C) Representative micro-CT 3D reconstruction of vasculature at the fracture site following EPO treatment. The specimens were harvested for micro-CT scanning at day 14 post-surgery. Con, non-treatment control. (D) Quantitation of vascular parameters including the total volume (TV), vessel volume (VV), vessel surface (VS), and vessel thickness (VTh) by micro-CT angiography analysis. ** $P<0.01$, $n=5$.

the fracture site was performed every other day from day 4 to day 12 post-surgery. At days 7 and day 14 post-surgery, cartilaginous callus formed at the fracture sites was visualized by Safranin O staining (Fig. 4A). Histomorphometry analysis of cartilaginous callus of the healing bones showed that callus size and cartilage area in the EPO treatment group were larger than that in the saline control group (Fig. 4A). Upon EPO treatment, the ratios of cartilage volume to the total tissue volume were 5% and 20% respectively at day 7 and day 14 post-surgery, while the saline control group only gave rise to the ratios of 1% and 8%, which were significantly lower than the former (Fig. 4B). This result demonstrated that EPO enhanced cartilaginous callus formation during the early stage of bone healing.

EPO stimulates angiogenesis *in vitro* and *in vivo*

Besides the cartilage callus formation, angiogenesis is also a crucial factor during bone regeneration. To examine the role of EPO in angiogenesis, we isolated metatarsal bones from E17.5 mouse embryos and performed the endothelial sprouting assay in an *in vitro* culture system. As a result, the endothelial sprouting area was significantly increased by 1.9-fold in metatarsals treated with EPO 40 ng/ml compared with that of non-treatment controls, though this effect was not as dramatic as that of VEGF treatment (Fig. 5A and B). These results suggests that EPO may play a similar role like VEGF in stimulating endothelial sprouting from the metatarsal bones to form vessel like structure *in vitro*.

To further determine the effect of EPO in angiogenesis *in vivo*, we performed microCT angiography analysis in the middle stage of bone healing following local delivery of EPO at the fracture site. 3D reconstruction of newly formed vasculature at the fracture site showed more vascularity in the group treated with EPO than that of the control group (Fig. 5C). Microstructure parameters of the newly formed vessels including vessel volume (VV), vessel surface (VS) and vessel thickness (VTh) were all significantly increased following EPO administration compared with that of the control (Fig. 5D). And these changes were associated with the significantly enlarged total volume of callus area. These data demonstrated that EPO functioned as a proangiogenic factor during bone repair.

EPO enhances consolidation of bony callus during fracture healing

The observed positive effects of EPO on the cartilaginous callus formation and angiogenesis in the early and middle stages of bone healing led to an enhanced bone consolidation during facture healing. At day 28 post-surgery, the femurs from EPO treated group showed increased bone mass and density of the bony callus compared with the control group as evaluated by X-ray examination (Fig. 6A). X-ray score of the bony callus was increased by 1.5-fold in the EPO administrated group than that of the controls (Fig. 6B). Micro-CT 3D reconstruction of the bony callus clearly revealed a more robust bone formation in the EPO treated group than that of the controls (Fig. 6C), with the bone microstructure parameters of bone volume (BV), bone volume/ total volume (BV/TV) and bone surface (BS) all significantly higher in the former than in the later (Fig. 6D). Further assessment of the biomechanical strength of the healing bones by three-point bending test showed that peak load, elastic modulus, bend strain at maximum, and bend strength at maximum were all significantly

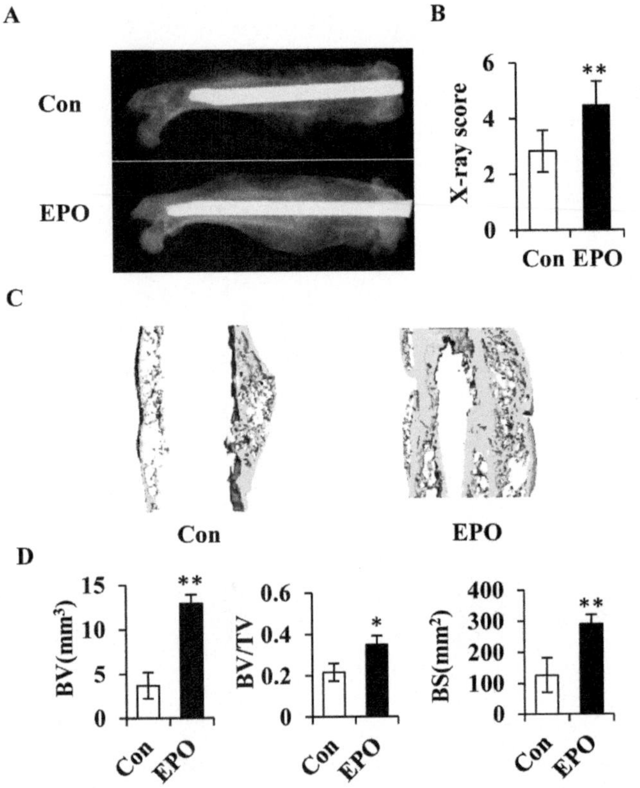

Figure 6. EPO increases the volume of the bony callus during consolidation of bone healing. (A) X-ray examination of the bony callus at day 28 post-surgery. Con, non-treatment control. (B) Quantitation of X-ray score of the bony callus at day 28 post-surgery. (C) Representative micro-CT 3D images of the new bone regenerates at day 28 post-surgery. (D) Quantitation of the bone microstructure parameters including bone volume (BV), bone volume/total volume (BV/TV), and bone surface (BS) by micro-CT analysis. $^*P<0.05$; $^{**}P<0.01$, $n=6$.

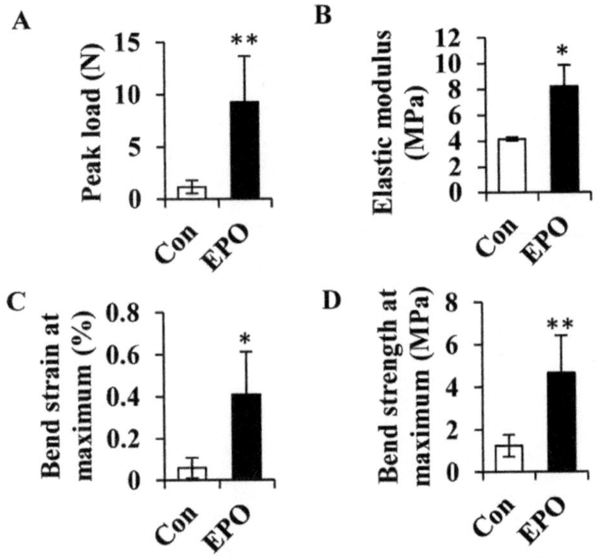

Figure 7. EPO improves biomechanical properties during consolidation of bone healing. Biomechanical parameters including peak load (A), elastic modulus (B), bend strain at maximum (C), and bend strength at maximum (D) were calculated at day 28 post-surgery. Con, non-treatment control. $^*P<0.05$; $^{**}P<0.01$, $n=3$.

increased in the group treated by EPO compared with the controls (Fig. 7A-D). Thus, local administration of EPO at the fracture site resulted in an increase in bony callus volume with improved biomechanical properties of the newly formed bone.

Discussion

Current procedures to promote skeletal regeneration include the applications of autografts, allografts, biocompatible implants, bioactive factors and mesenchymal stem cell-based therapy. However, the above approaches also face significant limitations due to insufficient supply, potential disease transmission, immuno-rejection, or less ability of functional engraftment. Thus, discovery of novel therapeutic approaches to improve skeletal repair and healing remains a great demand and clinical challenge in Orthopaedic regenerative medicine. In the present study, we demonstrated that local administration of EPO enhanced the consolidation and mechanical competence of the newly formed bone by promoting chondrogenic and angiogenic responses following injury, which can be explained by direct promotion effects of EPO on chondrocyte proliferation and differentiation, and on endothelial growth as shown in the *in vitro* studies. These findings expand the extent of EPO's tissue-specific functions and suggest that EPO may serve as a promising therapeutic agent for skeletal regeneration.

Previous study reported that EPOR was restrictedly expressed in hypertrophic chondrocytes during the cartilaginous callus stage of bone healing [45], and proposed that improved early endochondral ossification were mediated by EPO/EPOR signaling. In our study, knockdown of EPOR in primary chondrocytes resulted in a dramatic reduction of their responses to exogenous EPO in terms of cell proliferation (Fig. 2C) and chondrogenic marker genes expression upon chondrogenic differentiation (Fig. 3C). These evident reduction in EPO's effects on chondrocytes upon EPOR knockdown clearly demonstrated that EPO regulated the proliferation and differentiation of chondrocytes at least partially through EPOR.

Interestingly, EPO was also found to be present in chondrocytes in developing bones of new born mice as well as in newly formed cartilaginous callus of the healing bone in our study. Blockage of the endogenous EPO in primary chondrocytes using EPO block peptide impaired the chondrogenic differentiation, suggesting that endogenous EPO may function as an autocrine or paracrine factor for chondrocytes in normal bone development. Further clarifying the regulation of EPO production in chondrocytes in response to developmental and environmental cues will help better understanding its tissue-specific function in skeletal development and regeneration.

It is worthy to note that chondrocytes also produce VEGF [58,59], a well established angiogenic factor. Indeed, we observed a functional similarity of EPO and VEGF in the endothelial sprouting stimulation, indicating that both factors may exert overlapping but distinct roles in the angiogenic responses during bone healing. Given that EPO exerts versatile functions in varied tissues and cells and that bone regeneration is a complex process involving multiple cellular components or biological factors, the role of EPO in improving bone healing may also be versatile and complex. Direct and indirect signaling pathways may work coordinately to facilitate a better bone formation. For example, the increased volume of cartilaginous callus by EPO treatment may produce more VEGF and EPO to benefit angiogenesis and the increased vascularity by EPO administration may bring more blood and nutrient supply and osteoprogenitor cells to promote the consolidation of the healing bone. In addition, EPO may function as a coupling factor to coordinate haematopoiesis and the homeostasis of the skeleton, which deserves to be furthur defined.

In summary, EPO and EPOR are expressed in the neonatal developing growth plate and cartilaginous callus of healing bone. EPO may function as an autocrine or paracrine factor to regulate the spatial and temporal coordination among angiogenesis, chondrogenesis and osteogenesis during bone repair. EPO may serve as an effective agent to promote skeletal regeneration.

Acknowledgments

We are grateful for the assistance of the Core laboratories at School of Biomedical Sciences, the Chinese University of Hong Kong, and Small Animal Phenotyping Core at the University of Alabama at Birmingham.

Author Contributions

Conceived and designed the experiments: CW LW. Performed the experiments: LW FZ QH WPT CW. Analyzed the data: LW CW FZ QH. Contributed reagents/materials/analysis tools: LL QL ZW GQ GZ. Contributed to the writing of the manuscript: CW LW.

References

1. Einhorn TA (1995) Enhancement of fracture-healing. J Bone Joint Surg Am 77: 940–956.
2. Solomon DH, Patrick AR, Schousboe J, Losina E (2014) The Potential Economic Benefits of Improved Post-Fracture Care: A Cost-Effectiveness Analysis of a Fracture Liaison Service in the US Health Care System. J Bone Miner Res.
3. Hak DJ, Fitzpatrick D, Bishop JA, Marsh JL, Tilp S, et al. (2014) Delayed union and nonunions: Epidemiology, clinical issues, and financial aspects. Injury 45 Suppl 2: S3-7.
4. Richards JB, Rivadeneira F, Inouye M, Pastinen TM, Soranzo N, et al. (2008) Bone mineral density, osteoporosis, and osteoporotic fractures: a genome-wide association study. Lancet 371: 1505–1512.
5. Janghorbani M, Van Dam RM, Willett WC, Hu FB (2007) Systematic review of type 1 and type 2 diabetes mellitus and risk of fracture. Am J Epidemiol 166: 495–505.
6. Siddiqui NA, Owen JM (2013) Clinical advances in bone regeneration. Curr Stem Cell Res Ther 8: 192–200.
7. Wan C, Gilbert SR, Wang Y, Cao X, Shen X, et al. (2008) Activation of the hypoxia-inducible factor-1alpha pathway accelerates bone regeneration. Proc Natl Acad Sci U S A 105: 686–691.
8. Fassbender M, Strobel C, Rauhe JS, Bergmann C, Schmidmaier G, et al. (2011) Local inhibition of angiogenesis results in an atrophic non-union in a rat osteotomy model. Eur Cell Mater 22: 1–11.
9. Ferguson C, Alpern E, Miclau T, Helms JA (1999) Does adult fracture repair recapitulate embryonic skeletal formation? Mech Dev 87: 57–66.
10. Gerstenfeld LC, Cullinane DM, Barnes GL, Graves DT, Einhorn TA (2003) Fracture healing as a post-natal developmental process: molecular, spatial, and temporal aspects of its regulation. J Cell Biochem 88: 873–884.
11. Kanczler JM, Oreffo RO (2008) Osteogenesis and angiogenesis: the potential for engineering bone. Eur Cell Mater 15: 100–114.
12. Brandi ML (2013) Healing of the bone with anti-fracture drugs. Expert Opin Pharmacother 14: 1441–1447.
13. McKibbin B (1978) The biology of fracture healing in long bones. J Bone Joint Surg Br 60-B: 150–162.
14. Kolar P, Gaber T, Perka C, Duda GN, Buttgereit F (2011) Human early fracture hematoma is characterized by inflammation and hypoxia. Clin Orthop Relat Res 469: 3118–3126.
15. Sun H, Jung Y, Shiozawa Y, Taichman RS, Krebsbach PH (2012) Erythropoietin modulates the structure of bone morphogenetic protein 2-engineered cranial bone. Tissue Eng Part A 18: 2095–2105.
16. Kigami R, Sato S, Tsuchiya N, Yoshimakai T, Arai Y, et al. (2013) FGF-2 angiogenesis in bone regeneration within critical-sized bone defects in rat calvaria. Implant Dent 22: 422–427.
17. Warren SM, Steinbrech DS, Mehrara BJ, Saadeh PB, Greenwald JA, et al. (2001) Hypoxia regulates osteoblast gene expression. J Surg Res 99: 147–155.
18. Sheng MH, Lau KH, Baylink DJ (2014) Role of Osteocyte-derived Insulin-Like Growth Factor I in Developmental Growth, Modeling, Remodeling, and Regeneration of the Bone. J Bone Metab 21: 41–54.
19. Zelzer E, McLean W, Ng YS, Fukai N, Reginato AM, et al. (2002) Skeletal defects in VEGF(120/120) mice reveal multiple roles for VEGF in skeletogenesis. Development 129: 1893–1904.
20. Street J, Bao M, deGuzman L, Bunting S, Peale FV Jr, et al. (2002) Vascular endothelial growth factor stimulates bone repair by promoting angiogenesis and bone turnover. Proc Natl Acad Sci U S A 99: 9656–9661.
21. Wang Y, Wan C, Deng L, Liu X, Cao X, et al. (2007) The hypoxia-inducible factor alpha pathway couples angiogenesis to osteogenesis during skeletal development. J Clin Invest 117: 1616–1626.
22. Wan C, Shao J, Gilbert SR, Riddle RC, Long F, et al. (2010) Role of HIF-1alpha in skeletal development. Ann N Y Acad Sci 1192: 322–326.
23. Wu H, Liu X, Jaenisch R, Lodish HF (1995) Generation of committed erythroid BFU-E and CFU-E progenitors does not require erythropoietin or the erythropoietin receptor. Cell 83: 59–67.
24. Wu H, Klingmuller U, Besmer P, Lodish HF (1995) Interaction of the erythropoietin and stem-cell-factor receptors. Nature 377: 242–246.
25. Kertesz N, Wu J, Chen TH, Sucov HM, Wu H (2004) The role of erythropoietin in regulating angiogenesis. Dev Biol 276: 101–110.
26. Brines M, Grasso G, Fiordaliso F, Sfacteria A, Ghezzi P, et al. (2004) Erythropoietin mediates tissue protection through an erythropoietin and common beta-subunit heteroreceptor. Proc Natl Acad Sci U S A 101: 14907–14912.
27. Brines M, Cerami A (2006) Discovering erythropoietin's extra-hematopoietic functions: biology and clinical promise. Kidney Int 70: 246–250.
28. Tan CC, Eckardt KU, Ratcliffe PJ (1991) Organ distribution of erythropoietin messenger RNA in normal and uremic rats. Kidney Int 40: 69–76.
29. Fisher JW (1997) Erythropoietin: physiologic and pharmacologic aspects. Proc Soc Exp Biol Med 216: 358–369.
30. Yi C, Hak DJ (2012) Traumatic spinopelvic dissociation or U-shaped sacral fracture: a review of the literature. Injury 43: 402–408.
31. Tada H, Kagaya Y, Takeda M, Ohta J, Asaumi Y, et al. (2006) Endogenous erythropoietin system in non-hematopoietic lineage cells plays a protective role in myocardial ischemia/reperfusion. Cardiovasc Res 71: 466–477.
32. Kumral A, Tuzun F, Oner MG, Genc S, Duman N, et al. (2011) Erythropoietin in neonatal brain protection: the past, the present and the future. Brain Dev 33: 632–643.
33. Tsai PT, Ohab JJ, Kertesz N, Groszer M, Matter C, et al. (2006) A critical role of erythropoietin receptor in neurogenesis and post-stroke recovery. J Neurosci 26: 1269–1274.
34. Hak DJ, Makino T, Niikura T, Hazelwood SJ, Curtiss S, et al. (2006) Recombinant human BMP-7 effectively prevents non-union in both young and old rats. J Orthop Res 24: 11–20.
35. Acheson A, Richards JB, de Wit H (2007) Effects of sleep deprivation on impulsive behaviors in men and women. Physiol Behav 91: 579–587.
36. Cianferotti L, Brandi ML (2014) Muscle-bone interactions: basic and clinical aspects. Endocrine 45: 165–177.
37. Wright GL, Hanlon P, Amin K, Steenbergen C, Murphy E, et al. (2004) Erythropoietin receptor expression in adult rat cardiomyocytes is associated with an acute cardioprotective effect for recombinant erythropoietin during ischemia-reperfusion injury. FASEB J 18: 1031–1033.
38. Bernaudin M, Marti HH, Roussel S, Divoux D, Nouvelot A, et al. (1999) A potential role for erythropoietin in focal permanent cerebral ischemia in mice. J Cereb Blood Flow Metab 19: 643–651.
39. Sugawa M, Sakurai Y, Ishikawa-Ieda Y, Suzuki H, Asou H (2002) Effects of erythropoietin on glial cell development; oligodendrocyte maturation and astrocyte proliferation. Neurosci Res 44: 391–403.
40. Lee MY, Fukunaga R, Lee TJ, Lottsfeldt JL, Nagata S (1991) Bone modulation in sustained hematopoietic stimulation in mice. Blood 77: 2135–2141.
41. Takenaka T, Itaya Y, Ishikawa I, Kobayashi K, Tsuchiya Y (2003) Skeletal effects of erythropoietin in hemodialysis patients. Int Urol Nephrol 35: 407–413.
42. Singbrant S, Russell MR, Jovic T, Liddicoat B, Izon DJ, et al. (2011) Erythropoietin couples erythropoiesis, B-lymphopoiesis, and bone homeostasis within the bone marrow microenvironment. Blood 117: 5631–5642.
43. Shiozawa Y, Jung Y, Ziegler AM, Pedersen EA, Wang J, et al. (2010) Erythropoietin couples hematopoiesis with bone formation. PLoS One 5: e10853.
44. Garcia P, Speidel V, Scheuer C, Laschke MW, Holstein JH, et al. (2011) Low dose erythropoietin stimulates bone healing in mice. J Orthop Res 29: 165–172.
45. Holstein JH, Menger MD, Scheuer C, Meier C, Culemann U, et al. (2007) Erythropoietin (EPO): EPO-receptor signaling improves early endochondral ossification and mechanical strength in fracture healing. Life Sci 80: 893–900.
46. Mihmanli A, Dolanmaz D, Avunduk MC, Erdemli E (2009) Effects of recombinant human erythropoietin on mandibular distraction osteogenesis. J Oral Maxillofac Surg 67: 2337–2343.
47. Gosset M, Berenbaum F, Thirion S, Jacques C (2008) Primary culture and phenotyping of murine chondrocytes. Nat Protoc 3: 1253–1260.
48. Derks M, Sturm T, Haverich A, Hilfiker A (2013) Isolation and chondrogenic differentiation of porcine perichondrial progenitor cells for the purpose of cartilage tissue engineering. Cells Tissues Organs 198(3):179–189.
49. Ovchinnikov D (2009) Alcian blue/alizarin red staining of cartilage and bone in mouse. Cold Spring Harb Protoc 2009: pdb prot5170.
50. Lee YJ, Kong MH, Song KY, Lee KH, Heo SH (2008) The Relation Between Sox9, TGF-beta1, and Proteoglycan in Human Intervertebral Disc Cells. J Korean Neurosurg Soc 43: 149–154.

51. Enobakhare BO, Bader DL, Lee DA (1996) Quantification of sulfated glycosaminoglycans in chondrocyte/alginate cultures, by use of 1,9-dimethyl-methylene blue. Anal Biochem 243: 189–191.
52. Deckers M, van der Pluijm G, Dooijewaard S, Kroon M, van Hinsbergh V, et al. (2001) Effect of angiogenic and antiangiogenic compounds on the outgrowth of capillary structures from fetal mouse bone explants. Lab Invest 81: 5–15.
53. Cackowski FC, Anderson JL, Patrene KD, Choksi RJ, Shapiro SD, et al. (2010) Osteoclasts are important for bone angiogenesis. Blood 115: 140–149.
54. Lane JM, Sandhu HS (1987) Current approaches to experimental bone grafting. Orthop Clin North Am 18: 213–225.
55. Casazza K, Hanks LJ, Clines GA, Tse HM, Eberhardt AW (2013) Diabetes-related impairment in bone strength is established early in the life course. World J Diabetes 4: 145–150.
56. Akiyama H, Lefebvre V (2011) Unraveling the transcriptional regulatory machinery in chondrogenesis. J Bone Miner Metab 29: 390–395.
57. Akiyama H, Chaboissier MC, Martin JF, Schedl A, de Crombrugghe B (2002) The transcription factor Sox9 has essential roles in successive steps of the chondrocyte differentiation pathway and is required for expression of Sox5 and Sox6. Genes Dev 16: 2813–2828.
58. Haigh JJ, Gerber HP, Ferrara N, Wagner EF (2000) Conditional inactivation of VEGF-A in areas of collagen2a1 expression results in embryonic lethality in the heterozygous state. Development 127: 1445–1453.
59. De Spiegelaere W, Cornillie P, Van den Broeck W (2010) Localization of erythropoietin in and around growing cartilage. Mol Cell Biochem 337: 287–291.

23

Pullulan/dextran/nHA Macroporous Composite Beads for Bone Repair in a Femoral Condyle Defect in Rats

Silke Schlaubitz[1], Sidi Mohammed Derkaoui[2,3], Lydia Marosa[4], Sylvain Miraux[5], Martine Renard[1], Sylvain Catros[4,6], Catherine Le Visage[2,3], Didier Letourneur[2,3], Joëlle Amédée[4], Jean-Christophe Fricain[4,6]*

1 CIC 1401, University hospital of Bordeaux/Inserm, Bordeaux, France, **2** U1148, LVTS/Inserm, Paris, France, **3** Près Sorbonne Paris Cité, University of Paris Nord and University Paris Diderot, Paris, France, **4** U1026 Tissue Bioengineering, University of Bordeaux/Inserm, Bordeaux, France, **5** RMSB Center/UMR 5536, CNRS, Bordeaux, France, **6** Dental School, University of Bordeaux, Bordeaux, France

Abstract

The repair of bone defects is of particular interest for orthopedic, oral, maxillofacial, and dental surgery. Bone loss requiring reconstruction is conventionally addressed through bone grafting. Depending on the size and the location of the defect, this method has limits and risks. Biomaterials can offer an alternative and have features supporting bone repair. Here, we propose to evaluate the cellular penetration and bone formation of new macroporous beads based on pullulan/dextran that has been supplemented with nanocrystalline hydroxyapatite in a rat model. Cross-linked beads of 300–500 µm diameters were used in a lateral femoral condyle defect and analyzed by magnetic resonance imaging, micro-computed tomography, and histology in comparison to the empty defects 15, 30, and 70 days after implantation. Inflammation was absent for both conditions. For empty defects, cellularisation and mineralization started from the periphery of the defect. For the defects containing beads, cellular structures filling out the spaces between the scaffolds with increasing interconnectivity and trabecular-like organization were observed over time. The analysis of calcified sections showed increased mineralization over time for both conditions, but was more pronounced for the samples containing beads. Bone Mineral Density and Bone Mineral Content were both significantly higher at day 70 for the beads in comparison to empty defects as well as compared with earlier time points. Analysis of newly formed tissue around the beads showed an increase of osteoid tissue, measured as percentage of the defect surface. This study suggests that the use of beads for the repair of small size defects in bone may be expanded on to meet the clinical need for a ready-to-use fill-up material that can favor bone formation and mineralization, as well as promote vessel ingrowth into the defect site.

Editor: Dominique Heymann, Faculté de médecine de Nantes, France

Funding: This work is funded by ANR-07-TecSan-011-01 ITOV and ANR-10-EMMA-009-01 MATRI+ from Agence National de la Recherche: (http://www.agence-nationale-recherche.fr/) to JA and DL. The funders had no role in study design, data collection and analysis, decision to publish, or preparation of the manuscript.

Competing Interests: Although the authors Sidi Mohammed Derkaoui and Didier Letourneur are shareholders of the company IMMATIS for development and commercialization of the reported matrices.

* Email: jean-christophe.fricain@inserm.fr

Introduction

The repair of bone defects caused by trauma, surgery or due to cancer treatment is of particular interest for surgeons. Conventional bone grafting is still the gold standard, but depending on the size and the location of the defect, this method has limits and risks regarding the efficiency, possible infections and the manageable pain [1]. Biomaterials can offer an alternative and have osteoconductive [2,3] and/or osteoinductive [4–6] properties supporting bone repair while being biocompatible and biodegradable [7–12].

Bone substitute biomaterials are often based on calcium phosphates like hydroxyapatite (HA) [13], tricalcium phosphate (TCP) [13–15], biphasic calcium phosphates (BCP) [13,16,17], or coral [18] because of their biocompatibility due to a composition similar to mature bone, and their osteoconductive properties [2]. The use of calcium phosphate itself is limited to small defects, where biomaterials with osteoconductive properties are sufficient for bone reconstruction [5], or as a coating of other biomaterials [19], because those materials allow only limited neo-angiogenesis and are therefore not suitable for larger size defects.

Other groups of bone substitute biomaterials that promote vessel ingrowth are mainly based on polymers. The properties of natural polymers like collagen [20,21], dextran [22], chitosan [23], alginate/fibrin [24] or synthetic polymers like polyglycolic acid (PGA), polylactic acid (PLA), and poly(lactic-*co*-glycolic) acid (PLGA) among others [25,26] have been extensively studied in *in vitro* bone tissue engineering applications, mainly as delivery systems for encapsulated stem cells or growth factors. Polymer scaffolds can easily be generated in various 3D structures such as macroporous scaffolds, biospun scaffolds, micro beads, hydrogels, micro-molded matrices and nanoparticles [27]. Some polymers have little affinity with bone, but can easily be associated with cells or growth factors to promote bone tissue regeneration with angiogenic potential *in vivo* [28–32]. To combine properties favoring bone affinity and angiogenesis, specific composites of polymers and ceramics are being developed that have shown osteoinductive and osteoconductive properties [33]. Composite materials in different shape and sizes of scaffolds have been used in numerous *in vivo* investigations to promote bone healing [34–39], and can easily be associated with cells or growth factors to enhance osteoinductive and/or osteoconductive properties [40,41]. However the use of composite beads seems preferable for some clinical applications, because they could be injectable and therefore easy to handle and adapt to the morphology of any defect [42], as seen previously in a clinical trial [43].

Injectable beads have been studied *in vitro* as composite materials such as alginate/β-tricalcium phosphate [44], Chitosan-collagen/nano-hydroxyapatite [45], or fibrin/β-tricalcium phosphate [46], but *in vivo* studies have not been performed with those materials yet.

In the present study, a biomaterial based on a mixture of pullulan and dextran in association with nanocrystalline hydroxyapatite designed as cross-linked micro-beads was used as a scaffold. Previous experiments have shown the osteoconductive properties of the biomaterial when used as a massive macroporous scaffold [36]. In this study, the objective was to demonstrate for the first time that beads of a new ready-to-use fill-up composite material made of dextran/pullulan/nanocrystalline hydroxyapatite are suitable materials to activate and promote bone regeneration and mineralization in rat femoral condyle defects.

Materials and Methods

Preparation and characterization of the biomaterial

A nanocrystalline hydroxyapatite (nHA) solution was prepared by wet chemical precipitation using a 0.6 M solution of phosphoric acid (Prolabo, Paris, France) and a 1 M solution of calcium hydroxide (Alfa Aesar, Germany) [47,48]. The nHA powder was composed of 50–100 nm long rod-like crystals as observed by transmission electron microscopy. X ray quantitative micro analysis revealed a Ca/P ratio of 1.67 and FITR analysis confirmed the presence of phosphate, hydroxide and carbonate groups, as described previously [47].

Nanocrystalline hydroxyapatite-polysaccharide microparticles composite were obtained using water-in-oil (w/o) emulsification process. Briefly, 75% pullulan (MW 200000, Hayashibara Inc., Japan) and 25% dextran (MW 500000, Sigma, France) were dissolved in nHA suspension and NaCl as a porogen. The mixture was then dispersed in canola oil under mechanical stirring and polysaccharide beads were cross-linked by sodium trimetaphosphate at 50°C for 20 min. Resulting microbeads were extensively washed with 0.025% NaCl solution, and sieved, using a vibrating shaker (AS 200, Retsch, France) to obtain beads of 300–500 μm diameter that were freeze-dried [49].

Hydrated scaffolds were observed using environmental scanning electron microscopy (ESEM) with a Philips XL 30 ESEM-FEG (Eindhoven, The Netherlands) at an accelerating voltage of 15 keV and at a pressure of 3.5 Torr. Dry beads were observed by Back

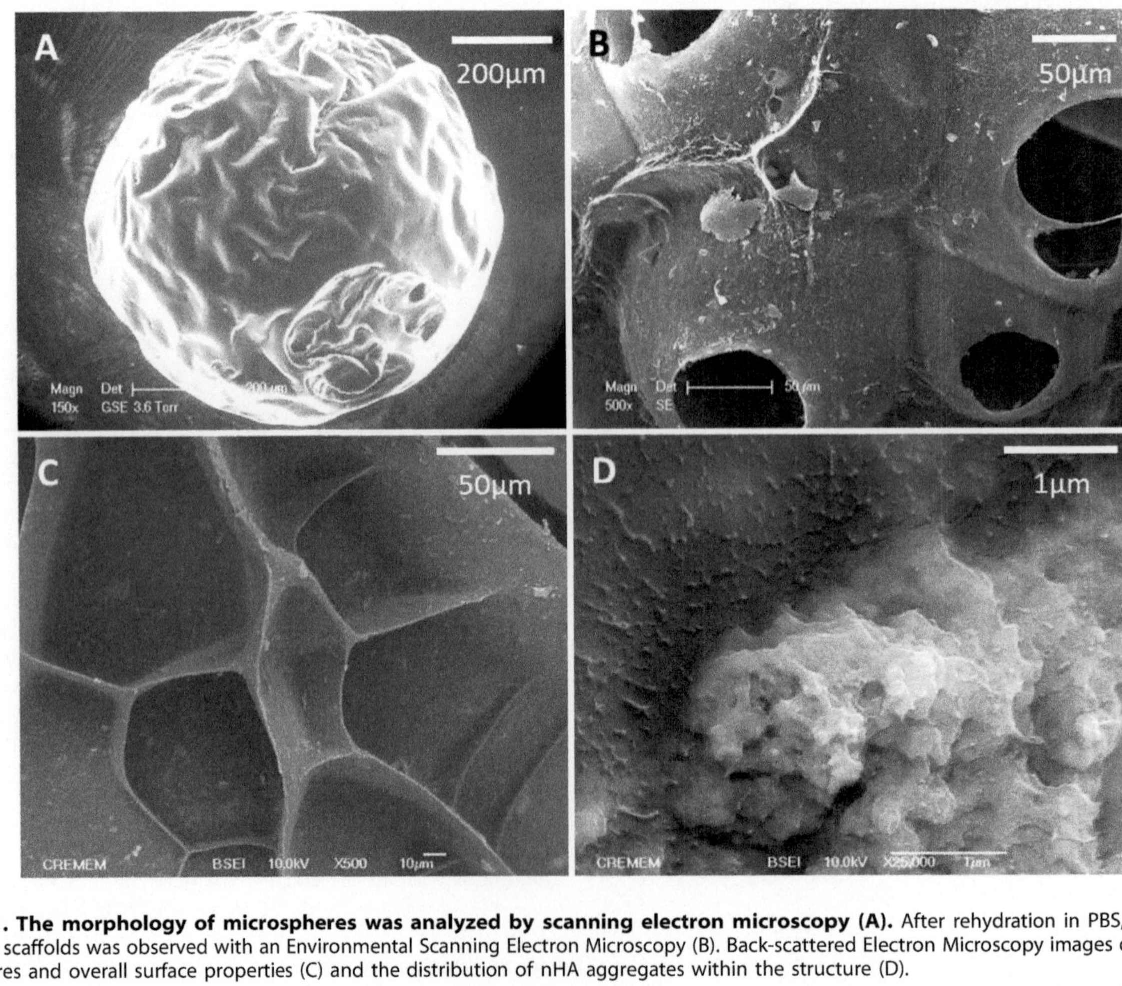

Figure 1. The morphology of microspheres was analyzed by scanning electron microscopy (A). After rehydration in PBS, porosity of hydrated scaffolds was observed with an Environmental Scanning Electron Microscopy (B). Back-scattered Electron Microscopy images of dry beads show pores and overall surface properties (C) and the distribution of nHA aggregates within the structure (D).

Scattered Electron Microscopy (BSEM) after gold sputtering on a 6700F electron microscope (JEOL, Peabody/MA, USA) working at 10 keV.

In vivo experiments

Animal experiments were performed in accordance with the "Principles of Laboratory Animal Care" recommended by the National Society for Biomedical Research in France. Interventions were carried out in an accredited animal facility (authorization n° A33-063-917) at the University of Bordeaux, under authorization n° B3310023 of the French Ministry of Agriculture and were approved by the Animal Ethic Committee of the University of Bordeaux.

Anesthesia was induced with a mixture of 4% isoflurane/Air 1–2 L/min (Baxter, Deerfield/IL, USA) and was maintained at 2% isoflurane/Air 0.8 L/min during the implantation. A stable body temperature was assured by the use of a heating device.

Medial defects of 3.5 mm diameter and 4 mm depth were introduced in left and right femoral condyles of 18 female Wistar RjHan rats at 10 weeks of age weighting 250–300 g (Janvier, Le Genest, France) using a dental microdrill (Thomas, France). Bone defects of about 38 mm^3 were rinsed with physiological solution NaCl 0.9% (w/v). The defect was either left empty or filled with 17±3 dry beads that were implanted into the site, leaving enough time for the beads to hydrate with the blood invading the defect and, as a consequence, to increase slightly in size. The scaffolds remained solid enough to stay inside the defect. Therefore, no membrane was needed to avoid leakage of the biomaterial. Absorbable Vicryl sutures were performed on lateral muscles before closing the cutaneous plan with non-absorbable prolene sutures and suture clips.

To assure analgesia, 0.3 mg/kg of buprenorphine (Vetergesic Multidose, Alstoe Veterinary, York, UK) was administered subcutaneously to each rat 30 min prior to the procedure as well as 24 hours afterwards. Additionally, animals were kept under free access to 0.2 mg/mL of Ibuprofen (Advil, Pfizer, Canada) 3 days prior to surgery and during 1 week after surgery through the drinking water. Twelve animals were euthanized by an overdose of CO_2 and the six animals that were followed longitudinally by MRI and therefore housed in a different facility, were euthanized by lethal injection (200 mg/animal) of sodium pentobarbital (Ceva, France) for the last time point when the regulator delivering the CO_2 was not available. The implants and the surrounding tissues were recovered 15, 30 and 70 days after surgery and fixed in 4% (w/v) paraformaldehyde for 4 days at 4°C. After rinsing in 0.1 M phosphate buffer pH 7.4, samples were processed for Micro-CT analysis and histology. For each time point, 6 condyles were left empty and 6 condyles were filled with the beads as matrices.

Magnetic Resonance Imaging

Immune response and degradation of the implanted scaffold was followed longitudinally in 6 rats by Magnetic Resonance Imaging (MRI). The rats were anaesthetized with 1–1.5% isoflurane/Air 0.8 L/min and maintained at a constant respiration rate of 75±15 respirations/min. Acquisitions at day 15, 30, and 70 after implantation were obtained with a 4.7T Biospec system (Bruker, Ettlingen, Germany) equipped with a 12 cm gradient system capable of 200 mT/m maximum strength. Measurements were performed with a Helmoltz coil (35/25 mm diameter) tuned to 200.3 MHz.

The animals were put in the prone position within the magnet, with the knee at the center of the NMR coil. A 3D TrueFISP imaging with alternating RF phase pulse method and sum of square reconstruction was used as described previously [50]. The aqueous volume was measured for the defect of each acquisition and the results are presented as the means of 6 samples with standard deviation.

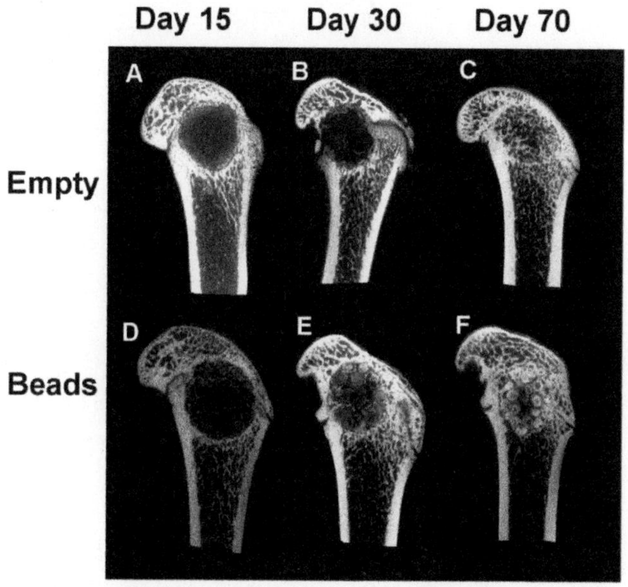

Figure 2. Representative 2D pictures of the median region of Micro-CT 3D reconstructed femoral condyles that were left empty (A–C) or received beads as implants (D–F). Mineralization around the beads is visible as early as 15 days after surgery (D). Empty defects show little mineralization within the defect 30 days after implantation (B), starting from the periphery of the defects. At day 70, mineralization is visible within the defect site for both conditions (C, F).

X-ray Micro-Computed Tomography (Micro-CT)

Three-dimensional images of the implants and surrounding tissue were produced by Micro-CT and used for quantification of the newly formed bone. *Ex vivo* acquisitions at 15 μm resolution were performed from 900 X-ray radiographs obtained on an Explore Locus SP X-Ray μCT device (General Electric, Milwaukee/WI, USA) with a source voltage of 80 kV, a current of 80 μA, and an exposure time of 3000 ms. Reconstruction of the region of interest was performed after correction of the center of rotation and calibration of mineral density. After calibration, three dimensional analyses were performed using Microview software (*GE Healthcare* Inc., Princeton/NJ, USA). The threshold for newly formed bone was determined for each scan individually. Quantification included Bone Mineral density (BMD), and Bone Mineral Content (BMC) as defined previously [51]. BMC values were analyzed from regions of interest (ROI) of a fixed volume. Six ROI throughout the defect were determined for each sample. The means of all ROI per sample were analyzed further to evaluate the means with standard deviation of six samples per condition at each time point. For the analysis of BMD, the entire defect site of six samples per condition was taken into account and the results of six samples per condition are shown as the means with standard deviation.

Histology

Each sample was cut median between the two femoral condyles. One half of each sample was decalcified for 7 hours in a commercially available decalcification solution (DC3, Labonord, France), dehydrated and embedded in paraffin, while the other

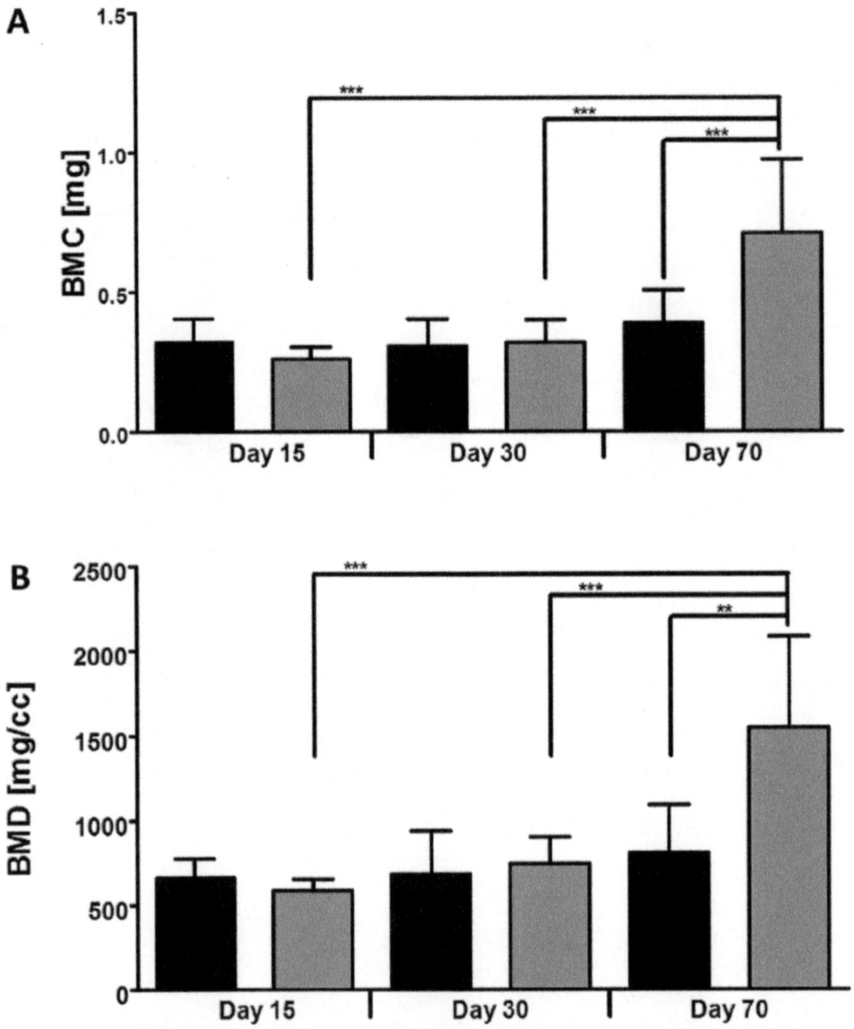

Figure 3. Ex *vivo* analysis of Bone mineral content (A) and Bone mineral density (B) by Micro-CT imaging. Regions of interest (ROI) were analysed in defects that were left empty (black columns) or received the beads (grey columns). Results are shown as means ± SD of 6 samples per condition. Significant differences are indicated with ** $p \leq 0.01$, and *** $p \leq 0.001$.

half was processed for resin inclusion in serial changes of 5% (w/v) Methyl benzoate (Sigma Aldrich), 35% (w/v) Butyl methacrylate (Sigma Aldrich), and 60% (w/v) Methyl methacrylate (VWR, Radnor/PA, USA) with increasing amounts of 4,N,N-Trimethylaniline (Sigma Aldrich, St. Louis/MO, USA).

Sections of 4–10 µm were obtained from each sample and stained with Masson's Trichrome (decalcified samples) or Von Kossa (calcified samples). Pictures were analyzed with an Eclipse 80i microscope light microscopy (Nikon, Japan) and captured using a DXM 1200C CCD camera (Nikon, Japan).

Immunohistochemistry

Infiltration of macrophages was evaluated by immunohistochemistry for transmembrane glycoprotein CD68, belonging to the lysosomal-associated membrane protein family. Vessel formation was investigated for the presence of the angiogenesis marker von Willebrand Factor, and the presence of osteoblast precursors was evaluated with immune-staining for BMP-2. Sections were deparaffinized in two changes of toluene for 5 min. Endogenous peroxidase was blocked by applying 3% (v/v) hydrogen peroxide in methanol for 10 min at −20°C. Antigen Retrieval was performed by applying Proteinase K (Invitrogen, Grand Island/NY, USA) for 10 min at room temperature. Endogenous biotin was blocked using an avidin/biotin blocking kit (Invitrogen, Grand Island/NY, USA), before blocking unspecific antibody binding using Histostain-SP kit (Invitrogen, Grand Island/NY, USA). Mouse monoclonal anti-rat Cluster of Differentiation 68 (CD68) antibody (AbD Serotec MCA341GA, Kidlington, UK; dilution 1:50), rabbit polyclonal anti rat Bone Morphogenetic Protein 2 (BMP2) antibody (Abcam 14933, Cambridge/MA, USA; dilution 1:250), and mouse monoclonal anti-rat von Willebrand Factor (vWF) antibody (DAKO A0082, Carpinteria/CA, USA; dilution 1:200) were all applied for 1 hour at room temperature. A biotinylated secondary antibody and the enzyme conjugate were applied for 10 minutes each, followed by 3 min with the AEC chromogen substrate (Histostain-SP kit, Invitrogen, Grand Island/NY, USA). Counterstaining was performed for 1 min with Mayer's hemalun (VWR, Radnor/PA, USA). Immune-staining was evaluated with an Eclipse 80i microscope light microscopy (Nikon, Tokyo, Japan).

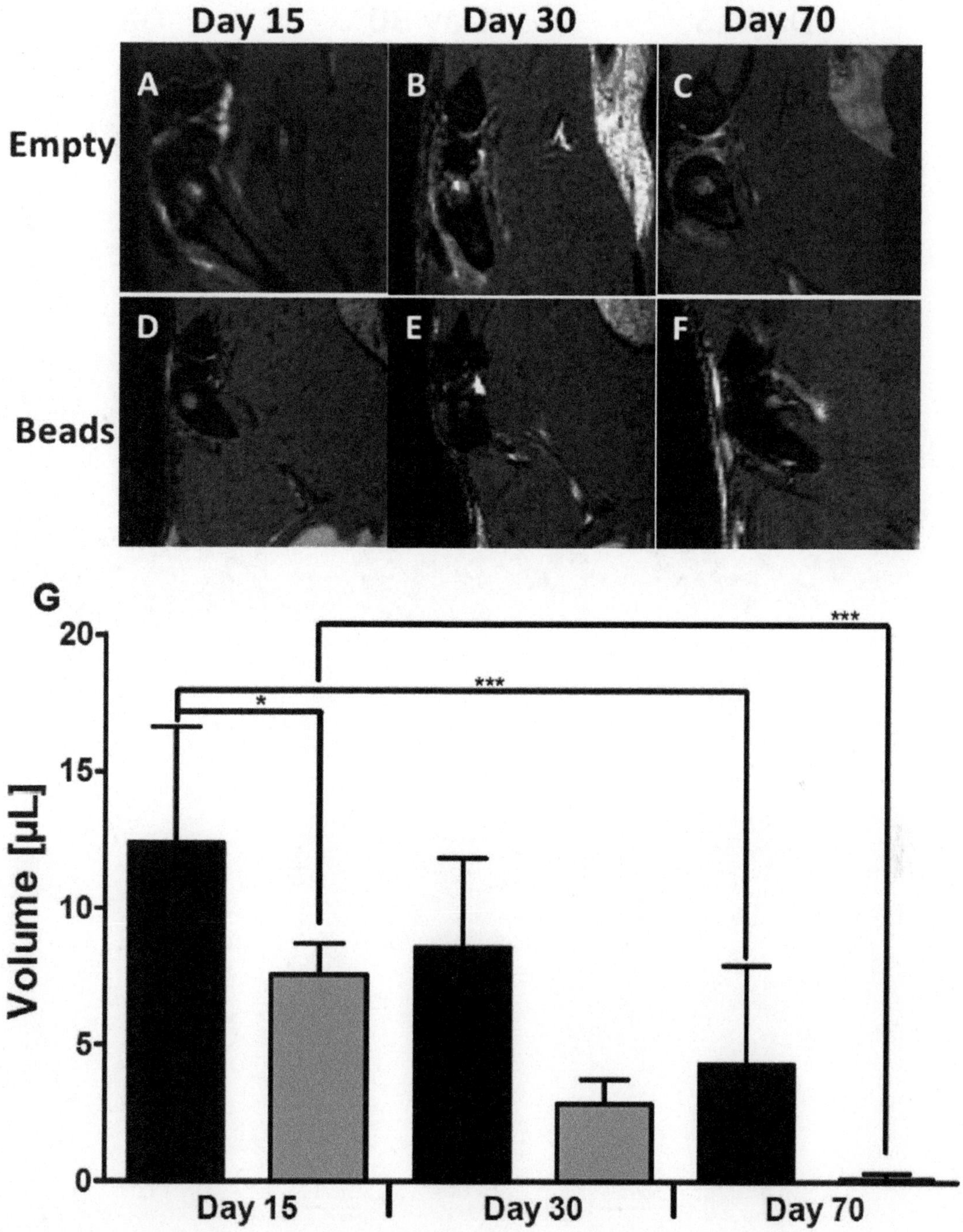

Figure 4. Representative images of MRI acquisition of condyles left empty (A–C) or after bead implantation (D–F) at 15 days (A, D), 30 days (B, E), and 70 days (C, F) after surgery. Quantification of the aqueous volume in µL of a fixed region of interest in defects that were left empty (black columns) or received the beads (grey columns), as obtained by longitudinal *in vivo* follow-up by Magnetic Resonance Imaging (G). Results are presented as means ± SD of 6 samples and significant differences are indicated with * $p \leq 0.05$, and *** $p \leq 0.001$.

Histomorphometry

The percentage of newly formed osteoid tissue in defects filled with beads was determined from histological paraffin sections using NIS-Elements software (Nikon, Japan). Osteoid formation that was stained in dark red by Trichrome's Masson staining protocol using 2 volumes of 1% (v/v) Fushine acid and 3 volumes of 1% (v/v) Xylidine Ponceau, was detected semi-automatically by the software. For samples that were left empty, the surface of osteoid was expressed as a percentage of defect surface. For samples that received the beads, two analyses were performed. Once, we performed the same analysis and once we took into account the invading tissue only, subtracting the surface of the beads from the defect surface. Histologically stained slides from three samples per condition were processed for analysis, and 12 to 19 sections were analyzed per condition. Results are shown as means with standard deviation per condition.

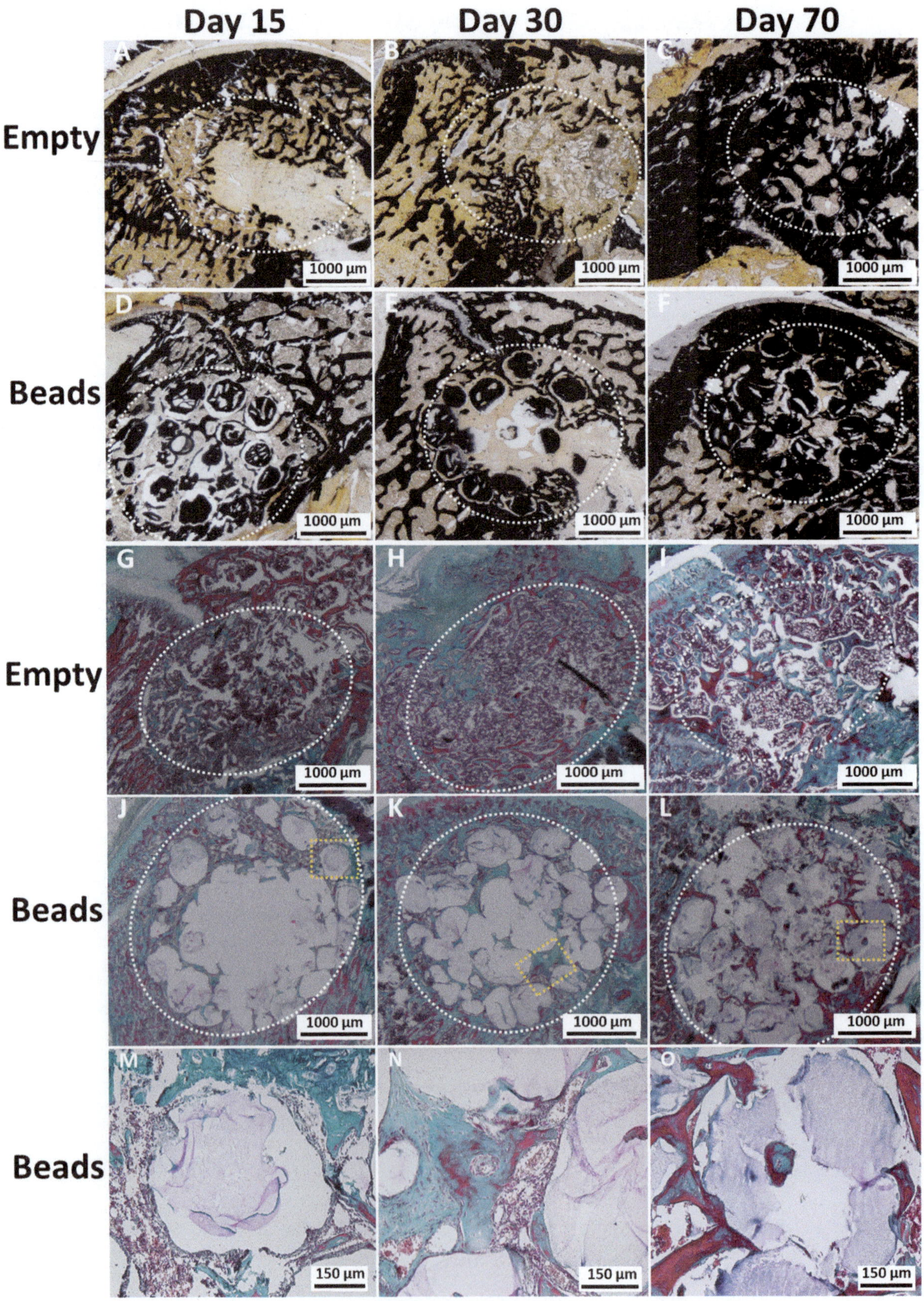

Figure 5. Representative images of histological staining of defects that were left empty (A–C, G–I) and for defects that received beads as implants (D–F, J–O). Calcified sections were stained with Von Kossa (A–F), while decalcified sections were stained with Masson's Trichrome (G–O). Increase of mineralization is visible over time when comparing sections obtained at day 15 (A, D, G, J) with sections of day 30 (B, E,

H, K) or those of day 70 (C, F, I, L). Areas of defects are marked with the dotted white line (A–L) and higher magnifications of the orange squares in J–L are shown in M–O.

Statistical analysis

Statistical significance was evaluated with a non-parametric "One-way Anova analysis of variance" followed by a Tukey's Multiple Comparison Test to compare all possible pairs of means independently, as provided by the GraphPad Prism Software (La Jolla/CA, USA). The significance level was set to alpha equal 0.05. Statistical significances are marked by stars with * indicating $p \leq 0.05$, ** $p \leq 0.01$, and *** $p \leq 0.001$.

Results

Chemical cross-linking with sodium trimetaphosphate of an alkaline solution containing NaCl as a porogen, nHA and a polysaccharide blend dispersed into canola oil under mechanical stirring allowed obtaining the beads. With this patented emulsification process [49], the resulting water-insoluble spherical beads were calibrated according to their size and then freeze-dried. The beads contained 2.8±0.1% (w/v) of nanocrystalline hydroxyapatite. Beads of 300–500 µm in diameter (Figure 1A) were observed by Back-scattered Electron Microscopy (BSEM), revealing micropores and a distribution of the nHA particles within the structure (Figure 1B–D).

2D images of 3D Micro-CT reconstructed femoral condyles after implantation of the beads in comparison with defects left empty revealed that mineralization occurred in both groups, empty defect and defect filled with beads. In the median of the defect, there was an increase in mineralized tissue over time of implantation (day 15 through day 70) (Figure 2) that seemed more pronounced and occurred faster for samples that received beads (Figure 2 D–F) than for defects that were left empty (Figure 2 A–C). At day 15, fine trabecular-like structures were only visible around the beads. These trabecular-like structures became more sophisticated over time. Empty defects showed little mineralization in the median of the defect after 30 days after implantation,

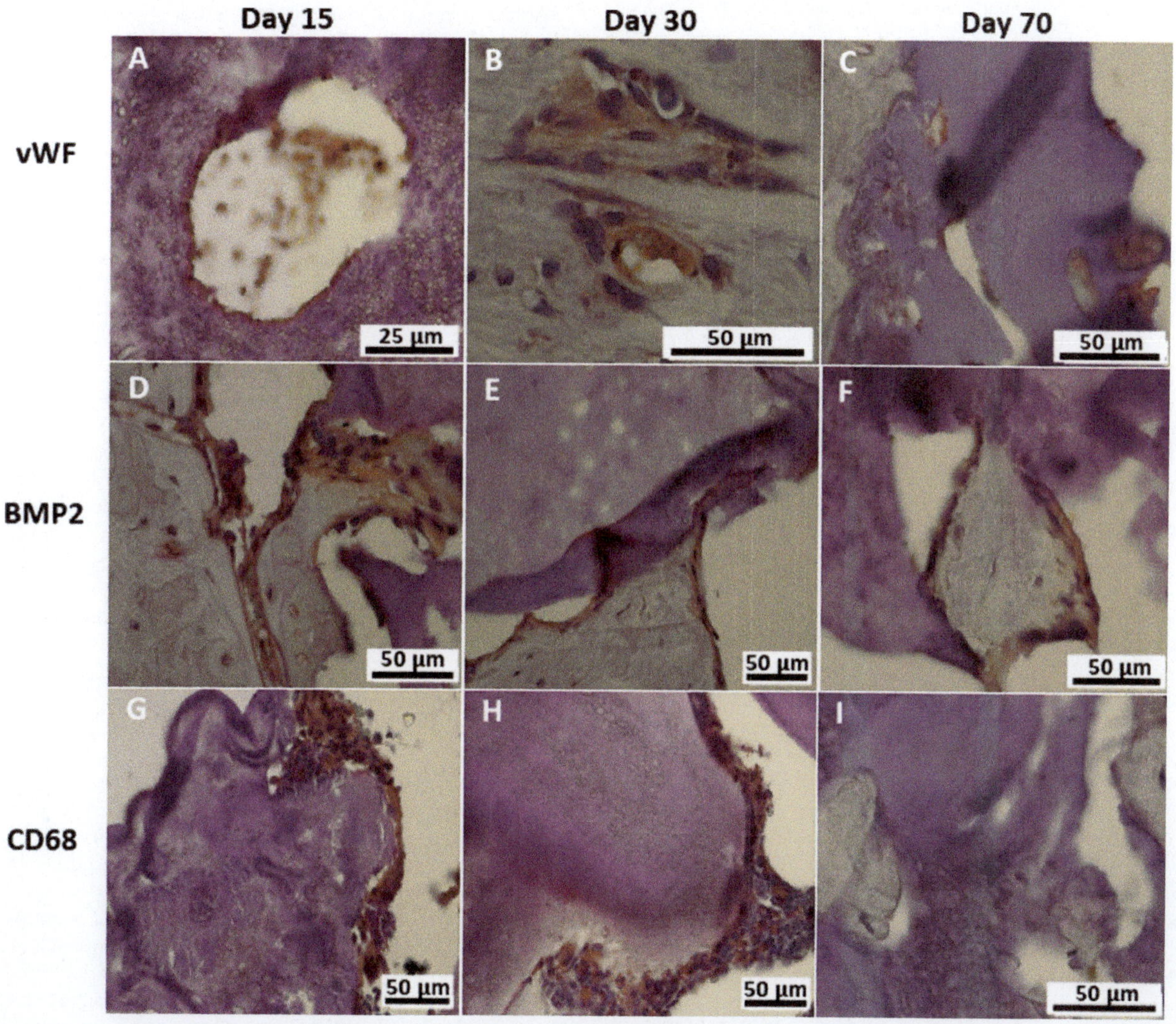

Figure 6. Representative images of immune-staining for cells in contact with the biomaterial using primary antibodies for von Willebrand Factor (A–C), Bone Morphogenetic Protein 2 (D–F) and CD 68 (G–I). Positive cells appear in brown and nuclei in dark blue.

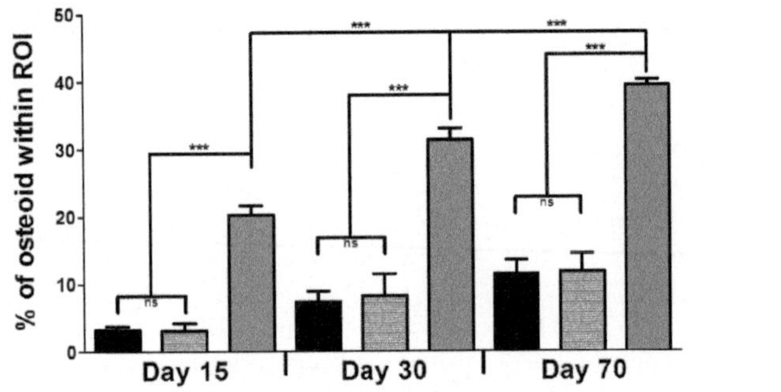

Figure 7. Histomorphometric analysis of newly formed osteoid in defects that were left empty (black columns) or received the beads (striped and grey columns). Osteoid surface over defect surface was expressed in percentage of osteoid within the region of interest (ROI), that was either the entire defect surface (black and striped columns) or the tissue surface around the beads (grey columns). Results are presented as means ± SD of 3 conditions and significant differences are indicated with *** $p \leq 0.001$.

starting from the periphery of the defects. At day 70, mineralization in form of trabecular structures was visible within the defect site.

When evaluating Bone Mineral density (BMD) and Bone Mineral Content (BMC), there were no statistically significant differences between the empty defects and the defects that received the beads at day 15 and day 30. Values were strongly increased at day 70 for samples treated with beads in comparison to the empty defects ($p \leq 0.01$) (Figure 3). When evaluating BMD and BMC for the samples that received beads, a significant increase was seen when comparing the two earlier with the latest time point.

Longitudinal *in vivo* follow-up by MRI did not reveal an inflammation in any of the conditions (Figure 4 A–F). The quantification of the aqueous volume showed a decrease for both conditions (Figure 4G). There were significant differences between the earliest and the latest time point for the two conditions ($p \leq 0.001$) and between the two conditions at day 15 ($p \leq 0.05$). Histological analysis did not reveal signs of inflammation at day 15 or at later time points (Figure 5). For defects that were left empty (Figure 5 A–C, G–I), cellularisation and mineralization started from the periphery of the defect. A similar process was observed with the beads, but cellular invasion also occurred within the defect (Figure 5 D–F, J–O).

Cellularisation of the material by endothelial cells forming vessels started within the first 15 days (Figure 6 A). Vessels were detected by vWF immune-staining in the trabecular-like structures (Figure 6 B) as well as within the material (Figure 6 A, C). BMP-2 positive cells secreting extracellular matrix were present at any time point, lining the trabecular-like structures, as well as in contact with the material (Figure 6 D–F). CD68 positive cells occurred mainly at the two earlier time points (Figure 6 G, H), while there was little presence of those cells at the latest time point (Figure 6 I). CD68 positive cells were seen in direct contact with the material.

Cellularisation was fully completed by day 70 for both conditions (Figure 5 I, L), but with different cellular structures. For the samples implanted with beads, cellular structures filled out all spaces between the beads with increasing interconnectivity and trabecular-like organization over time (Figure 5 D–F, J–L). Empty defects at day 15 after implantation showed few interconnected structures (Figure 5 A, G) and fibrosis that was still present at day 30 (Figure 5 H). At day 70, connective tissues were still visible, but most of the defect was filled with mineralized, trabecular structures (Figure 5 C, I). As it was seen in Von Kossa stained sections, the beads themselves, as well as the trabecular structures mineralized over time (Figure 5 D–F). Histomorphometric analysis of the newly formed tissue within the defect showed no significant difference at all time points between the two conditions when the percentage of osteoid surface was directly calculated within the surface of the entire defect (Figure 7). However, there was a significantly higher percentage of osteoid tissue formation at each time point when the surface of the beats was first subtracted from the defect surface in comparison to the empty defects (Figure 7). For the two calculations concerning the beads, there was a significant increase over time, while the increase in osteoid formation in empty defects was non-significant (not indicated in Figure 7).

Discussion

In the present study, macroporous cross-linked beads based on a mixture of pullulan and dextran [49,52] in association with nHA were used as a scaffold. This new scaffold, with injectable properties, was evaluated in a non-critical size bone defect, matching most clinical needs for small size defects.

Although most biomaterials are tested in critical-size defects, surgeons are often in need of materials to simply fill-up a small size defect that may not always be of a critical size [53]. The material tested in this experiment was previously implanted in the form of cylinders of 5 mm diameter and 6 mm depth in a critical size defect in rat femoral condyles and showed osteoconductive properties [36]. The goal of the present study was to investigate whether the material could modulate bone formation in a spontaneous bone regeneration model i.e. non-critical size defect to guide and activate bone mineralization and bone regeneration. The material was tested in the form of beads of 300–500 μm in diameter (Figure 1) to adapt to small size defect.

To fit specific needs for small size defects, the use of beads seems preferable. Scaffolds can be produced in any shape, but the advantage of small size beads is their capability to entirely fill up bone defects. The presented beads are sieved and can be produced at any desired diameter. In a previous study, the presented composite materials were used in the form of macroporous 3D cylinders [36], that showed limited access to invading cells and was therefore less cellularized than the material in the form of beads.

Although mineralization seemed to increase visually over time (Figure 2), it did not progress in the same way for the two conditions. It is known that defects left empty progress in bone repair from the periphery [54]. For that reason, the defects stayed rather empty in the median plan for the first 30 days (Figure 2 A, B). The presence of the beads seemed to allow a mineralization even within the defect; because trabecular-like structures were visible as early as 15 days after implantation (Figure 2 D). Thus, the material was used as a support for the invading cells, allowing a faster ingrowth of trabecular-like structures. Although those structures were less present within defects that were left empty, there was no significant difference for the BMC and the BMD in comparison with defects loaded with the material at day 15 and day 30. This is due to the fact that the entire defect was taken into account for the analysis and the defects left empty still repaired from the periphery. At day 70, bone repair was completed for the two conditions and BMC and BMD were significantly higher in the defect loaded with the beads. Overall, these results indicate that mineralization was delayed in empty defects in comparison with the condition that received the material. This indicates that beads of pullulan-dextran-nHA are suitable for a non-critical size defect and that mineralization was favored in the presence of the material.

As shown by histology, invading cells penetrated the scaffold within the first 15 days (Figure 5 J, M). Although pore sizes of the material were not investigated in this study, the beads allowed an attachment of invading cells, as cells, including vWF and BMP-2 positive cells, were visible in direct contact with the material at all time points (Figure 5 M–O, Figure 6). At day 30, Masson's Trichrome stained sections (Figure 5 H) showed the presence of fibrous tissue that was not seen at any time point with the beads, allowing a better cellularisation of the defect. Similar results concerning tissue preservation and bone formation were observed with Bio-Oss® collagen (Geistlich, Wolhausen, Switzerland) that contains demineralized bovine bone, considered as the gold standard biomaterial for alveolar sockets implantations to promote bone formation and ridge preservation [55]. In that study, non-critical-size defects in the extraction sockets of dogs were either filled with the material or left empty. Although the material did not enhance new bone formation, the profile of the ridge was better preserved with the graft.

As seen by immune-staining with a macrophage marker, CD68 positive cells were mainly seen at the two earlier time points (Figure 6 G, H). This is due to the cascade of events that is involved in inflammatory and wound healing responses following biomaterial implantation [56]. Directly after the implantation, polynuclear cells, monocytes and lymphocytes invade the defect site. The presence of a biomaterial as a foreign body provokes the infiltration with macrophages that differentiate and fuse to giant cells like osteoclasts at the end of the acute phase of the inflammation. At day 70, those processes are finished and CD68 positive cells are therefore no longer present.

MRI acquisition indicated a decrease of aqueous content over time for the two conditions (Figure 3 G), probably due to an increasing mineralization of the defect site over time, as seen by Micro-CT analysis. Although indicated in the graph, a direct comparison of the two conditions should be avoided, since the offset for the aqueous volume was not comparable for the two conditions. We did not measure the volume immediately after implantation because the animals were not transportable due to ethical reasons.

When analyzing Bone mineral density (BMD) and Bone mineral content (BMC), either the full defect or an area of interest, the distinction between newly formed bone and the biomaterial itself was difficult, since most micro-CT software choose thresholds representing the mineralized tissue. In the case of a biomaterial made of calcium phosphate containing hydroxyapatite, thresholding methods also capture the scaffold material in addition to the surrounding bone, as the densities of the bead material overlaps the heterogeneous densities found in bone and forming bone. We therefore decided to perform a histomorphometric analysis based on decalcified histological sections stained for osteoid tissue whose overall percentage was analyzed for the surface of the defect. While BMD and BMC values indicated an overall trend when using CaP based biomaterials, the histomorphometric analysis allows a more precise view on cellular processes. The main interest in performing this study was the evaluation of the increasing mineralized tissue surrounding the beads. Increasing osteoid formation, as analyzed by histomorphometric measurements, confirmed the increasing mineralization determined by Micro-CT analysis. As mentioned for the interpretation of the MRI results, a direct comparison of the two conditions seemed difficult, because the offset is not the same. Therefore, two series of measurements were performed. When the osteoid formation was expressed as percentage of the defect surface, there was no significant difference between the two conditions. But when the surface of the beads was first subtracted from the defect surface, the percentage of osteoid formation was significantly higher in samples that received beads (Figure 7). This result shows that beads have strong osteoconductive properties. The increasing presence of forming osteoid around the beads also indicates that the overall mineralization within the defect was not only due to the increased mineralization of the biomaterial itself as was shown before in an ectopic site [36].

While dextran is already used as a biomaterial in the form of hydrogels [57,58] to deliver proteins and its synthetic derivatives can control the biological activity of growth factors [59], pullulan-based scaffolds have been evaluated more recently and studied as a support for smooth muscle cells [60]. Cylinders, disks or electrospun fibers of pullulan and dextran were evaluated *in vitro* as a composite matrix for endothelial progenitor cells [61], human dermal fibroblast [62], human bone marrow stromal cells [63], and human adipose derived stem cells [64]. The composition of the scaffold studied in the form of cylinders has shown abilities for mineralization and formation of a dense mineral collagenous tissue in both an ectopic site and a critical-sized orthotopic defect [36]. Here, we demonstrated the *in vivo* potential of pullulan-dextran-nHA beads for bone repair. It is known that materials based on polymers often need to be associated with cells or growth factors to achieve osteoconductive properties [65]. In this study, potentially injectable cell-free beads have been tested in a rat femoral medial-epicondyle defect of 3.5 mm diameter and 4 mm depth, and showed osteoconductive properties as shown by μCT, histology and histomorphometric analysis.

It is known that materials based on polymers often have inflammatory properties.

Regarding *in vivo* applications, the host response to the material is therefore an important parameter to look at [66,67]. Polymers have been studied for their inflammatory properties and i.e. PLA or chitosan are long known to enhance the functions of inflammatory cells such as macrophages [68,69], and recent studies focused on the evaluation of the influence of different acetylation degrees [70], as well as the 3D structure [71] on the inflammatory response to chitosan. Similar studies have been performed for hydroxyapatite, suggesting an influence of the material shape, size and sintering temperature on the inflammatory response [72]. The composite beads did not show an obvious inflammatory response, as investigated by MRI and histology (Figure 4 and 5), but CD68 positive cells were present as a consequence of the biomaterial implantation. A loss of aqueous volume for the two conditions was observed over time (Figure 4G). In case of a chronic inflammation, the aqueous loss would not decrease, but stay stable or even increase.

Although the present study demonstrated non-inflammatory and osteoconductive properties of the new injectable macroporous composite, improvements regarding its biodegradability, bone tissue invasion, and injectable properties are needed and ongoing. Since a cellularisation of the defect was visible and happened quite fast after implantation, it would be preferable to have beads of an injectable size that are resorbing over this time frame, to allow the replacement of the biomaterial itself by cells and extracellular matrix secreting cells. It is likely that the abundant vascularization observed inside the defect would allow a continuous infiltration of the site and a progressive replacement of the scaffold to achieve complete bone regeneration.

Conclusion

Bone formation and mineralization for the defects filled with these beads were increased in comparison to empty defects. Cellular infiltration of the defect was well organized in trabecular-like structures, suggesting the use of beads for bone repair of small size defects. The beads are of an injectable size and can therefore be used to fill-up any type of bone defect of variable size and should become useful for surgeons in clinical applications.

Acknowledgments

The authors would like to thank the French Research National Agency and the institutions of Inserm (National Institute for Health and Medical Research), University of Bordeaux, Universities of Paris 7 and Paris 13 for financial support.

Thanks to the *Laboratory Animal Care Facility* for housing and taking care of the rats. The help of Letitia Medan, Myriam Touati and their co-workers is highly acknowledged.

The authors also would like to thank *The Resource Center of Electron Microscopy and Microanalysis* (CREMEM) at the University of Bordeaux for BSEM observations.

Special thanks to Brian Christopher Dawson for proofreading the manuscript.

Author Contributions

Conceived and designed the experiments: SS SMD SM CLV DL JA JCF. Performed the experiments: SS SMD LM SM MR SC. Analyzed the data: SS SMD SM. Contributed reagents/materials/analysis tools: SS SMD SM SC. Contributed to the writing of the manuscript: SS SMD SM SC CLV DL JA JCF.

References

1. Seiler JG, Johnson J (2000) Iliac crest autogenous bone grafting: donor site complications. J South Orthop Assoc 9: 91–97.
2. LeGeros RZ (2002) Properties of osteoconductive biomaterials: calcium phosphates. Clin Orthop Relat Res 395: 81–98.
3. Stodolak-Zych E, Szumera M, Blazewicz M (2012) Osteoconductive Nanocomposite Materials for Bone Regeneration. Materials Science Forum 730–732: 38–43.
4. Barradas AMC, Yuan H, van Blitterswijk CA, Habibovic P (2011) Osteoinductive biomaterials: current knowledge of properties, experimental models and biological mechanisms. Eur Cell Mater 21: 407–429.
5. Yuan H, Fernandes H, Habibovic P, de Boer J, Barradas AMC, et al. (2010) Osteoinductive ceramics as a synthetic alternative to autologous bone grafting. Proc Natl Acad Sci U S A 107: 13614–13619.
6. Habibovic P, de Groot K (2007) Osteoinductive biomaterials-properties and relevance in bone repair. J Regen Med Tissue Eng 1: 25–32.
7. Ji W, Sun Y, Yang F, van den Beucken JJJP, Fan M, et al. (2011) Bioactive electrospun scaffolds delivering growth factors and genes for tissue engineering applications. Pharm Res 28: 1259–1272.
8. Liu J, Xu L, Li Y, Ma J (2011) Temporally controlled multiple-gene delivery in scaffolds: A promising strategy to enhance bone regeneration. Med Hypotheses 76: 173–175.
9. Porter JR, Ruckh TT, Popat KC (2009) Bone tissue engineering: a review in bone biomimetics and drug delivery strategies. Biotechnol Prog 25: 1539–1560.
10. Zhao X, Kim J, Cezar CA, Huebsch N, Lee K, et al. (2011) Active scaffolds for on-demand drug and cell delivery. Proc Natl Acad Sci U S A 108: 67–72.
11. Catros S, Guillemot F, Nandakumar A, Ziane S, Moroni L, et al. (2012) Layer-by-layer tissue microfabrication supports cell proliferation in vitro and in vivo. Tissue Eng Part C Methods 18: 62–70.
12. Garg T, Singh O, Arora S, Murthy R (2012) Scaffold: a novel carrier for cell and drug delivery. Crit Rev Ther Drug Carrier Syst 29: 1–63.
13. Bose S, Tarafder S (2012) Calcium phosphate ceramic systems in growth factor and drug delivery for bone tissue engineering: a review. Acta Biomater. 8: 1401–1421.
14. Uchida A, Nade S, McCartney E, Ching W (1985) Bone ingrowth into three different porous ceramics implanted into the tibia of rats and rabbits. J Orthop Res3: 65–77.
15. Uchida A, Nade SM, McCartney ER, Ching W (1984) The use of ceramics for bone replacement. A comparative study of three different porous ceramics. J Bone Joint Surg Br. 66: 269–275.
16. Castellani C, Zanoni G, Tangl S, van Griensven M, Redl H (2009) Biphasic calcium phosphate ceramics in small bone defects: potential influence of carrier substances and bone marrow on bone regeneration. Clin Oral Implants Res 20: 1367–1374.
17. Garrido C, Lobo SE, Turíbio FM, Legeros RZ (2011) Biphasic calcium phosphate bioceramics for orthopaedic reconstructions: clinical outcomes. Int J Biomater 2011: 129727.
18. Fricain JC, Bareille R, Ulysse F, Dupuy B, Amedee J (1998) Evaluation of proliferation and protein expression of human bone marrow cells cultured on coral crystallized in the aragonite of calcite form. J Biomed Mater Res 42: 96–102.
19. Junker R, Dimakis A, Thoneick M, Jansen J (2009) Effects of implant surface coatings and composition on bone integration: a systematic review. Clin Oral Implants Res 20 Suppl 4: 185–206.
20. Oh, Lee, Lee JH, Kim, Jang, et al. (2012) Collagen three-dimensional hydrogel matrix carrying basic fibroblast growth factor for the cultivation of mesenchymal stem cells and osteogenic differentiation. Tissue Eng Part A 18: 1087–1100.
21. Ferreira AM, Gentile P, Chiono V, Ciardelli G (2012) Collagen for bone tissue regeneration. Acta Biomater 8: 3191–3200.
22. Chen F, Wu Z, Wang Q, Wu H, Zhang Y, et al. (2005) Preparation of recombinant human bone morphogenetic protein-2 loaded dextran-based microspheres and their characteristics. Acta Pharmacol Sin 26: 1093–1103.
23. Costa-Pinto AR, Reis RL, Neves NM (2011) Scaffolds based bone tissue engineering: the role of chitosan. Tissue Eng Part B Rev 17: 331–347.
24. Zhou H, Xu HHK (2011) The fast release of stem cells from alginate-fibrin microbeads in injectable scaffolds for bone tissue engineering. Biomaterials 32: 7503–7513.
25. Kretlow JD, Mikos AG (2007) Review: mineralization of synthetic polymer scaffolds for bone tissue engineering. Tissue Eng 13: 927–938.
26. Dhandayuthapani B, Yoshida Y, Maekawa T, Kumar DS (2011) Polymeric Scaffolds in Tissue Engineering Application: A Review. Int J Polym Sc 2011: 1–19.
27. Mallick KK, Cox SC (2013) Biomaterial scaffolds for tissue engineering. Front Biosci 5: 341–360.
28. Borden M, Attawia M, Khan Y, El-Amin SF, Laurencin CT (2004) Tissue-engineered bone formation in vivo using a novel sintered polymeric microsphere matrix. J Bone Joint Surg Br. 86: 1200–1208.
29. Dragoo JL, Choi JY, Lieberman JR, Huang J, Zuk P, et al. (2003) Bone induction by BMP-2 transduced stem cells derived from human fat. J Orthop Res 21: 622–629.
30. Cho MH, Kim KS, Ahn HH, Kim MS, Kim SH, et al. (2008) Chitosan gel as an in situ-forming scaffold for rat bone marrow mesenchymal stem cells in vivo. Tissue Eng Part A 14: 1099–1108.
31. Grellier M, Granja PL, Fricain JC, Bidarra SJ, Renard M, et al. (2009) The effect of the co-immobilization of human osteoprogenitors and endothelial cells within alginate microspheres on mineralization in a bone defect. Biomaterials 30: 3271–3278.
32. Kolambkar YM, Dupont KM, Boerckel JD, Huebsch N, Mooney DJ, et al. (2011) An alginate-based hybrid system for growth factor delivery in the functional repair of large bone defects. Biomaterials 32: 65–74.
33. Swetha M, Sahithi K, Moorthi A, Srinivasan N, Ramasamy K, et al. (2010) Biocomposites containing natural polymers and hydroxyapatite for bone tissue engineering. Int J Biol Macromol 47: 1–4.
34. Cao H, Kuboyama N (2010) A biodegradable porous composite scaffold of PGA/beta-TCP for bone tissue engineering. Bone 46: 386–395.
35. Winter GD, Simpson BJ (1969) Heterotopic bone formed in a synthetic sponge in the skin of young pigs. Nature 223: 88–90.
36. Fricain JC, Schlaubitz S, Le Visage C, Arnault I, Derkaoui SM, et al. (2013) A nano-hydroxyapatite–pullulan/dextran polysaccharide composite macroporous material for bone tissue engineering. Biomaterials 34: 2947–2959.
37. Zheng H, Bai Y, Shih, Hoffmann C, Peters F, et al. (2014) Effect of a β-TCP collagen composite bone substitute on healing of drilled bone voids in the distal femoral condyle of rabbits. J Biomed Mater Res B Appl Biomater 102: 376–383.
38. Kim, Ahn, Park MS, Lee, Choi CY, et al. (2007) A poly(lactide-co-glycolide)/hydroxyapatite composite scaffold with enhanced osteoconductivity. J Biomed Mater Res A 80: 206–215.
39. Barbieri D, Renard JS, de Bruijn JD, Yuan H (2010) Heterotopic bone formation by nano-apatite containing poly(D,L-lactide) composites. Eur Cell Mater 19: 252–261.
40. Tsai C, Chou M, Jonas M, Tien Y, Chi EY (2002) A composite graft material containing bone particles and collagen in osteoinduction in mouse. J Biomed Mater Res 63: 65–70.
41. Wu D, Hao A, Zhang C, Cui F, Wang X, et al. (2012) [Promoting of angiogenesis and osteogenesis in radial critical bone defect regions of rabbits with nano-hydroxyapatite/collagen/PLA scaffolds plus endothelial progenitor cells]. Zhonghua Yi Xue Za Zhi 92: 1630–1634.
42. Daculsi G, Uzel AP, Weiss P, Goyenvalle E, Aguado E (2010) Developments in injectable multiphasic biomaterials. The performance of microporous biphasic calcium phosphate granules and hydrogels. J Mater Sci Mater Med 21: 855–861.

43. Weiss P, Layrolle P, Clergeau LP, Enckel B, Pilet P, et al. (2007) The safety and efficacy of an injectable bone substitute in dental sockets demonstrated in a human clinical trial. Biomaterials 28: 3295–3305.
44. Matsuno T, Hashimoto Y, Adachi S, Omata K, Yoshitaka Y, et al. (2008) Preparation of injectable 3D-formed beta-tricalcium phosphate bead/alginate composite for bone tissue engineering. Dent Mater J 27: 827–834.
45. Chen Y, Huang Z, Li X, Li S, Zhou Z, et al. (2012) In Vitro Biocompatibility and Osteoblast Differentiation of an Injectable Chitosan/Nano-Hydroxyapatite/Collagen Scaffold. J Nanomater 2012: 1–6. doi:10.1155/2012/401084.
46. Zhao H, Ma L, Gao C, Wang J, Shen J (2009) Fabrication and properties of injectable β-tricalcium phosphate particles/fibrin gel composite scaffolds for bone tissue engineering. Mater Sci Eng C Mater Biol Appl 29: 836–842.
47. Catros S, Guillemot F, Lebraud E, Chanseau C, Perez S, et al. (2010) Physico-chemical and biological properties of a nano-hydroxyapatite powder synthesized at room temperature. IRBM 31: 226–233.
48. Afshar a, Ghorbani M, Ehsani N, Saeri M, Sorrell C (2003) Some important factors in the wet precipitation process of hydroxyapatite. Mater Des 24: 197–202.
49. Letourneur D, Le Visage C, Derkaoui SM (2012) Crosslinked Polysaccharide Beads and their biomedical Uses. Available: http://patentscope.wipo.int/search/en/detail.jsf?docId=WO2012028623&recNum=195&maxRec=19887&office=&prevFilter=&sortOption=&queryString=calcitonin*+or+parathyroid*+or+pth+or+thrombomodulin*+or+milnacipran*+or+naftopidil*+or+fusudil*+or+mizoribin*+or+bredinin*&tab=PCT+Biblio. Accessed: 2012 March 08.
50. Miraux S, Massot P, Ribot EJ, Franconi, Thiaudiere E (2008) 3D TrueFISP imaging of mouse brain at 4.7T and 9.4 T. J Magn Reson Imaging 28: 497–503.
51. Parfitt AM, Drezner MK, Glorieux FH, Kanis JA, Malluche H, et al. (1987) Bone histomorphometry: standardization of nomenclature, symbols, and units. Report of the ASBMR Histomorphometry Nomenclature Committee. J Bone Miner Res 2: 595–610.
52. Abed A, Assoul N, Ba M, Derkaoui SM, Portes P, et al. (2011) Influence of polysaccharide composition on the biocompatibility of pullulan/dextran-based hydrogels. J Biomed Mater Res A 96: 535–542.
53. Bongio M, van den Beucken JJJP, Leeuwenburgh SCG, Jansen JA (2012) Preclinical evaluation of injectable bone substitute materials. J Tissue Eng Regen Med doi: 10.1002/term.1637.
54. Monfoulet L, Rabier B, Chassande O, Fricain JC (2010) Drilled hole defects in mouse femur as models of intramembranous cortical and cancellous bone regeneration. Calcif Tissue Int 86: 72–81.
55. Araújo MG, Lindhe J (2009) Ridge preservation with the use of Bio-Oss collagen: A 6-month study in the dog. Clin Oral Implants Res 20: 433–440.
56. Anderson JM, Rodriguez A, Chang DT (2008) Foreign body reaction to biomaterials. Semin Immunol 20: 86–100.
57. Van Tomme SR, Hennink WE (2007) Biodegradable dextran hydrogels for protein delivery applications. Expert Rev Med Devices 4: 147–164.
58. Rekha MR, Sharma CP (2007) Pullulan as a Promising Biomaterial for Biomedical Applications: A Perspective. Trends in Biomater Artif Organs 20: 111–116.
59. Degat, Dubreucq G, Meunier A, Dahri-Correia L, Sedel L, et al. (2009) Enhancement of the biological activity of BMP-2 by synthetic dextran derivatives. J Biomed Mater Res A 88: 174–183.
60. Autissier A, Letourneur D, Le Visage C (2007) Pullulan-based hydrogel for smooth muscle cell culture. J Biomed Mater Res A 82: 336–342.
61. Thébaud, Pierron D, Bareille R, Le Visage C, Letourneur D, et al. (2007) Human endothelial progenitor cell attachment to polysaccharide-based hydrogels: a pre-requisite for vascular tissue engineering. J Mater Sci Mater Med 18: 339–345.
62. Shi L, Le Visage C, Chew SY (2011) Long-term stabilization of polysaccharide electrospun fibres by in situ cross-linking. J Biomater Sci Polym Ed 22: 1459–1472.
63. Guerrero J, Catros S, Derkaoui SM, Lalande C, Siadous R, et al. (2013) Cell interactions between human progenitor-derived endothelial cells and human mesenchymal stem cells in a three-dimensional macroporous polysaccharide-based scaffold promote osteogenesis. Acta biomater 9: 8200–8213.
64. Lalande C, Miraux S, Derkaoui SM, Mornet S, Bareille R, et al. (2011) Magnetic resonance imaging tracking of human adipose derived stromal cells within three-dimensional scaffolds for bone tissue engineering. Eur Cell Mater 21: 341–354.
65. Janicki P, Schmidmaier G (2011) What should be the characteristics of the ideal bone graft substitute? Combining scaffolds with growth factors and/or stem cells. Injury 42 Suppl 2: S77–81.
66. Franz S, Rammelt S, Scharnweber D, Simon JC (2011) Immune responses to implants - a review of the implications for the design of immunomodulatory biomaterials. Biomaterials 32: 6692–6709.
67. Babensee J, Anderson J, McIntire L, Mikos A (1998) Host response to tissue engineered devices. Adv Drug Deliv Rev 33: 111–139.
68. Porporatto C, Bianco ID, Riera CM, Correa SG (2003) Chitosan induces different l-arginine metabolic pathways in resting and inflammatory macrophages. Biochem Biophys Res Commun 304: 266–272.
69. Vasconcelos DP, Fonseca AC, Costa M, Amaral IF, Barbosa M, et al. (2013) Macrophage polarization following chitosan implantation. Biomaterials 34: 9952–9959.
70. Barbosa JN, Amaral IF, Aguas AP, Barbosa MA (2010) Evaluation of the effect of the degree of acetylation on the inflammatory response to 3D porous chitosan scaffolds. J Biomed Mater Res A 93: 20–28.
71. Almeida CR, Serra T, Oliveira MI, Planell J, Barbosa M, et al. (2014) Impact of 3-D printed PLA and chitosan-based scaffolds on human monocyte/macrophage responses: Unraveling the effect of 3-D structures on inflammation. Acta biomater 10: 613–622.
72. Laquerriere P, Grandjean-Laquerriere A, Addadi-Rebbah S, Jallot E, Laurent-Maquin D, et al. (2004) MMP-2, MMP-9 and their inhibitors TIMP-2 and TIMP-1 production by human monocytes in vitro in the presence of different forms of hydroxyapatite particles. Biomaterials 25: 2515–2524.

Permissions

All chapters in this book were first published in PLOS ONE, by The Public Library of Science; hereby published with permission under the Creative Commons Attribution License or equivalent. Every chapter published in this book has been scrutinized by our experts. Their significance has been extensively debated. The topics covered herein carry significant findings which will fuel the growth of the discipline. They may even be implemented as practical applications or may be referred to as a beginning point for another development.

The contributors of this book come from diverse backgrounds, making this book a truly international effort. This book will bring forth new frontiers with its revolutionizing research information and detailed analysis of the nascent developments around the world.

We would like to thank all the contributing authors for lending their expertise to make the book truly unique. They have played a crucial role in the development of this book. Without their invaluable contributions this book wouldn't have been possible. They have made vital efforts to compile up to date information on the varied aspects of this subject to make this book a valuable addition to the collection of many professionals and students.

This book was conceptualized with the vision of imparting up-to-date information and advanced data in this field. To ensure the same, a matchless editorial board was set up. Every individual on the board went through rigorous rounds of assessment to prove their worth. After which they invested a large part of their time researching and compiling the most relevant data for our readers.

The editorial board has been involved in producing this book since its inception. They have spent rigorous hours researching and exploring the diverse topics which have resulted in the successful publishing of this book. They have passed on their knowledge of decades through this book. To expedite this challenging task, the publisher supported the team at every step. A small team of assistant editors was also appointed to further simplify the editing procedure and attain best results for the readers.

Apart from the editorial board, the designing team has also invested a significant amount of their time in understanding the subject and creating the most relevant covers. They scrutinized every image to scout for the most suitable representation of the subject and create an appropriate cover for the book.

The publishing team has been an ardent support to the editorial, designing and production team. Their endless efforts to recruit the best for this project, has resulted in the accomplishment of this book. They are a veteran in the field of academics and their pool of knowledge is as vast as their experience in printing. Their expertise and guidance has proved useful at every step. Their uncompromising quality standards have made this book an exceptional effort. Their encouragement from time to time has been an inspiration for everyone.

The publisher and the editorial board hope that this book will prove to be a valuable piece of knowledge for researchers, students, practitioners and scholars across the globe.

List of Contributors

Chunlan Huang, Ming Xue, Hongli Chen, Regis J. O'Keefe and Xinping Zhang
Center for Musculoskeletal Research, University of Rochester, School of Medicine and Dentistry, Rochester, New York, United States of America

Jing Jiao and Harvey R. Herschman
Department of Molecular and Medical Pharmacology, David Geffen School of Medicine, University of California Los Angeles, Los Angeles, California, United States of America

Albrecht W. Popp, Helene Buffat and Kurt Lippuner
Department of Osteoporosis, Inselspital, Berne University Hospital and University of Berne, Berne, Switzerland

Ursula Eberli, Manuela Ernst, R. Geoff Richards, Vincent A. Stadelmann and Markus Windolf
AO Research Institute Davos, Davos, Switzerland

Yi-Jie Kuo
Department of Orthopaedic, Taipei Medical University Hospital, Taipei, Taiwan, Republic of China
Institute of Clinical Medicine, National Yang Ming University, Taipei, Taiwan, Republic of China

Fon-Yih Tsuang
Division of Neurosurgery, Department of Surgery, National Taiwan University Hospital, Taipei, Taiwan, Republic of China

Jui-Sheng Sun
Department of Orthopaedic Surgery, National Taiwan University Hospital-Hsin Chu, Hsin-Chu, Taiwan, Republic of China
Graduate Institute of Clinical Medicine, College of Medicine, Taipei Medical University, Taipei, Taiwan, Republic of China

Chi-Hung Lin and Chia-Hsien Chen
Institute of Microbiology and Immunology, National Yang Ming University, Taipei, Taiwan, Republic of China

Jia-Ying Li and Wei-Yu Chen
Department of Biology and Anatomy, National Defense Medical Center, Taipei, Taiwan, Republic of China

Yi-Chian Huang
Institute of Anatomy and Cell Biology National Yang Ming University, Taipei, Taiwan, Republic of China

Chin-Bin Yeh
Department of Psychiatry, Tri-Service General Hospital, Taipei, Taiwan, Republic of China Abstract

Jia-Fwu Shyu
Department of Biology and Anatomy, National Defense Medical Center, Taipei, Taiwan, Republic of China
Department of Psychiatry, Tri-Service General Hospital, Taipei, Taiwan, Republic of China Abstract

Nicolas Bonnet and Serge Ferrari
Division of Bone Diseases, Department of Internal Medicine Specialties, Geneva University Hospital, Geneva, Switzerland

Jean Louis Saffar
Laboratoire Pathologies, Imagerie et Biothérapie de l'organe dentaire EA 2496, UniversitéParis Descartes, Faculté de Chirurgie Dentaire, Paris, France

Philippe Lesclous
Laboratoire Pathologies, Imagerie et Biothérapie de l'organe dentaire EA 2496, Université Paris-Descartes, Faculté de Chirurgie Dentaire, Paris, France
INSERM-UMRS 791, LIOAD: Laboratoire d'Ingénierie Ostéo-Articulaire et Dentaire, STEP: Skeletal Tissue Engineering and Physiopathology group, Nantes University, School of Dentistry, Hôtel Dieu Hospital, LUNAM Université, Nantes, France

David L. Boyle, Deepa Hammaker, Meghan Edgar and Gary S. Firestein
Medicine, University of California San Diego, La Jolla, California, United States of America

Mario M. Zaiss
Global Health Institute, École Polytechnique Fédèrale de Lausanne, Switzerland

Stefan Teufel and Jean Pierre David
Institute of Osteology and Biomechanics, University Medical Center Hamburg-Eppendorf, Hamburg, Germany

Georg Schett
Department of Internal Medicine 3,University of Erlangen-Nuremberg, Friedrich Alexander University, Erlangen, Germany

Xiaohua Wu, Shi Chen, Yongzheng He, Xiaohong Li, Xianlin Yang, Li Jiang, D. Wade Clapp and Paige Snider
Department of Pediatrics, Indiana University School of Medicine, Indianapolis, Indiana, United States of America
Herman B Wells Center for Pediatric Research, Indiana University School of Medicine, Indianapolis, Indiana, United States of America

Steven D. Rhodes
Herman B Wells Center for Pediatric Research, Indiana University School of Medicine, Indianapolis, Indiana, United States of America
Anatomy and Cell Biology, Indiana University School of Medicine, Indianapolis, Indiana, United States of America

Alexander G. Robling
Anatomy and Cell Biology, Indiana University School of Medicine, Indianapolis, Indiana, United States of America

Khalid S. Mohammad and Theresa A. Guise
Endocrinology and Metabolism, Department of Internal Medicine, Indiana University School of Medicine, Indianapolis, Indiana, United States of America

Simon J. Conway and Feng-Chun Yang
Department of Pediatrics, Indiana University School of Medicine, Indianapolis, Indiana, United States of America
Herman B Wells Center for Pediatric Research, Indiana University School of Medicine, Indianapolis, Indiana, United States of America
Anatomy and Cell Biology, Indiana University School of Medicine, Indianapolis, Indiana, United States of America

Grzegorz Nalepa
Department of Pediatrics, Indiana University School of Medicine, Indianapolis, Indiana, United States of America

Herman B Wells Center for Pediatric Research, Indiana University School of Medicine, Indianapolis, Indiana, United States of America
Pediatric Hematology-Oncology, Indiana University School of Medicine, Indianapolis, Indiana, United States of America

Jeong-Tae Yeon, Kwang-Jin Kim and Young-Jin Son
Research Institute of Basic Science, Sunchon National University, Suncheon, Republic of Korea

Sik-Won Choi and Byung Jun Ryu
Laboratory of Translational Therapeutics, Pharmacology Research Center, Division of Drug Discovery Research, Korea Research Institute of Chemical Technology, Daejeon, Republic of Korea

Seong-Hee Moon
Laboratory of Translational Therapeutics, Pharmacology Research Center, Division of Drug Discovery Research, Korea Research Institute of Chemical Technology, Daejeon, Republic of Korea
Department of Biology, Chungnam National University, Daejeon, Republic of Korea

Young Sik Park
Herbal Medicine Research Division, National Institute of Food & Drug Safety Evaluation, Cheongwon, Republic of Korea
Graduate School of New Drug Discovery and Development, Chungnam National University, Daejeon, Republic of Korea

Seong Hwan Kim
Laboratory of Translational Therapeutics, Pharmacology Research Center, Division of Drug Discovery Research, Korea Research Institute of Chemical Technology, Daejeon, Republic of Korea
Graduate School of New Drug Discovery and Development, Chungnam National University, Daejeon, Republic of Korea

Jaemin Oh
Department of Anatomy & Institute for Skeletal Diseases, School of Medicine, Wongkwang University, Iksan, Republic of Korea

Min Seuk Kim and Munkhsoyol Erkhembaatar
Department of Oral Physiology, School of Dentistry, Wongkwang University, Iksan, Republic of Korea

Elizabeth Rendina, Kelsey D. Hembree, McKale R. Davis, Stephen L. Clarke, Edralin A. Lucas and Brenda J. Smith
Department of Nutritional Sciences, Oklahoma State University, Stillwater, Oklahoma, United States of America

Denver Marlow
Comparative Medicine Group, Kansas State University, Manhattan, Kansas, United States of America

Bernard P. Halloran
Veterans Affairs Medical Center, University of California San Francisco, San Francisco, California, United States of America

Laufey Steingrimsdottir and Thorhallur I. Halldorsson
Unit for Nutrition Research, University of Iceland and Landspitali University Hospital, Reykjavik, Iceland

Kristin Siggeirsdottir, Berglind O. Einarsdottir, Gudny Eiriksdottir and Sigurdur Sigurdsson
Icelandic Heart Association Research Institute, Kopavogur, Iceland

Lenore J. Launer and Tamara B. Harris
Intramural Research Program, Laboratory of Epidemiology, Demography and Biometry, National Institute of Aging, Bethesda, Maryland, United States of America

Mary Frances Cotch
Division of Epidemiology and Clinical Applications, National Eye Institute, Bethesda, Maryland, United States of America

Vilmundur Gudnason and Gunnar Sigurdsson
Icelandic Heart Association Research Institute, Kopavogur, Iceland
University of Iceland, Reykjavik, Iceland

Fiona E. McGuigan
Clinical and Molecular Osteoporosis Research Unit, Department of Clinical Sciences, Lund University, Sweden

Maria Swanberg
Clinical and Molecular Osteoporosis Research Unit, Department of Clinical Sciences, Lund University, Sweden

Neurodegeneration and Inflammation Genetics Unit, Department of Experimental Medical Science, Lund University, Sweden

Kaisa K. Ivaska
Department of Cell Biology and Anatomy, Institute of Biomedicine, University of Turku, Turku, Finland

Paul Gerdhem
Department of Clinical Science, Intervention and Technology, Karolinska Institute, Stockholm, Sweden, Department of Orthopaedics, Karolinska University Hospital, Stockholm, Sweden

Kristina Åkesson
Clinical and Molecular Osteoporosis Research Unit, Department of Clinical Sciences, Lund University, Sweden
Department of Orthopaedics, Skåne University Hospital, Malmö, Sweden

Satya S. Varanasi and Harish K. Datta
Musculoskeletal Research Group, Institute of Cellular Medicine, Medical School, Newcastle University, Newcastle Upon Tyne, United Kingdom

Ole K. Olstad
Department of Clinical Biochemistry, Oslo University Hospital, Ullevål, Norway

Daniel C. Swan
Bioinformatics Support Unit, Institute for Cell and Molecular Biosciences, Medical School, Newcastle University Newcastle Upon Tyne, United Kingdom

Paul Sanderson
Department of Orthopaedic Surgery, Newcastle General Hospital, Newcastle Upon Tyne, United Kingdom

Vigdis T. Gautvik and Sjur Reppe
Department of Clinical Biochemistry, Oslo University Hospital, Ullevål, Norway
Institute of Basic Medical Sciences, University of Oslo, Oslo, Norway

Roger M. Francis
Institute for Ageing and Health, Newcastle University, Newcastle Upon Tyne, United Kingdom

Kaare M. Gautvik
Department of Clinical Biochemistry, Oslo University Hospital, Ullevål, Norway
Institute of Basic Medical Sciences, University of Oslo, Oslo, Norway
Department of Clinical Chemistry, Lovisenberg Deacon Hospital, Oslo, Norway

Hila Haskelberg, Janaki Amin and Sean Emery
The Kirby Institute, University of New South Wales, Sydney, Australia

Nicholas Pocock and Andrew Carr
St. Vincent's Hospital, Sydney, Australia

Peter Robert Ebeling
North West Academic Centre, University of Melbourne, Melbourne, Australia

Marlène Gallet, Juliette Sailland, Julie Carnesecchi, Violaine Tribollet, Bruno Barenton, Christelle Forcet and Jean-Marc Vanacker
Institut de Génomique Fonctionnelle de Lyon, Université de Lyon, Centre national de la recherche scientifique UMR5242, Ecole Normale Supérieure de Lyon, Lyon, France

Soraya Saïdi, Eric Haÿ, Caroline Marty and Martine Cohen-Solal
Institut National de la Santé et de la Recherche Médicale U606, Hôpital Lariboisière, Paris, France

Johann Photsavang and Olivier Chassande
Institut National de la Santé et de la Recherche Médicale U1026, Bordeaux, France

Marie-Christine Birling and Tania Sorg
Institut Clinique de la Souris, Illkirch-Graffenstaden, France

Nathalie Saulnier, Soizic Guihard, Vincent Feuillet, Françoise Porteu and Murielle Gaudry
Institut Cochin, Université Paris Descartes, Sorbonne Paris Descartes, CNRS (UMR 8104), Paris, France
Inserm U1016, Paris, France

Xavier Holy
Service histologie et réparation tissulaire, IRBA/IMASSA, Brétigny-sur-Orge, France

Elodie Decembre and Pierre Jurdic
Institut de Génomique Fonctionnelle de Lyon, Université de Lyon, Université Lyon 1, CNRS, INRA, Ecole Normale Supérieure de Lyon, Lyon, France

Denis Clay
Inserm U972, Institut André Lwoff, Hôpital Paul Brousse, Villejuif, France

Gilles Pagès and Jacques Pouysségur
Institut de recherche Signalisation, Biologie du Développement et Cancer, Université de Nice, France

Jerald Silverman
Department of Animal Medicine, University of Massachusetts Medical School, Worcester, Massachusetts, United States of America

Gregory Hendricks
Department of Cell Biology, University of Massachusetts Medical School, Worcester, Massachusetts, United States of America

Kenneth E. S. Poole and Paul M. Mayhew
Department of Medicine, University of Cambridge, Cambridge, Cambridgeshire, United Kingdom

Graham M. Treece and Andrew H. Gee
Department of Engineering, University of Cambridge, Cambridge, Cambridgeshire, United Kingdom

Jan Vaculík and Pavel Dungl
Department of Orthopaedics, Faculty of Medicine, Charles University Prague and Bulovka Hospital, Prague, Czech Republic

Martin Horák
Department of Radiology, Homolka Hospital, Prague, Czech Republic

Jan J.Štěpán
Department of Rheumatology, Faculty of Medicine 1, Charles University Prague and Institute of Rheumatology, Prague, Czech Republic

Masashi Muramatsu
Laboratory of Genomics and Proteomics, National Center for Geriatrics and Gerontology (NCGG), Aichi, Japan

Sawako Moriwaki and Shumpei Niida
Laboratory of Genomics and Proteomics, National Center for Geriatrics and Gerontology (NCGG), Aichi, Japan
Biobank Omics Unit, National Center for Geriatrics and Gerontology (NCGG), Aichi, Japan

Keiko Suzuki
Department of Pharmacology, School of Dentistry, Showa University, Tokyo, Japan

Atsushi Nomura and Fumihide Inoue
Nihon Seiyaku Kogyo, Co., Ltd., Aichi, Japan

Takeshi Into
Department of Oral Bacteriology, Division of Oral Infections and Health Sciences, Asahi University School of Dentistry, Gifu, Japan

Yuji Yoshiko
Department of Oral Growth and Developmental Biology, Hiroshima University Graduate School of Biomedical Sciences, Hiroshima, Japan

Sam Van Wassenbergh
Department of Biology, Universiteit Antwerpen, Antwerpen, Belgium
Department of Biology, Ghent University, Gent, Belgium

Billy Dries
Department of Biology, Universiteit Antwerpen, Antwerpen, Belgium
Department of Veterinary Medical Imaging and Small Animal Orthopaedics, Ghent University, Merelbeke, Belgium

Anthony Herrel
Department of Biology, Universiteit Antwerpen, Antwerpen, Belgium
Department of Biology, Ghent University, Gent, Belgium
Département d'Ecologie et de Gestion de la Biodiversité, Centre National de la Recherche Scientifique/Muséum National d'Histoire Naturelle, Paris, France

Hiromu Ito, Toshiyuki Kitaori, Koichi Murata, Hideyuki Shibuya, Takayuki Fujii and Shuichi Matsuda
Department of Orthopaedic Surgery, Kyoto University Graduate School of Medicine, Kyoto, Japan

Masahiro Ishikawa and Moritoshi Furu
Department of Orthopaedic Surgery, Kyoto University Graduate School of Medicine, Kyoto, Japan
Department of the Control for Rheumatic Disease, Kyoto University Graduate School of Medicine, Kyoto, Japan

Hiroyuki Yoshitomi
The Center for Innovation in Immunoregulative Technology and Therapeutics, Kyoto University Graduate School of Medicine, Kyoto, Japan

Koji Yamamoto
Center for the Promotion of Interdisciplinary Education and Research, Kyoto University, Kyoto, Japan

Hui-Tzu Yu
Department of Food Science and Biotechnology, National Chung Hsing University (NCHU), Taiwan, R.O.C.

Shen-Shih Chiang and Jeng-Leun Mau
Department of Food Science and Biotechnology, National Chung Hsing University (NCHU), Taiwan, R.O.C.
NCHU-UCD Plant and Food Biotechnology Center, NCHU, Taiwan, R.O.C.

Shin-Yu Chen
Department of Food Science and Biotechnology, National Chung Hsing University (NCHU), Taiwan, R.O.C.
NCHU-UCD Plant and Food Biotechnology Center, NCHU, Taiwan, R.O.C.
Agricultural Biotechnology Center, NCHU, Taiwan, R.O.C.

Ju-Po Kao and Chung-Chun Yang
Veterinary Medical Teaching Hospital, College of Veterinary Medicine, NCHU, Taiwan, R.O.C.

Darya O. Mishchuk
Department of Food Science and Technology, University of California Davis, Davis, California, United States of America

Carolyn M. Slupsky
Department of Food Science and Technology, University of California Davis, Davis, California, United States of America

Department of Nutrition, University of California Davis, Davis, California, United States of America

Randa Al-Fotawei and Ashraf F. Ayoub
University of Glasgow, Glasgow, United Kingdom

Neil Heath
Oral & Maxillofacial Radiology, Glasgow University Dental Hospital & School, Glasgow, United Kingdom

Kurt B. Naudi
Oral Surgery, Glasgow University Dental Hospital & School, Glasgow, United Kingdom

K. Elizabeth Tanner
Biomedical Materials, School of Engineering, University of Glasgow, Glasgow, United Kingdom

Matthew J. Dalby
Centre for Cell Engineering, University of Glasgow, Glasgow, United Kingdom

Jeremy McMahon
Oral & Maxillofacial Surgery, Southern General Hospital, Glasgow, United Kingdom

Lin Wan
Ministry of Education Key Laboratory for Regenerative Medicine, School of Biomedical Sciences, Faculty of Medicine, The Chinese University of Hong Kong, Hong Kong SAR, China

Fengjie Zhang, Wing Pui Tsang and Chao Wan
Ministry of Education Key Laboratory for Regenerative Medicine, School of Biomedical Sciences, Faculty of Medicine, The Chinese University of Hong Kong, Hong Kong SAR, China
School of Biomedical Sciences Core Laboratory, Shenzhen Research Institute, The Chinese University of Hong Kong, Shenzhen, China

Qiling He
Departments of Microbiology and Pathology, University of Alabama at Birmingham, Birmingham, Alabama, United States of America

Li Lu and Qingnan Li
Ministry of Education Key Laboratory for Regenerative Medicine, School of Biomedical Sciences, Faculty of Medicine, The Chinese University of Hong Kong, Hong Kong SAR, China
Guangdong Key Laboratory of Pharmaceutical Bioactive Substances, New Drug Function Research Center, School of Life Science and Biopharmacy, Guangdong Pharmaceutical University, Guangzhou, China

Zhihong Wu and Guixing Qiu
Department of Orthopaedics, Peking Union Medical College Hospital, Peking Union Medical College and Chinese Academy of Medical Sciences, Beijing, China

Guangqian Zhou
The Center for Anti-Ageing and Regenerative Medicine, Medical School, Shenzhen University, Shenzhen, China

Silke Schlaubitz and Martine Renard
CIC 1401, University hospital of Bordeaux/Inserm, Bordeaux, France

Sidi Mohammed Derkaoui, Catherine Le Visage and Didier Letourneur
U1148, LVTS/Inserm, Paris, France

Près Sorbonne Paris Cité, University of Paris Nord and University Paris Diderot, Paris, France

Lydia Marosa and Joëlle Amédée
U1026 Tissue Bioengineering, University of Bordeaux/Inserm, Bordeaux, France

Sylvain Miraux
RMSB Center/UMR 5536, CNRS, Bordeaux, France

Sylvain Catros and Jean-Christophe Fricain
Dental School, University of Bordeaux, Bordeaux, France

Index